UCL INSTITUTE OF ARCHAEOLOGY PHD SERIES

VOLUME 9

Urbanism and its Impact on Human Health

A long-term study at Knossos, Crete

ANNA C. MOLES

BAR INTERNATIONAL SERIES 3130 | 2023

BAR
PUBLISHING

Published in 2023 by
BAR Publishing, Oxford, UK

BAR International Series 3130

UCL Institute of Archaeology PhD Series, Volume 9
Urbanism and its Impact on Human Health

ISBN 978 1 4073 6035 5 paperback
ISBN 978 1 4073 6036 2 e-format

DOI https://doi.org/10.30861/9781407360355

A catalogue record for this book is available from the British Library

COVER IMAGE *The sorting of commingled and fragmentary remains from KMF/78 Tomb 311 during the skeletal analysis at the Knossos Stratigraphical Museum of the British School at Athens. Photo: Anna Moles.*

BAR
PUBLISHING

BAR titles are available from:

BAR Publishing
122 Banbury Rd, Oxford, OX2 7BP, UK
info@barpublishing.com
www.barpublishing.com

UCL INSTITUTE OF ARCHAEOLOGY PHD SERIES

A specialist sub-series in the BAR Series

Series Editor: Ruth Whitehouse (Chair of the IoA Publications Committee)

The aim of this series is to offer rapid publication of largely unaltered PhD theses. It covers the full range of subject areas studied at the Institute, including world archaeology, archaeological science, cultural heritage, conservation and museum studies. It makes data, analyses and interpretation available promptly to a wide audience.

The UCL Institute of Archaeology is one of the oldest, largest and most prestigious archaeology research facilities in the world. Its extensive publications programme includes the best theory, research, pedagogy and reference materials in archaeology, cultural heritage and cognate disciplines. Through its publications, which also include a General Series and a Critical Cultural Heritage Series, and a number of associated journals, the Institute brings together key areas of theoretical and substantive knowledge, improves archaeological and heritage practice and brings archaeological findings to the general public, researchers and practitioners.

Titles in the UCl Institute of Archaeology PhD Subseries

Pattern and Process in the Material Culture of Anglo-Saxon Non-elite Rural Settlements
Hana Lewis
BAR British Series **649** | 2019 — Volume 1

Ancient Maya Settlement and the Alacranes Bajo
Landscape and Communities in the Three Rivers Region, Northwestern Belize
Gail A Hammond
BAR International Series **2956** | 2019 — Volume 2

A Consideration of Gender Roles and Relations in the Aegean Bronze Age Interpreted from Gestures and Proxemics in Art
Susan E. Poole
BAR International Series **2980** | 2020 — Volume 3

On the Hunt for Medieval Whales
Zooarchaeological, historical and social perspectives on cetacean exploitation in medieval northern and western Europe
Youri van den Hurk
BAR International Series **2988** | 2020 — Volume 4

Land, People and Power in Early Medieval Wales
The cantref of Cemais in comparative perspective
Rhiannon Comeau
BAR British Series **659** | 2020 — Volume 5

Of Related Interest

The Funerary Landscape at Knossos
A diachronic study of Minoan burial customs with special reference to the warrior graves
Madelaine Miller
BAR International Series **2201** | 2011

Archaeology of a World of Changes. Late Roman and Early Byzantine Architecture, Sculpture and Landscapes
Selected Papers from the 23rd International Congress of Byzantine Studies (Belgrade, 22–27 August 2016) – In memoriam Claudiae Barsanti
Edited by Dominic Moreau, Carolyn S. Snively, Alessandra Guiglia, Isabella Baldini, Ljubomir Milanović, Ivana Popović, Nicolas Beaudry and Orsolya Heinrich-Tamáska
BAR International Series **2973** | 2020

The Collapse of Palatial Society in LBA Greece and the Postpalatial Period
Guy D. Middleton
BAR International Series **2110** | 2010

Rhadamanthys
Studi di archeologia minoica in onore di Filippo Carinci per il suo 70° compleanno/Studies in Minoan archaeology in honour of Filippo Carinci on the occasion of his 70th birthday
Holly Alane Raab
BAR International Series **984** | 2001

Rural Settlement in Hellenistic and Roman Crete
The Akrotiri Peninsula
Holly Alane Raab
BAR International Series **984** | 2001

Death Management and Virtual Pursuits: A Virtual Reconstruction of the Minoan Cemetery at Phourni, Archanes
Examining the use of Tholos Tomb C and Burial Building 19 and the role of illumination in relation to mortuary practices and the perception of life and death by the living
Constantinos Papadopoulos
BAR International Series **2082** | 2010

Continuity and Destruction in the Greek East
The Transformation of Monumental Space from the Hellenistic Period to Late Antiquity
Edited by Sujatha Chandrasekaran and Anna Kouremenos
BAR International Series **2765** | 2015

Minoan Kato Zakro: A Pastoral Economy
Judith Reid
BAR International Series **1713** | 2007

The Aegean and its Cultures
Proceedings of the first Oxford-Athens graduate student workshop organized by the Greek Society and the University of Oxford Taylor Institution, 22-23 April 2005
Edited by Georgios Deligiannakis and Yannis Galanakis
BAR International Series **1975** | 2009

Bronzeworking on Late Minoan Crete
A diachronic study
Lena Hakulin
BAR International Series **2980** | 2004

Cretan Locations
Discerning site variations in Iron Age and Archaic Crete (800-500 B.C.)
Lena Sjögren
BAR International Series **1185** | 2003

For more information, or to purchase these titles, please visit **www.barpublishing.com**

Acknowledgments

This book stems from my PhD research, completed in 2019 at University College London. I would like to thank my PhD supervisors Todd Whitelaw and Simon Hillson for their guidance, advice and feedback from the conception of this project through to completion. I would particularly like to thank Todd for sharing his endless knowledge of Knossos and for his detailed feedback on my draft chapters. Simon, I am grateful to for his assistance with developing my initial methodology, sharing his database and helping with adjusting it to the needs of my project, and for crucial assistance and feedback on aspects of data analysis and statistics.

A special thank you goes to the British School at Athens (BSA) and the Crete Committee for giving me the opportunity to study the skeletal material from past BSA excavations at Knossos. I am grateful to Matthew Haysom, who as Knossos Curator was the initial contact to support my interest in studying the material from Knossos. Thanks also goes to the interim curators Anthoulla Vassiliades and Caroline Thurston, and to the current Knossos Curator, Kostis Christakis, who has been extremely supportive of my work and whose assistance in securing my permit for sampling for stable isotope analysis was crucial. I would also like to thank Tania Gerousi at the BSA for her assistance in the permit application process, and the Heraklion Museum and Heraklion Ephoreia for granting the permit and supervising the sampling.

A very special thank you goes to Rebecca Sweetman who has been an inspirational mentor since my undergraduate days and without whose encouragement, I would never have started the PhD. Her support has been motivational throughout and I cannot thank her enough for going above and beyond in reading my work and for her invaluable advice.

I would like to thank Rhiannon Stevens for supervising the stable isotope analysis aspect of my project, Hazel Reade for providing additional advice and assistance in this process, and Anne-Lise Jourdan for her supervision and guidance in the BEIF lab, and for analysing the samples in the mass-spectrometer. I am grateful to Amy Bogaard for her advice on isotope controls and for sharing her unpublished paper on the isotopic analysis of plant remains from Knossos with me.

My thanks go to the London Arts and Humanities Partnership for the provision of the AHRC funding during the PhD, as well as to the British School at Athens (Richard Bradford McConnell School Studentship) and the Onassis Foundation for each funding six months of my final writing up year. I would like to thank John Bennet, not only for his support in my capacity as BSA School Student, but also for supervising my Onassis Fellowship.

I am incredibly grateful to Penny Wilson, Sandra Pepelasis and Amalia Kakissis for their assistance in the BSA Library and Archives and as my long-time friends and colleagues for their support, encouragement and all-important writing breaks in the library office. A special mention must also go to the smallest member of the library team, Bouboulina, who was first to greet me each morning at the BSA and always willing to provide a diversion from work.

In addition to the Knossos curators, I must also extend an important thank you to the Curation Project team, Flora Michelaki, Céline Murphy and Hannah Gwyther, not only for their assistance and company in the Stratigraphical Museum at the Knossos Research Centre, particularly in the cold and quiet winter months. Special thanks must also be extended to Hannah, for her eternally enthusiastic encouragement that helped see me through to the end of this research.

I am grateful to have had useful and insightful conversations with or advice from Tamara Dijkstra, Emma-Jayne Graham, Conor Trainor, Borja Legarra Herrero, and Caroline Carrier. Thanks also to Tamara for proofreading sections of this manuscript.

Finally, I want to say thank you to my friends and family for their support, encouragement, understanding, and tolerance, and to the London family for housing me during my time in London.

Contents

Appendices are available online at:
Appendix A: Catalogue of Skeletal Units - doi.org/10.30861/9781407360355-AppendixA
Appendix B: Demography Results - doi.org/10.30861/9781407360355-AppendixB
Appendix C: Stable of Isotopes - doi.org/10.30861/9781407360355-AppendixC
Appendix D: Activity Results - doi.org/10.30861/9781407360355-AppendixD

List of Figures

List of Tables

Abstract

This book demonstrates how social, economic and political changes impacted the everyday lives of the people of Knossos, in terms of their health and diet, during the Hellenistic, Roman and Late Antique periods. Knossos, in north-central Crete, was an important site in Aegean and Mediterranean networks throughout this timespan, though the city experienced cycles of urban development and decline. As an extensively studied and well-documented site, it provides a unique opportunity to study long-term phenomena associated with its varied past. The present osteological research is contextualised using previous work on material culture and textual sources.

The skeletal material was mostly fragmentary and commingled, its poor condition exacerbated by excavation techniques and storage conditions. It was necessary to develop a methodology to work around these limitations. A palaeoepidemiological approach was adopted and recording by element rather than individual was necessary. A selection of skeletal and isotopic analyses was conducted in order to investigate the demography, diet, development, and activity documented by the assemblage, as broad indicators of health.

The results of this systematic study demonstrate that changes were not only manifested in the political administration, cultural tastes, and urban fabric of the city but also filtered down into the everyday lives of people, affecting their fundamental wellbeing and way of life. Changes occur in diet, activity and living conditions between the Hellenistic and Roman assemblages, and an inactive elite class is distinguishable from the (osteo)archaeological record. The later transition into Late Antiquity is a more gradual socio-economic change and this is also reflected in the less substantial differences in health and lifestyle indicators. However, there is a general picture of an improvement in living conditions alongside the reduction in population size, with less pressure on food resources and suggestion of a less hierarchical society.

1

Introduction[1]

This book demonstrates how social, cultural, economic and political changes – framed within the context of urbanism at the site – impacted the everyday lives of the people of Knossos, in terms of their health and diet, during the Hellenistic, Roman and Late Antique periods. This study is primarily based on the analysis of the human skeletal remains but it strives to integrate the available archaeological and historical evidence and bring in comparative studies, contextualising Knossos within the wider temporal and geographic setting.

1.1. The site

The site of Knossos in north-central Crete (Figure 1.1) was a significant centre through most of its nearly eight millennia of occupation. One of the earliest Neolithic settlements in Europe, founded c. 7000 BC, it developed into the earliest known urban centre in Europe c. 2000 BC. It is most famous for its Bronze Age 'Minoan' palatial society, due to over a century of intensive archaeological investigation and the plethora and wealth of finds. However, it remained a significant centre throughout much of its history through to AD 800, though it experienced cycles of urban development and decline. Following a significant decline at the end of the Bronze Age, Knossos was one of the first Greek city-states to develop early in the first millennium BC. Traditionally it was thought that there was another urban collapse, referred to as the 'Archaic Gap', due to the complete absence of burials assignable to the 6th or 5th centuries BC and relatively little evidence of occupation (Coldstream *et al.* 1999). However, the recent work by the Knossos Urban Landscape Project paints a picture of gradual expansion through the Archaic and Classical periods (Whitelaw *et al.* 2017; Trainor 2019). Knossos became one of the major Aegean centres during the Hellenistic period and one of a small number of dominant centres on Crete. It continued as a significant urban centre following the Roman conquest of Crete and was formally refounded as a Roman colony in 27 BC,[2] flourishing for several centuries as the subject of public and private building works. After the 2nd century AD there is less evidence for significant new building projects (other than the basilica churches of the 5th and 6th centuries), though with only limited excavations, understanding of this period is restricted and occupation is known to have continued at the site. There was a continual contraction of the city limits and reduction of population at the site, until it was eventually reduced to nothing more substantial than a small village by the end of the 7th century AD (Sweetman 2004a; Trainor 2019).

The site has been intensively investigated since 1900, with major excavations focusing on the Bronze Age occupation at Knossos (Hogarth 1900; Evans 1906; Hood and Smyth 1981). This focus on the prehistoric phases, particularly the later prehistoric, palatial periods, has created long-term biases in the investigation of the site. While excavations and surveys have covered all phases of occupation in the city and the extensive cemeteries surrounding it, there has been no systematic programme of investigation of the post-Bronze Age city. There has been relatively little study and publication of these later remains, and those that do exist have largely focused on ceramics or on a few specific excavations (for example: Wardle 1972; Carington Smith 1982; Hayes 1983; 2001; Paton 1991; 1998; Sackett *et al.* 1992; Carington Smith and Wall 1994; Cavanagh and Curtis 1998; Coldstream *et al.* 2001; Cadogan *et al.* 2004; Sweetman and Becker 2005; Sweetman and Grigoropoulos 2010; Trainor 2021).

The aim of this study is to investigate how these changes in the urban environment and the associated social, political and economic factors affected the health, diet and lifestyle of the population at Knossos. It focuses on the later phase of urban development and decline using a study of the human skeletal remains from Hellenistic, Roman and Late Antique tombs from British School at Athens (BSA) excavations. This time span extends from the Early Hellenistic period when the site was at its maximum extent (c.120 ha.) since the Bronze Age 'Neopalatial' period, followed by a contraction in the Late Hellenistic, with the thinning or even cessation of habitation from the Gypsades hill to the south of the city (Paton 1994; Trainor 2019; Whitelaw *et al.* 2019). This appears to have been prior to the Roman invasion of 69–67 BC which served as a further blow to the city which had put up some of the greatest resistance to the Roman presence on Crete (Paton 1994; de Souza 1998; Sweetman 2007; Trainor 2019). Though the city does not appear to have expanded or the population to have grown substantially after the establishment of the Roman colony, it certainly prospered economically as demonstrated by the monumental architectural remains, elaboration of domestic spaces with mosaics, frescos and imported stone, increased diversity and monumentality in the burial sphere, and evidence for trade connections (Paton

[1] Appendices mentioned in the text, with supplementary data, have been made available to download - refer to table of contents for DOIs

[2] This date is not certain but the discussion of its likelihood is summarised by Paton (1994, 143), Baldwin Bowsky (2002, 77) and more recently by Carrier (2018, 697–98), referencing Cassius Dio (XLIX.14.5), Velleius Paterculus (II.81.2), Svoronos (1890), Grant (1946, 55, 180, 262–63), Brunt (1971, 599), Hood and Smyth (Hood and Smyth 1981), Engels (1990, 18), De Caro (1993, 310), Spawforth (1996, 169) and Rizakis (1997, 15). The absence of Knossos from the *Res Gestae* and the name *Colonia Iulia* suggest a Caesarean date, but the coinage suggests a later date and Crete being under the jurisdiction of Mark Antony from 42 BC indicates a date after the Battle of Actium. It may have been a proposal by Caesar carried out by Augustus (Baldwin Bowsky 2002, 77).

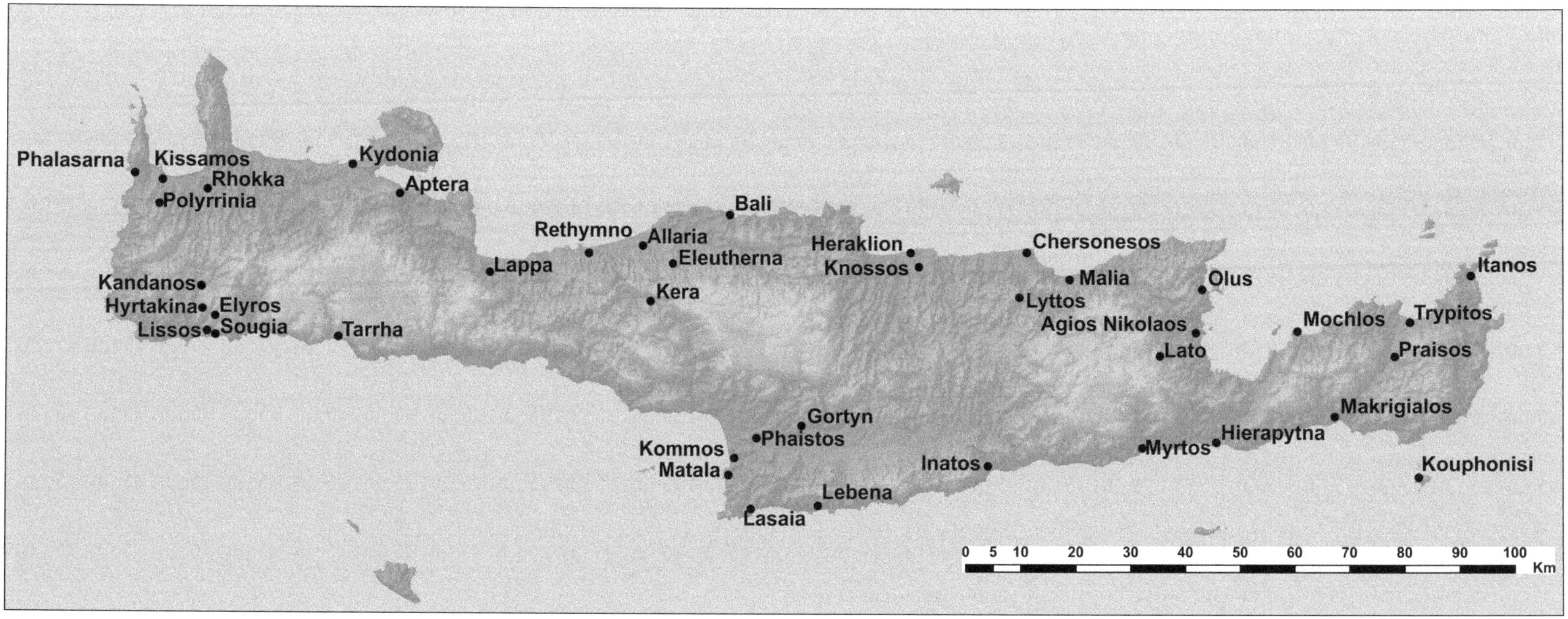

Figure 1.1. Map of Crete indicating Knossos and other important Hellenistic, Roman and Late Antique sites. Basemap: James Herbst, American School of Classical Studies at Athens (CC BY-SA 4.0).

1994; Sweetman 2006; 2007). There is little evidence for monumental public architecture (other than the Christian basilica churches), luxury elements in private dwellings,[3] monumental tombs (discussed further in Section 3.5) or the same levels of activity in trade networks beyond the 4th century AD. There also appears to be a gradual decline in population from about the 3rd century onwards when coastal Heraklion begins to grow as a more significant centre (Whitelaw *et al.* 2019). This could be linked to the disturbances at this time referred to as the 'third century crisis' which led to a period of economic decline across the Roman Empire (Hekster *et al.* 2007; Jongman 2007a). There was a shift in the economic focus of Crete towards the eastern Mediterranean at this time, though this does not appear to reflect decline with evidence for increased imports at some sites in the later Roman period (Gallimore 2016). There was also climatic change that manifested as a period of prolonged cold and aridity beginning in the 3rd century causing landscape desiccation throughout Crete and the southwest Aegean, which may have resulted in food shortages (Moody 2016, 67, 72). These grand scale changes across these time periods, in terms of political administration, economic productivity and prosperity, intra- and off-island connectivity, population size and diversity, environmental conditions, settlement size, urban planning, and investment in infrastructure and monumentality, represent significant changes that would have impacted on the population of Knossos in a variety of ways. This project aims to demonstrate how these changes affected the lives of the inhabitants in terms of health, diet, longevity, activity, and – by inference – wellbeing and lifestyle.

1.2. The main questions

Using materials and methods that have rarely or never been applied to this time period on Crete, this study aims to answer questions that have thus far eluded scholars of Hellenistic, Roman and Late Antique Crete, and add to the discussion of what life was like during these centuries of change, including the nature and extent of the changes and their impact on people's lives. Much of the value of this study comes from its contribution of new material to the fields of post-prehistoric[4] studies of Knossos and Crete, as well as adding to the growing scholarship on human remains in historic periods in Greece (Bourbou 2005; 2009; Roberts *et al.* 2005; Bourbou 2010; Lagia 2014; 2007; Tritsaroli and Valentin 2008; Papageorgopoulou and Xirotiris 2009; Vika *et al.* 2009; Bourbou and Niniou-Kindeli 2009; Bourbou and Tsilipakou 2009; Hillson *et al.* 2009; Bourbou and Themelis 2010; Vika 2011; Lagia *et al.* 2014; Tritsaroli 2014; 2020; Tritsaroli and Karadima 2017; Dotsika *et al.* 2018; Nikita *et al.* 2019; Vergidou *et al.* 2021; 2022; Karligkioti *et al.* 2023). This project works with problematic legacy material and accompanying archival records from old excavations and in doing so creates a model for other studies in demonstrating how much can be done with legacy material (a valuable but neglected and under-exploited resource). Scholars should feel a moral obligation to study and publish legacy material and data rather than allowing such information and cultural heritage to be lost, forgotten about or potentially even destroyed in storerooms. Not only does this study use this approach to bring new data to the discussion of these later time periods Crete, that have been side-lined due to a preference in focus on their prehistoric, and particularly Bronze Age Minoan and Mycenaean, counterparts, but it has used methods that have not previously been applied to Cretan studies of these time periods. This creates a more interdisciplinary discussion to the understanding of life and society in these periods on Crete.

Hellenistic Crete has been depicted as a place rife with conflict, wars, social disorder, piracy, and was an important supplier of mercenaries to the armies of the Hellenistic world by the accounts of several ancient authors[5] (Hatzfeld 1919, 28–38, 157–60; de Souza 1998; Marshall and Towner 1999, 202; Perlman 1999; Chaniotis 2005, 108). At the same time, Knossos was considered a major Aegean centre and a key player in the Cretan *koinon* (Perlman 1992; Ager 1994). This raises the question of what the balance was between the images of war and turmoil, versus political and social stability, structure and functionality. The written sources may have exaggerated anti-Cretan biases and created stereotypes due to the conceptually marginalised position of Crete in Greek thought (Perlman 1999, 133–34; Erickson 2010, 14). A break-down of administrative order and political control in times of war can lead to interruptions in trade networks and supply chains, as occurred during the third century crisis in the Roman Empire (Nappo 2007, 237). It is not clear what the repercussions of the Hellenistic Cretan wars would have been. There are plentiful inscriptions referring to intra-island trade during this period, as well as to taxes and restrictions on trade relating to the relationship between particular poleis and often with clauses for tax exemptions between allies (Perlman 1999; Viviers 1999, 228). This would suggest that there may not have been any full interruptions to supply chains. Chaniotis (1999, 200) argues that the majority of intra-island trade was conducted by sea during the Hellenistic period. However, just as the settlement pattern through the Ierapetra isthmus supports overland trade as an important feature of the economy on the island, so too does the Mesara corridor linking Knossos with the south coast (Perlman 1999, 146–47, 149; Vogeikoff-Brogan 2004, 219; Gallimore 2015, 265). These accounts suggest that trade and communications remained successful. However, this may only have been for the larger centres while smaller settlements may have been more affected by the turmoil of wars and changing alliances. An example of this may be

[3] There is little exposure of domestic evidence after the 3rd century so little can be said about this absence of evidence.

[4] i.e. 'historic'. Post-prehistoric is a necessarily convoluted term used to highlight how focused the scholarship has been to date on the prehistory of Crete, at the expense of the later time periods.

[5] Strabo 10.4.9-10; Polybius 6.46.9, 6.47.5, 8.16.4-7, 33.16.4; Plutarch *Moralia* 490B, 761D; Diodorus Siculus 30.13; Homer *Odyssey* 19.173 ff.; *Anthologia Palatina* 7.654.

the short-lived settlement at Mochlos, which was occupied only for a matter of decades from the late 2nd to early 1st century. However, it is likely that there were at least short-term set-backs to trade and civic order caused by these wars which often required external arbitration to resolve (de Souza 1998, 112; Viviers 1999, 223). Disruption in the production of coinage can be observed at Knossos in c.220–140 BC due to the frequent conflicts with Gortyn (Carrier 2018, 564).

A study of the skeletal material has the potential to offer independent evidence for conflict, an exodus of the prime age males (as mercenaries), and the degree of social (dis)order these may have caused at Hellenistic Knossos. Unreliable access to food and adequate nutrition, which could have resulted from these conflicts and disruptions, can be detected by stable isotope analysis (Chapter 5) and stunted growth (Chapter 8), while types of foods being consumed can be additionally investigated in dental diseases (Chapter 6). Similarly, a lack of waste management, and poor upkeep of sewage systems, waste disposal, and water sources results in unsanitary living conditions and the proliferation of infectious diseases, detectable by increased mortality (Chapter 4), and increased morbidity can also be detected through shorter bone lengths being attained (Chapter 8).

Although the major trade centres of Hellenistic Crete were along the south coast, Knossos was nevertheless a major power within Hellenistic Crete, well connected physically through overland trade via the Mesara with these southern ports as well as through treaties (Chaniotis 1999; Perlman 1999). It is still uncertain how significant the change was between these periods in connectivity within wider networks, as determined by the material culture, architecture, and written record. The study of the diet of Hellenistic population may contribute to knowledge of connections with Knossos. The detection of new and distinctive foodstuffs, such as millet or fish, being incorporated into the diet could indicate an expansion of trade, knowledge or technology surrounding food. There are also cultural factors that may have resulted in a change in both food types consumed and the adequacy of nutrition. For example, the *syssitia* (communal meals) are attested to have existed in Hellenistic Crete, which may have influenced what foods were available to different segments of society (such as by age, sex, citizen status, social affiliation or lineage) (Chaniotis 1999, 193–94; Lewis 2015, 19).

A question that has long been at the centre of discussions of Crete in this time period, is how Crete changes (if at all) on becoming part of the Roman Empire, and specifically, how (and whether) Knossos changes with its formal refoundation as a Roman colony (Paton 1994; 2004; Baldwin Bowsky 1995; 2004b; 2006; 2011; Sweetman 2007). Crete was an important acquisition for Rome, with its strategic position for shipping networks and with a diversity of tradeable resources, including herbs, wine, honey, cypress wood and purple dye (Sanders 1982; Marangou-Lerat 1995; Haggis 1996; Francis 2016). The mythical past of Knossos may also have been incentive to found a colony there, renaming it the *Colonia Iulia Nobilis Cnosus* to make connections to that glorious past as a sort of vanity project. Internal peace and cooperation amongst the cities and the quashing of piracy were assured by Crete's incorporation into the Empire after the conquest of the island by Metellus (69–67 BC), thus enabling Crete's harbours and resources to be capitalised on (Blackman and Branigan 1975; de Souza 1998). Crete was able to thrive as a commercial centre and Knossos, along with many other cities experienced a period of economic prosperity.

Roman intervention in most cities was unlikely to have been very pervasive; a governor would have been installed to ensure the system already in place for running the city was successful and that taxes were paid (Sanders 1982; Sweetman 2013). There were visible changes to the cities of the island, in terms of the forms of houses, appearance of mosaics, investment in public buildings, cemetery locations, tomb forms and types and provenance of imports. These changes are initially seen in the port cities along the south coast due to the intensified trading connections along the Alexandria-Rome grain route, but the changes gradually spread throughout the island during the 1st century AD (Sanders 1982; Baldwin Bowsky 1994; Gallimore 2015). The earliest of the new style of built barrel-vaulted style tombs are known from Lissos, Sougia, Lasaia and Ierapetra, demonstrating changes in burials along the south coast from the 1st century BC (Savignoni 1901, 443–48; Davaras 1968, 405; Markoulaki 1996; Apostolakou 1997, 1047; 2011; Guyon 2008, 112). There is real evidence of prosperity during the 2nd century, with a booming trade in local imitation wares, elaborate polychrome mosaics, major investment in public buildings, infrastructure and private houses, dedications and honorific inscriptions attesting to a variety of achievements from infrastructural development to athletic success (Hayden 2005, 58; Sweetman 2013, 142). This evidence comes from many centres on the island, including Knossos, Chania, Kissamos, Ierapetra, Eleutherna, Gortyn, Chersonissos, and many more, demonstrating that change throughout the 1st century and prosperity in the 2nd century was an island-wide phenomenon and not a Knossos-specific development due to its colony status. Details of the changes at Roman Knossos and across Crete are outlined in Section 2.2.

While changes can be detected in the architecture and material culture, the question remains to what the extent this new type of urban status – with its external connections, integral position within the Roman Empire, and economic prosperity – impacted on people's lifestyles. An investigation of mortality, morbidity and developmental conditions (Chapters 4 and 8) can give insight into living conditions and act as a basic proxy of wellbeing. A study of diet (Chapters 5 and 6) can demonstrate whether the socio-economic changes on the island extended to the choice of foodstuffs being imported or grown. The economic prosperity and increased trade connections in the early Roman period are likely to have affected what types of food were consumed and in what quantities foodstuffs were readily available. Evidence for luxury additions to the diet and a consideration of tomb type as a proxy for social status could demonstrate the levels of inequality in society at this time. There is evidence for such items in the Spanish garum amphorae (Hayes 1983, 146) and a total of fifty different types of amphorae from the Villa Dionysus excavations, a good representation of amphorae found on Crete in c.150–250, from various Eastern and Western locations including Gaul, Northern Italy, Spain, North Africa, Upper Egypt, as well as local types demonstrating the strong export market (Hayes 1983, 140). The export trade would have required a significant increase in production of items such as wine and honey which may have resulted in these items being more readily available locally as well as for export. The observation of activity levels (Chapter 7) and patterns can demonstrate changes in physical labour levels and diversity or division of labour in aggregate terms. In addition to the changes in health and diet over time, differences between demographic (age, sex) and social sub-groups of the population may be distinguishable. Identifying how socio-economic conditions may have affected, for example, females and males differently in the different time periods, can enable changes in societal attitudes to be identified. Changes in the distribution of wealth in the population can be identified from a comparison of the health profile and diet of different social groups (using tomb type and cemetery as a potential proxy for social status) and demonstrate whether there was 'extensive' or 'intensive' economic growth (Scheidel 2009b).[6] The latter is the expectation for the Roman Empire as numerous sources attest to social inequality (Huskinson 2000; Griffin *et al.* 2011; Garnsey and Saller 2014), therefore an elite group may be identifiable through distinguishing differences in life expectancy, diet, stature or activity between their different social groups identified from the burial contexts.

As the only formal colony on Crete, the question is what the significance was of having colony status and to what extent Knossos differed from other major centres on Crete which also had a Roman presence. An important consideration that has caused great consternation in the past for scholars of Roman Crete is whether there is any evidence of changing populations at Knossos with the foundation of the colony. The names of *Duoviri* (magistrates) on coin legends and a small number of official inscriptions in Latin (Svoronos 1890; Guarducci 1935; Chapman 1968; Sanders 1982) attest to at least a small number of colonists seeing to the official running of the colony, though it is also likely that there was some Latinising of names (Baldwin Bowsky 1999; 2004b). The archaeological evidence known to date cannot identify a substantial influx of settlers at Knossos (Sweetman 2011a, 2). In the private sphere a preference for Greek was maintained in the inscriptions and there appear to be fewer Latin inscriptions than would normally be expected of a colony (Baldwin Bowsky 2004b). There was no new investment in monumental architecture for about a century after the foundation of the colony, though this has also been observed at the colonies at Catania and Syracuse in Sicily, with others seeing a shorter delay in such investment, such as approximately 30 years at Corinth (Korhonen 2011; Scotton 2011; Sweetman 2011a). Additionally, there were no changes in burial architecture identified until the second half of the 1st century AD and the Roman practice of cremation is never adopted, nor are the affiliated architecture and accoutrements, such as *columbaria* and cinerary urns (Dijkstra and Moles forthcoming). *Columbaria* were not common outside the city of Rome but they were present at the colonies of Patras and Corinth (Walbank 2005, 255–56; Rife 2007, 114; Borbonus 2014, 146; Dijkstra 2015, 167; 2019). There was evidence of increased contacts with Rome, such as a short-lived (late 1st century BC-mid 1st century AD) increase in preference for Italian sigillata as opposed to eastern tablewares (Eiring 2004; Baldwin Bowsky 2011), but this was evident in many cities throughout the provinces and is not a distinctive sign of colonists or even colonial identity. Additionally, the adoption of Roman material culture was less evident at Knossos than at Gortyn, which had been more accepting than Knossos of being incorporated into the Empire from the outset, but Gortyn had also already had a considerable resident population of Roman merchants prior to the Roman invasion (Baldwin Bowsky 2004a; Chevrollier 2016; Lippolis 2016).

Ideally, a study of non-metric traits, aDNA, or strontium and oxygen isotope analysis would be undertaken to identify migrants. This would require the clear identification of the remains of first-generation migrants, which are not easily identifiable from the available evidence in the present sample. However, a comparison of the health and dietary status with other sites on Crete for which there are studies of contemporary skeletal remains could help assess the impact of Knossos' colonial status and in comparison with other cities on Crete. A further comparison with other colony sites is needed, particularly with Corinth where mortuary and skeletal research has been conducted (Wesolowsky 1973; Fox Leonard 1997; Barnes 2003; Fox 2005; Kyle McIllvaine 2012; Kennedy 2016; Kyle McIllvaine *et al.* 2016; Slane 2017; Petry 2020), and in the future with Dion, where research is currently being carried out (Tritsaroli 2020). A broader comparison of the available archaeological evidence from a range of Roman colonies would also enable further discussion of what it meant to be a colony and the impact of colonisation on people's lives.

There is an expectation of urban decline in the Late Antique period in line with the economic depression and constant threats to security from invading forces across the Empire from the 3rd century onwards, but this is not easily discernible at Knossos or elsewhere in Crete from

[6] Extensive economic growth would mean increased income and prosperity relatively equally throughout the population. Intensive economic growth would mean the creation of greater differences in wealth and consequently in social standing.

the evidence. Is there any indication of urban decline at Knossos beyond the absence of substantial signs of new civic buildings or private dwellings? Alternatively, can a dwindling urban centre be substantiated by the available evidence? The absence of settlement evidence led Sanders to conclude that the site must have been abandoned in the 4th century AD after the earthquake of 365 (Sanders 1982). Sadly Ian Sanders (1949–1977) did not live to see the 1978 excavation of the Knossos Medical Faculty (KMF) basilica church, constructed in the early 5th century, and the associated tombs of the North Cemetery, dating from the 5th–7th centuries. Prior to this discovery, the Sanatorium basilica (constructed in the early 6th century), another basilica church below the modern church of Agia Sofia, and the KFF/74 osteotheke (likely dating to the 7th or even 8th century) were considered extra-urban features of the settlement at Heraklion. There is also now evidence for habitation which proves that Knossos continued to be a prosperous centre throughout the 4th and 5th centuries. This presumably continued into the 6th century, given that there were the incentive and means to construct a new martyrium basilica while the nearby earlier basilica continued in its function as a mortuary church as well as a martyrium into the 7th century. There is now substantial evidence for new 4th and 5th century constructions and occupation into the 6th century in the area around and to the south of the Villa Dionysus (Hayes 1983, 99; French 1994, 75; Tomlinson 1996, 41; Sweetman 2004b, 483; Forster 2009, 230–36), described in further detail in Section 2.3. The recent intensive urban survey documents continued occupation with a gradual contraction of the settlement. The survey evidence suggests that Knossos remained a substantial settlement until the 7th century, but fewer than ten sherds have been identified as dating to the 8th century (Whitelaw *et al.* 2017, 12). Not only did the city continue to exist but, from the evidence of mosaics and religious architecture, it also appears to have prospered. The presence of over 90 basilicas, many luxuriously decorated, across Crete demonstrates the security and prosperity on the island, in at least some social spheres. For the first time the mosaics demonstrate conformity with fashion and even innovation, particularly in the case of the KMF basilica, rather than lagging behind much of the rest of the Empire as had sometimes been the case in earlier Roman times (Sweetman 2004b, 485). With the introduction of Christianity, known at Knossos from the 2nd century AD (Eusebius *Historia Ecclesiastica* iv.21 and 23.7, discussed in Frend and Johnston 1962, 186; Sweetman 2004a, 315), though not monumentally commemorated at Knossos or elsewhere in Crete until the 5th century, the strict regimens of the religion may have influenced dietary practices.

There is no clear division between the Roman and Late Antique periods, but the archaeological evidence suggests a shift in focus of investment in art and architecture from the private to the public sphere and from the secular to the religious realm (Sweetman 2004b, 487). There is this image of an economically secure and thriving Crete, and of a prosperous Christian community at Knossos, but there is also a clear and significant long-term trend of people leaving Knossos for coastal Heraklion throughout the later Roman and Late Antique periods (Whitelaw *et al.* 2019). Was prosperity enjoyed by all or only by certain members of society? The available evidence gives us little insight into the private sphere and everyday lives of the people of Knossos, which can be investigated through the present study of health status. Changes to diet (Chapters 5 and 6), activity (Chapter 7), and the environmental conditions affecting childhood development and life expectancy (Chapters 4 and 8) can elucidate how these social, economic and religious changes impacted people's lifeways in comparison with the preceding Roman period. This can indicate whether the people's wellbeing prospered alongside the religious investment. It may also be possible to discern socio-economic differences within the society, such as identifying an elite class or clergy.

1.3. Urbanism and its impact on human health

Urbanism is referred to in both the title and introductory paragraph of this book, but what is meant by 'urbanism'? Defined as a way of life associated with living in cities in geographical and social science disciplines, urbanism encompasses everything from the social elements, including the nature of the social bond, the impersonal nature of urban social life, human nature's need for power divisions leading to hierarchical power structures, through to the urban planning and the physical divisions of land-use, with residential, political, religious, commercial and civic foci (Wirth 1938; Bridge 2009). For this study of urbanism and its impact on human health, a broad meaning of the term is applied. These include the more obvious impacts from the urban environment, such as population size, housing density, economic connectivity and movement of people with trade and migration, but also the more indirect environmental factors, such as natural disasters. The effects of such environmental factors are not exclusive to an urban environment but their impact on the population of an urban environment is different to that of a rural environment, where the population tends to be more self-sufficient. Natural disasters can lead to a breakdown of networks, secondary effects can include resource deficits, famines, disease and social conflict which are more easily initiated and spread in crowded living conditions (Scheidel 2009a; 2013).

For this study urbanism is used to mean characteristics or processes within the urban environment with a direct or indirect impact on human health, that could leave any physical markers or indicators in the human skeletal record. It is the relationship between the physical environment and its exploitation, and the economic, political, social and cultural institutions that create the urban environment that people interact with and live in. Urban planning can have a very direct impact on health as it defines the density of living conditions and can control access to a clean and adequate water supply and an efficient waste disposal or sewage system. These are all important factors in the occurrence and spread of disease.

Infectious diseases could always pose a risk to life and impact health but with urbanism and its associated population growth, higher density living conditions, changes in food production, poor community hygiene, and a lack of knowledge of the causation of disease, the manifestation and spread of disease were more pervasive than in rural populations, impacting heavily on urban communities and even capable of causing major social changes. Rapid population growth could increase pressure on resources, while increased density of living conditions could result in deteriorating hygiene and the easier spread of disease. Although Knossos was large, it was not an exceptional urban centre and does not appear to have had a dramatic influx of newcomers during the period under study. It is, therefore, unlikely to have experienced the demographic stress of Imperial Rome which suffered from seasonal diseases and epidemic outbreaks which could in some extreme cases have killed a significant proportion of the urban population, in the region of hundreds of thousands of lives (Scheidel 2009a, 7). Similarly, the studies of the expansion of the cities of medieval Europe demonstrate the pressures imposed and the toll taken on human health and diet (Bassett 1992). The analysis of the skeletal remains of its residents can determine whether urbanisation at Knossos would have levied similar costs.

2

Knossos in Context

Crete has always played an important role in the movement of materials, people and ideas in wider Aegean and Mediterranean networks due to its strategic position. This is the major reason for why it has been occupied by foreign powers for much of its history through to relatively modern times. Across the time periods covered by this study, Knossos was one of the foremost cities of the island, maintaining the dominance in north coastal Crete that it had throughout later prehistory and the Early Iron Age through Classical periods. As an important and well-connected city, the grand-scale changes occurring in the Hellenistic world with the expansion of the Roman Empire and Crete's incorporation into the Empire, were felt at Knossos, though material changes were not immediate. As a Roman colony and major centre, it continued to be impacted by the evolution of the Empire, with the spread of Christianity and the division of the Empire into West and East. In the Late Antique period, Crete was at the boundary of these two halves of the Empire, with its political and religious jurisdictions separately controlled by the East and West respectively. As an island, and with its proximity to many diverse regions reducing its reliance on a close relationship with Rome, it also was somewhat insulated from certain problems that plagued Rome and the Empire, such as economic crises, invasion from foreign forces, and indeed, plague epidemics.

At Knossos, although the archaeological focus has been on the Bronze Age, the intensive investigation of the site has enabled a great deal of evidence from the later time periods to also be collected. A large area of land around Knossos is now a protected zone, but already Agios Ioannis (Figure 2.1) and the neighbouring Heraklion suburbs had encroached upon the extended archaeological area (particularly the extensive cemeteries) to the north of the site.

2.1. Hellenistic Knossos

2.1.1. Dysfunctional conflict or functional koinon*? The political and economic situation*

The traditional image of Hellenistic Crete, created by an account by Polybius,[7] is one of warring cities, home to pirates and mercenaries, and a place of excess, greed and savagery (Ager 1994). However, this portrayal of a dysfunctional and primitive society has been negated by studies of the epigraphy and material culture of Hellenistic Crete. Epigraphic sources suggest that Knossos was one of the most important cities in Hellenistic Crete and that it headed a large network of allied cities (Guarducci 1935, 46–53 (*IC I*); Callaghan 1992, 134; Carrier 2018, 466). When Knossos and Gortyn were at peace there was a Cretan league or federation that united the island. The attestation of a Cretan *koinon* (federation of city states) in the epigraphic record demonstrates that although inter-polis wars were common. At times there was unity and a functional tribunal (*koinodikion*) operating under the leadership of Knossos and Gortyn (Ager 1994), though it is suggested that when these two key centres were at war, these institutions collapsed. Rome was involved in Cretan affairs sporadically from 195 BC in its capacity as an external mediator between some Cretan states, demonstrating the difficult relations on the island which were not resolved in any lasting way until the Roman conquest (Sweetman 2013, 7). Politically, Crete was inclined to support the Aetolian League in its efforts to oppose Macedon and by the end of the 3rd century, Cretan cities had joined an anti-Macedonian alliance. At a similar time, Ptolemaic troops that had been stationed at Itanos withdrew to Egypt, allowing for the increased involvement of Rome in Cretan affairs (Spyridakis 1992, 133). This would have affected its position in the networks of the Hellenistic world, its wider connections, and potentially, its economic prosperity.

The main attraction of Crete for the Romans, and the reason cited for the invasion of 69–67 BC, was likely to have been its geographical location and its potential to be exploited as an economic resource (de Souza 1998, 112). De Souza also suggests that the Cretan aristocracy would have accumulated much of their wealth in material goods (de Souza 1998, 114), but this is certainly not evident from the burial record at Knossos (Moles forthcoming; Dijkstra and Moles forthcoming), nor is it particularly manifest in the public or private sphere throughout Crete (Chaniotis 2005, 109). However, there has been relatively little excavation of Classical-Hellenistic levels to enable a clear archaeological perspective on the subject. There is evidence for a small number of gold objects and other prestigious items from tombs at Knossos and other sites in Crete (Guyon 2008, 129–41). Chaniotis (1999) argues that Crete had a subsistence economy with no evidence for substantial exports, but that it was nevertheless active in trade networks in exploiting its location for 'transit trade'. It appears to have had important links with Rhodes, Egypt, Asia Minor and the Levant due to its important position along nautical networks (Spyridakis 1970), and at least by the late Hellenistic period, the increased scale of amphora production and occasional finds of Cretan stamped amphora handles at Alexandria suggests that Crete was beginning to engage more in export activities (Empereur *et al.* 1992, 640; Cankardeş-Şenol 2007, 44–45; Gallimore 2015, 269–75). There was also evidence for some imports including wine and sculpture, and exchange activity involving slaves and luxury objects which likely came to the island as war spoils (Chaniotis 1999, 184; 2005, 107).

[7] Polybius on Crete: iv 8.11; xi 46.2–3; xi 46.9; xi 47.5; ii 4.3.

2.1.2. The archaeological evidence for life at Hellenistic Knossos

There have been few coherent contexts excavated from the Classical-Hellenistic centre of Knossos, with much of the evidence for the habitation of this period coming from ceramic fills and insubstantial remnants of walls. This is because many rescue excavations stop at the uppermost levels, once they have established there is archaeological material in the plot, and construction is halted, but also because digging for stone-robbing and rubbish pits, such as those observed in the 'Unexplored Mansion' excavations (Figure 2.1), have disturbed the stratigraphy down to Minoan levels (Sackett 1992, 3). It is supposed that the earlier public centre (agora) lay below the Roman city and that stone-robbing for the construction of the Roman public buildings and digging down to Minoan levels for this purpose were the reason for the lack of physical remains from this time period (Eiring 2001). There was a building constructed of large ashlar blocks close to the Villa Dionysus which may have been a Hellenistic public building, but nothing further is known about it (*KS2*:114[8]; Hood and Smyth 1981, 19; Raab 2001, 12). Unlike the preceding Archaic and Classical periods – for which there is scant evidence for burials – graves have been excavated from Hellenistic Knossos. The majority of these known graves are from the extensively explored North Cemetery area. Given the documented continuity in cemetery use, it is possible that Hellenistic burials also took place in other (as yet unknown) Archaic and Classical cemeteries. Early excavations also neglected the pottery of this time period and much of the study that has been conducted has focused on defining the typology and stylistic sequence of the finewares (Callaghan 1978; 1980; 1981; Eiring 2001), though some efforts have been made that begin to redress the balance (Coldstream 1999; Coldstream *et al.* 2001; Eiring 2001; Trainor 2019; 2021). Key remains from the Hellenistic city include residential and industrial areas to the south of the centre, including houses and roads in the area of the 'Unexplored Mansion', a wine press in the area of the modern Upper Village, and a number of kilns and cisterns in this same region (Homann-Wedeking 1950; Sackett 1992; Carington Smith and Wall 1994).

Evidence for cult activity has been found at a number of locations around Knossos. A hero-shrine attributed to Glaukos was likely founded in the Archaic period and appears to have remained in use at least until the time of the Roman conquest (Callaghan 1978; *KS2*:197, Hood and Smyth 1981, 22). A temple dedicated to Rhea on the palace site was first suggested by Arthur Evans, and although the dedication is uncertain the finds confirm a sanctuary in this area (Evans 1928, 5–6;1930, 4; Popham 1978, 185–87; Hood and Smyth 1981, 16, 20; Sporn 2002; Prent 2005, 514). The discovery of huge marble foot, and terracotta figurines and lamps dating from 600–200 BC indicate a temple dedicated to Zeus and Hera may have been located on the northern 'acropolis' (Monastiriako Kephali hill) (Payne 1935, 168; *KS2*:136, Hood and Smyth 1981, 20). A sanctuary of Demeter was excavated by Coldstream from 1957–1960 on the Lower Gypsades hill which may have been founded in the Protogeometric period and endured beyond the Roman conquest until the 2nd century AD (Coldstream 1973; *KS2*:286). There have been additional scattered finds that indicate further temples, sanctuaries and shrines from a variety of locations at Knossos (Hood and Smyth 1981). To the north, there was a Late Classical or Early Hellenistic hill-top tower (Figure 2.1), which may have been part of more extensive fortifications and is the only evidence for a defensive structure from any time period at the site (*KS2*:37; Hood and Boardman 1957; Kotsonas 2016).

2.1.3. Hellenistic burial practices at Knossos

The North Cemetery of Knossos, located in the area of the modern Venezelion Hospital and University Medical Faculty, is the main burial area known for the Hellenistic period. This is the only cemetery from which there was human skeletal material available for study, which comes from the KMF/78 and VNP/76 British School at Athens excavations. More recent excavations conducted by the Greek Archaeological Service have continued to reveal more pit, tile and cist graves dating to the Hellenistic period in this area (Grammatikaki 1991; 2006; Rousaki *et al.* 2019; 2020). In addition, small numbers of simple Hellenistic graves have been identified on all sides of the settlement, though they are often not fully studied and occasionally only described generally as 'Graeco-Roman' (Hood and Smyth 1981). As well as the more recent discoveries by the Greek Archaeological Service, there may be rock-cut chambers and cist graves among those graves not studied. The likelihood of cemeteries from the Hellenistic period existing in this area is supported by occasional discoveries of graves or finds suggestive of tombs in the area (Hutchinson and Boardman 1954, 216; Boardman 1967, 57; *KS2*:6).

The majority of grave goods from the known burials do not display substantial evidence for the ostentatious wealth that might be expected as a result of piracy or mercenary activities and as described by de Souza (1998, 114). A small number of graves did contain gold items, such as a pair of earrings, some rings, and a gold-leaf *epistomion*. The evidence from the rest of Crete includes some displays of wealth from funerary contexts with a total of fifteen gold wreaths known from tombs at Kissamos, Chania, Gortyn, Chersonissos and Lato, though the type and density of the leaves varied (Guyon 2008, 129). This is a Hellenistic practice and may reflect a practice of wreaths of real foiliage in graves. It endures into the Roman period but does not appear to continue beyond the 2nd century AD (Guyon 2008, 131). There were examples of rings (of gold and silver inset with stones, though more commonly iron or bronze bands), earrings

[8] *KS2* numbers refer to the Hood and Smyth (1981) survey; an interactive version of the survey map (Figure 2.1) is available online through the British School at Athens' website: https://digital.bsa.ac.uk/hood.php (last accessed 12 December 2022).

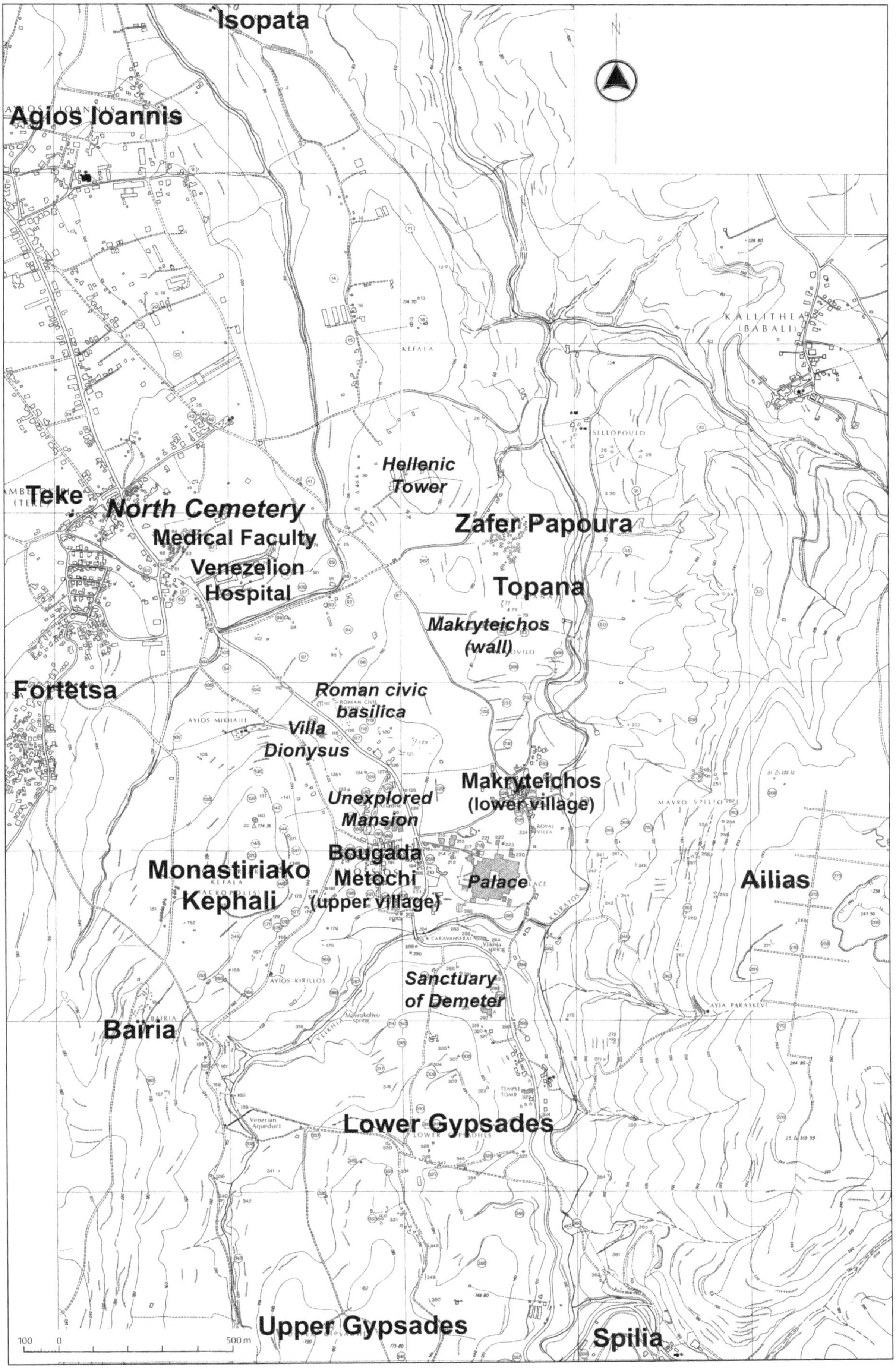

Figure 2.1. Map of the Knossos area with some key sites and locations. After Hood and Smyth (KS2) 1981.

(uncommon and found alongside necklaces and rings), necklaces (beads, chains and pendants in a variety of materials), gold-leaf *epistomia*, terracotta jewellery, coins, bronze mirrors, terracotta figurines and reliefs, and a wide range of clay vessels found in tombs across the island (Guyon 2008). While some of these finds, such as the ten gold beads from a *hypogeum* tomb at Chania, reflect displays of wealth, these are relatively uncommon finds (Guyon 2008, 138). Such displays of wealth, with large amounts of gold adornment, are better known from graves on mainland and northern Greece. Within the Hellenistic pit and tile graves at Knossos, there were usually either no associated burial goods (meaning the dating is unsure) or one or two poorly fired unguentaria of a soft, grey, friable fabric, and sometimes with a black glaze. Other shapes, including lamps, cups, lekythoi and thymiateria, were also occasionally present (Callaghan n.d.; Rousaki *et al.* 2020). Non-pottery grave goods were rarer but included coins, gold jewellery, bronze jugs (*prochous*), strigils, glass vessels, terracotta figurines, protomes and Dionysiac masks, and an incised carnelian gemstone with the image of Perseus (Grammatikaki 1991, 392). Green staining on mandibles from 'Charon's obol'[9] is found in both the Hellenistic and Roman periods at Knossos.

2.2. Roman Knossos

2.2.1. Roman conquest of Crete and cultural change

Though the Roman conquest of Crete was a forceful affair met by opposition from many Cretan cities, taking two years from invasion to conquest, the cultural and material changes that came with becoming a Roman province were slow to manifest themselves. Crete had been connected with Rome during the Hellenistic (Roman Republican) period via shipping routes and Roman merchants were living in some Cretan cities. Rome had started to become involved in Cretan affairs, acting as a mediator in disputes between different city states, since the early 2nd century BC. The port cities along the south coast, that had already been linked to Rome along its grain shipping route from Alexandria, were the first to show signs of change in their architecture and material culture. One of the first areas showing evidence of such change along the north coast was around the Mirabello Bay, with evidence of change in material culture spreading across the narrowest point between the north and south coasts of Crete from Ierapetra, illustrating the commercial context of this cultural spread (Hayden *et al.* 1992, 333; Haggis 1996; Gallimore 2015, 282). It was also noted in this corridor and across Crete that there was an increase in numbers of sites in the early Roman period as it became safer to live outside of the cities (Sanders 1982; Hayden *et al.* 1992). The island not only witnessed a spread of Roman culture and material culture, but the presence of eastern and African material culture and potential architectural influences demonstrate an intensification of trade and connectivity throughout the Mediterranean. Lissos and Sougia, on the south-west coast, have barrel-vaulted *opus incertum* tombs appearing potentially from the late 1st century BC which may have had had precursors in both Asia Minor and Italy (Moles forthcoming). Monumental above-ground burial structures, such as the free-standing mausolea in ashlar masonry at Knossos, Gortyn and Kissamos, are rare before the middle of the 1st century AD (Grammatikaki and Litinas 2000; Grammatikaki 2004; Vasilakis 2004; Lippolis *et al.* 2015; Skordou 2016). During this century, the south coast had a wider range of imports with large quantities of Arretine, African and Cypriot red slipped wares and smaller amounts of Çandarli ware and Italian sigillata (Eiring 2004; Baldwin Bowsky 2011). By the end of the 1st century AD, eastern sigillata B dominated across the island and general change across the north coast was widespread by this time. There were new cemeteries, public buildings and houses at many sites, the first mosaics at Knossos and Chania, and a number of expanded ports including at Tholos and Bali (Haggis 1996; Sweetman 2013, 142; Gallimore 2015).

2.2.2. The evolving urban landscape at Knossos

According to the Knossos Urban Landscape project, the settlement size was reduced during the Hellenistic period with a contraction of the city occurring prior to the Roman conquest, seen through the lack of evidence for Late Hellenistic pottery on the Lower Gypsades hill (Trainor 2019; Whitelaw *et al.* 2019). There may have been setbacks to urban development caused by the frequent disputes between poleis and the Roman invasion. The city, however, flourished as a thriving and connected centre of trade and, with the establishment of the colony, saw investment in new infrastructure and buildings. Knossos was re-founded as a civilian colony, thought to have had a Campanian, if not specifically Capuan, contingent, and was the only Roman colony in Crete. Farming lands to the south were granted to Capua to gain an income from (rather than necessarily to settle) after the Battle of Actium in 31 BC, as compensation for Capuan lands in Italy being granted to Octavian's soldiers from Sicily. It is in these years following the Battle of Actium, and probably after the settlement of the province in 27 BC, that the *Colonia Julia Nobilis Cnossus* is likely to have been established. It may have been excluded from the *Res Gestae* due to its original conception by Augustus' adoptive father, Julius Caesar, for whom the colony was named (Paton 1994, 143). The centre of the Roman city lay to the north of the Minoan Palace at Knossos, the ruins of which would presumably still have been visible at this time. A fascination with the city's mythical past is attested to in the Augustan coins which feature the Labyrinth of King Minos and in the Emperor Galba's claim to descent from the fabled Minoan royal family (Paton 1994, 144; 2004, 454; Alcock 2002, 123–30, 179–80). Kotsonas (2018) demonstrates that this fascination was not new in the Roman period, with the numismatic, literary and epigraphic sources of the Hellenistic period showing an interest in the epic myths.

[9] A custom originating in Classical Greece, but common across the Greek world and Roman Empire, where a bronze coin was placed in the mouth of the deceased to pay the boat fare to the underworld.

The new public buildings known from the colony include the theatre (*KS2*:110), the vast, barrel-vaulted civic basilica (*KS2*:112), and the remains of possibly two or three public baths, at least one of which was substantial in size (Hood and Smyth 1981; French 1994; Tomlinson 1996; Whitelaw and Trainor 2016). The *Makryteichos* (*KS2*:86) is a large concrete structure, thought potentially to have been a stoa (Hood and Smyth 1981; Sweetman 2004b). Regarding other public works, the Roman roads and property lines of known houses, in a small excavated area of the 'Unexplored Mansion', appear to follow the same lines as their Hellenistic predecessors (Sackett 1992, 18), and an aqueduct was built, which is thought to have been started in the 2nd century though there is no dating evidence for its initial construction (Hood and Smyth 1981; Sackett *et al.* 1992, 47; Kelly 2013, 135). The sanctuary of Demeter to the south, on Lower Gypsades hill, continued in use during the earlier Roman period, while the so-called Shrine of Glaukos, at the south of the Roman city in the modern upper Knossos village, may have gone out of use with the Roman conquest (Callaghan 1978). The cult of a local hero associated with military training was perhaps not favoured by the Roman authorities (Callaghan 1978; Hood and Smyth 1981), though the assignation of the shrine to Glaukos and the dating of its abandonment may be erroneous (Trainor, pers. comm.). Other possible temples, including one possibly dedicated to Rhea on the Palace site and another potentially of Zeus and Hera at the northern end of the Acropolis hill may also have continued in use but too little is preserved of their deposits to document continuity (Hood and Smyth 1981). Recent excavations have uncovered a temple dedicated to Zeus and Artemis from the 2nd century AD on the Anetakis plot in the upper Knossos village (Kanta and Serpetsidaki 2015). There is also epigraphic and sculptural evidence for the imperial cult, a temple of Asclepius, and possibly also for the cults of Isis and Serapis (Paton 2004, 453). The sculpted blocks from a 2nd century Corinthian porticoed building of Pentelic marble were preserved by their reuse in a 5th century built tomb (KMF78, Tomb 244) in the region of the North Cemetery. This may have been a temple, heroön or a grand mausoleum originally (Paton 1994, 149). There is evidence for both change and continuity in the buildings and religion but the evidence for change is largely coming from the 2nd century AD and later.

Wealth among some of the colony's inhabitants is attested by the 2nd century grand houses, including the Villa Dionysus, with its impressive collection of fine mosaics, imported-marble veneered walls and frescos. The House of the Diamond Frescos had walls of painted plaster mimicking coloured marble and decorative architectural mouldings in stucco, demonstrating the illusion of grandeur, though a cheaper alternative to the 'real thing'. There was scattered evidence throughout the Roman city for the use of exotic stones used as flooring and veneering (Paton 1994, 148; 2004, 454; Paton and Schneider 1999). Mosaics known from excavations and mosaic tesserae and marble veneers recorded during the urban survey are prevalent across the whole northern area, covering approximately two-fifths of the city, suggesting a widespread affluent district (Sweetman 2003; Trainor 2019).

2.2.3. The presence of colonists

During the first decades of the colony's existence, there is not a great deal of change evident from either the architecture, as discussed above, or the material culture. Pottery styles initially appear to continue in the local Hellenistic tradition. The introduction of stamped Italian sigillata fine wares at Knossos can be interpreted as a gradual process (there are no early Augustan stamps known from the colony) of local elite tastes selectively integrating aspects of Roman culture with their own as they redefined their position in the Roman world (Eiring 2004, 71; Baldwin Bowsky 2011, 117). In the Augustan period, eastern sigillata A, Cypriot sigillata and in particular eastern sigillata B were popular tablewares at Knossos, as at other sites in the Greek East. A shift in balance from these eastern regional tablewares towards the Italian sigillatae occurred in the mid-late Augustan period; however, the Italian sigillatae are estimated to have been less significant than the eastern sigillatae generally across time at Knossos and their popularity was short-lived (Eiring 2004, 71; Poblome 2004, 18, 22). The production of both strictly local shapes and copies of international shapes continued at Knossos during the Roman period (Eiring 2000, 197).

Changes are noted in the epigraphic record with the introduction of Latin, however, this does not occur on the scale that would be expected for a colony (Baldwin Bowsky 2004b; Dijkstra and Moles forthcoming). It has been noted that the names of most magistrates and priests known to us were Latin, though Greek inscriptions are more common than Latin outside the administrative sphere (Sanders 1982; Baldwin Bowsky 2004b; 2006; 2011; Sweetman 2007). Strong links are also attested between Knossos and Campania from inscriptions in the 1st century AD and the abundant presence of Campanian pottery from the 1st–3rd centuries, though it is difficult to tell if these links were due to the original colonists or simply due to a more widespread trading pattern throughout Crete (Paton 1994, 143). Baldwin Bowsky (2011, 117) also suggests that there is onomastic evidence to suggest that, as well as the presence of Italian and specifically Campanian names, the presence of the colony (a 'little Rome') at Knossos also attracted new people from elsewhere in Crete. The 1st or early-2nd century Poseidon mosaic from Knossos was signed by the artist (ΑΠΟΛΛΙΝΑΡΙϹ ΕΠΟΙΕΙ) in Greek, though he had a Roman name that frequently appeared in Campanian inscriptions (Alexiou 1968, 126; Sweetman 2013, 118). There appears to have been a good deal of mixing of names, with, for example, a Roman family name and a Greek personal name potentially indicating newly-attained Roman citizenship, thus making it impossible to judge the scale of in-migration from the onomastic evidence (Baldwin Bowsky 1999). The new building types, such as baths, may have been a requirement for incoming colonists or migrants from Italy, though these do not appear to have been built until the 2nd century AD, more than a century after the initial establishment of the colony (Kelly 2013).

Unlike Corinth, which was established as a colony for the purpose of re-housing many people, mainly ex-slaves, from Rome, it seems that Knossos had a presence of Campanian settlers, particularly in official administrative roles but perhaps did not receive huge numbers of incomers to dominate the local population. Having put up a great resistance to the original Roman conquest in 67 BC, the establishment of the colony and presence of Roman officials, may have been partially to ensure that the was no further trouble from Knossos, and, in terms of the lack of imposing Roman cultural features (such as language and burial practices) on the local population. It may have been the case that as long as Knossos was not causing trouble, there was no need for the Romans to enforce further changes on the city, other than those that occurred as a process of acculturation or 'globalisation' (Sweetman 2007). This process of change was gradual throughout Crete.

2.2.4. Knossos, a cultural melting pot

Baldwin Bowsky (2011, 129) describes the evolving mix of tablewares over time at Knossos as representing a long-term process of 'normalisation' (rather than Romanisation), essentially meaning acculturation or what Sweetman (2007) refers to as 'globalisation'. These are ways of describing the processes of cultural exchange that occurred due to the increased contact and interaction of peoples throughout the Empire, in Rome and the provinces. Though there was a brief increased preference for Italian finewares, various eastern finewares were more popular during the Roman period (Coldstream *et al.* 2001; Eiring 2004; Poblome 2004). A range of new tomb types at Knossos have earlier parallels at sites in Italy, Egypt, the Aegean islands, Cyprus, Asia Minor and the East (Toynbee 1971; Empereur and Nenna 2001; Venit 2002, 37–65; Empereur and Nenna 2003; Hellmann 2006, 296–99; Guyon 2008; Guimier-Sorbets and Michaelides 2009; Nenna 2009; Brandt *et al.* 2017). At Knossos, society was a constantly evolving in terms of its identity, finding a balance between its position both as a Roman colony, with Roman houses and public spaces, and as an Aegean city with a taste for regionally-produced fine wares, a preference for the Greek language and a maintenance of inhumation burial rites throughout. While Knossos was well-integrated within the networks of the Empire it retained a strong local cultural identity within the province (Sweetman 2007). Though the process of cultural alterations at Knossos seems much slower than comparable cities in the Greek east, such as Gortyn, Corinth and Sparta, especially when taking into account the initial investment that must have been made in the colony. Gradual change has been noted at colonies in the western Empire, at Lyon and Nyon (Sweetman 2007). The term Romanisation should be rejected for these processes, as it does not account for the range of diverse reactions to similar processes in different cities and in different contexts, and it certainly does not cover the intensification of trade and connectivity involving Crete in the Mediterranean network which resulted in a melting pot of cultures – alongside a maintenance of local characteristics – visible in the material remains.

2.2.5. The burial evidence

Cist, tile and pit graves remain common features of the burial landscape and are likely to have remained the dominant (if not only) burial types in the Early Roman period up to the mid-1st century AD, but there is a move towards more elaborate architecture and greater variety in tomb types. From the mid-1st century AD, there is the appearance of monumental built tombs or mausolea (masonry tombs with various features, including visible structures of large cut-stone blocks, barrel-vaulted roofs, and subterranean chambers), and rock-cut chamber tombs (with *arcosolia* usually on three sides, often with small niches cut in their walls and *klinai* (funerary couches) with hewn 'pillow' for the head of the deceased, and an entranceway with short dromos on the fourth side). In the Mid-Late Roman period (3rd–4th centuries), stone-lined (sometimes referred to as built) tombs or cist graves (see discussion on the distinction in Section 3.5) are the most widely attested tomb types and a walled and paved funerary enclosure was uncovered during the Sanatorium Basilica excavations (Frend and Johnston 1962, 204). This array of built and rock-cut chamber tombs, alongside the stone-lined and brick cist, tile and pit graves, is very common throughout Roman Crete, with parallels for these tomb types in both the eastern and western Empire (Moles forthcoming; Sanders 1982; Guyon 2008). None of the distinctive Campanian funerary stelae have been discovered at Knossos. These were sculpted in high relief depicting the dead person and their family within a shrine or *aedicula*, and were common in Capua and neighbouring towns (Frederiksen 1984, 287). Their absence has been used in the past to refute the idea that the colonists came from Campania, the supposition being that they would have brought their burial customs with them (Paton 1994, 144). However, the more widespread lack of Roman or Italian burial customs by the colonists, including the rite of cremation, may be indicative of an abandonment of some of these 'home' traditions in favour of adopting features of the local funerary rites or wholly new ones. Another possibility is that there were not many incomers or that they were buried in distinct cemeteries that have not yet been encountered.

While there are changes in the funerary landscape at Knossos in the Roman period, in both burial location and tomb types (see Chapter 3), there does not appear to be a transferral of many common Roman – nor any specifically Campanian – burial customs. The most notable of these is the complete absence of any cremated remains discovered for this time period anywhere at Knossos, or the associated burial architecture, such as *columbaria*, and this pattern prevails across all of Crete. While it cannot be stated with certainty that there were no cremation burials in Roman

Crete, if it existed it was a rare, minority custom. It is completely unattested in the archaeological record for the Roman period, and only a single possible example is known from the Hellenistic period, in the case of a 3rd century BC amphora in a pit grave at Rhokka in west Crete (Gondicas 1984, 302; Guyon 2008, 177). However, it is possible that this is a grave offering rather than a cinerary urn. Cremation cannot be seen solely as a Roman rite, however, as it had been a minority practice in regions of the Greek world in the preceding periods, including in the Peloponnese and Asia Minor (Spanu 2000, 174; Dimakis 2016, 38). Its usage does, however, increase dramatically at sites such as Patras in the Early Roman period suggesting a direct link with the presence of colonists (Dijkstra 2015; 2019). It was a short-lived phenomenon for most cities in Greece that had adopted cremation in the Early Roman period and it went out of use at most sites throughout the Empire in the course of the 3rd century AD (Faber *et al.* 2007). Cremation was an expensive process, with inhumation often being considered the more primitive or lower status option in the Roman Empire (Toynbee 1971). However, the absence of cremation at Knossos cannot be explained by a lack of wealth, but rather it was a conscious decision to maintain the traditional burial custom.

Though inhumation occasionally appears alongside cremation in Republican Rome, and was notably favoured by some families, such as the Gens Cornelia, these were unusual cases, remarked upon by Pliny and Cicero for going against the grain (Toynbee 1971, 39). It was not until during the reign of Hadrian, in the 2nd century AD, that a gradual but steady increase in numbers of inhumations replacing cremations is seen (Toynbee 1971, 40). Such examples demonstrate that within the Empire, with its well-connected networks and cultural infusion, new practices were adopted in Rome as well as throughout the provinces. This is the product of increased contact and the manifestation of the processes of globalisation that occurred across the Empire. The sarcophagus, an eastern form of burial container already popular in Asia Minor in the Hellenistic period, was still considered a foreign marvel in Rome at the end of the 1st century AD (Spanu 2000, 173). Stone sarcophagi were a new burial feature on Crete in the Roman period, though there were some terracotta sarcophagi known from the Hellenistic period. The 1st century AD sculpted marble 'Polybos sarcophagus' from Knossos was an early example of the stone sarcophagi (Alexiou 1968; Sanders 1982), and of the more than sixty examples known from Crete, the majority were of 2nd or 3rd century date (Guyon 2008, 119).

In the Roman period, the burial goods are both more plentiful and varied. Besides pottery, common finds include glass and stone vessels (such as perfume bottles and bowls), coins, jewellery, other metal objects such as mirrors, probes and spoons, metal fittings for wooden caskets and boxes, terracottas and figurines (Cavanagh 1978; Carington Smith 1982; Wardle and Wardle 2004; Rousaki *et al.* 2016). Theatrical masks were found in three chamber tombs, dating in use from approximately AD 50 to 150 (Paton 1994, 152). The Greek and local custom of placing a coin in the mouth of the deceased continued but it is not found in any studied skeletal material or published reports after the 2nd century AD.

2.3. Late Antique Knossos

2.3.1. Dates and terminology

The transition from the Roman to Late Antique period (5th–7th centuries) Knossos is less well defined than that between the Hellenistic and Roman periods, in name as well as socio-politically. As 'Late Antique' encompasses a period of time that can either be referred to as Late Roman or Early Byzantine, it was decided that this term would be employed to avoid the confusion of which is more applicable and because it carries fewer cultural inferences, in line with Sweetman's discussion of terminology for the period (Sweetman 2004a, 317). 'Early Christian', which has previously been used at Knossos for this time period (Catling *et al.* 1976; Hayes 2001), was also rejected due to the cultural and religious implications of the term, as well as the fact that there is actually evidence for Christianity at Knossos as early as the second century AD (Paton 1994, 148). It would have been convenient for comparative purposes to use the same ceramic-based date ranges and terms as the Knossos Urban Landscape Project (KULP), Early Roman (1st century BC-1st century AD), Middle Roman (2nd–3rd centuries), Late Roman (4th–5th centuries, and Late Antique (6th–7th centuries), but as some of the tomb groups that are the focus of this study were in use from the 1st–2nd centuries and others bridged the 3rd–4th centuries, these ranges were often unsuitable. Even the KULP authors have ended up using a selection of terms for the Late Antique years and any discussion of this period inevitably ends up reaching back into the earlier Roman centuries as the contraction of the city and the diminishing evidence for new building projects was a continuous and gradual process from the 3rd to 7th centuries (Whitelaw *et al.* 2007; 2012; 2016; 2017; 2019; Whitelaw and Trainor 2016; Trainor 2019).

2.3.2. Urban contraction and evidence for gradual change

The gradual transition and lack of a clear socio-political or cultural division between the Roman and Late Antique periods is evident in the continued use of areas of the city and the staggered abandonment of others. There appears to have been a contraction of the city from the 2nd century onwards particularly in the southwest of the city, though there is abundant evidence for continued prosperity in the public and private spheres through to the 3rd century AD (Whitelaw *et al.* 2017, 12). By the 4th century the settlement was significantly reduced in size, though it is uncertain how long many of the public buildings constructed in the 2nd and 3rd centuries (e.g. the civic basilica, baths, theatre) remained in use. There are concrete ruins and a concentration of coloured glass tesserae to the north of the Roman civic basilica (*KS2*:94) that indicate a major, probably Late Antique, monumental building and the recent KULP survey also observed many mosaic tesserae in this area (Whitelaw pers. comm.). There is some suggestion of maintenance of the aqueduct into the Late Antique period (Whitelaw pers. comm.). The recent survey evidence reinforces the scattered excavated deposits in suggesting the continued contraction of the settlement during this period in the northern area of the Greco-Roman city (Whitelaw and Trainor 2016; Trainor 2019).

Findings in the areas of the Unexplored Mansion and Villa Dionysus demonstrate some evidence of destruction and abandonment during the 3rd and 4th centuries (Hayes 1983; Sackett 1992, 25; Paton 1998, 127). However, while the Villa Dionysus itself had only evidence of 'squatter occupation' after its destruction towards the end of the 2nd century (Paton 1998, 127), two mosaics to the south of the Roman civic basilica and east of the modern road demonstrate 4th century habitation in this area, with one (KS2:117) being constructed at this time and the other (KS2:119) having a coin of Theodosius directly on top of it demonstrating its continued use into this period (Sweetman 2004b, 483). Extensive 4th and 5th century ceramic evidence from the 'Knossos 2000' (K2K) excavation demonstrate habitation to the west of the road and south of the Villa Dionysus (Forster 2009). This excavation also produced evidence of new buildings being constructed into the 4th century, with activity continuing in the area into the 6th century (French 1994, 75; Tomlinson 1996, 41; Forster 2009), and there were late 4th and/or early 5th century minor walls and drains found on the Villa Dionysus site (Hayes 1983, 99). The House of the Diamond Frescos on the Unexplored Mansion site was damaged in the 2nd century and rebuilt before further destruction and abandonment in the 3rd century. The whole area was said to have been abandoned in the 4th century, likely after the AD 365 earthquake, when evidence of destruction was attested across sites in Crete. However, there was 4th century pottery in wash levels across the site indicating some level of continued activity in the area, and it is possible that they dug through late levels with only mud-brick architecture, as was found in the K2K trenches, but failed to recognise it. There was later evidence from the nearby sites, with clear indications of 4th century occupation in the Royal Road area and some limited evidence for 5th–6th century occupation from the Stratigraphic Museum Extension excavation (Sanders 1982; Warren 1988; Sackett 1992). The KULP survey also observed 5th–6th century material in this area, flanking the modern road (Whitelaw, pers.comm.) The evidence for the continued vitality of Knossos (and Crete) into at least the 6th century AD, despite the contraction of the city, has been discussed in Section 1.2.

2.3.3. The religious architecture and burial evidence

The evidence for Late Antique Knossos comes largely from the three basilica churches, the North Cemetery Basilica, the nearby Sanatorium Basilica, and a third unexcavated and undated example below the modern church of Agia Sofia in Makryteichos (lower Knossos) village, and from burials, which were located largely in the North Cemetery. Though Christianity is known to have been present on Crete since the 2nd century, the 5th century saw the beginning of its monumentalisation with the appearance of over 90 basilica churches across Crete. This indicates the economic security of the island, which was due to its agricultural produce and location along the Alexandria to Constantinople grain route (Sanders 1982; Sweetman 2017). Like at Knossos, there is relatively little domestic evidence at any site across the island from the late 3rd century onwards, nor is there substantial evidence for other monumental public buildings (Sweetman 2013, 9, 144). This suggests a change in focus in the expression of wealth and in art and architecture from the secular to the religious and from the private to the public spheres (Sweetman 2004b, 487). However, at most sites in Crete, excavations have not focused on Roman or later levels, and Byzantine-focused excavations have been primarily concerned with churches until very recently, therefore post-Roman (and often Roman) levels have received little or no attention. Gortyn and Kissamos are the only sites where there has been an explicit focus on Roman levels and both sites have produced substantial amounts of Roman and Late Antique material (Pologiorgi 1985; Stiros and Papageorgiou 2001; Ortolani 2004; di Vita 2010; Giorgi 2016; Theodoulou *et al.* 2018).

The construction of the North Cemetery (or KMF) Basilica has been dated to the early 5th century and there is evidence to suggest it was both a martyrium and a mortuary or cemetery church (Megaw 1984; Sweetman 2004a; 2011b; Sweetman and Becker 2005). It was innovative in its use of wall mosaics, demonstrating that Knossos continued to be a well-connected and important centre that still attracted craftspeople. The Sanatorium Basilica was constructed in the early 6th century, while the earlier basilica was still in use. It was also likely to have been a martyrium due to its positioning over the earlier 3rd–4th century cemetery and in particular, its incorporation of one particular tomb into the narthex of the church, with a hole and inset Minoan stone bowl in the cover slabs, presumably for pouring libations or some other ritual surrounding the relics interred within (Frend and Johnston 1962). Little is known of the plan or date of the Agia Sofia basilica due to its inaccessibility below the later church. There are also smaller churches or chapels known at Agios Kyrillos (*KS2* map D7, standing ruin 80m downslope of where it was marked by Hood and Smyth 1981) and two east of the modern road, north-east and south of the civic basilica (*KS2*:96 and 111 respectively), but these have not been dated and could be of any period from Roman to Medieval (Whitelaw, pers. comm.).

The majority of tombs known for the Late Antique period come from the North Cemetery, surrounding the KMF Basilica and excavated at the same time (KMF/78 and 79, *KS2*:64; Hayes 2001; Sweetman and Becker 2005). There have also been a small number of graves assigned to a Late Antique or Byzantine date at various other locations. In fairly close proximity to the North Cemetery, the Fortetsa

Fork osteotheke (KFF/74, *KS2*:59) was a similar sort of construction to the KMF osteothekai and contained more burials than any other tomb known from Knossos (Catling *et al.* 1976). The northern contraction of the settlement, indicated in the survey results and the limited evidence from excavated abandonment deposits, is also supported by the scattered and largely undated 'Roman' burials, such as the cist and tile graves to the west of the palace (*KS2*:211 and 212, and KOP/79), the cist grave (*KS2*:209, Skeletal Unit 105) which can be dated to the 4th century (Hutchinson 1936), and two rock-cut rectangular graves, one of which had large cover slabs, of 5th or 6th century date (*KS2*:183 Alexiou 1966, 325), perhaps suggesting a similar date for the other graves in this area. There was also the KEP/79 stone- and tile-lined tomb excavated on the lower northern slopes of Gypsades (Sweetman and Grigoropoulos 2010). Tile graves north-east of the Villa Dionysus, near the Ariadne nightclub and in the upper Knossos village are all thought likely to be Late Antique (Sweetman and Grigoropoulos 2010). The location of these burials suggests that this area was otherwise no longer inhabited, though intramural burials had become acceptable by this time period as Christians looked to be buried on sacred land associated with churches (Ivison 1996, 102).

The diversity of tomb forms decreased in the later Roman period and into Late Antiquity with all the tombs known from this period being some form of stone-lined cutting in the earth, whether cist grave or osteotheke, slab-lined or masonry built. Grave goods were extremely rare and generally coincidental trappings rather than intentional offerings, as was standard in Christian graves.

3
Material

Skeletal remains offer a fundamental source of information for the study of health and diet. However, they should not be relied upon in isolation and should be considered alongside their archaeological context, comparative evidence, and any available historical resources. Although the skeletal remains can offer a broad range of evidence derived from past contexts, supplementary information helps to depict a more complete picture.

The human skeletal material available for this study comes from excavations undertaken by the British School at Athens (BSA) at Knossos from the 1930s to 1970s. It spans the time periods from the Hellenistic period to Late Antiquity, approximately 323 BC to 800 AD. A catalogue detailing the contextual information for the skeletal units studied appears in Appendix A.[10]

3.1. Previous studies on the Knossos skeletal material

Some of the material studied for this book has previously been looked at to provide a basic skeletal report for the publication of the excavation of the specific tomb or cemetery. This includes the report by Marshall Becker for the Late Antique North Cemetery material (Sweetman and Becker 2005, 370–83) and that by Jonathan Musgrave for the Late Antique Fortetsa Fork osteotheke (Catling *et al.* 1976, 40–46). Musgrave has also conducted the skeletal analysis of the Early Iron Age North Cemetery burials which were largely cremations and some other Early Iron Age and Bronze Age assemblages (Sackett and Musgrave 1976; Callaghan, Coldstream, *et al.* 1981; Musgrave and Evans 1981; Wall *et al.* 1986; Coldstream and Catling 1996). Argyro Nafplioti has also studied some Bronze Age skeletal assemblages from the Sellopoulo, Ailias and Mavrospelio Middle-Late Minoan chamber tombs and the Lower Gypsades tholos tomb of a similar date, though the publications from this work are thus far limited to isotopic analyses looking at both migration and diet (Nafplioti 2007; 2008; 2015; 2016). The dietary isotope work is particularly relevant for the present project as it enables diet to be traced at Knossos from approximately 1900 BC to AD 800, with a gap in the middle from Protogeometric to Classical times due to the skeletal material being cremated or absent entirely in the archaeological record.

3.2. Recovery, preservation and sample condition

The condition of the material, the excavation methods for its initial retrieval, and the recording and preservation of contextual information were often not optimal. Many excavated burial contexts from Knossos have produced very poorly preserved skeletal material, often to the extent that it preserved no diagnostic elements for study, including the Marathaniou Lakkos (ML/70) and Monastiriako Kephali (KLT/78) chamber tombs.[11] This may also be why no bones have been kept from some excavations despite being mentioned in excavation notes (Curator's Logbook, BSA Archive). The bones have suffered from poor excavation due to the lack of value attributed to the material at the time. Throughout the 20th century osteoarchaeology was a slowly developing discipline which only really took off in the last quarter of that century. The excavation and retention of skeletal material became an essential part of excavations, with specialists ensuring the proper excavation of the remains as well as carrying out post-excavation studies using the standard methods that now exist (Armelagos and Gerven 2003; Roberts *et al.* 2005; Buikstra and Beck 2006; Lagia *et al.* 2014; Larsen 2018). For the different contexts and excavations which produced material for this study, differing degrees of care were afforded to the retrieval and preservation of skeletal elements. Excavation was often quite coarse, using hand picks rather than trowels, particularly for rapid rescue excavations. Recovery was almost always by hand in the trench, with no sieving, which would have resulted in the loss of small bones and fragments. Numerous fresh breaks, scratches and trowel marks were observed on the bones during the analysis. This exacerbates the already general poor condition of the bones and fragmentation from natural taphonomic processes for the majority of contexts. Some contexts were eliminated from the macroscopic analysis for this study because all that survived were small fragments of bone shafts with poor surface condition and no diagnostic pieces, such as joint surfaces, or teeth that were so degraded that it would not be possible to accurately score any sort of lesion or attrition.

Commingling was a cultural pattern with many of the studied tombs being collective burials, with reorganisation and displacement of bones to make space for later burials and potentially secondary re-burial in the osteothekai.

[10] Appendix A can be accessed at https://doi.org/10.30861/9781407360355-AppendixA

[11] Many of the North Cemetery Hellenistic/Early Roman pit graves (KMF/78) were also too poorly preserved for study. The bones from Spilia Tomb E also fell into this category and only the teeth from this tomb were studied.

However, the analysis of the material is further complicated due to poor storage resulting in a loss of contextual information. This can happen due to a lack of understanding of human skeletal anatomy at the excavation stage with groups of bones being wrongly attributed to specific individuals. There were incidences, for example, where a bag labelled 'Skeleton 2' contained a random selection of elements from a minimum number of three individuals, and cases of wrong labelling, such as a navicular (foot bone) being labelled 'Skull', perhaps being confused for an orbit by an untrained eye. Following this, there were further problems caused for the material situation in the loss of contextual information (however little or much was recorded at the time) due to conditions in the apotheke where they were stored for the past c.40–80 years and the inadequate materials used to contain them. Cardboard boxes had become weak and disintegrated in the damp, paper bags and labels had been eaten away by rodents and insects, sunlight had faded some external labels of boxes, and poor-quality plastic bags had cracked and split. Thus, the material became even more commingled in storage and while for most at least some contextual information could be retrieved, for a few it was entirely lost. For some there was little information other than an excavation code attributed to a box of commingled bones with no attempt even to designate so much as areas of the tomb, bone groupings or individual skeletons. In cases like this, where a mass of bones was left loose in the box, they have also suffered from further fragmentation and attrition.

The material was never cleaned, significantly slowing the analytical processing and demonstrating the lack of depth that some of the previous published studies went into with the skeletal material. Although cleaning can damage delicate specimens, particularly cleaning with water as they often crack as they dry, without some careful cleaning diagnostic surfaces are not visible. Even elements such as skulls and complete long bones which were glued back together, as was often done, with a particular focus on skulls, for metrical studies in the 20th century (Musgrave and Evans 1981), were not cleaned prior to glue being applied.

3.3. Topography

3.3.1. Hellenistic cemeteries

While scant evidence survives for Hellenistic cemeteries on all sides of the settlement (Figure 3.1), the area that has become known as the North Cemetery area has produced the greatest numbers of burials by far, compared to the rest of the Knossos valley. In the Teke area, immediately north of the Medical Faculty site, tile and cist graves were noted by Sara Paton, Sinclair Hood and David Smyth in 1976, and by Alexandra Karetsou in 1979 (*KS2*:43–45). Further graves have continued to be uncovered in the North Cemetery area over the last forty years, beginning with four tombs reported by Catling in 1982 and many more excavated by the Greek Archaeological Service (Catling 1983, 51; Grammatikaki 1991, 391–92; 1997, 987–89; Serpetsidaki 1994, 698–99; Banou 1997, 985; 2002, 307–14; Ministry of Culture (ΥΠΠΟ) 1997, 124; Guyon 2008). These have largely been the narrow pit graves but some tile and cist graves have also been discovered, as well as a small number of large rectangular rock-cut pits (Grammatikaki 1991).

To the north-east of the settlement, at Topana, two Hellenistic/Roman 'rock-cut shaft graves'[12] were excavated by Cressida Ridley and Mark Cameron in 1968 (KS2:78; Fraser 1969, 34). These are the same sort of narrow pit graves known abundantly from the North Cemetery (Curator's Logbook). To the east of the settlement on slopes of the Ailias hill (north of the earlier Mavrospelio cemetery), six tombs were excavated which were said to date to the end of the 4th century BC. The tomb type was not described but they contained spindle-shaped unguentaria and one grave had a burial with a coin that had been placed in the mouth of the deceased (*KS2*:238; Alexiou 1957, 342; Hood 1957, 24).

Hellenistic graves were identified in the Fortetsa Cemetery, which was predominantly Early Iron Age graves (Brock 1957). As the focus of the publication was on the Early Iron Age cemetery, there was very little description of the later graves, but they appear largely to have been pit graves, referred to as inhumation graves or occasionally cists.[13] Burial goods were similar to those of the North Cemetery, simple and few, often restricted to a single grey fusiform unguentarium. Other finds mentioned include lamps, jugs, a lekythos, coins, a silver ring and a bronze ring covered in gold leaf with an impression of a charging bull on the bezel (Brock 1957).

Over 50 'Greco-Roman' rock-cut tombs were visible at the southern end of the acropolis on the Baïria hill (*KS2*:154). Four were excavated in 1968 by Popham, Cameron and Ridley though they were thought likely to date to the beginning of the Roman period (KS2:157; Fraser 1969, 33). Two more were investigated in 1977 by Jill Carington Smith which were both Roman, but it is possible there were also earlier tombs here (Catling 1977b, 61). The same applies to the rock-cut chamber tombs on Monastiriako Kephali, often originally described as Greco-Roman (Platon 1947, 632). All tombs of this type, with rock-cut niches and *klinai*, that have been investigated more recently have proved to be Roman in date (Carington Smith 1982; Wardle and Wardle 2004; Guyon 2008) and those investigated by Hogarth near Zafer Papoura were all dated to the 2nd-3rd centuries with coins of A. Severus,

[12] These are rock cut pit or tile graves, similar to those in the North Cemetery. One has gabled *kalyvitis* tiles covering it and contained a Roman lamp (Topana 1968 Photo IV [BSA Archives]; Curator's Logbook, 32). *AR* 1968–69 calls these graves 'Roman', but *KS2*:78 says 'Hellenistic (?)' and the entry in the Curator's Logbook (p.32) says 'probably Hellenistic'. The rock cut pit graves next to these were dated to the 2nd-3rd century AD by coins (*KS2*:77; Hogarth 1900, 82).

[13] From a closer look at the terminology, it appears these are not stone-lined cists, as was originally assumed, but are more likely to be the common type of pit graves cut into the soft kouskouras rock (Brock 1957, 85, 99).

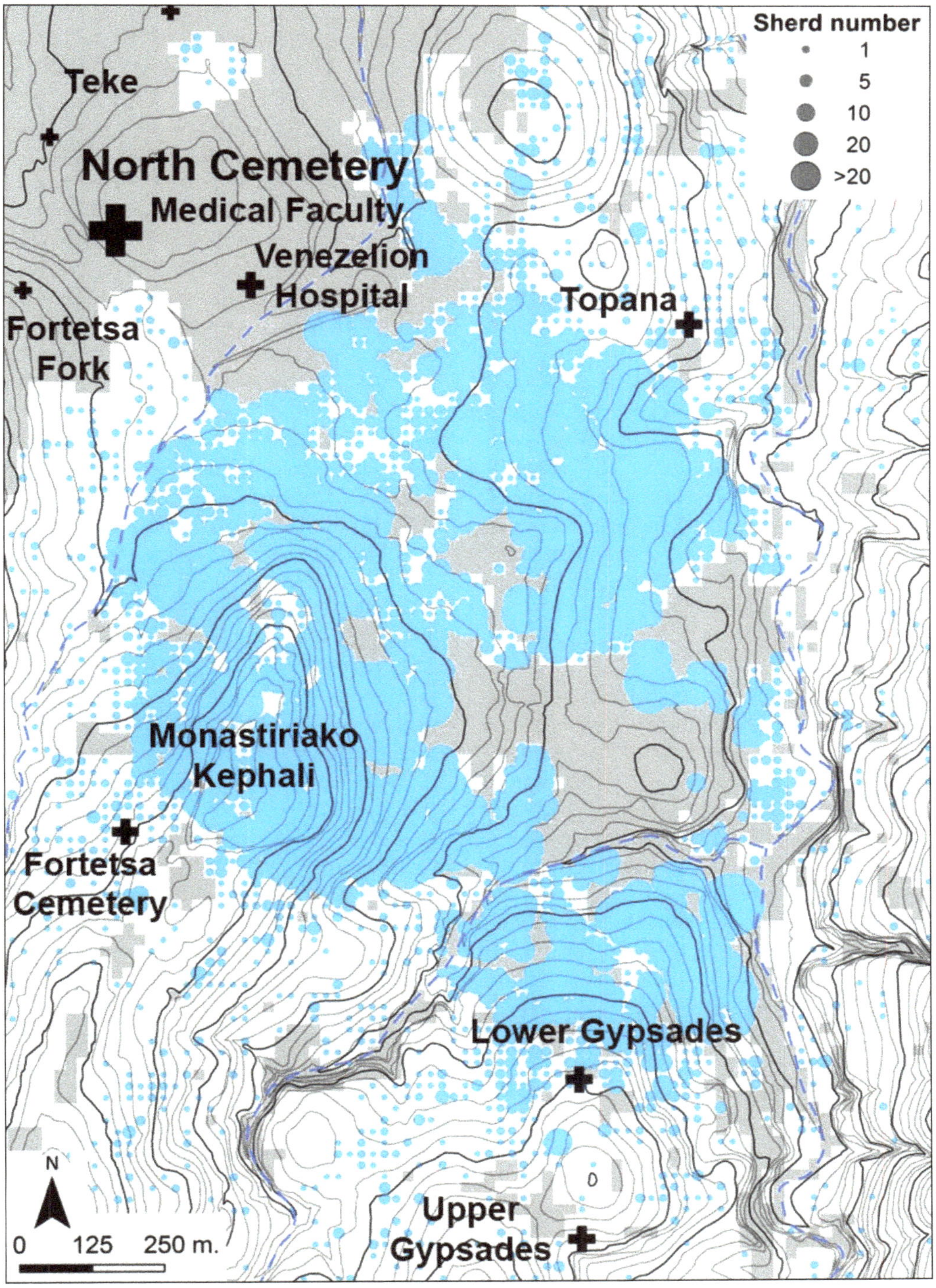

Figure 3.1. 'Hellenic' (Classical-Hellenistic) sherds (blue dots) from the Knossos Urban Landscape Project (KULP) and known tombs of this period (black crosses). Grey squares are unsurveyed area. Map: Todd Whitelaw.

Gordian and Julia Mammaea (Hogarth diary 25/04/1900; Hogarth 1900).

An inscribed tombstone was observed on the Gypsades hill in 1947, potentially indicating tombs in this area (*KS2*:334; Jeffery 1949, 37), which was confirmed by the discovery of two cist graves in the area, dating to the Late Hellenistic period and containing lamps, lekythoi, glass and ceramic unguentaria and bronze coins and further pit graves cut into the LMIIIB chamber tombs on the south slope of Lower Gypsades (Grammatikaki 1993, 448–49; 2006). There were also Early Roman 'poor' tile graves found here by Hogarth, some of which Callaghan claims were Hellenistic due to the 3rd-2nd century pottery (*KS2*:305; Hogarth 1900, 70). Further south-east at Seragia, near Spilia, two rectangular rock-cut tombs were excavated and thought to date to the 3rd century BC due to the black fusiform unguentarium placed on the legs of one individual (*KS2*:366; Alexiou 1967, 486; Megaw 1967, 20). These were a similar length to the pit graves of the North Cemetery (170cm and 180cm) but were much wider at 100cm and 130cm respectively, compared to the standard 50cm of most of the pit graves.

There was a 4th century *hypogeum* excavated at Katsambas, east of Heraklion (Alexiou 1969). This is the only more monumental tomb known from the wider area, though it was not as elaborate as the only other known examples of *hypogea* on Crete, at Chania (Markoulaki and Niniou-Kindeli 1982; 2009). These in turn were much less elaborate than the examples known from Egypt and the Near East, such as at Alexandria and Dura Europos (Empereur and Nenna 2001; 2003; Venit 2002; Konrad 2007). No *loculi* are mentioned for the Katsambas tomb, though due to its depth below the surface (the chamber floor was 5.3 metres below the present surface), with the presence of a dromos it was termed a *hypogeum* (Guyon 2008, 694), and its chamber was much larger than any of the rectangular pits, rock-cut or built chamber tombs known from Hellenistic or Roman Knossos at 2.95 by 4.1 metres.

It is not only the lack of study that makes some of these tombs difficult to date but even those that have received some attention cannot be closely dated due to the continuity in pottery in both fabrics and repertoire of shapes across the transition in political status between the Classical and Hellenistic and again between Hellenistic and Early Roman periods (Eiring 2001, 1). The only skeletal material available to study from the Hellenistic period was from the North Cemetery, from the Knossos Medical Faculty excavations (KMF/78, *KS2*:62) and two tile graves from the Venizelion North Perimeter excavations (VNP/76, *KS2*:63) as displayed in Figure 3.2. Of the c.163 KMF/78 graves assigned to a Hellenistic (or probable Hellenistic) date, 59 had skeletal material that was preserved well enough to merit study. These were largely simple pit graves cut into the soft kouskouras rock with few or no burial goods. An elaboration on the representativeness of the skeletal material can be found in section 3.6.

3.3.2. Roman cemeteries

The distribution of known Roman tombs is mapped in Figure 3.3. The North Cemetery continued to be an important burial area during the Roman period and with its position along the main road out of the city towards Heraklion and the north coast, it attracted many of the grandest monumental built tombs (mausolea). As well as these conspicuous built tombs, pit, tile, and – to a lesser extent – cist graves all continued in the area and there were also a small number of rock-cut chamber tombs discovered. Dozens of excavations during over a century of investigation have continued to unearth tombs in this area. There have been a number of extensive excavations in connection with the development of the hospital that have produced large numbers of Roman graves of various forms (built mausolea, rock-cut chambers, brick and stone cists, pit and tile graves, sarcophagi). These include the Sanatorium (de Jong in 1951, and KSM 1953–60), Pediatric Clinic (KPC/78) and Medical Faculty (KMF/78) excavations by the BSA (*KS2*:72, Cook 1952; *KS2*:74, Frend and Johnston 1962; *KS2*:62, Catling 1979; Catling *et al.* 1982), and various excavations by the Greek Archaeological Service, particularly the 118 Hellenistic and Roman tombs unearthed in 1991 (Vasilakis 1988; Grammatikaki 1991; 1992; 1996; 1997; Banou 1997; 2002; Grammatikaki and Litinas 2000), and including more recent excavations yet to be fully studied (Rousaki *et al.* 2016; 2019a; 2019b; 2020). The Roman skeletal remains from this region that were analysed for this study come from the KSM/53–60 and KMF/78 excavations. Besides those investigated as part of these larger excavation programmes, there have also been a number of built mausolea reported over the years, including one reported by Platon in 1957 and the so-called 'Tomb of Caiaphas' reported by early travellers (*KS2*:48, 57). A rock-cut chamber tomb was reported in the Teke 'Kambon' area by Xanthoudides (1918).

Tile graves have been discovered sporadically in and around the university and hospital sites. One tile grave was cleared by de Jong in 1950 (*KS2*:52), another one by Hood in 1958 (*KS2*:42), a further one in 1963 just west of the hospital (KS2:55; Coldstream 1968), and one containing two pots and a bronze mirror by McFadzean in 1970 (*KS2*:61). Alexiou discovered two 2nd-3rd century tile graves in 1973 (*KS2*:72; Alexiou 1973, 464), others were excavated alongside the Late Antique osteotheke near the Fortetsa Fork (*KS2*:59), and several more were excavated in the second half of this decade (*KS2*:43, 44, 45, 68; Lembessi 1977, 315; Karetsou 1978, 358). Two graves with Laconian tiles but no grave goods were discovered on the pediatric clinic site of the hospital in 1978 (Catling *et al.* 1982). In 1983, eight tile graves were reported by Rethemiotakis containing a clay prochous, a silver pin, glass unguentaria, bronze beads and coins (Rethemiotakis 1983, 354). Towards what may have been the northern end of the North Cemetery (to the extent it is known), off Nathenas street on the neighbouring Skoulas and Vorvoris plots, 26 tile graves were excavated, alongside one poorly preserved cist grave (Grammatikaki 1991, 393; 1992, 557; Blackman 1997, 106; Blackman *et al.* 1998, 114). On the Markomanolaki plot, west of the university, Banou (2002) excavated a tile grave alongside two mausolea. There have also been a smaller number of pit and cist graves excavated in isolation (rather than as part of more extensive excavations), including a small rock-cut pit excavated by Karetsou (*KS2*:69; Karetsou 1976, 359), a cist excavated by Hood in 1958 (*KS2*:42) and three cists excavated alongside a mausoleum by Grammatikaki (1996, 624–30).

Built and rock-cut chamber tombs have also been discovered at Topana which may represent a stand-alone cemetery or may represent a near-continuous burial area spread across this entire northern end of the valley from Teke to Topana. The former suggestion is supported by the division created by the river and finds suggesting

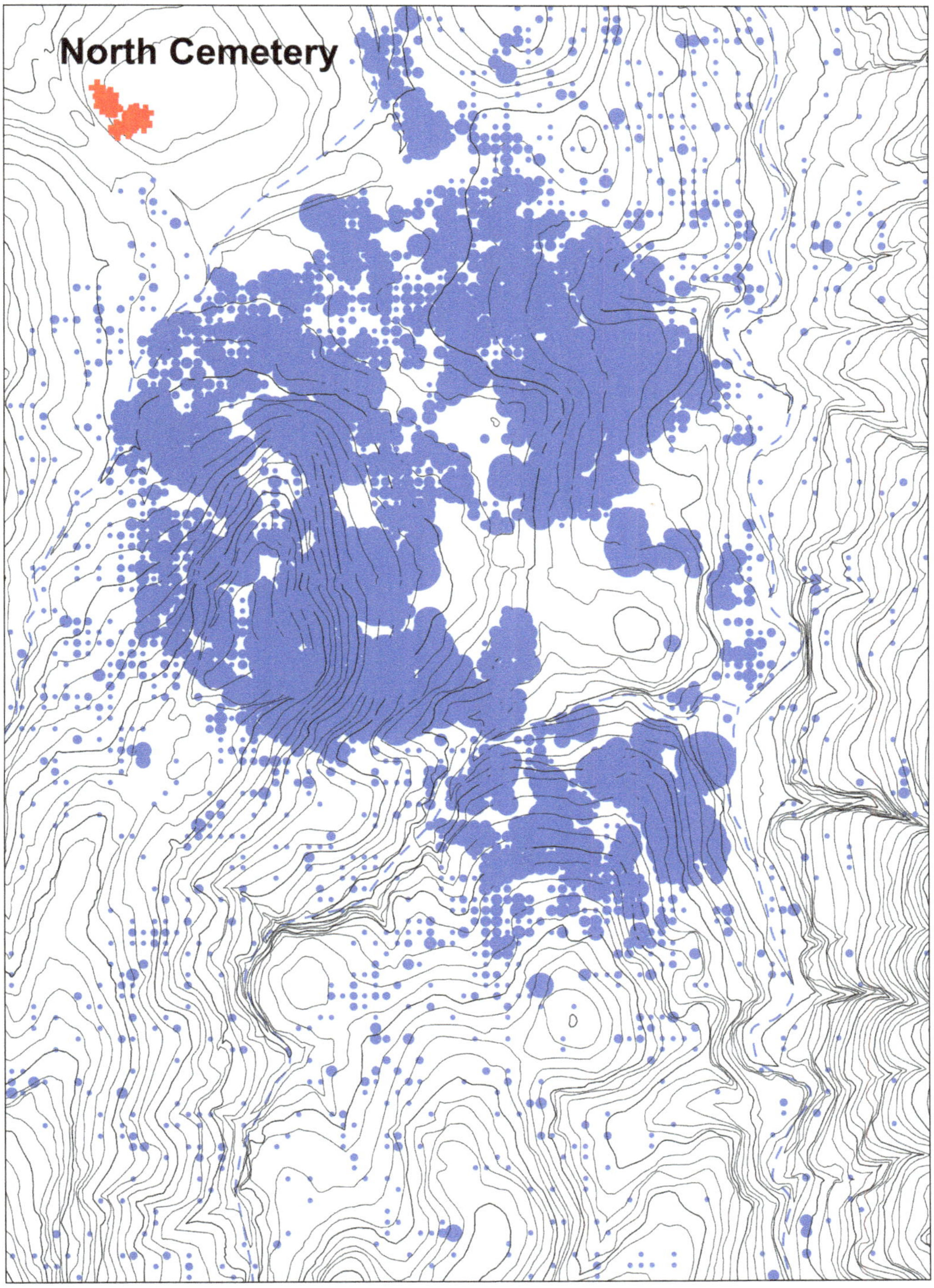

Figure 3.2. Hellenistic tombs (red crosses) with skeletal material studied for this project, plotted on map of 'Hellenic' KULP survey sherds within the Knossos area. Map: Todd Whitelaw.

civic (e.g. the *Makryteichos* wall at *KS2*:86) or religious buildings (potential evidence of a temple at *KS2*:76 and 87) standing between the furthest east burials of the North cemetery and the Topana cemetery. With a Roman bridge crossing the Kairatos river known just to the east of the Topana cemetery, it is possible that this flanked another main road out of the city (*KS2*:81). Human skeletal remains have been included in this study from one of these large, well preserved barrel-vaulted built tombs, which dated to the second half of the 1st century AD (Hood 1962). There was a similar tomb destroyed in 1935 for the construction of a house (*KS2*:83), 2nd-3rd century rock-cut pit graves (*KS2*:77; Hogarth 1900, 82, cf. *KS2*:78), and other tombs without any description discovered in 1958 (*KS2*:82).

Rock-cut chamber tombs were more common to the south of the city where the soft kouskouras slopes of the surrounding hillsides accommodated vast numbers

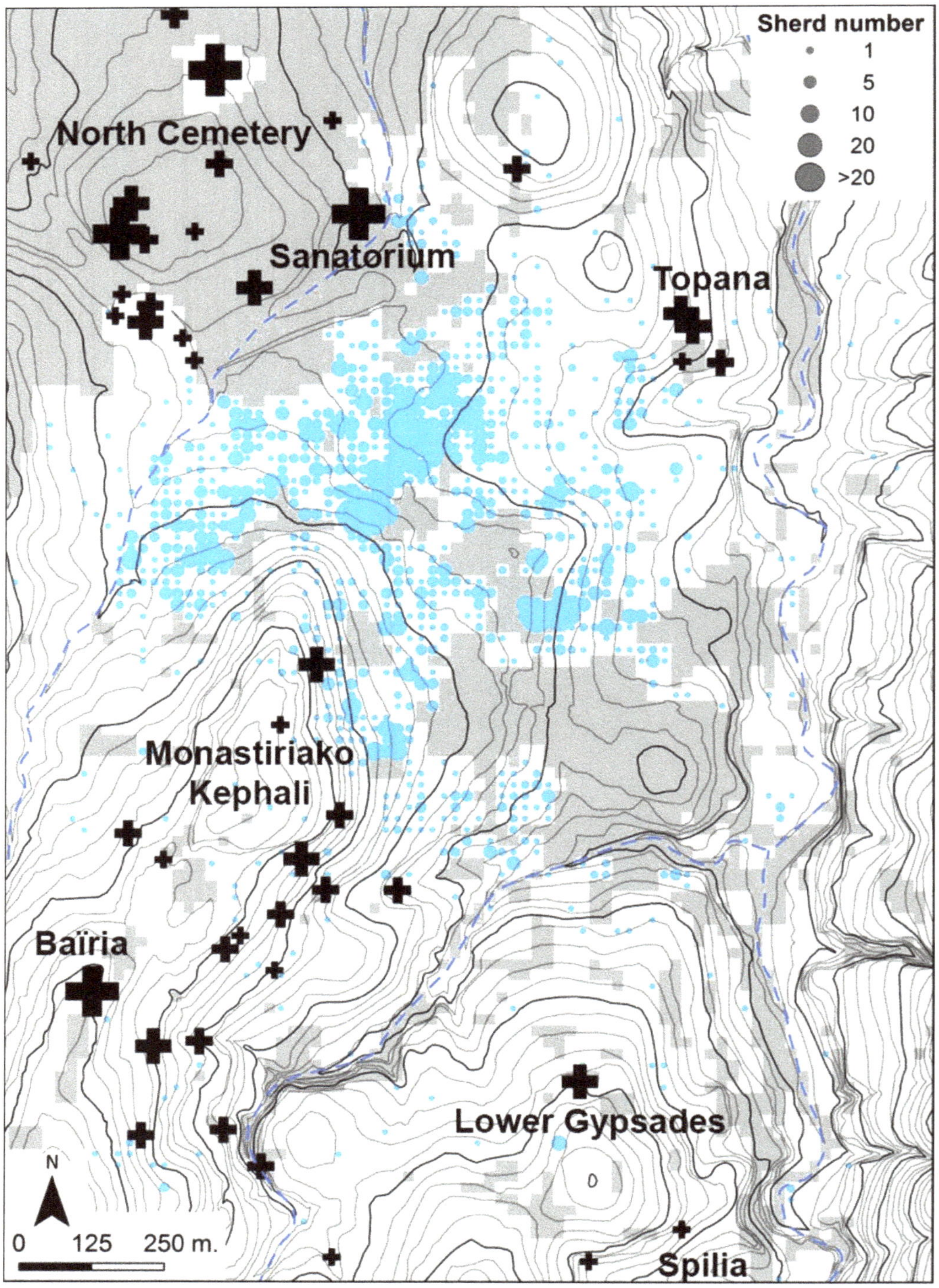

Figure 3.3. Early-Middle Roman sherds (blue dots) from the KULP survey and known tombs of this period (black crosses). Grey squares are unsurveyed area. Map: Todd Whitelaw.

of these tombs, many of which would also have been prominently visible in the landscape along and above the southern route out of the city. These were cut into the slopes of the Monastiriako Kephali (acropolis), Baïria and Spilia hills around the west and south sides of the valley. The first proper excavations[14] of these rock-cut chamber tombs began at the end of the 19th century (*KS2*:142; Hogarth 1900, 81); while Evans investigated the palace, Hogarth sought out the associated 'royal Minoan' tombs (Evans 1906). Another early excavation of one of these tombs was reported by Hutchinson in 1936 (*KS2*:143). Graves of undescribed form were also excavated in the Fortetsa cemetery and there was another rock-cut tomb (unknown whether pit or chamber) just to the east of here (*KS2*:151–152; Brock 1957). In 1966, Alexiou

[14] These tombs were frequently looted or used as shelters for people and livestock due to their continued visibility in the landscape.

reported the excavation of a child's tomb, its form was not described, near Agios Kirillos (*KS2*:166; Alexiou 1966, 325). Popham excavated four rock-cut chamber tombs in 1968 to the south of this area at Baïria (*KS2*:157, Fraser 1969, 33; Wardle and Wardle 2004). Several more were excavated in the Monastiriako Kephali region and extending south to Baïria throughout the 1970s. On the lower slopes at Marathianou Lakkos, Wardle dug two rock-cut chamber tombs of the standard form, with a dromos and chamber with three *klinai* under *arcosolia* and niches in the wall of each, dating from the late 1st to early 2nd century (*KS2*:170; Wardle 1972; Wardle and Wardle 2004). Several more were excavated by Howell in 1976 as part of the water mains trench excavations (*KS2*:156, 159, 164, 165; Knossos Logbook 1976; Catling 1977a, 22) as well as a group of 1st century AD tile graves (*KS2*:171; Catling 1977a, 10). Jill Carington Smith excavated two of a group of seven visible chamber tombs at Baïria in 1977 (*KS2*:155) and one tomb in the larger Baïria cemetery where over 40 tombs were known (*KS2*:154). There were also groups of tombs visible just north of Agios Kirillos (*KS2*:167–168), further south near the Venetian aqueduct (*KS2*:158) and further south again (*KS2*:342). Carington Smith excavated the southernmost of a group of five tombs in a row next to the road; the other four in this group had lain open for many years (*KS2*:168; Carington Smith 1982). There are other chamber tombs marked on the survey map but unnumbered (north of *KS2*:161) which are still visible in the slopes below the road today, some of which show signs of recent use as shelters.

On the Lower Gypsades hill, Hogarth put test trenches into an extensive Roman cemetery of 1st century AD graves, one of which was noted as visible in 1957, though Callaghan suggests that there must also have been Hellenistic graves in this area due to the presence of 3rd-2nd century pottery (*KS2*:305; Hogarth 1900). There were also reports of two built tombs higher up on the Gypsades hill to the south, which were apparently plundered by local inhabitants before the Second World War according to Spiro Vasilakis in 1957 (*KS2*:326–327). Concrete structures above the Sanctuary of Demeter and Hogarth's Houses sites were thought to have been Roman built tombs but were thought likely to have been from late in the period (*KS2*:286,297; Coldstream 1960, 265). Evidence of tombs at Spilia had been observed by several early travellers. Eight of these rock-cut chamber tombs were excavated by Karetsou and Howell as part of the 1976 water mains trench excavations, including Tomb E which was an interesting variation on the standard three-*arcosolia* form, with a stone sarcophagus in an *arcosolium* opposite the chamber entrance (*KS2*:361–362; Karetsou 1976, 358–59). There was also a rectangular rock-cut chamber tomb, classified by Guyon as a *hypogeum* due to its depth below the surface, with a dromos of three irregular steps, excavated by Lembessi and Dimopoulou in 1975. Containing Knossian coins of Augustus, Tiberius, Claudius-Messalia, and Nero, it was dated to the 2nd half of the 1st century AD (*KS2*:361; Lembessi 1975c, 199; 1975a, 342; 1975b, 518–20).

Large numbers of Roman tombs have been excavated from Knossos and this extensive description lists all the published references to excavated and observed tombs. The skeletal assemblage studied covers most regions and tomb types, though there were considerable limitations to how extensively some of these were represented due to the availability and preservation of the material (Figure 3.4). Five rock-cut chamber tombs from the Monastiriako Kephali region are represented in the assemblage: three from Popham's 1968 excavation, dated to between the mid-1st and mid-2nd centuries (*KS2*:157 Fraser 1969, 33; Wardle and Wardle 2004), and two from Howell's 1976 excavations, one excavated in April and dated to the 2nd century and the other on the Hadzimanolis plot in September (*KS2*:156; Knossos Logbook 1976; Catling 1977a, 22). Five built tombs from the KMF/78 excavations in the North Cemetery are represented, four dating to the 1st or 2nd centuries, and Tomb 33 dated to the 2nd-3rd centuries (*KS2*:62; KMF Excavation Notebooks [BSA Archives]; Catling 1979). Five tile graves and one pit grave were also uncovered during the KMF/78 excavations.

3.3.3. Late Antique cemeteries

Due to the lack of artefacts accompanying the burials found in Christian graves, it is likely that some of these tombs have been misidentified as Roman (or Graeco-Roman) or missed entirely, but those that can be identified with certainty have been plotted in Figure 3.5. Such misidentification probably accounts for a number of graves from the 'Royal Road' area, just northwest of the palace site. These cist and tile graves have been reported as Hellenistic or Roman (*KS2*:209, 211 and 212; Megaw 1936, 150; Platon 1959, 385; 1973, 464), but this area would have been within the settlement during the Hellenistic and early Roman periods. A later Roman or Late Antique date for these tombs is confirmed by an unpublished report mentioning the coins from the Krevatina cist grave (*KS2*:209) and assigning this tomb to the 4th century AD (Hutchinson 1936 reports, BSA Archives). There is also a Late Antique cist grave (or 'stone-lined' tomb) further west of these graves, upslope and west of the modern upper village (Bougada Metochi), on the Panagiotakis (KOP/79) plot (Sweetman and Grigoropoulos 2010). Another cist grave was excavated on the Sevastakis field on Monastiriako Kephali, dated to 'late Roman or early Christian' times (Grammatikaki 1991, 393). The continued northward contraction of the Late Antique centre closer to the basilica churches, around the late 4th or 5th century, is supported by the discovery of 'Roman' tile graves in the areas of the modern upper Knossos village, the Ariadne nightclub (southeast of the Roman civic basilica), and the area northeast of the Villa Dionysus during the DEYAH 1992–1993 rescue excavations for the laying of water pipes (Sweetman and Grigoropoulos 2010). These are almost certainly Late Antique graves.

The main known Late Antique burial area is within the North Cemetery area, where a large number of osteothekai and some cist graves were discovered in association

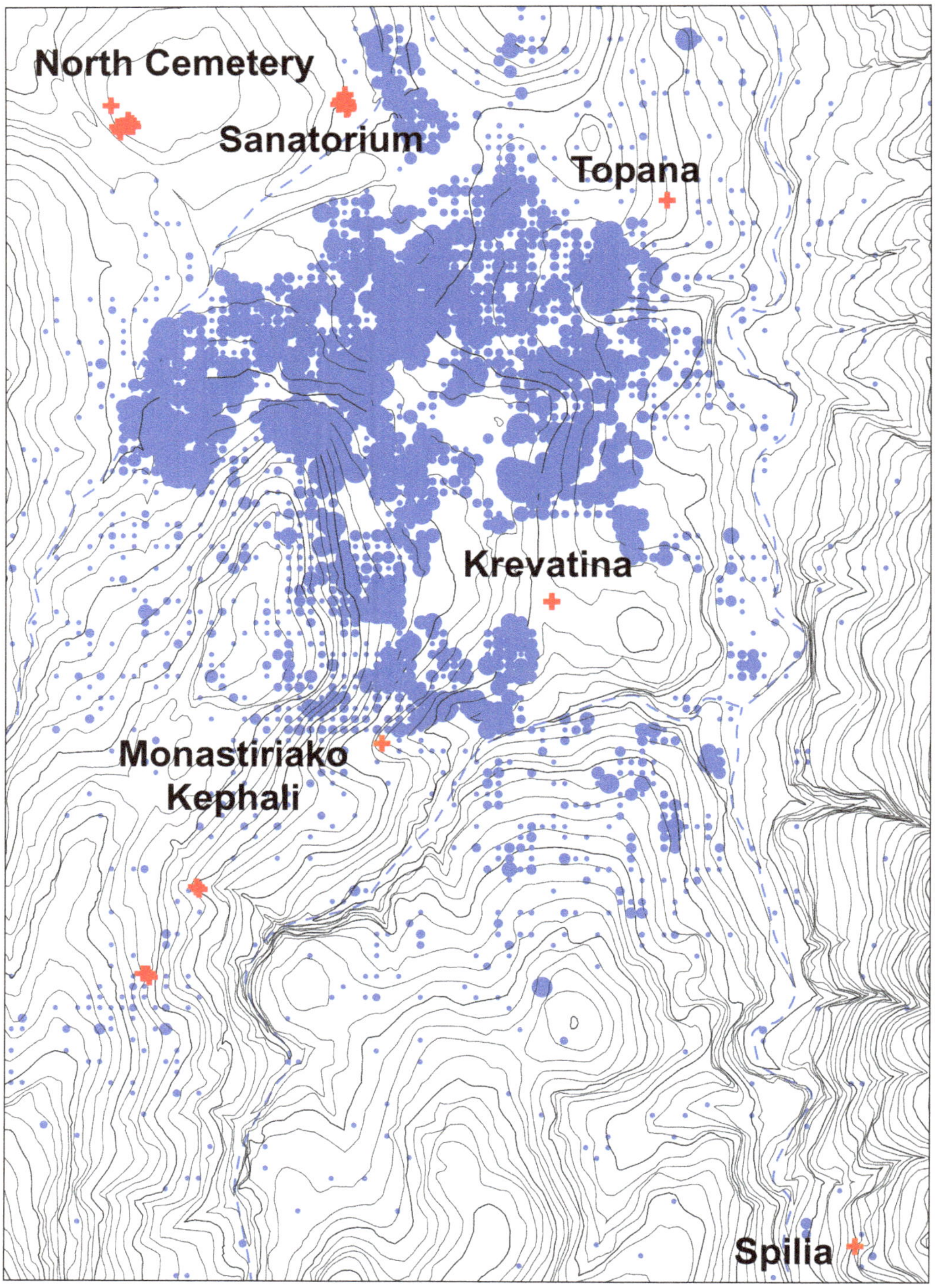

Figure 3.4. Roman tombs (red crosses) with skeletal material studied for this project, plotted on map of Early-Middle Roman KULP survey sherds within the Knossos area. Map: Todd Whitelaw.

with the KMF basilica church on the university Medical Faculty site (*KS2*:64; Sweetman and Becker 2005). The majority of these tombs lie within the *peribolos* wall of the basilica but some were outside, though still within close proximity to this precinct. A little to the west, at the fork in the road towards Fortetsa village ('Fortetsa Fork'), another similar osteotheke was excavated in 1974 (KFF/74, *KS2*:59; Catling *et al.* 1976), which was dated to the 7th or 8th century due to comparative evidence from the Athenian agora for the six jugs included within the tomb (Robinson 1959, 121–22; KS2:59; Catling *et al.* 1976, 39).

While the latest evidence for burials in the area of the Sanatorium basilica dates to the 4th century, this cemetery was still recognised when the 6th century basilica was constructed, particularly Tomb 8 which was venerated by its incorporation into the nave of the church, likely as a martyr's tomb (Frend and Johnston 1962, 197). There

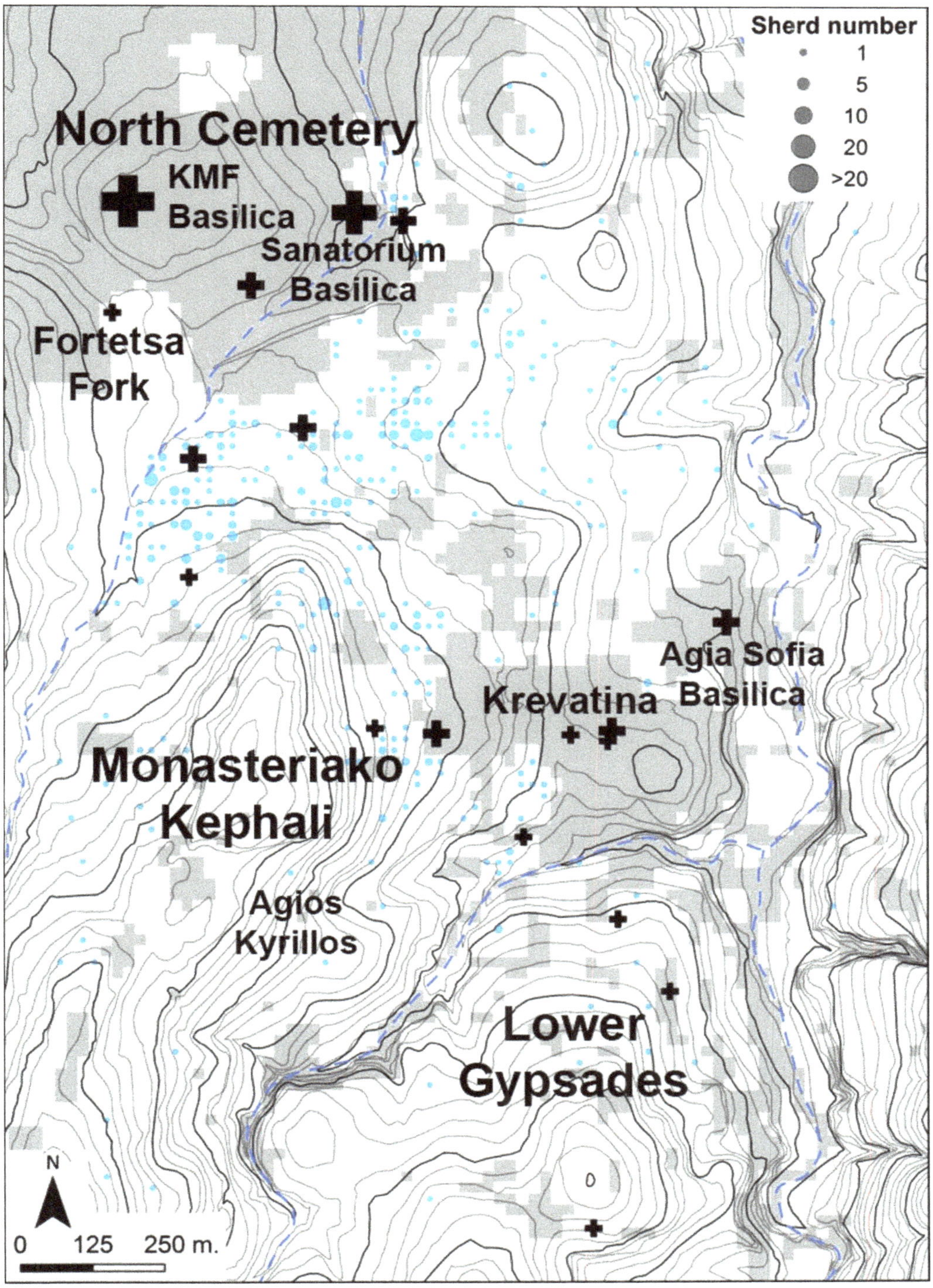

Figure 3.5. Late Roman- Late Antique sherds (blue dots) from the KULP survey and known tombs of this period (black crosses). Grey squares are unsurveyed area. Map: Todd Whitelaw.

was a Late Antique tomb discovered just east of here on the east side of the original streambed and diversion in 1951 (*KS2*:75). While the descriptions of both this tomb and many of the Sanatorium tombs are limited, it seems this was a similar form to some of the tombs from the Sanatorium cemetery. It was double-chambered, built of coursed rubble with heavy cover slabs, with a niche in the back wall and a marble grille floor with a cross engraved on it (Cook 1952, 108).

There have been further occasional finds of Late Antique tombs, with two 'Roman or Byzantine' graves excavated south-west of the modern Agios Mikhaili cemetery church (*KS2*:108; Hood 1958, 21) and two others in the modern upper Knossos village discovered in 1966 on the Froudharakis plot and assigned to a 5th or 6th century date (*KS2*:183; Alexiou 1966, 325). Further tombs known from the south-east of the settlement, close to the Late Antique Agia Sofia basilica church in the Makryteichos village

(*KS2*:235) and across the river, further south in the ravine below the modern Agia Paraskevi church (*KS2*:279), may date to later Byzantine times but could also be earlier. They certainly appear to be Christian graves due to their associations with churches and their east-west orientation. Two tombs on the south slopes of Lower Gypsades, the KOP/79 stone-lined tomb with a single individual and the KEP/79 stone-and-tile-lined tomb, were thought to be isolated tombs according to the excavator who saw no evidence in the area for a cemetery (Sweetman and Grigoropoulos 2010). The KULP survey collected fragments of human bone from Agios Kyrillos, indicating a potential cemetery of Late Antique date associated with the church (Whitelaw, pers.comm.).

The majority of tombs that had skeletal material available for this study were from the KMF/79 excavation, next to the basilica church in the North Cemetery, but the large quantities of skeletal remains from the KFF/74 Fortetsa Fork osteotheke were also included, as was the individual skeleton from the KOP/79 tomb. The tombs studied are mapped in Figure 3.6.

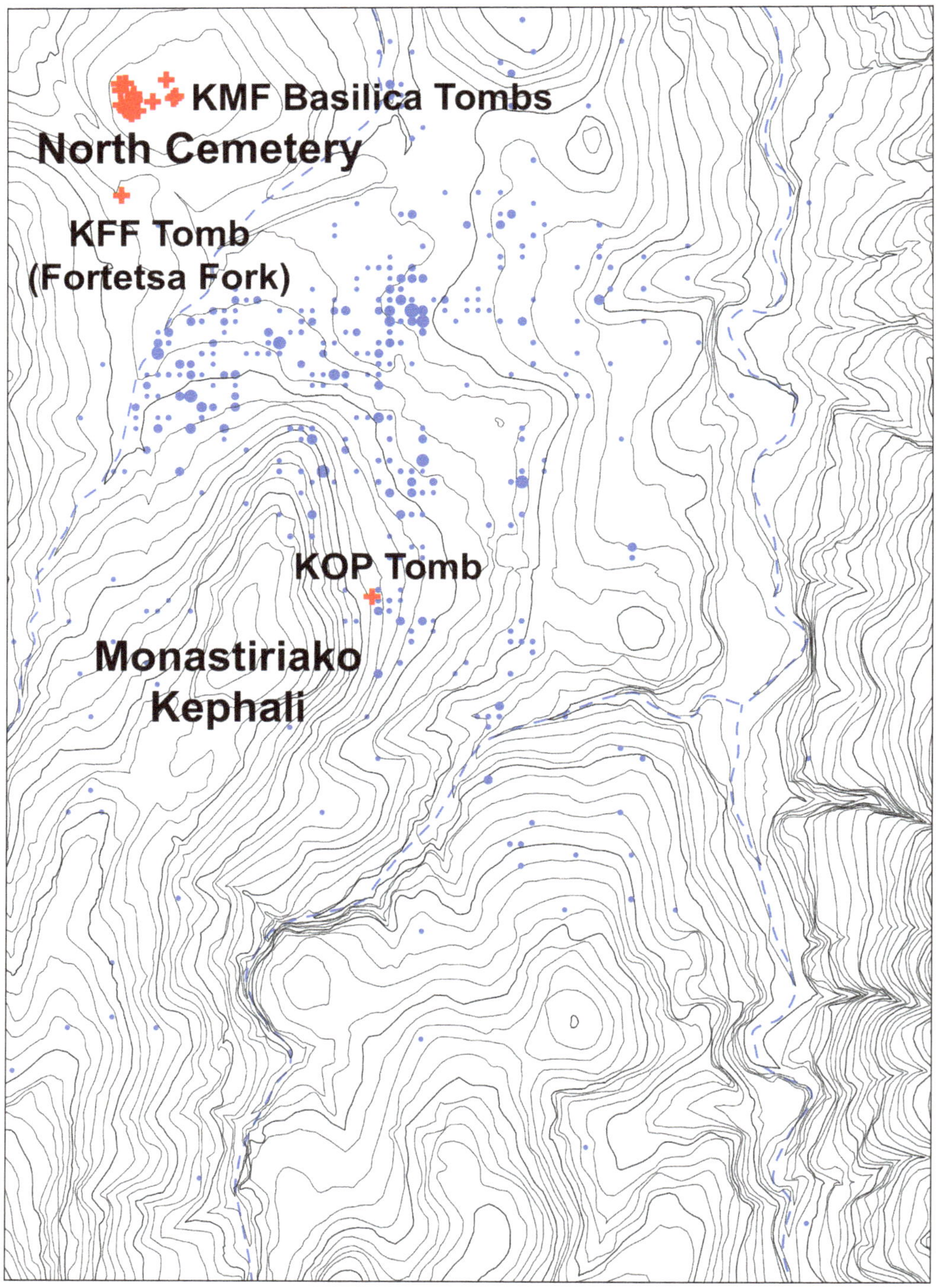

Figure 3.6. Late Antique tombs (red crosses) with skeletal material studied for this project, plotted on map of Late Roman-Late Antique KULP survey sherds within the Knossos area. Map: Todd Whitelaw.

3.4. Social status of the dead

The tomb types present at Knossos form an important element of this study in acting as a proxy for social status for the investigation of differential health and diet in the population. This use of the tomb types comes with the established caveats that 'the dead do not bury themselves' and there is no guarantee that an individual's social status or wealth is reflected in their funerary architecture (Morris 1992, 1; Parker Pearson 1999, 3). The visibility of a tomb, the investment of time and materials, and evidence for continued commemoration in terms of access and revisiting the grave for further burials or funerary activities, reflect the priorities of those burying the dead. These reflect the status which the burying group wishes to reflect on the deceased and often depend on the social group of which both the deceased and individuals organising the burial are a part. Grave goods and treatment of the body can also play into this discussion but due to the unknown extent of looting and disturbance in some of the graves, and the state of preservation and methods for retrieval during excavation (such as sieving), these have not been systematically considered.

For this study tombs were divided into eight categories: monumental built tombs (mausolea), rock-cut chamber tombs, osteothekai, stone-lined tombs, cist graves, sarcophagi, tile graves, and pit graves. But these are by no means homogenous categories as there are different construction types and materials used and the categories could in some cases be further sub-divided. In other cases, it is likely certain categories (particularly the stone-lined and cist graves) could be merged together, particularly in light of the lack of detailed understanding or description for some tombs. In many cases, it was deemed pertinent to default to the excavator's terms, under the assumption that distinctions between different terms and tomb types were meaningful in some way that had not been fully described.

The cist graves, stone-lined tombs and osteothekai are all dug into the earth and usually have stone slabs as flooring and to cover the tomb (entry is from above). Sometimes there were no floor slabs and the body would have been laid on the earth or rock floor, or sometimes there was a floor of pebbles or *opus signinum*. The walls can either be lined with stone slabs or bricks, or built of substantial blocks or rough masonry, smaller stones and rubble. The walls were also sometimes lined with mortar or plaster. It has been attempted to distinguish the more substantial stone-lined tombs from the simpler stone-lined graves by referring to them as 'stone-lined tombs' and 'cist graves' respectively, acknowledging the greater investment of labour in constructing the former. These tombs vary greatly in size, but this does not appear to be a defining characteristic in their terminology. Tomb 244 was the largest (6.05m × 5.40m) and most prominently situated tomb, built of reused architectural blocks from a monumental Corinthian-style Roman building (Paton 1991). It was followed in size by its neighbouring osteotheke, Tomb 243 (3.95m x 3.90m), but the osteothekai ranged down to much smaller tombs, such as Tomb 254 (2.00m x 1.10m), Tomb 300 (1.94m x 0.88m) and Tomb 311, with a width of only 0.50m (Sweetman and Becker 2005). Cist grave, Tomb 309 (2.20m x 1.40m), and stone-lined, grave Tomb 12 (2.00m x 1.10m), have intermediate dimensions compared to the range of measurements for the osteothekai. The osteothekai are differentiated from the other stone-lined tombs due to their perceived role as secondary burial receptacles. They are all of 5th-8th century date and are largely associated with the KMF Christian basilica church. The numbers of individuals in the osteothekai ranged from 3 to 54 and did not always correspond with tomb size, indicating intended and eventual uses may not have been the same. It is possible that there was a social difference between osteothekai made of rubble and small stones, and those made of large dressed blocks, though this may also be a temporal difference, with architectural blocks from Roman buildings more readily available earlier in the use of the burial precinct (Sweetman and Becker 2005, 365). Additionally, as these large stone blocks were robbed from earlier buildings, this would have been an economical reuse of building materials. Nevertheless, it is visually more impressive than some of the rougher-built tombs and would have involved a greater investment of labour to manoeuvre the large blocks.

Regarding the terminology, osteotheke implies that these tombs were ossuaries for the secondary interment of bones after they had lost their flesh and connective tissue. It was assumed this differentiated them from other stone-lined tombs or cist graves (as they were referred to at the time of excavation), with KMF Tomb 309 (Figures 3.7–9), for example, identified as a cist (KMF 1978–1979 Excavation Notebooks [BSA Archives]; Sweetman and Becker 2005). However, it is unclear why the majority of these are 'osteothekai' while Tomb 309 is a 'cist', Tomb 311 is an 'osteotheke but very narrow', and Tombs 12 (Figure 3.10), 158, 172 and 173 are stone-lined graves (Sweetman and Becker 2005). Several osteothekai descriptions, in addition to Tomb 158, mention articulated or partially articulated skeletal material indicating primary burials, therefore the term 'osteotheke' is not being used as synonymous with 'ossuary', which would indicate a place for bone storage as part of a secondary burial practice. Despite two articulated burials being identified in Tomb 309, the bones from earlier burials are also identified as subject to a degree of sorting. The assumption that it was not an osteotheke cannot have been based on the dimensions of the tomb, because at 2.20m by 1.40m it was larger than some of the tombs referred to as osteothekai. The only factor that appears to differentiate this tomb from the other stone-lined tombs or osteothekai was the construction materials. Cut slabs of a poor quality stone made up the floor, walls and covering, with the cracks between mortared with a sandy plaster (Sweetman and Becker 2005, 362). Descriptions of all these tomb types suggest they are cut into the kouskouras and lined with various sorts of stones, including reused blocks, cut blocks, fieldstones, rubble packing or a mixture of materials. It seems likely that the

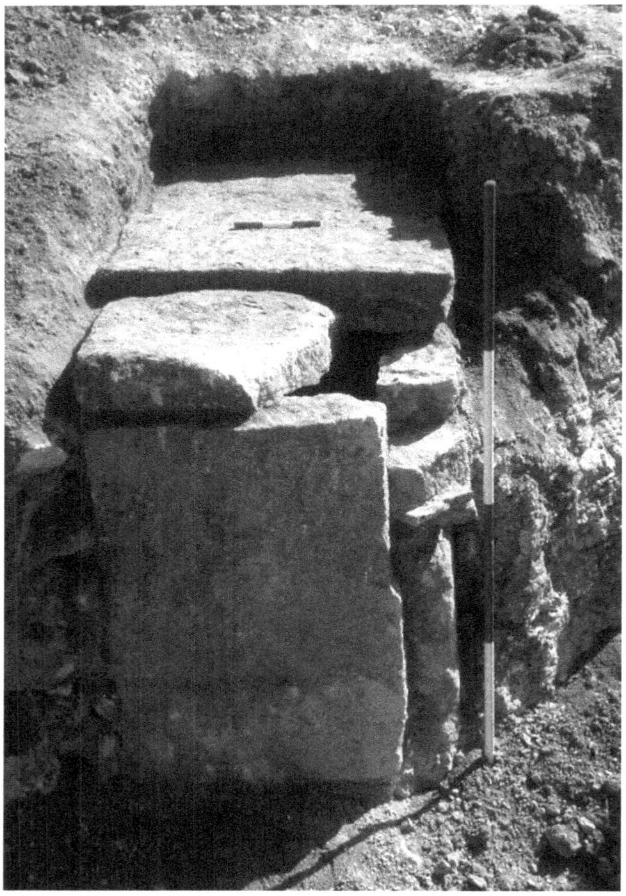

Figure 3.7. 'Cist grave' KMF Tomb 309 (Unit 91) external view from northwest with cover slabs in place. Photo: BSA Archive.

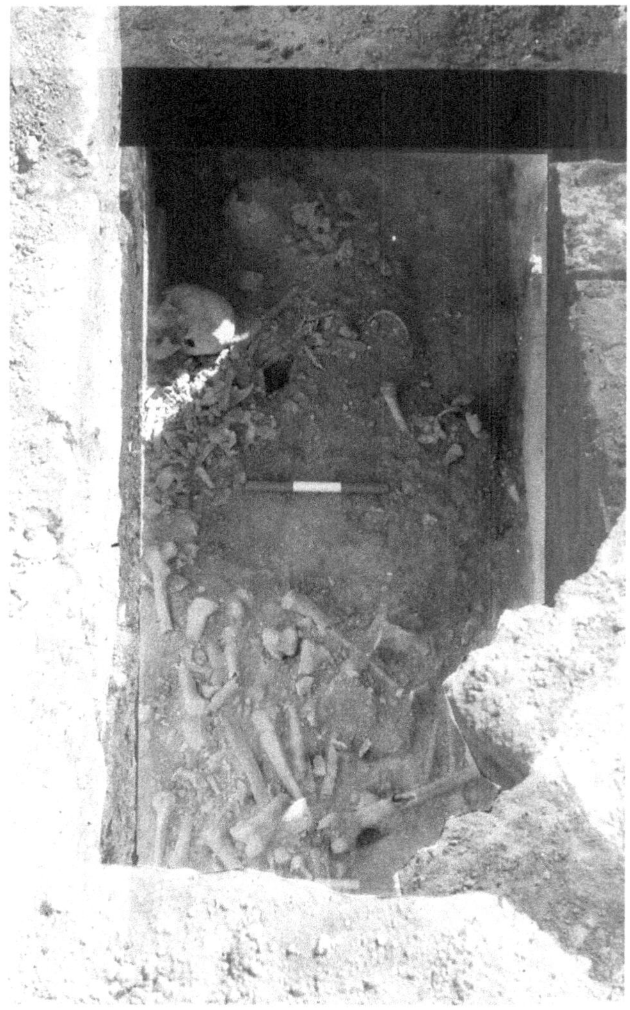

Figure 3.8. 'Cist grave' KMF Tomb 309 contents showing remains of multiple individuals, view from southeast. Photo: BSA Archive.

differences in terminology may just be inconsistencies between different excavators, but because the excavators were not involved in the publication, Sweetman has simply replicated the tomb descriptions from the excavation notebooks, though in some cases questions the assignation of the term 'osteotheke', as is the case with Tomb 297 which appears to have one burial pushed to the side for a second interment (Sweetman and Becker 2005, 354). With the hasty rescue excavation of these tombs, limited documentation, and lack of a human osteoarchaeologist present at the time of excavation the assumptions made about whether tombs contained primary or secondary burials cannot be considered fully reliable.

Different building materials and construction styles were also used for the monumental built tombs. Most of the built tombs known from Knossos were constructed of dressed blocks of ashlar masonry or mortared stones (regular and *opus incertum*) similar to contemporary examples from elsewhere on Crete (Guyon 2008, 112, 114–15). There are also some remnants of *opus caementicium* (concrete) mausolea at Knossos which may originally have had stone facings. The full range of monumental built tombs known from Hellenistic and Roman Crete is categorised by Guyon (2008), following the definitions by Moretti (2006) for tombs throughout Greece. This includes those dug into the ground (*hypogea* and rock-cut chamber tombs both entered by a dromos), those partially cut into the rock (rock-cut chamber tombs with a crypt that were never fully buried and with a vaulted roof appearing at ground level, semi-interred built chamber tombs, built chamber tombs backed into the rocky slope, and the single case of a conical-shaped rock-cut tomb at Elyros), and those built at ground level and above (mausolea, the single case of an altar tomb from Knossos (T.52, Grammatikaki 2004) and the single case of a heroön tomb of impressive size with pedestals inscribed with heroic dedications from Aptera (Niniou-Kindeli 2004; 2008)). It is impossible to categorise these tombs in a way that will incorporate all their features and therefore within each of these categories there tends to be a degree of architectural diversity, in the type of stones used, whether there was stone veneering or plastered walls, the types of covers and roofing, the form of the entrance, and the presence of additional extra features such as an antechamber, niches, pits, benches, *klinai*, and *arcosolia*.

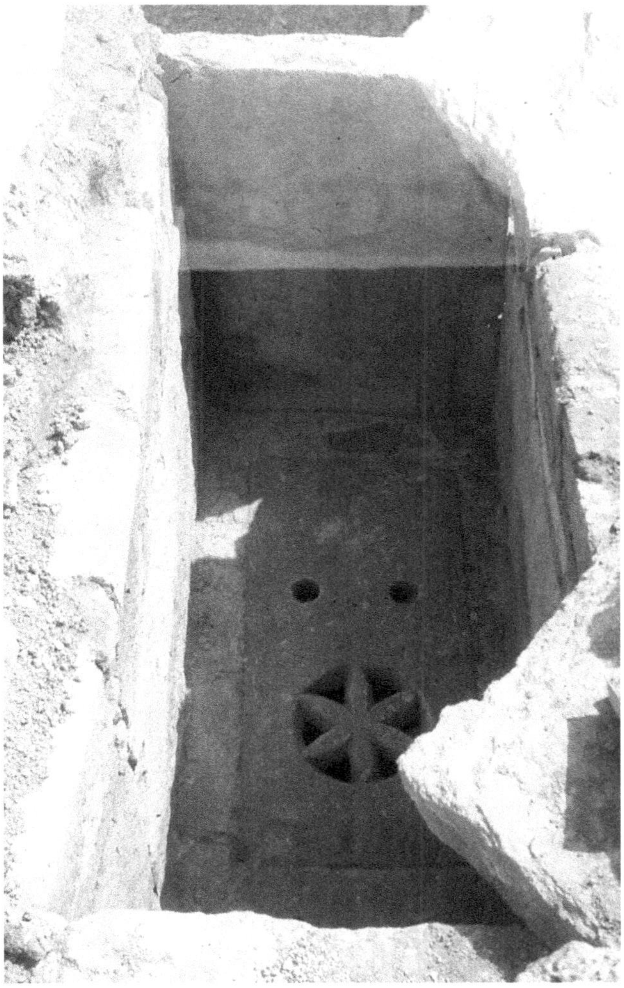

Figure 3.9. 'Cist grave' KMF Tomb 309 cleared revealing a re-used Roman drain cover used as a floor slab, view from southeast. Photo: BSA Archive.

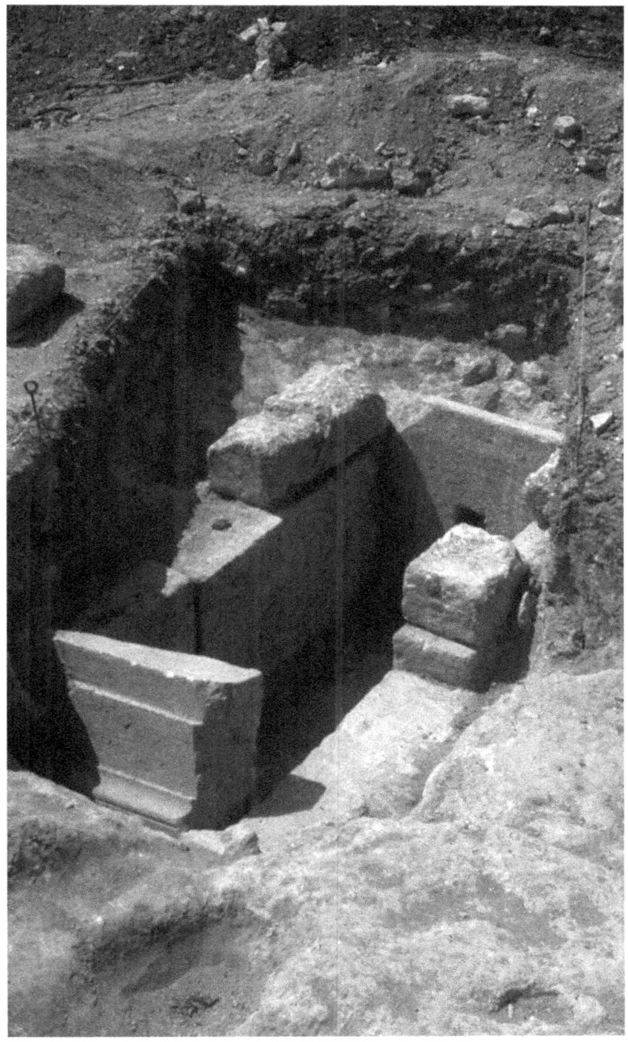

Figure 3.10. 'Stone lined grave' KMF Tomb 12, cut into the bedrock and lined with spolia blocks, including a column shaft. Photo: BSA Archive.

Additionally, depending on the state of preservation, it can be difficult to determine a tomb's exact form and features. However, the Knossos built tombs appear to largely be those dug down into the ground with a barrel-vaulted roof above ground, or above-ground, free-standing structures (sometimes with an additional underground chamber) and designed for the burial of multiple individuals.

Certain built tombs are similar in form to the rock-cut chamber tombs which are fairly standardised with a limited range of variations. This potentially suggests that the same degree of monumentality and visibility was achieved aesthetically but with less investment of materials, as the natural rock-face was simply carved out rather than having to quarry, cut and transport building stone. These rock-cut tombs consisted of a rectangular burial chamber which was approached by a short dromos or sometimes an antechamber with low rock-cut benches along the sides (Figure 3.11). The entrance was either a rock-cut opening or formed by monolithic jambs and a lintel (Figure 3.12). In most cases at Knossos, the three walls, other than the one featuring the entrance, had *arcosolia* and *klinai*, often with a rock-cut pillow at one end for the head and a niche in the back wall (Figure 3.13). Instead of *klinai* there were sometimes pits cut into the floor for inhumations, which were covered by stone slabs. It is possible that some tombs also had *klinai* made from organic materials. In one case at Knossos (Spilia 1976 Tomb E), there was a sarcophagus under the one *arcosolium* in the tomb, opposite the entrance (Figure 3.14). The barrel-vaulted built chamber tombs, such as MK/61 Tomb 1 (Figure 3.15), Sanatorium 1951 Roman vaulted tomb (Figure 3.16) and KMF/78 Tomb 33 (Figure 3.17), are of a similar form, with a dromos leading to a doorway of monolithic jambs and lintel, and a rectangular burial chamber containing niches in the walls. The built chambers were generally slightly larger, but without the additional space created by the *loculi* this may have allowed for coffins or *klinai* of organic materials to be placed along the sides of the chamber.

In considering the very simplest grave types known from Knossos, the pit graves, even these involved a degree of

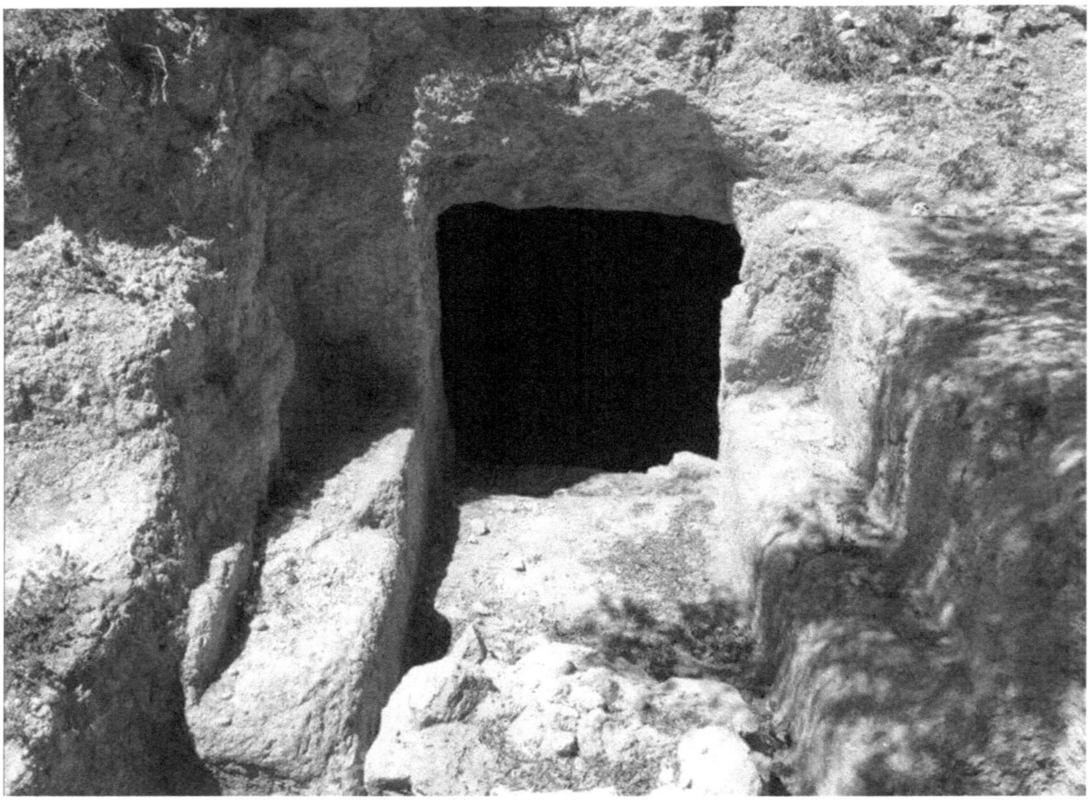

Figure 3.11. Rock-cut benches along the sides of the antechamber or dromos leading to a rock-cut square doorway into the burial chamber of a tomb at Baïria (below the road, north of KS2:161). Photo: Anna Moles.

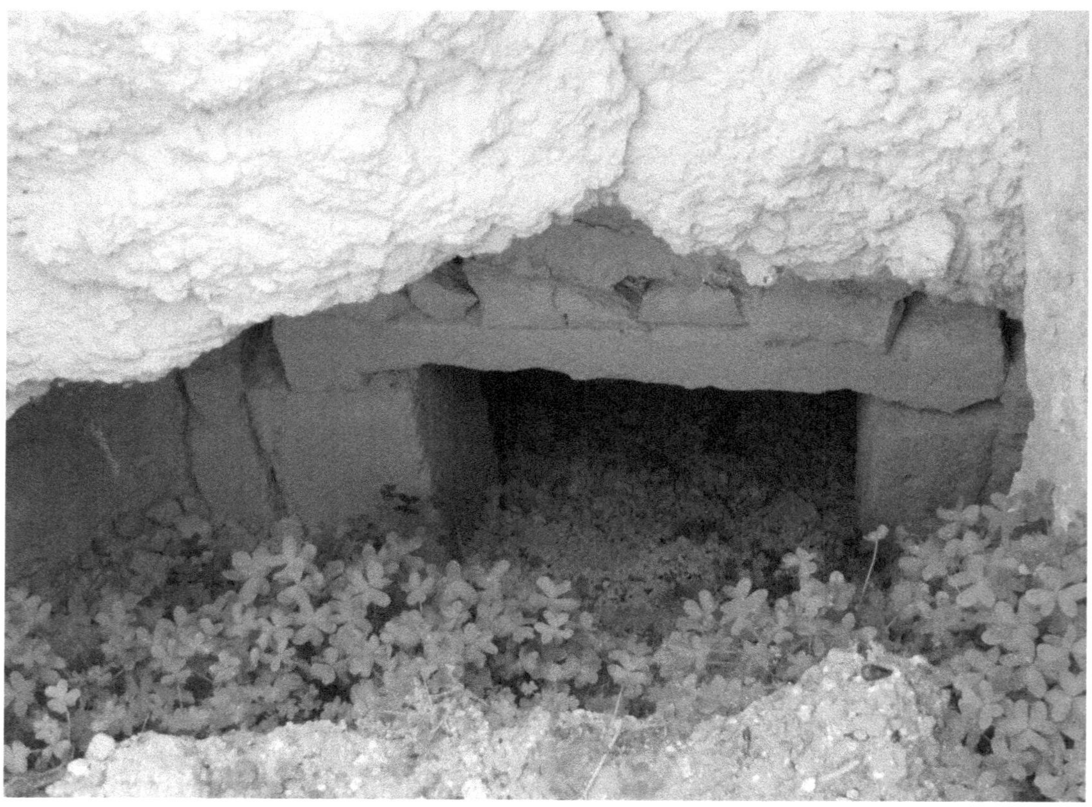

Figure 3.12. Monolithic door jambs and lintel of one of the rock-cut chamber tombs at Monastiriako Kephali (KS2:168), visible next to the road. Photo: Anna Moles.

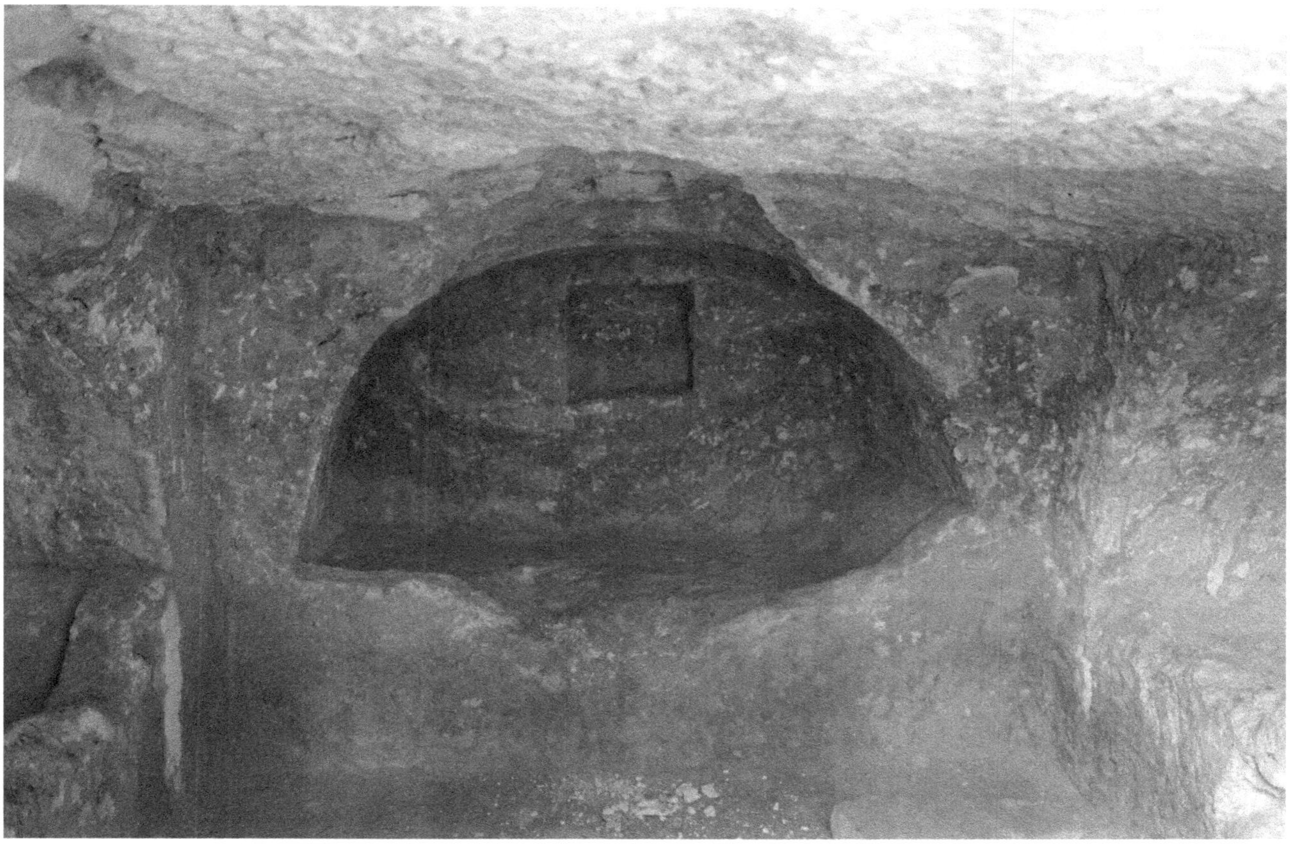

Figure 3.13. Rock-cut chamber tomb at Baïria (below the road, north of KS2:161), featuring an arcosolium, a *klinē* with rock-cut pillow, and a niche. Photo: Anna Moles.

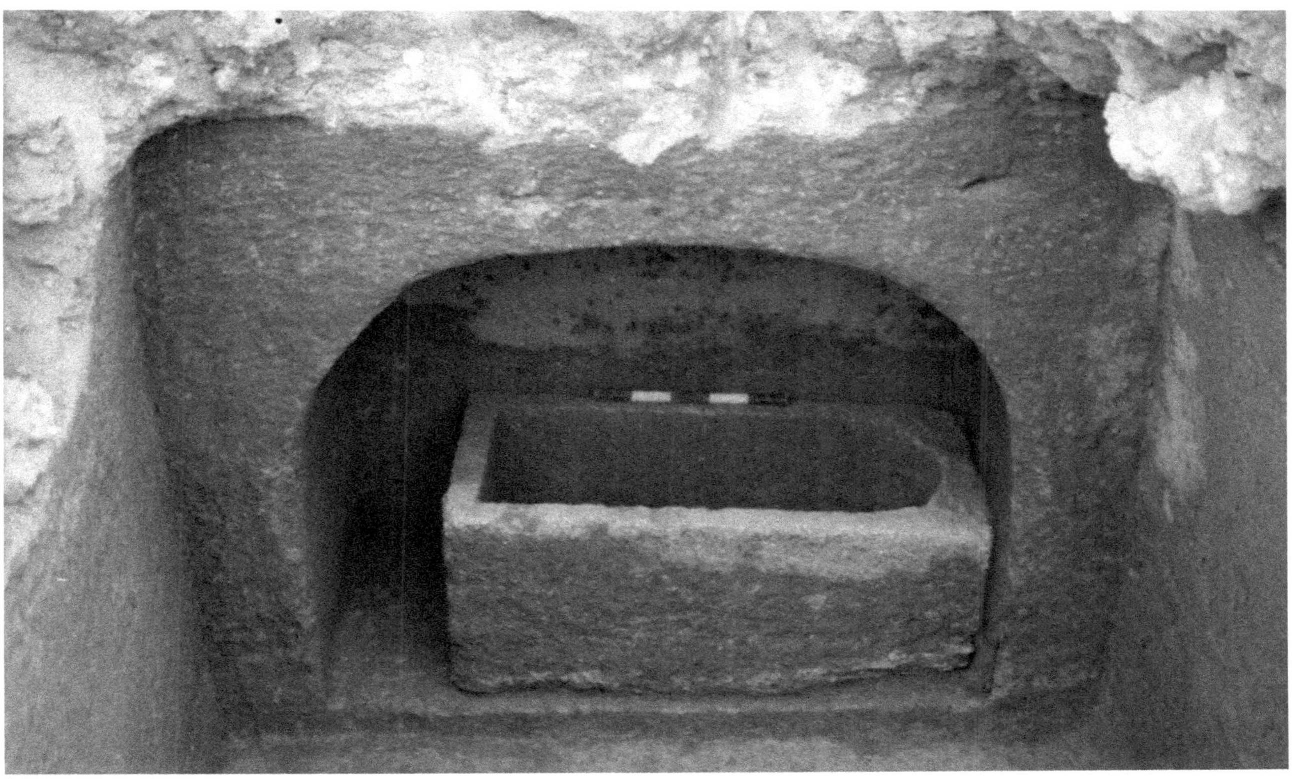

Figure 3.14. Tomb E, Spilia 1976 (Unit 109), cleared by Roger Howell as part of the water mains trench excavations. Photo: BSA Archive.

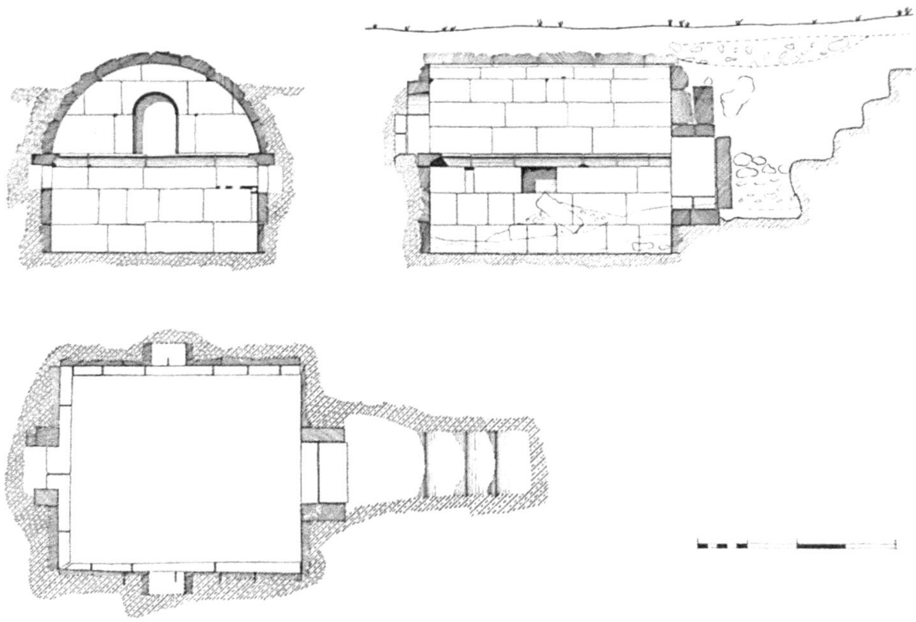

Figure 3.15. Plan and section drawings of MK/61 Tomb 1 (Unit 104). BSA Archive.

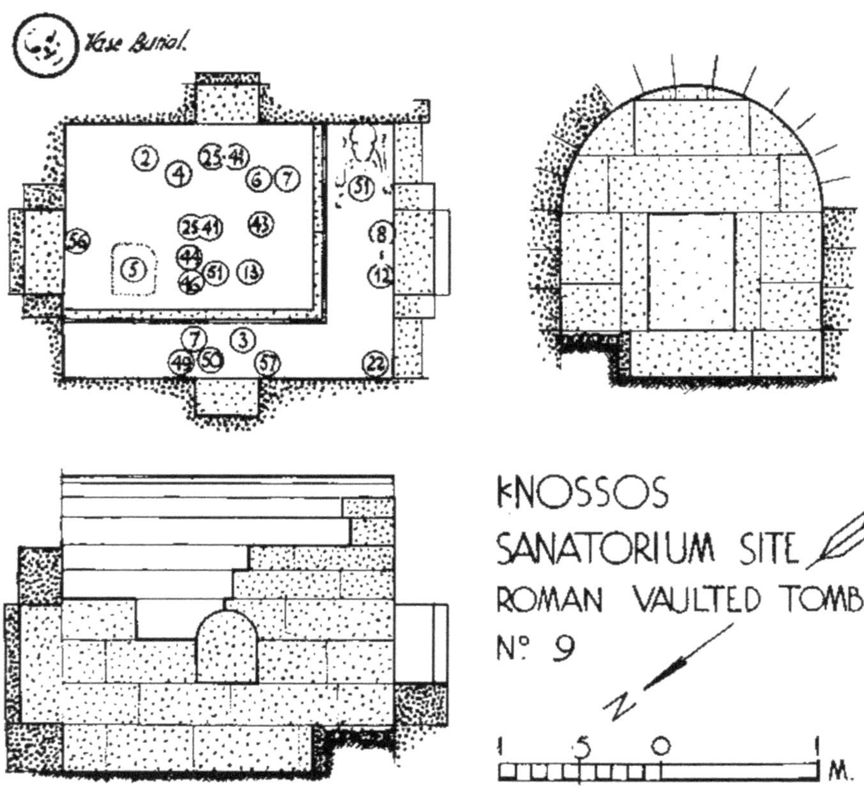

Figure 3.16. Plan and section drawings of Sanatorium 1951 Roman vaulted tomb. BSA Archive.

labour beyond a shallow earth dug grave as they had been cut into the soft kouskouras bedrock. These are the most common burial type known on the island (Guyon 2008, 99). They also exist on a continuum of grave types from simple to monumental, as several large rectangular cuttings are of a size comparable to a chamber tomb but lack any further elaboration. A tile grave is usually similar to the standard pit grave in dimensions but has the additional elaboration of tiles used either as cover slabs or to create a gabled cover over the burial (*kalyvitis* tiles, e.g. KMF T.46,

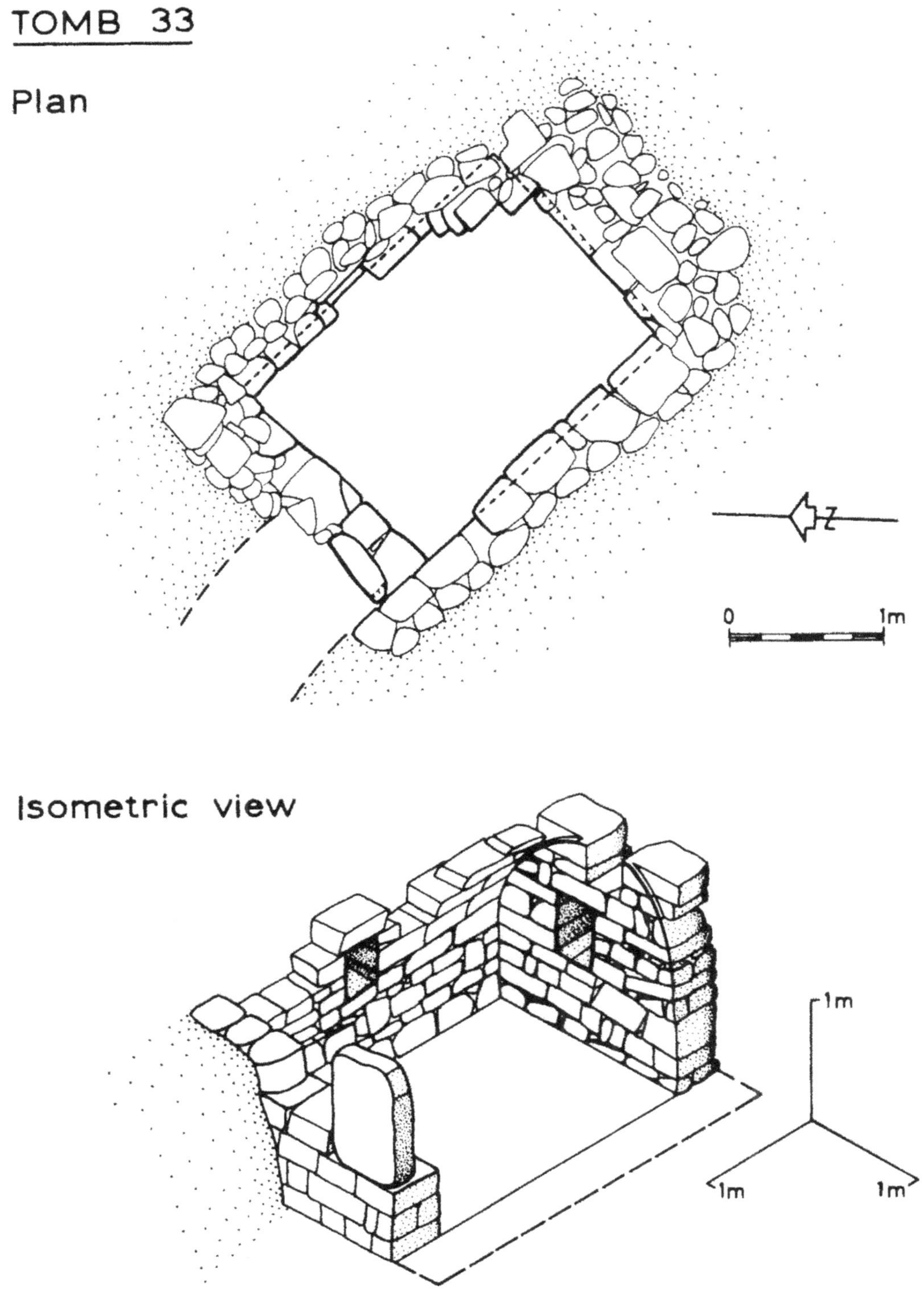

Figure 3.17. Plan and isometric view drawings of KMF/78 Tomb 33 (Catling 1979, Fig. 43).

Figure 3.18). As discussed above, cist graves can range from narrow pits with unworked stone slabs or bricks lining the walls and cover slabs to much more significant constructions not dissimilar to some of the built tombs (missing only the dromos, (more or less) monumental doorway, and built roof). An additional problem is caused by the fact that many of these tombs are not found intact, and therefore we are often not presented with the full array of original features in the archaeological context.

Another factor in considering the social significance of the tomb is the number of individuals it housed. The

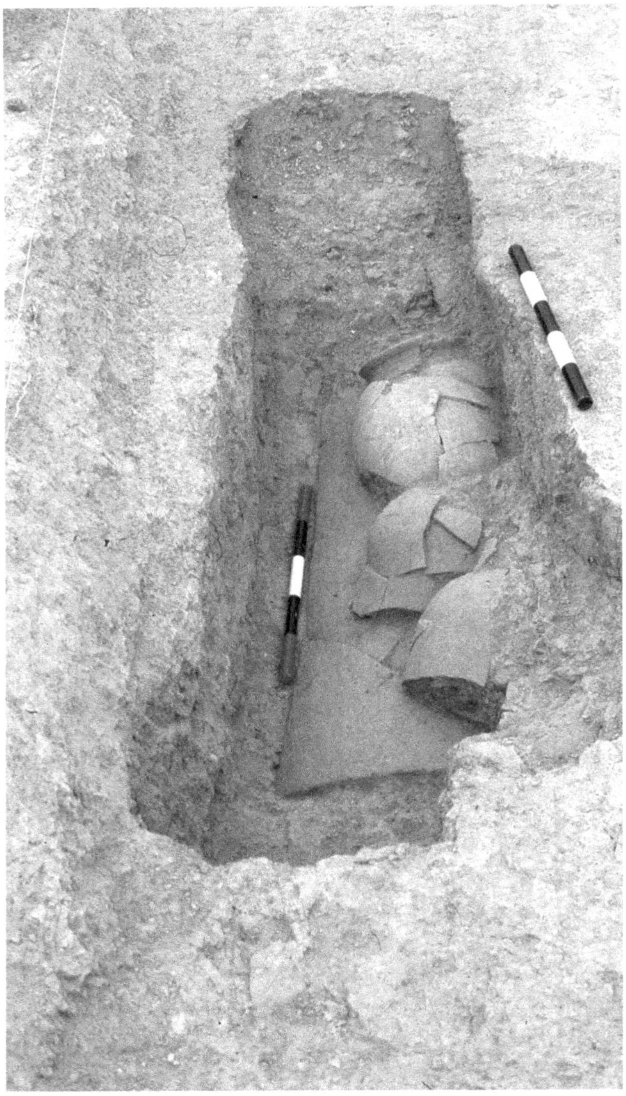

Figure 3.18. KMF T.46 tile grave, seemingly with *kalyvitis* tiles and large pot fragments. Photo: BSA Archive.

Late Antique KOP/79 tomb (Figures 3.19–20) was a well-constructed stone-lined tomb which contained a single inhumation. In comparison with the contemporary osteothekai, such as KFF/74 Tomb 1 (Figures 3.21–22) built of irregular stones of different sizes or KMF/78 Tomb 244 (Figures 3.23–3.24), which were estimated to have contained 54 and 28 individuals respectively, KOP/79 is a substantial construction for a single individual. The same applies to the Roman built tombs. MK/61 Tomb 1 and KMF/78 Tomb 33 have a similar chamber form and number of individuals (estimated at nine and ten respectively), though the former was built from ashlar blocks while the latter was of rougher masonry. The built tomb KSM Tomb 1a, on the other hand, was estimated to contain the remains of 42 individuals, though its exact structure is little known due to destruction for the basilica tower (Frend and Johnston 1962, 202, 206), but there does not appear to be a correlation between tomb size or monumentality of structure and numbers of interments. However, the intended and actual uses of a tomb may have been different, and the perceived prestige of a tomb may have changed over time. KMF Tomb 124 was of an unusual form, with two shallow sarcophagi surrounded by a substantial ashlar '*peribolos*'[15] (Figures 3.25–26) and had a minimum number of individuals of eight comparable to the barrel-vaulted built tombs. Several of the other monumental built tombs, for which skeletal material has been analysed to give an estimated number of individuals, contained very small numbers of burials. KMF Tomb 58 (structure unknown with only three large, well-dressed blocks in situ; Figure 3.27) and KMF Tomb 156 (also poorly preserved but built of large, worked blocks and smaller stones) each contained two individuals, while KMF Tomb 239 (Figure 3.28) had three occupants. However, considering the state of destruction of some of these tombs and the speed of excavation, it is possible the numbers of individuals are under-represented, a problem that is further discussed in Chapter 4. It is also possible that tombs were not intended for only one or two burials but went out of use or collapsed before further individuals could be interred.

Using tomb types as a proxy for social status presents many problems both in knowing how to interpret the known features and in not knowing what additional features would have been present. Whether the presence or absence of door jambs and a lintel in the rock-cut chamber tombs would have been significant in terms of social status cannot be known. Was the use of large and ornate blocks of spolia considered more or less distinguished than other cut stone blocks? Was it more prestigious to lay the dead on *klinai* under *arcosolia* than in pits in the floor or simply on the chamber floor? It is likely that some of these characteristics depended on personal taste, practical factors – such as the workability of the rock or time constraints – and for how long the tomb was expected to and remained in use and how many individuals it received. Many of the tombs, whether rock-cut, of dressed stone masonry or in rough uncut stones, had their walls and ceilings plastered so it may be the case that the stonework of these tombs was not as significant to the onlooker as it appears in the surviving architectural remains. In some situations, the type of tomb appears to have been dictated by the topography of the valley. The steep slopes of soft kouskouras could have large (monumental?) chamber tombs easily dug into the hillsides. This would save both material resources and construction time compared to the built mausolea, which are largely known from the flatter northern region and some on the gentle slopes of lower Gypsades. The question remains whether the more modestly built tombs and rock-cut chamber tombs carried the same level of social prestige. However, it is likely that all built tombs were not equal and the ashlar masonry, above-ground, free-standing mausolea were built to accommodate the highest status members of society. Each

[15] It is unclear why this is referred to as a *peribolos* (Catling 1978, 52) rather than as the lower courses of a tomb built of ashlar masonry, considering the large numbers of fallen blocks and rubble stones referred to in the fill in the excavation notebook (KMF Notebook 22, BSA Archive).

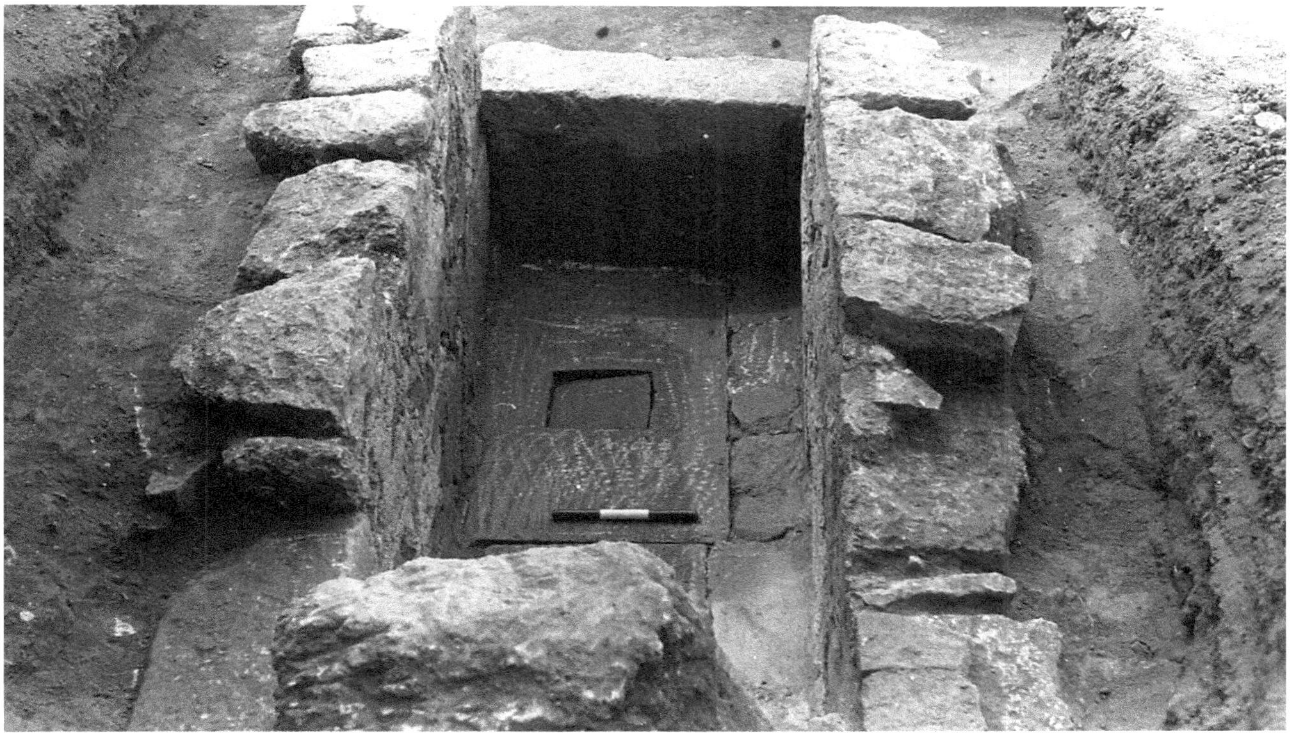

Figure 3.19. KOP/79 stone-lined tomb. Photo: BSA Archive.

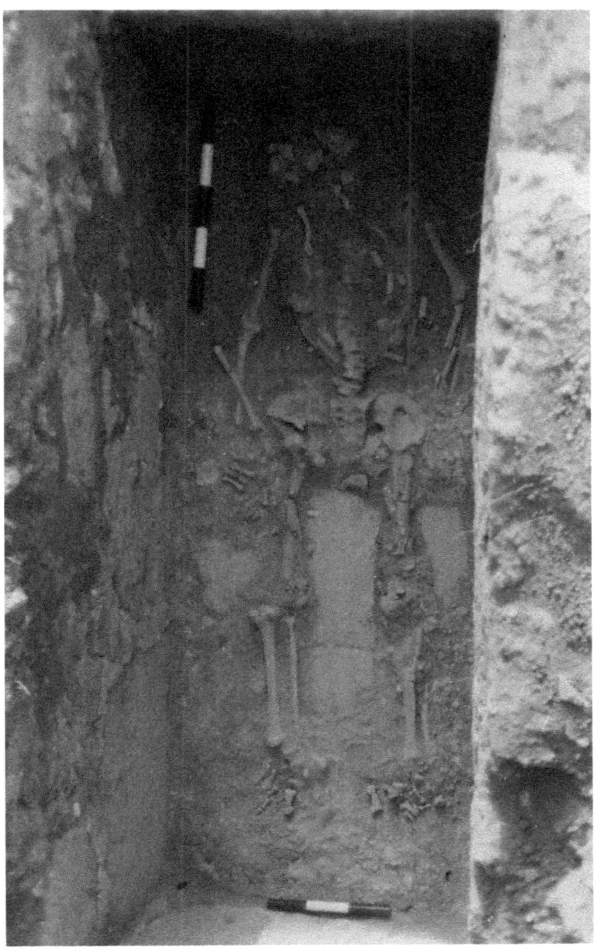

Figure 3.20. KOP/79 stone-lined tomb. Photo: BSA Archive.

investment of additional resources, whether of materials or time and labour, and each effort towards an elaborate appearance and prominent visibility, are assumed to be meaningful because these decisions were made to do more than simply dispose of a corpse in the simplest fashion possible.

3.5. Grave goods and identity

Grave goods were not used as an indicator of social status on a categorical level for a comparison of the skeletal analyses for this study due to the large numbers of disturbed and looted graves. A tomb with no (or few) burial goods cannot be said to be a tomb of low social standing. Items may have been lost to the archaeological record through decay or looting and there may be numerous other reasons besides wealth or status for a lack of grave goods being interred with the deceased. However, where there is positive evidence, a certain amount can be deduced from this record and these artefacts can assist in the discussion of the socio-economic significance of the tomb types, as well as being important for dating purposes. Grave goods are particularly unhelpful for the late Roman and Late Antique Christian graves which tended to have very few or no associated artefacts.

The majority of known Hellenistic graves were narrow rock-cut pits and the notion that these were simple, non-elite graves would seem to be supported by the poverty of grave goods in both quantity and quality. However, a comparison with burials elsewhere on Crete indicates there was relatively little differentiation in burial type, and grave goods tended to be modest in the majority of

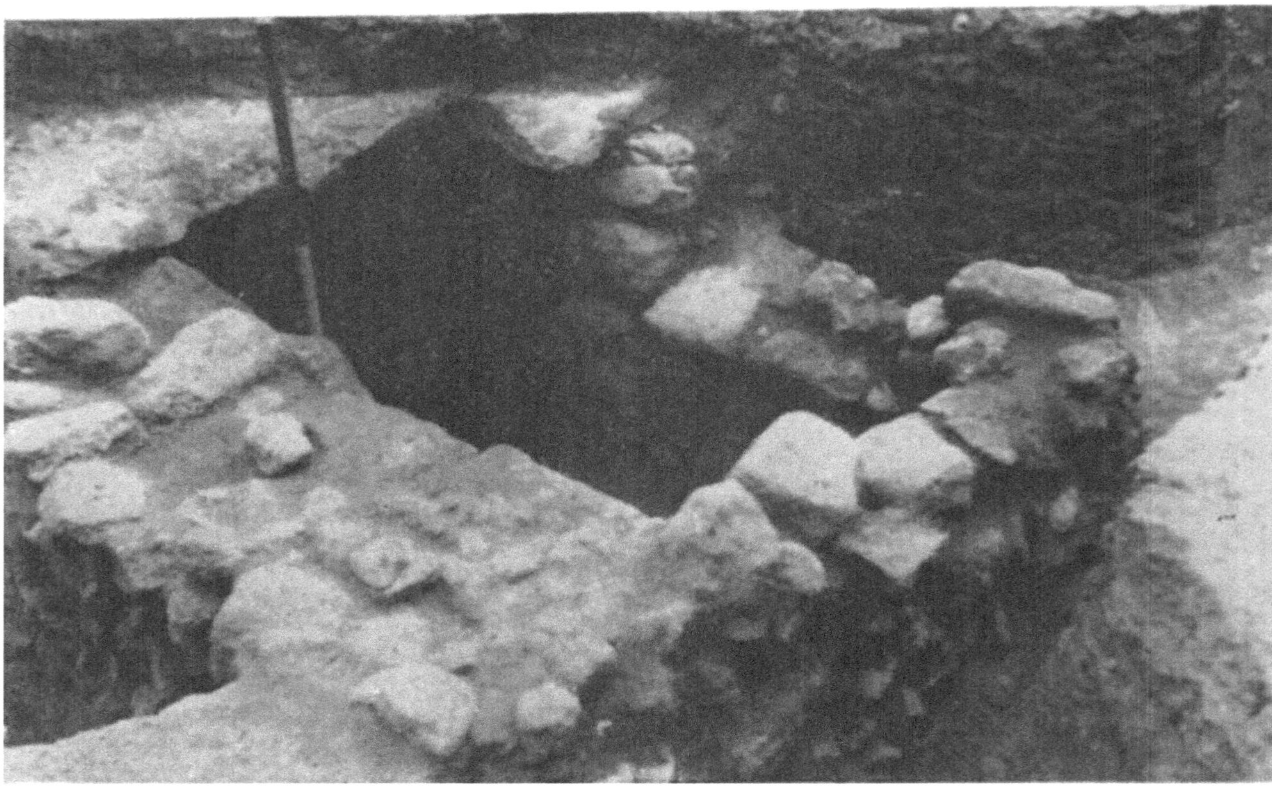

Figure 3.21. KFF osteotheke (Unit 4). Photo: Catling *et al.* 1976 Pl.4b.

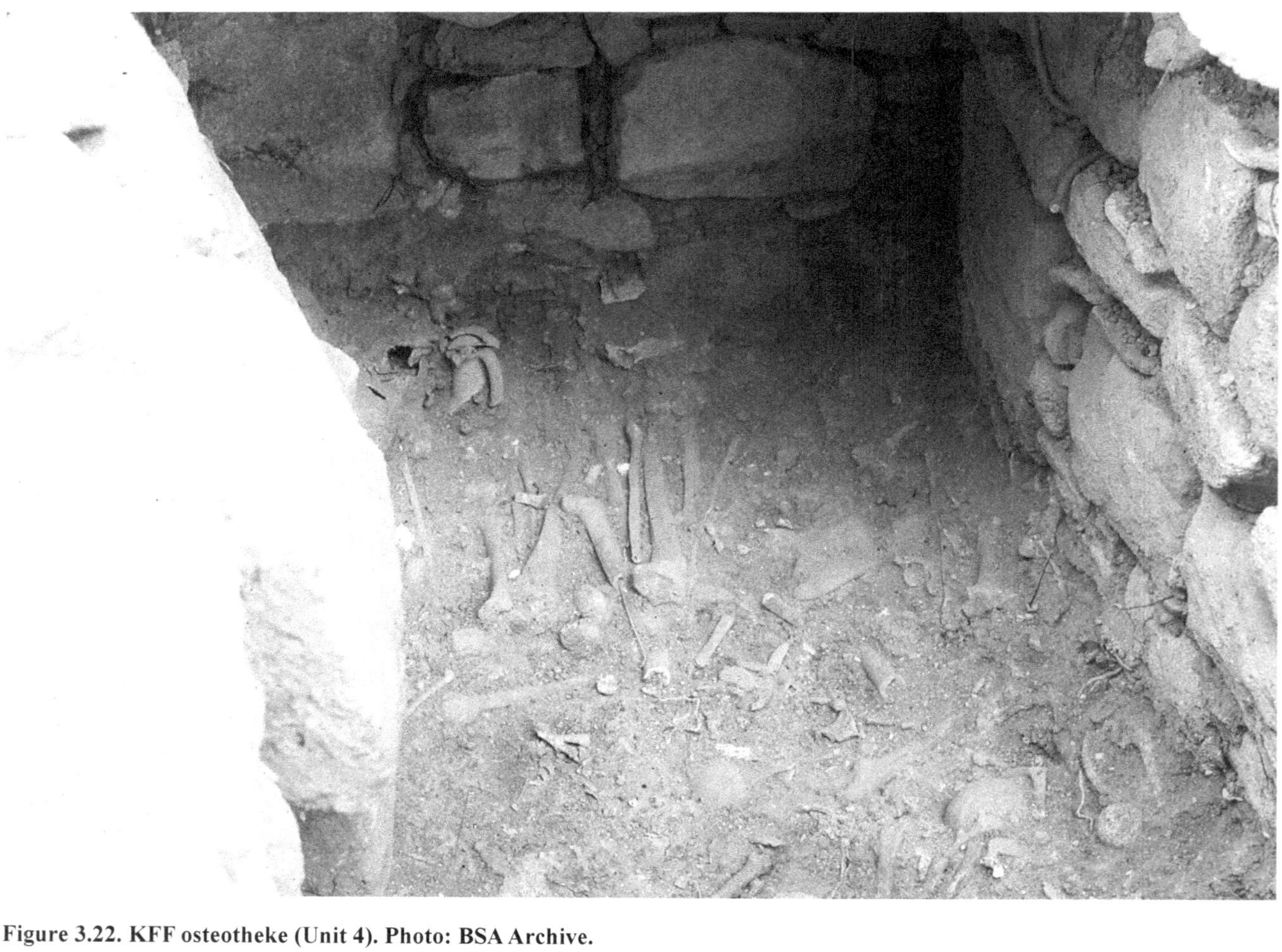

Figure 3.22. KFF osteotheke (Unit 4). Photo: BSA Archive.

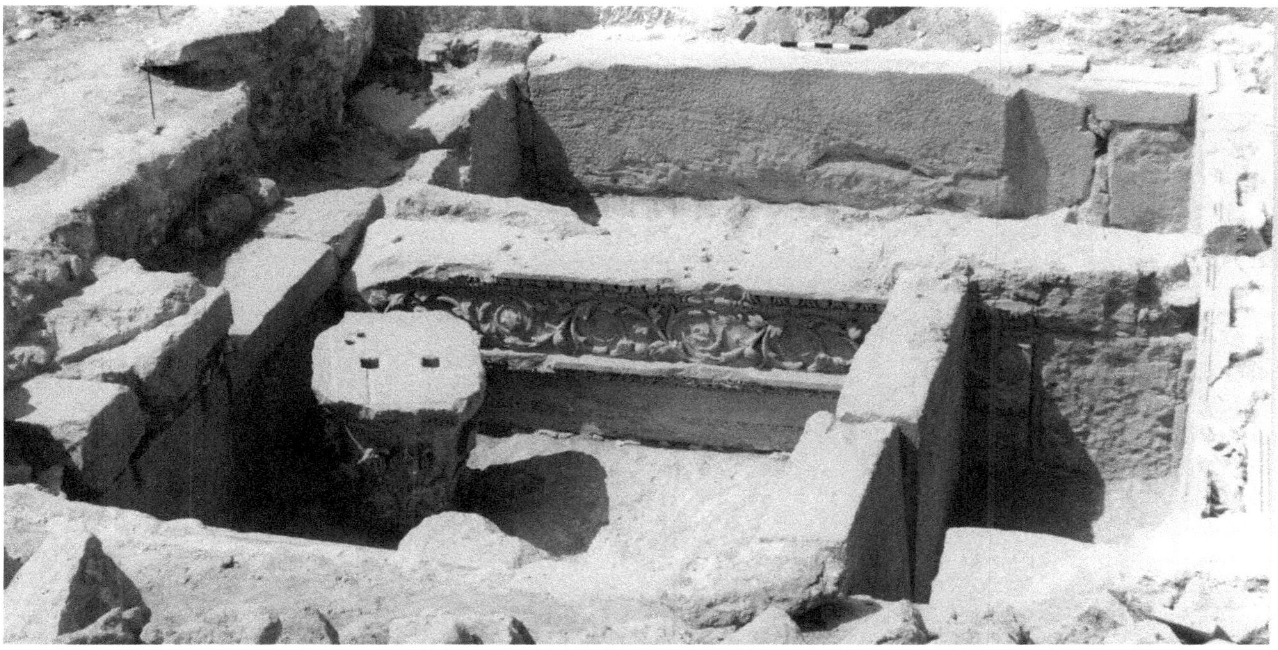

Figure 3.23. KMF Tomb 244 (Unit 84). Photo: BSA Archive.

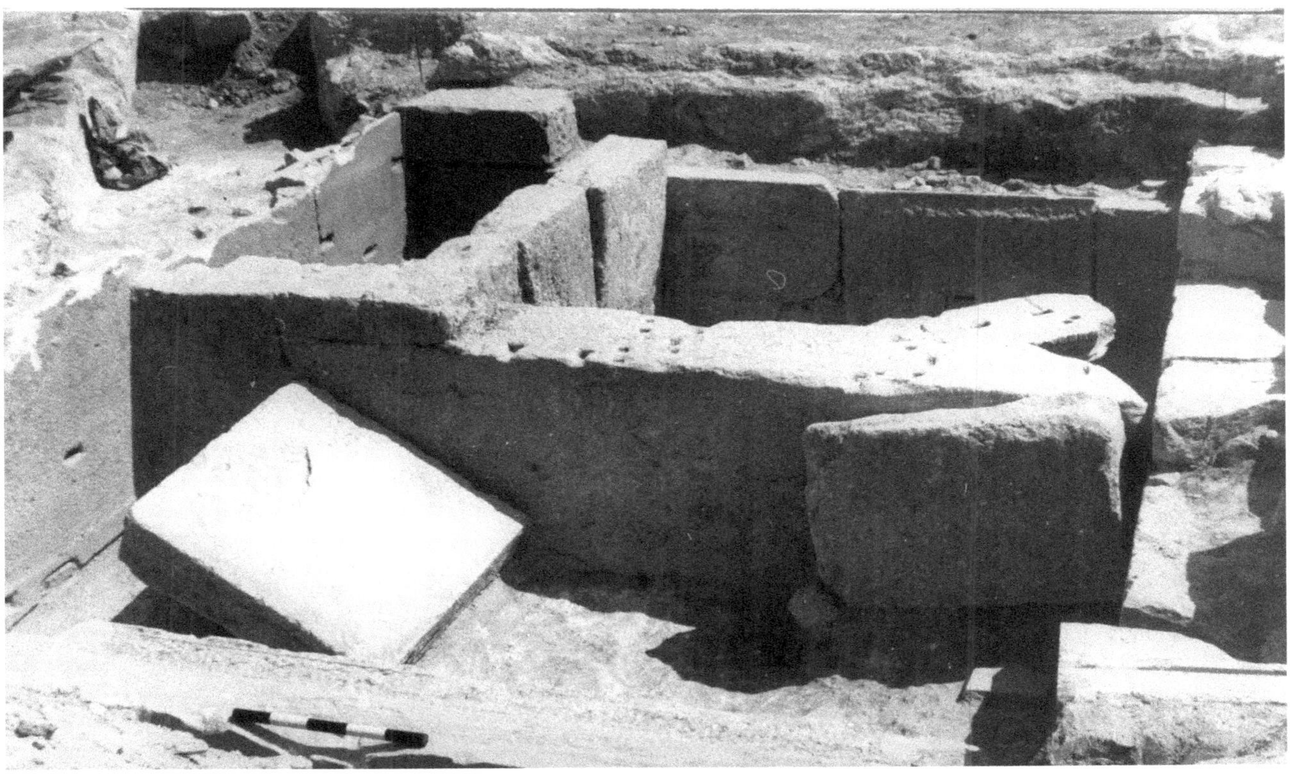

Figure 3.24. KMF Tomb 244 (Unit 84). Photo: BSA Archive.

contexts. Small numbers of more elaborate graves are known, such as the *hypogeum* chamber tombs with *loculi* at Chania. These contained larger numbers of offerings, though there were also larger numbers of interments, which included coins, lamps, clay unguentaria, cups and jugs, glass unguentaria and jugs, iron strigils, bronze pyxides and mirrors, terracotta figurines, glass beads, a gold epistomion, gold and silver rings and earrings, gold-coated clay jewellery, and a gold necklace (Markoulaki and Niniou-Kindeli 1982; 2009; Tsigkou 2004; 2009; Niniou-Kindeli 2009). There are also a number of more elaborate offerings from simple graves, such as the gold

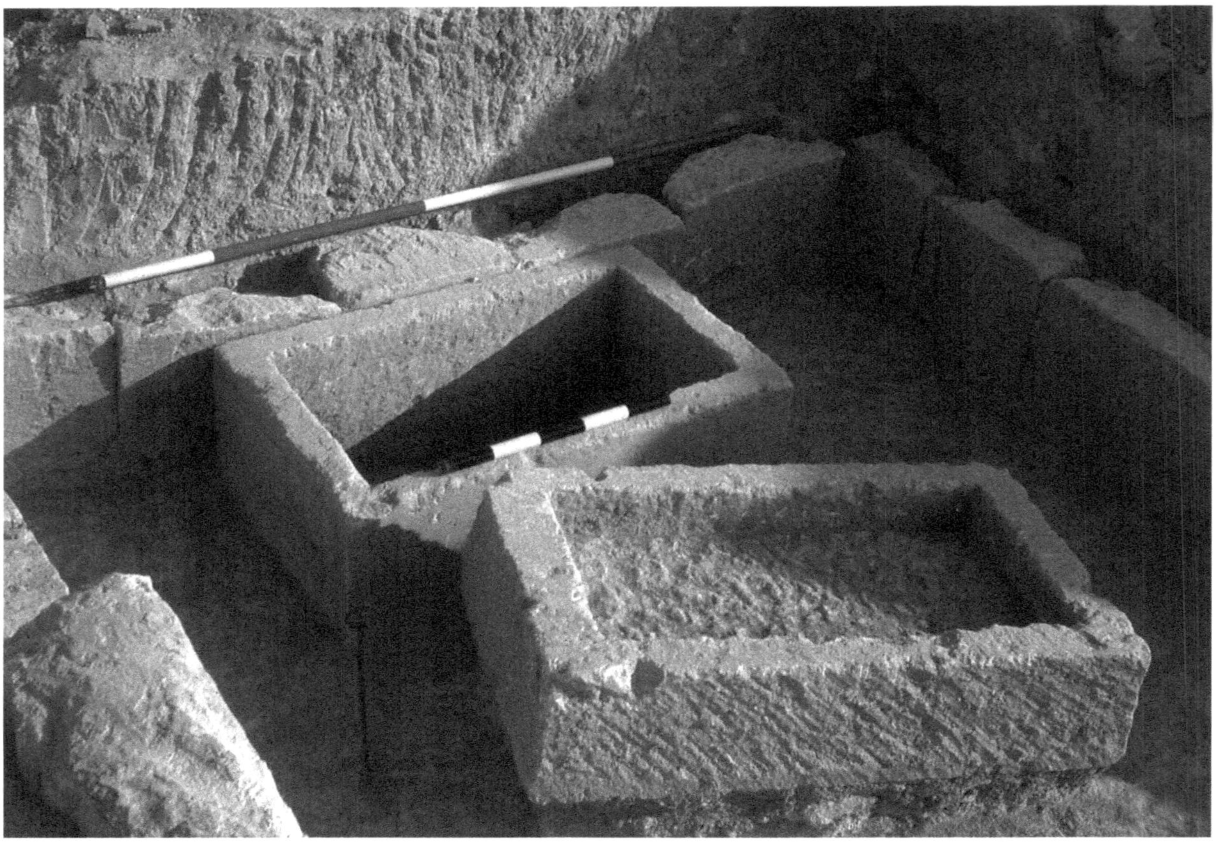

Figure 3.25. KMF Tomb 124 (Unit 71) sarcophagus and '*peribolos*', view from south-west. Photo: BSA Archive.

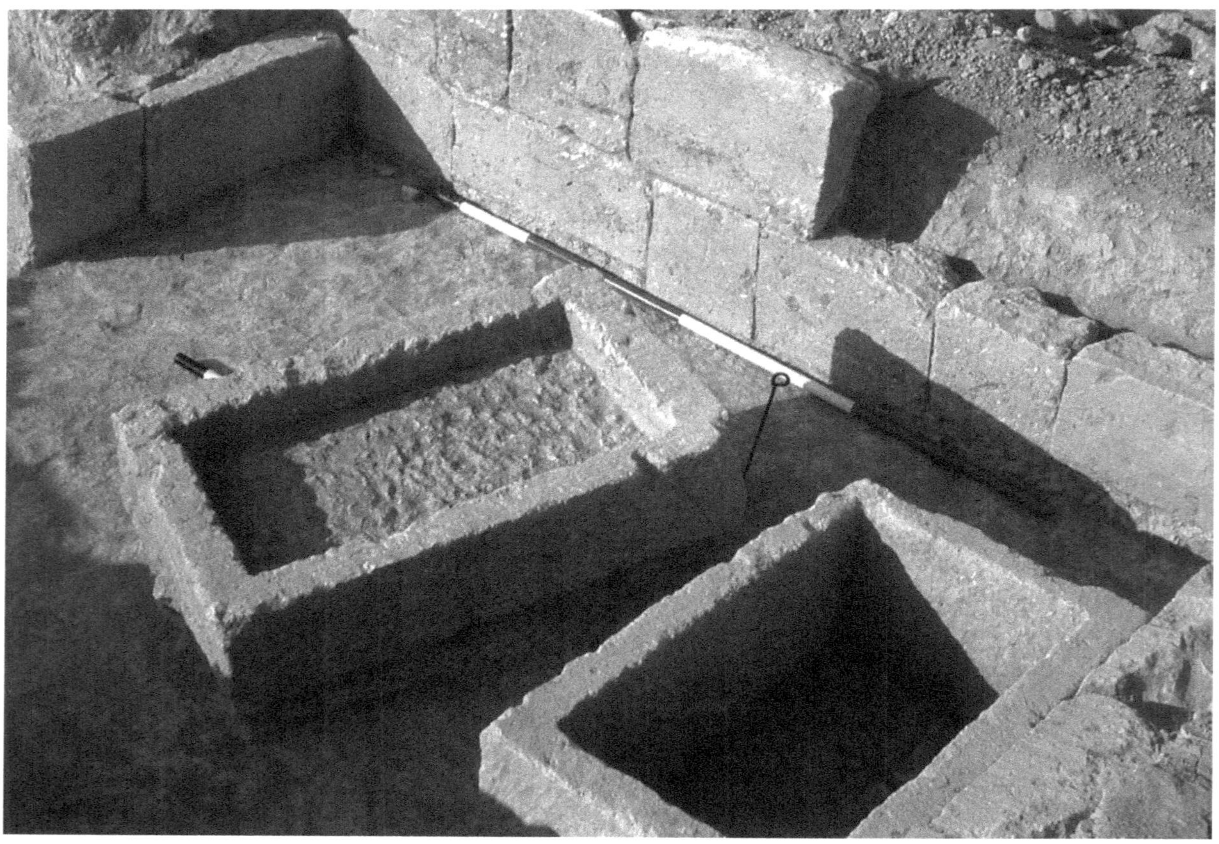

Figure 3.26. KMF Tomb 124 (Unit 71) sarcophagus and '*peribolos*', view from north-east. Photo: BSA Archive.

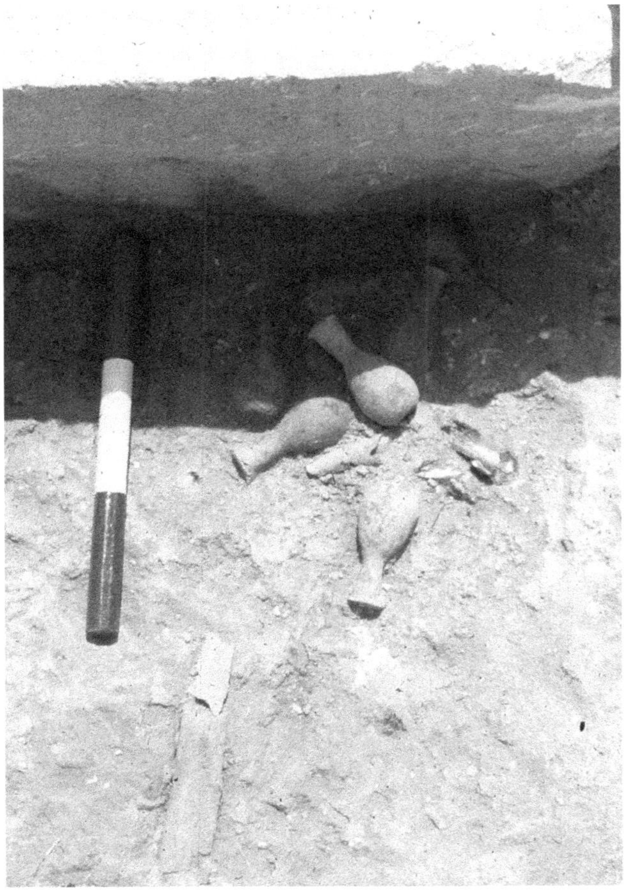

Figure 3.27. KMF Tomb 58 (Unit 70), showing finds next to one of the three surviving dressed stone blocks along the south wall. Photo: BSA Archive.

wreaths known from tombs at Kissamos, Chania, Gortyn, Chersonissos and Lato (Guyon 2008, 129). Many of the Knossos burials had no accompanying items surviving (though organic offerings cannot be excluded) or often one or two poorly-fired unguentaria of a local grey fabric (Coldstream *et al.* 2001). However, there were other pottery shapes present in these graves, including cups, jugs, lekythes, thymiateria, and lamps. There were also coins, occasionally metal objects or glass vessels. Infrequently there was jewellery discovered, such as the gold earrings from the late 3rd century BC KMF Tomb 143 which also contained a gold coin and lamp (Figure 3.29) and the gold-coated bronze and silver rings from the Fortetsa cemetery (Brock 1957, 59, 100). This raises the question of whether individuals buried with finer, more elaborate, or simply more (in terms of quantity) grave goods had been higher status individuals in life. Such items are rare finds from Hellenistic graves in Crete. A description of grave goods by Guyon (2008) did not often distinguish between the Hellenistic and Roman periods, but this identified only 30 earrings from Crete between the 2nd century BC and 2nd C AD, and of the 80 iron, bronze, silver and gold rings identified (the most common type of jewellery find) he states that the majority of simple iron and bronze rings were in graves of late 4th-early 3rd century BC graves, and while some of the gold and silver rings came from Hellenistic graves, the majority date to the 1st-2nd century AD (Guyon 2008, 136). The only significantly more elaborate tomb known from near Knossos was the 4th century *hypogeum* at Katsambas (Alexiou 1969). As this was pillaged in antiquity, there are no finds reported other than black-glazed sherds. The looting and disturbance

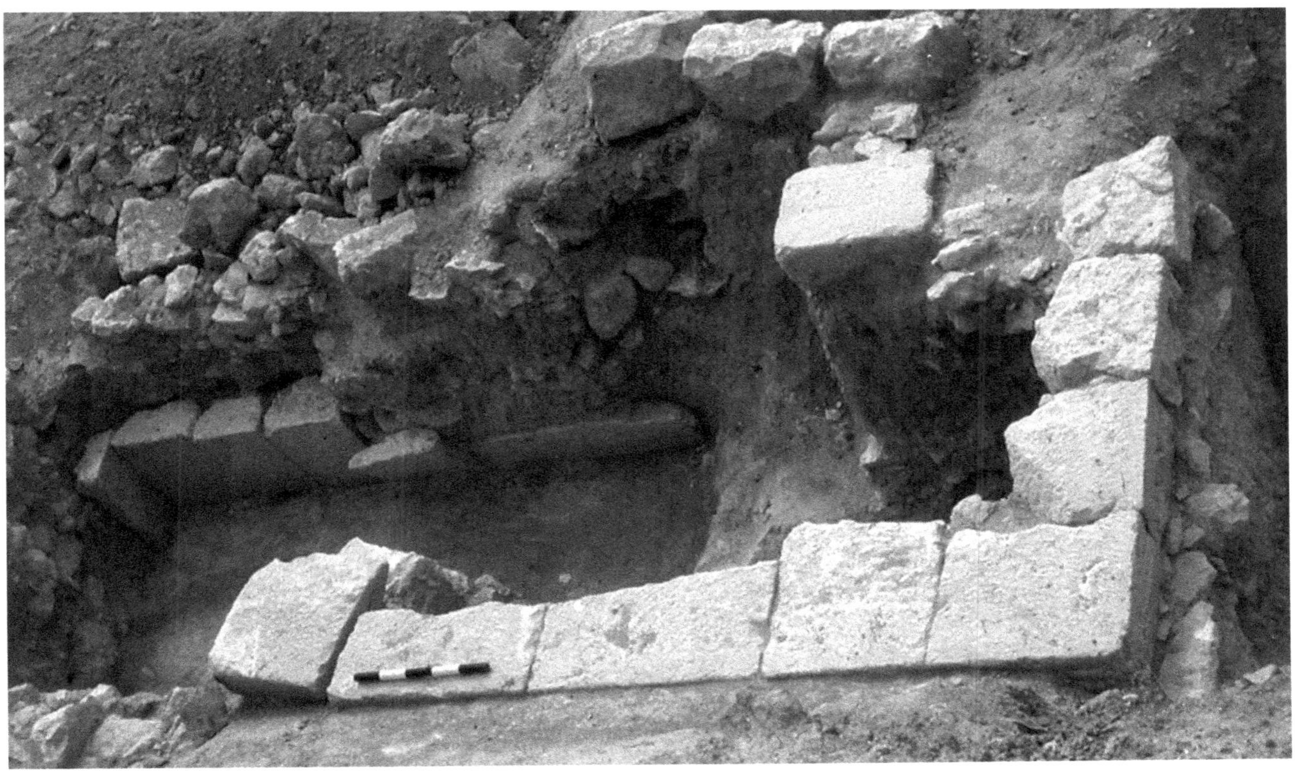

Figure 3.28. KMF Tomb 239 (Unit 73), view from east, Roman vaulted (collapsed) built tomb. Photo: BSA Archive.

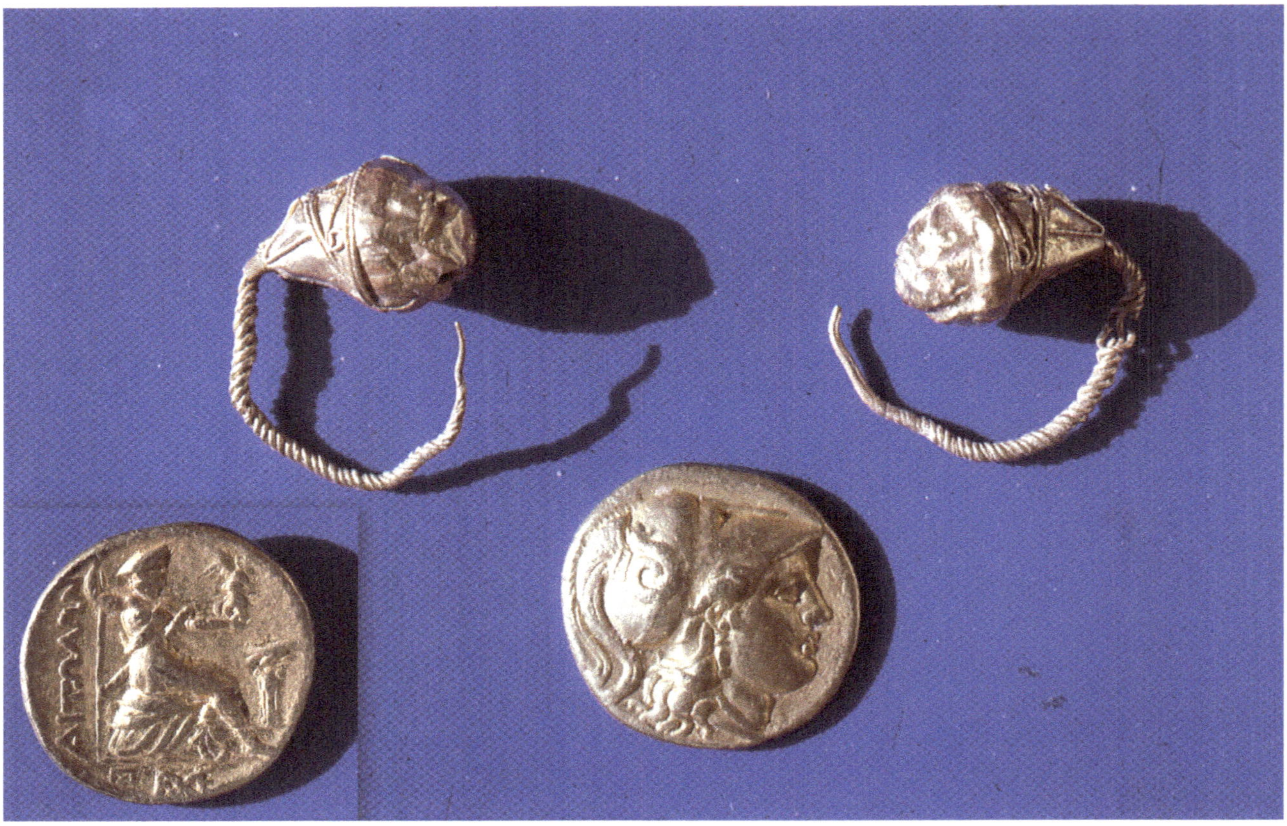

Figure 3.29. Gold earrings featuring lions' heads and gold Aetolian stater (c.250–200 BC) from KMF Tomb 143 (Unit 31), the obverse depicting Athena in a Corinthian helmet pictured with the earrings and the inset showing the coin reverse with Aetolia holding a Nike and spear. Photos: BSA Archive.

of graves (both in antiquity and recent times), as well as disintegration of organic offerings, mean that the archaeological record does not present a complete picture of the offerings deposited in a grave.

The same problem is relevant to the Roman tombs. The barrel-vaulted built KMF Tomb 33, though surviving fairly intact structurally, was thought to have been looted, leaving only a bronze mirror and bronze coin, the latter found with a mandible fragment stained green by the coin (Figure 3.30). The 1st century AD vaulted ashlar-built MK/61 Tomb 1 had large numbers of offerings, to accompany the large number of individuals buried, but these were not particularly rich or elaborate objects, being limited to glass ungentaria, clay lamps and bronze coins (Hood 1962, 29). On the other hand, gold items were found in some of the mausolea of the North Cemetery including jewellery, *epistomia*, rosettes and remnants of gold thread and gold leaf. A 1st-2nd century vaulted built tomb excavated by Grammatikaki (1996) had been partially pillaged but the finds included the remains of fabric with gold thread and little stars, three lead urns, six glass unguentaria, a clay unguentarium, two lamps (with images of sirens and animals), a silver pyxis, gold olive leaves (probably the remnants of a crown wreath), gold rosettes, bone beads, bronze studs and a bronze chain. The rock-cut chamber tombs to the south of the valley showed a similar variation in the presence and variety of burial goods. The 1st century KLT/78 rock-cut chamber tomb, excavated by Carington Smith (1982), contained a large number of items including pottery, lamps, glass vessels, Dionysiac masks, terracotta figurines, plaques and protomes, coins, a gold earring, gold and silver rings, bone pins, bronze, iron and lead items, and a silver spoon and stylus. The contemporary Marathaniou Lakkos tombs nearby contained only glass vessels, clay lamps and the second of the two tombs excavated in 1970 also contained two clay theatrical masks (Wardle 1972;

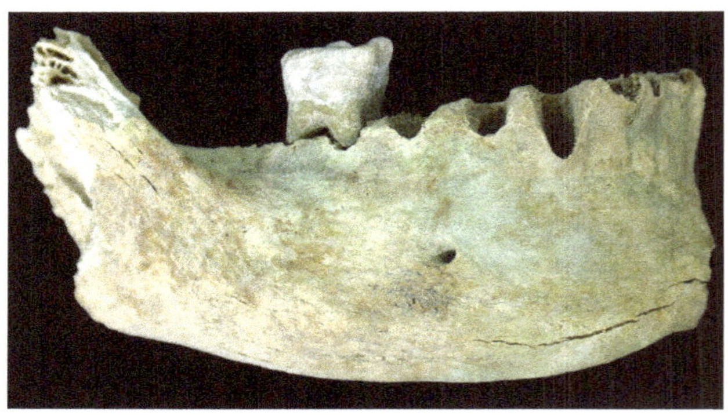

Figure 3.30. Mandible fragment from KMF Tomb 33 (Unit 68, Ind.128) showing green staining from a bronze coin. Photo: Anna Moles.

Wardle and Wardle 2004). Many other rock-cut chamber tombs were completely looted and retained no artefacts.

The later Roman and Late Antique graves generally only contained incidental items of dress or body ornament, such as buckles, fastenings and jewellery, but even these were few. Occasionally, pottery was found, as was the case of the six jugs in the KFF/74 tomb which enabled it to be dated to the 7th or 8th century (Catling *et al.* 1976). Infrequent pottery finds also enable dates to be assigned to several of the KMF tombs including T.199, T.223, and T.296 (Hayes 2001). Sherds in the fill of Tombs 244 and 245 gave a *terminus ante quem* and potentially represented the latest burials in these tombs (Sweetman and Becker 2005). Coins found in several of the KMF osteothekai also enabled some tombs to be dated (Sweetman and Becker 2005).

3.6. Representativeness of material

The skeletal assemblage for Hellenistic Knossos comes from a single cemetery and consists solely of basic pit and tile graves, therefore it is unlikely that a complete cross-section of society is represented. However, these are the most common burial type on Crete and the burial sphere does not appear to show great differentiation in tomb form or grave goods. There are small numbers of more elaborate tombs but these are largely the *hypogea* rock-cut *loculi* tombs from Chania and a built 'funerary monument' from Phaistos (Markoulaki and Niniou-Kindeli 1982; 2009; Hatzi-Vallianou 1989; Tsigkou 2004; 2009; Andreadaki-Vlazaki 2009; Niniou-Kindeli 2009). Small numbers of rock-cut chamber tombs are also reported as being Hellenistic from Polyrhenia and Phaistos and, although these were said to have been pillaged, few or no grave goods were recovered (Savignoni 1901; Hatzi-Vallianou 1995; Guyon 2008, 107). Hellenistic cist graves on Crete also contained modest offerings (e.g. Karetsou 1974). The range of burial goods in the Knossos graves represented by the assemblage, from none or a single poorly fired unguentarium to gold earrings and a gold coin indicates that quite a broad representation of society may be represented, as these finds are across the expected range of grave goods for most contexts from Hellenistic Crete (see catalogue of graves in Appendix A for further details). However, with a precedent set for more elaborate tombs by those at Chania and Phaistos, it is possible that small numbers of more elaborate tombs are missing from the archaeological record at Knossos. The burial situation on Crete in this time period is different to the Peloponnese, Northern Greece, Cyprus, Rhodes, Asia Minor or Egypt, all of which had greater monumentality in tomb form for the elite members of society and, in many cases, a greater wealth of grave goods, particularly in the inclusion of gold items (Andronikos 1984; Karageorghis 1985; Fedak 1990; Themelis and Touratsoglou 1997; Empereur and Nenna 2001; 2003; Nenna 2009; Guimier-Sorbets and Michaelides 2009; Lilimbaki-Akamati and Akamatis 2014; Dimakis 2016; Brandt *et al.* 2017; Dijkstra 2019). This indicates that Hellenistic Crete remained culturally independent of its neighbours, at least in how they buried their dead and suggests that inferences drawn from the skeletal study are likely to only be applicable to Crete rather than representing wider-scale patterns.

The Roman tombs at Knossos show the greatest architectural diversity of the periods included in this study, potentially suggesting the best representation of a complete cross-section of society. However, it is also evident that there was a greater emphasis on the burial sphere as a means of self-representation (or representation of the deceased) and expression of social status, and potentially that there was a more hierarchical society and established elite presence at the site in the Early-Middle Roman period. The increased monumentalisation of tomb forms is a widespread pattern across the island, with large numbers of built and rock-cut chamber tombs, though pit graves remain the most common grave type, as would be expected from a hierarchical society where the wealth, power and high social status belong to a very small percentage of the population. The simplest grave types are severely underrepresented by the skeletal assemblage (no pit and only six tile graves) and by the excavation record at Knossos in general. This may indicate that the lower echelons of society are underrepresented (if present at all) in the skeletal assemblage. However, it is not always the case that larger, communal tombs are only for the wealthy and high status members of society. The widespread parallels for tomb form (as well as in other architecture and material culture) found throughout the Mediterranean area, from Italy, Greece, North Africa and Asia Minor, indicate the better connectedness of Knossos and Crete within networks during the Roman period (Moles forthcoming). With this increased connectivity and contact throughout the Roman Empire (and particularly the Mediterranean in relation to Knossos), the changes that are observed from the skeletal analysis may have broader implications throughout the wider region.

Tomb forms become increasingly homogenous in the later Roman and Late Antique periods, with almost all graves being a form of stone-lined tomb. The small number of tile graves known at Knossos are not represented in the skeletal assemblage and it is assumed there would have been many more basic pit and tile graves which have not been detected archaeologically, as these remain a common grave type on Crete (di Vita 2010, 347). The diversity of sizes and stone types used for the Late Antique graves may represent differing social status, but, like the Roman period, it may the case that the lower status members of society are largely missing from this study. Although the intense level of connectivity involving Crete in wider networks may have decreased in the Late Antique period, imports remain common (Hayes 2001; Gallimore 2016), mosaics are innovative and demonstrate contacts with mainland Greece, Asia Minor and the East (Sweetman 2004a, 316) and stone-lined tombs (sometimes built with *spolia* from Roman buildings) have parallels with mainland Greece and Asia Minor in this time period (Poulou-Papadimitriou *et al.* 2012; Lightfoot 2017; Wenn *et al.* 2017). It is possible therefore than the conclusions drawn from the Knossos skeletal material may have broader implications within Greece and the Eastern Mediterranean.

Recognising the problems of the assemblage and addressing its representativeness are important for the interpretation of the results of the skeletal analysis. This study in turn has the potential to give further insights into how well society is represented by identifying differences in health and diet among different groups of the population and between the time periods.

4

Demography

4.1. Introduction

"Palaeodemography is the field of inquiry that attempts to identify demographic parameters from past populations derived from archaeological contexts" (Hoppa 2002, 9). The age-at-death and sex determinations of individuals, as well as estimations of numbers of individuals, form a fundamental first step in the investigation of any skeletal assemblage as they provide a core of palaeodemographic data important for all further analyses. They are important for understanding past population dynamics and can inform on aspects of society. Age-at-death, in particular, can be important for understanding many of the variations in the prevalence of diseases and other conditions that leave a mark on the skeleton. It can demonstrate the simple age-progressive nature and cumulative effect of pathological conditions, but can also provide a fundamental indication of well-being, just as life expectancy is used today in living populations as a standard of health and well-being (Larsen 2015, 402). Consequently, this chapter's contribution to the study of lifeways at Knossos is two-fold. The understanding of the age and sex structure of the skeletal assemblage provides variables for the analysis of diet and disease, for the study of variation within the population. Concurrently, age-at-death gives a very approximate indication of life expectancy (only by broad age category) of the ancient Knossians which is investigated for variation across the time periods and between different demographic and social sub-groups within the population.

To consider how representative a death assemblage is, there is a need to overcome the shortcomings of age estimation techniques and recognise the problems of an archaeological death assemblage, one key point being that although a death assemblage is drawn from a population, it is never a sample of one. These include differential mortuary treatment for different demographic sub-groups of the population, preservation and recovery methods that affect both the representativeness of the assemblage and the ability to age and sex elements or individuals, and the inherent bias of an archaeological death assemblage in the variation in probability of death across different age classes (Jackes 2011; Larsen 2015). Some of these issues are side-lined by the simple recognition that mean age-at-death does not reflect life expectancy and is more strongly influenced by fertility than mortality (Wood *et al.* 1992). Mean age-at-death can be seen as the inverse of birth rate, thus if mean age-at-death declines, it is likely that birth rate is increasing (Larsen 2015, 411). This, however, does not circumvent the problem of inaccuracy of ageing techniques. Age-at-death estimation methods based on reference collections (Todd 1920; McKern and Stewart 1957) can be too heavily influenced by the known ages-at-death of the reference collection. Solutions to this problem have included using multiple age indicators (Lovejoy *et al.* 1985), dental wear seriation (Miles 1963), and progressive cranial suture closure (Meindl and Lovejoy 1985). Many characteristics become increasingly uninformative for assessing age-at-death in the later years of life but using a combination of skeletal characteristics that undergo progressive age changes and employing broad age categories (e.g. young, middle and old adults) rather than precise age estimates can demonstrate the progressive transitions of ageing most successfully (Bocquet-Appel and Masset 1982; Van Gerven and Armelagos 1983; Chamberlain 2006; Bocquet-Appel 2008; Milner and Boldsen 2012; Larsen 2015).

The issue of how representative a skeletal assemblage is of a living biological population is a problem for both palaeodemography and palaeoepidemiology. The mortality sample (skeletal assemblage) is never the same as a sample of living people because mortality is selective and the most vulnerable people at each age are the ones who die. In 'The Osteological Paradox', Wood *et al.* (1992) outlined three fundamental problems for the interpretation of statistics calculated from archaeological skeletal assemblages: demographic non-stationarity, selective mortality, and unmeasured, individual-level heterogeneity in the risks of disease and death. A population in reality is never likely to be in a stationary state, which would be a population closed to migration, with constant age-specific fertility and mortality, zero growth rate, and an equilibrium age distribution. Selective mortality refers to the fact that a skeletal sample can never include all of the individuals who were at risk of disease and death at a specific age, but only those who actually died, and as such the sample of any specific age is not representative. The hidden heterogeneity in risks within the population, meaning that the population from which the assemblage is drawn consisted of an unknown mixture of individuals who varied in their underlying susceptibility to disease and death, could be due to genetic causes, socio-economic differentials, microenvironmental variation, or even temporal trends in health. Therefore, even if an excavated assemblage recovered every person born into an ancient society, the skeletal record would still be biased, relative to the living population at any point in time. This is built on another important point, that the observation of healed bone lesions is more indicative of an increased ability to withstand disease rather than of ill-health. In observing those in the assemblage with and without a particular pathological lesion, the skeletons without the lesion can come from two groups, those who have never been exposed to the disease or were strong enough to fight it off before the bone was affected, and those who were unable to put up any resistance to the disease and died quickly before there was any bony response.

Taphonomic processes dictate the state in which an archaeological assemblage is found, and this influences how the assemblage should be recorded and studied. Taphonomy is the study of "the physical and chemical processes (induced by human, animal, or natural agents) that modify an organism after its death and through which it is incorporated into geological deposits" (LaMotta and Schiffer 2005). An understanding of the depositional context and taphonomic processes can help in the interpretation of the representativeness of the assemblage compared to that originally deposited. Fragmentation and commingling pose a problem for analysing multiple ageing or sexing traits in the same individual, as well as many other analyses that would benefit from being able to identify intact individuals. There are a number of indices for the quantification of commingled and fragmentary remains, including the minimum number of individuals (MNI), most likely number of individuals (MLNI), minimum number of elements (MNE) and the Lincoln Index (LI) for estimating population size (Adams and Konigsberg 2004; 2008). For fragmentary assemblages or where retrieval of elements has been poor, these cases are not suited to meaningful attempts to quantify the original number of individuals represented by the skeletal assemblage. The MNI technique can only conduct counts within the bounds of the recovered assemblage but is the most useful technique to employ with the caveat that it may not represent the actual numbers of dead originally buried. However, an assessment of the relative preservation of different bones, metric pair-matching of bones and taking into account the demographic composition of the assemblage where possible can help demonstrate how likely it is that the minimum number is close to the actual number.

4.2. Methodology

4.2.1. Data Collection and Recording

One of the main challenges in creating a methodology and recording system for the Knossos assemblage was dealing with the condition of the material, which was fragmentary and commingled. In zooarchaeology, this is frequently the inherent nature of the material, as animal remains are often excavated from rubbish dumps having been processed for human consumption (i.e. as individual bones or small numbers of associated bones from joints of meat). The bones have been chopped, cut, cooked and gnawed and are therefore fragmentary even at the point of initial deposition before further taphonomic processes start to act on them (Reitz and Wing 1999; O'Connor 2004; Peres 2010). The use of recording by diagnostic zones, rather than the whole bone as an individual element, aids in recording what is actually present in the assemblage and in counting zones of elements which enables estimates of minimum numbers of individuals (MNI). This is a flexible system used frequently by zooarchaeologists and increasingly also applied to human osteology (Knüsel and Outram 2004). It is easily adaptable to the assemblage by adjusting the size of the zone being used, depending on various factors such as the degree of fragmentation, the archaeological importance of the assemblage, the nature of the research questions and the skill and experience of the zooarchaeologist (Dobney and Reilly 1988; Ringrose 1993; Marean *et al.* 2001). For this project, documentation by many small diagnostic zones is not likely to aid in a more accurate estimation of numbers of individuals, nor does it assist in answering the research questions, but would be more likely to slow down and complicate the recording process for little or no gain. Therefore key diagnostic zones, such as joint surfaces, were designated as separate from the main shaft or body of the bone. Thus, long bones are assessed in three zones, distal, shaft and proximal, with the distal and proximal zones being the focus of attention. Irregular bones have more varied numbers of zones, such as the manubrium, carpals and tarsals being recorded as a single zone, while the scapula has four zones, with the glenoid and acromion as the important zones for diagnosis and the coracoid and spine/superior border/lateral border/ body simply recorded as present, absent or fragmented. For a zone to be recorded as present and included in the MNI count, it must be largely complete (>50%) to avoid any double recordings of a zone or element.

Terminology for recording:

- a **unit** is a unique number to identify the material deposited in a single burial.
- an **individual** is a group of elements that make up a single skeleton.
- an **element** is a bone, a fragment or a group of anatomically associated fragments.

When recording the skeletal material in the Microsoft Access database, originally designed for the Çatalhöyük Research Project by Hillson *et al.*[16] (Hillson *et al.* 2013; Boz and Hager 2014), and adapted by Hillson in 2015 to suit the present project's research questions and recording methods, each unit is numbered and recorded separately. Within a unit, the material can be recorded as an individual, an element or associated elements. There is a choice of three skeletal recording forms, adult, sub-adult (for adolescents, children and infants), and neonate. There are also associated forms for recording age-at-death and sex, deciduous and permanent dentition, measurements, and entheseal changes. Recording of joint disease is integrated into the main adult skeletal recording form and the dental form includes options for recording attrition, caries,

[16] The database was developed by the human remains team of the Çatalhöyük Research Project between 2008 and 2009. The authors are Simon Hillson, Sarah Jones, Basak Boz and Lori Hager. It was transformed into a standalone database by Sarah Jones in 2009 and further modified for the Astypalaia Bioanthropology Project by Simon Hillson in 2010. The general version was created by Simon Hillson in 2014.

calculus and periodontal disease. Other pathological lesions can be included in the notes section of the skeletal recording form.

As the recording of material was done either by individual (for identifiable individual skeletons or associated elements) or by element (for commingled material), this made the comparison of the single or double Hellenistic burials (largely the former recording method) to the Roman and Late Antique large communal tombs of commingled remains (recorded largely by element) difficult. However, by excluding the vast numbers of unaged elements from a comparison of the age profiles of the population over time by element and by calculating the minimum numbers of individuals (MNI) for each age group for comparing the different time periods, this problem can be circumvented. Due to the limitations of adult ageing techniques and the inherent difficulty of linking skeletal morphology to chronological age (Hoppa and Vaupel 2002, 5), broad adult age categories of Young, Middle and Old were employed.

4.2.2. Minimum numbers of individuals (MNI)

In calculating the MNI for each tomb (Appendix B[17]), occasionally the MNI for each adult age category will not add up to the same as the overall total of adults as they are calculated separately, and it was deemed prudent to retain this discrepancy as it can occur either as an over- or under-counting of the 'true' MNI. Over-counting in the different age categories can occur if different elements from the same individual fall either side of the age category borderline (i.e. the auricular surface might suggest a Middle Adult while the dental wear might indicate a Young Adult). However, in an assemblage such as this where element retrieval is not always good, under-counting in the overall MNI can occur. It may be the case that when counting numbers of each element, only one adult is identified but on closer inspection of the demographic identifiers any particular element, both a Middle Adult and Young Adult (or a Male and a Female) could be identified. This sort of double counting can also occur between the different sub-adult categories close to the category divisions, but as sub-adult ageing can be executed more accurately, this is less likely to occur amongst sub-adults.

In Appendix B: Table 1, counts of individuals of indeterminate sex are included in parentheses where it is deemed likely that indeterminate elements may belong with other male or female elements and that these should therefore not be factored in to the overall MNI count. Where indeterminate counts are included without parentheses, these individuals are likely to be represented across a range of elements or represented in the same element as the identified males and females (e.g. there is an overall MNI of 9 adult individuals in a tomb represented by the left mastoid process with 4 female, 1 indeterminate and 4 male, and no other element counts any more than 4 females or 4 males). Although in the tables these discrepancies are retained, in the following presentation of total MNI and for the graphs and statistics, the smaller number (i.e. the more certain minimum number) is used unless dealing with specific age categories.

4.2.3. Age-at-death

Adult age-at-death estimates are often overly ambitious in their attempts to assign a specific number or narrow age range. While this need for an accurate chronological age may be important for forensic studies, which have pushed techniques to be more specific, as it is necessary for the accurate identification of individuals, it is often not necessary to have such a degree of specificity for archaeological questions. The standard techniques for ageing adult skeletons rely on the degeneration of certain joint surfaces, giving a biological age which can vary depending on environmental and genetic factors (Garvin *et al.* 2012). Rather than attempting to estimate the chronological age from the biological age, broad age categories were assigned to the phases of degeneration, dividing adults into Young, Middle and Old. These fit the age ranges of 18–30 years for Young Adults, 31–45 years for Middle Adults, and >45 years for Old Adults, but these ageing techniques become less reliable with increased age and the confidence intervals for the mean age of each phase become increasingly wide for the older categories.

Using the Suchey-Brooks pubic symphysis method, Phases 1 and 2 were assigned Young Adult, Phases 3 and 4 as Middle Adult and Phases 5 and 6 as Old Adult. Using the Lovejoy *et al.* (Lovejoy, Meindl, Pryzbeck, *et al.* 1985) auricular surface method, Phases 1–2 were named Young Adult, Phases 3–5 as Middle Adult and Phases 6–8 as Old Adult. Tooth wear was also widely used for estimating age at death. However, the established techniques focus either on the molars or require relatively complete dentition to be present (Miles 1963; Lovejoy 1985; Brothwell 1989). Tooth wear was recorded using the Smith (1984) method and cross referencing these wear stages with the aforementioned Miles, Lovejoy and Brothwell ageing systems. Smith wear stage 1 was assigned as Child/Adolescent (with dental development providing more detailed sub-adult ages), stages 2–4 as Young Adult, 5–6 as Middle Adult and 7–8 as Old Adult.

Sub-adult (referring to all pre-adult age categories) ageing can be estimated more accurately as it is based on development, which proceeds at a more predictable rate than degeneration, though is still variable depending on environmental and genetic factors. Though closer chronological ages can be estimated from epiphyseal fusion and tooth formation and eruption, sub-adults are also recorded by age categories of neonate (at/around birth), infant (c. >0 to 3 years), child (c. >3 to 12 years), and adolescent (c. >12 to 20 years). The methods for estimating age from epiphyseal fusion were collated and summarised by Schaefer *et al.* (2009) and

[17] Appendix B can be accessed at https://doi.org/10.30861/9781407360355-AppendixB

the Schour-Massler (1941) technique was used for ageing from the development of teeth.

4.2.4. Sex

Biological sex, as defined by Walker and Cook (1998) as entirely distinct from gender (an aspect of social identity), was estimated using a variety of standard techniques using the morphological traits of the skull and os coxae (pelvis), as illustrated and described by Buikstra and Ubelaker (1994) and in *The Human Bone Manual* (White and Folkens 2005). Growth changes during adolescence result in distinctive differences in the female and male os coxae, as the female pelvic outlet widens for the purposes of birthing, while the male pelvic growth generally follows a trajectory to meet the demands of locomotion (Buikstra and Ubelaker 1994, 16; White and Folkens 2005, 246, 394).

The Phenice (1969) method for sexing from the pubic symphysis uses the presence or absence of the ventral arc, subpubic concavity and inferior ramus ridge. These refer to the posterior-inferior aspect of the pubic bone and ischio-pubic ramus. The greater sciatic notch is the other pelvic feature scored systematically (Buikstra and Ubelaker 1994; White and Folkens 2005). The scoring of the greater sciatic notch follows the illustrations by Walker in Buikstra and Ubelaker (1994, 18) on a five-point scale as Female (1), Female? (2), Indeterminate (3), Male? (4), and Male (5), with females having a much wider angle than males. When multiple features score differently an average was generally taken but following the recommendations of the Phenice method, if a feature does not obviously sex the specimen, it can be discarded as a criterion. If there is ambiguity in one or two of the criteria (most common for the medial aspect of the ischiopubic ramus, and least common for the ventral arc) usually the remaining criteria were clearer in attributing a sex category (White and Folkens 2005). There were also the more subjective features of the male and female os coxae that these scores could be checked against, such as the expectation that female pelvic bones are smaller and less robust and have longer pubic portions than males (to allow for the wider pelvic outlet/birth canal).

For the skull the morphology of the occipital protuberance, nuchal crest, mastoid prominence (accounting for volume, projection and height/length), mastoid breadth, supramastoid crest, supraorbital margin and glabella (Nemeskéri and Acsádi 1970; Buikstra and Ubelaker 1994; White and Folkens 2005). These morphological traits of the skull are scored on a five-point scale as Female (1), Female? (2), Indeterminate (3), Male? (4), and Male (5), with a score of 1 being a typical female morphology and a score of 5 being a typical male shape. Generally, these features consist of the female features being smaller and more gracile, while the male features are more robust and protruding. The five-point scoring of these features used the illustrations by Walker in Buikstra and Ubelaker (1994, 20), alongside the accompanying descriptions. Mastoid prominence and width are recorded as separate categories in an attempt to encompass the different dimensions of the mastoid, which Petaros *et al.* (2015, 5) point out are not captured by the two-dimensional images in Buikstra and Ubelaker (1994). The supramastoid crest, as described by Bass (1995, 86), was an additional criterion added to the sex estimation analysis. For the mandible, the mental eminence was scored on the five-point scale following the illustrations and description in Buikstra and Ubelaker (1994, 20), from the minimal expression in females (1) to the massive protrusion occupying most of the anterior part of the mandible in males (5). Ramus breadth, ramus flexure, body depth and gonial flare were also scored on this five-point scale though they are not described in this way in any standards but rather based on several studies which have investigated their sexual dimorphism. Ramus breadth and body depth of the mandible were much wider (or deeper) in males than in females (White and Folkens 2005, 386; Abu-Taleb and El Beshlawy 2015; Sairam *et al.* 2016). Ramus flexure is the distinct angulation of the posterior border of the mandibular ramus at the level of the occlusal surface of the molars in males, while this border of the ramus in females was straight (Loth and Henneberg 1996; Kemkes-Grottenthaler *et al.* 2002). Gonial flare or eversion is found in male mandibles with the outward turn of the gonial angle, while for females this tends to be straight or even in-turning (Meindl *et al.* 1985; St Hoyme and İşcan 1989, 74; Kemkes-Grottenthaler *et al.* 2002; White and Folkens 2005, 386).

4.3. Results

4.3.1. Minimum numbers of individuals (MNI)

In the 109 tombs studied, there was an MNI of 537: 347 adults (Old: 17, Middle: 65, Young: 131, Unaged: 134), 43 adolescents, 86 children, 43 infants and 18 neonates (Appendix B Table 4, with Tables 1–3 demonstrating the breakdown for each unit of how the final MNI was calculated). Within the adults, 134 individuals fall into this 'unaged' adult category as they can be identified as adult but there are no further ageing criteria available. The MNI in any individual tomb ranged from 1 to 54, with 1 individual in many of the North Cemetery Hellenistic graves (KMF/78, KS2:62) to 54 in the Late Antique Fortetsa Fork osteotheke (KFF/74 Tomb 1, Unit 4, *KS2*:59) with the second largest MNI of 42 coming from the Roman built tomb at the Sanatorium Basilica (KSM/60 Tomb 1a, Unit 94, *KS2*:74).

The Hellenistic assemblage consisted of an MNI of 82 from 61 graves. If calculated within the individual adult age categories the MNI was 85, and this number was used for calculating the percentage that each age category contributes to the total MNI (Figure 4.2 and Appendix B: Table 5). 48 of the Hellenistic graves contained a single individual, while 7 were double burials, 5 graves contained 3 individuals and 1 had 5 individuals (3 adults, 1 child and 1 neonate). There are substantially more female individuals identified than males (see results section 4.3.3 and Figure 4.8) and relatively few sub-adults (see results section 4.3.2 and Figure 4.2). There were only three sub-adult individual burials: KMF/78 Tomb 99 (Unit 23), KMF/78 Tomb 20 (Unit 34), and KMF/78 Tomb 215 (Unit 51). These were all older adolescents and likely to have been considered socially as adults, even if not yet biologically mature. All other sub-adults were interred with adults.

For the Roman period there were 29 tombs and a total MNI (not counting all adult age categories separately) of 231 (Appendix B: Table 6). The MNI for each individual age category is presented in Figure 4.3, which added up to a total MNI of 238. The numbers of individuals in Roman tombs ranged from 1 to 42, with a mean MNI of 8. This would be expected from the diverse range of tomb forms, with individual burials in the tile graves to large numbers of burials in the chamber and built tombs. In some tombs there are fewer burials than might be expected considering the scale of the tomb, such as KMF/78 Tomb 156 (Unit 72), a peribolos built tomb, with an MNI of only 2 and MK/68 Tomb 5 (Unit 2), a rock-cut chamber tomb, with an MNI of 1. The small number of elements retained from both of these tombs indicate poor survival or retrieval rates from these tombs making it possible that the MNI underestimates the original number of individuals interred in the tombs, particularly in the case of MK/68 Tomb 5 where preservation appears to have been very poor, though it was chosen to be included in the study due to the survival of a mandible with teeth. Alternative explanations for KMF/78 Tomb 156 include that the young adult and c.7-year-old child merited an important burial or that the tomb went out of use before further individuals could be interred.

There were 19 tombs studied from the Late Antique period with an overall MNI (not separating the adult age categories) of 223. The MNI for each tomb is presented in Appendix B: Table 7. The MNI for each age category is presented in Figure 4.4, which add up to an MNI of 227. There was one stone-lined tomb studied which was a single inhumation (KOP/79, Unit 108). The other Late Antique tombs, which were all some form of built or stone-lined tomb, varied in MNI from 2 to 54 with an average of 12. Most of these are osteothekai (ossuaries) and are interpreted as secondary burials, but in some cases it seems they also contained primary burials. All tombs with an MNI greater than 3 contained both adults and sub-adults. Only 3 of the tombs studied from this time period did not contain any evidence of sub-adult burials all of which had an MNI of either 2 or 3. This demonstrates that all age groups are represented in the burial record. KMF/78 Tomb 223 (Unit 81) has a particularly interesting demographic composition with 2 adults (both Middle Adult, one female and the other of unknown sex), and 15 sub-adults (4 adolescents, 9 children, 1 infant and 1 neonate).

4.3.2. Age-at-death

Figure 4.1 shows the total MNI counts for each age category by time period, while Figures 4.2–4 demonstrate the proportions (i.e. each age category as a percentage of the total MNI for each time period), making the different time periods more directly comparable. All age groups are represented in all time periods, other than no neonates in the Hellenistic period. The Young Adult age category has the largest number of individuals for every time period. This suggests that life expectancy was not very high in any of these periods, though there may be a degree of under-ageing inherent in certain age estimation techniques.

The majority of adult ageing was done from dental wear, with 697 adult individuals or individual loose teeth aged in this way, compared to just 18 adults that were aged from either the auricular surface or pubic symphysis of the pelvis. There is some indication that the methods for the pelvis tend to produce older ages-at-death than the dental method, with the pelvis methods (n=18) placing 22.2% of adults in the Young category, 66.7% in the Middle category and 11.1% in the Old category, while the dental method (n=697) placed 73.5% of adults in the Young category, 22.4% in the Middle category and 4.2% in the Old category. However, the number of adults ageable from pelvic methods was extremely small and there were very few incidences were both pelvis and dental methods could be employed on the same individual. Those incidences that do exist are listed in Table 4.1 and the two methods frequently produce the same age category, and when they do not, it is often because the individual appears to be close to the division between Young and Middle adult. However, invariably when there was a difference, the dental method aged individuals as younger than the pelvis methods. Dental wear as an ageing technique can be highly variable between and within populations due to differences in the coarseness of diet (food types, preparation, and grit inclusions), non-masticatory uses of the teeth (including the use of the teeth as tools and bruxism), prevalence of dental diseases (particularly caries), patterns of malocclusion, and eruption times of teeth (Kieser *et al.* 1983; Walker *et al.* 1991; Hillson 2005; Clement and Hillson 2012).

The most noticeable difference between the time periods is that there are relatively few sub-adults in the Hellenistic period, representing only 14% of all individuals, compared to 37% in the Roman sample and 39% in the Late Antique assemblage (Table 4.2). Of the 61 Hellenistic graves, 48 were single-individual burials, but there were no sub-adult individual burials, other than the aforementioned three adolescent burials, and these individuals were likely to have been considered as adults by society. The suggestion of a bias in age category of those being buried in the North Cemetery for the Hellenistic assemblage makes it harder to compare to the other time periods, but the adult death profiles can still be compared (Table 4.3; Figures 4.5–7).

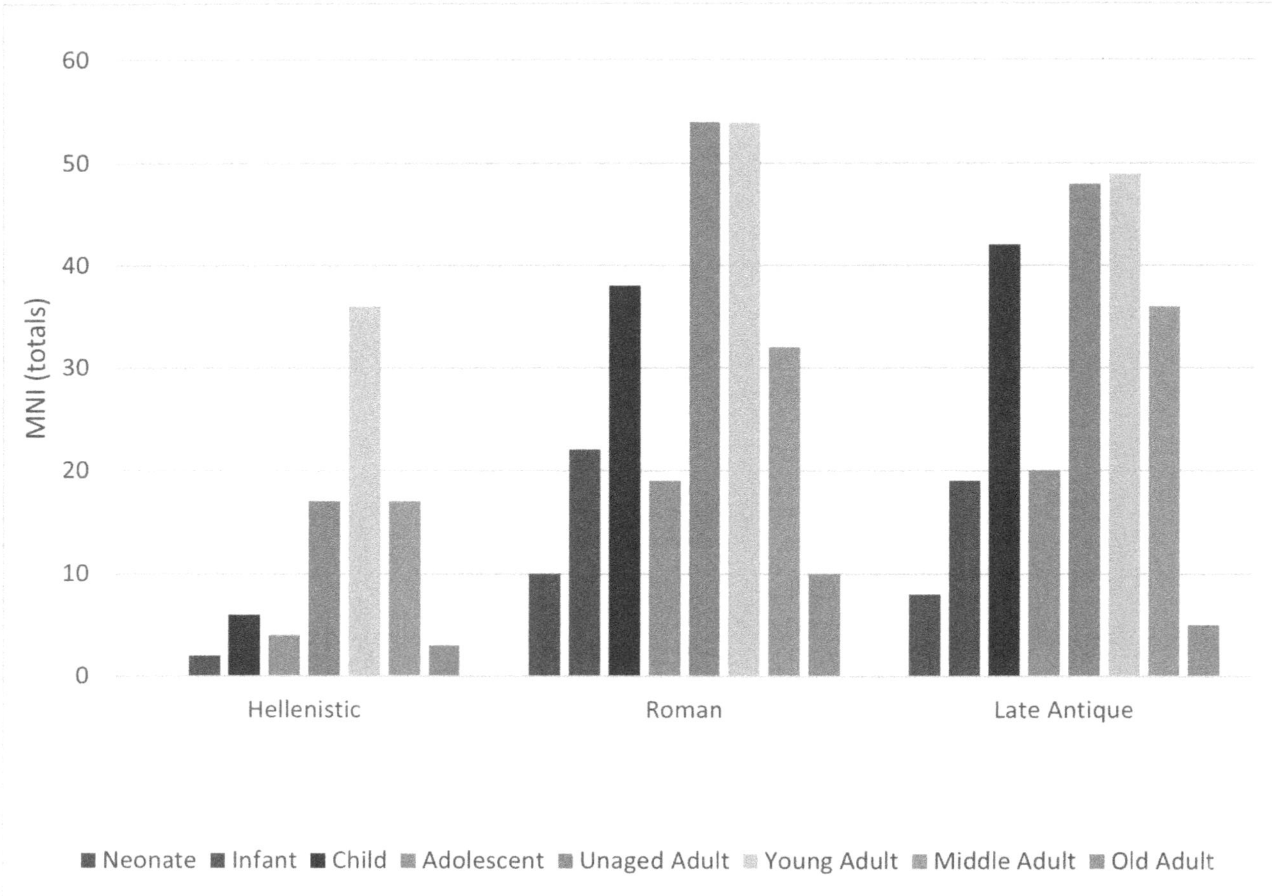

Figure 4.1. Bar chart demonstrating total MNI counts for each age category in each time period.

Table 4.1. List of individuals with multiple ageing criteria, using both dental wear and the degenerative traits of the pelvis (auricular surface and/or pubic symphysis), and the age categories each method placed them in: YA (Young Adult), MA (Middle Adult), and OA (Old Adult).

Unit	Individual	Pelvis age category	Dental age category
4	609	MA	MA
7	2	MA	YA/MA
38	1	YA	YA
41	3	OA	OA
48	1	MA	YA/MA
67	1	MA	YA
73	1	MA	YA
93	1	MA	YA
105	1	MA	YA
105	2	MA	MA
105	3	MA	MA
105	4	YA	YA
108	1	YA	YA

The Roman and Late Antique assemblages are more directly comparable as they appear to be more representative of a complete cross-section of the population (as it tends to be seen in the burial record), and were recorded in the same fashion, as most were large, commingled burials with an MNI of up to 54 individuals. The Roman period has the largest proportion of adults making it to Old adulthood with 4.2% compared to 2.2% in the Late Antique, or even the

Table 4.2. Percentage of adults and sub-adults that compose the total MNI for each time period. For adults this includes the 'true' MNI (Adults, any age), which is the count of adult elements regardless of age or sex, and the 'maximum' MNI (Adults, combined total), which is the combined total for the counts for each adult age category (old, middle, young and unaged). The sub-adult (all) category represents the combined sub-adult age categories (adolescent, child, infant and neonate).

Time Period	Adults (any age)	Adults (combined total)	Sub-adult (all)
Hellenistic	85.4%	85.9%	14.1%
Roman	61.9%	63.0%	37.0%
Late Antique	60.1%	60.8%	39.2%

Table 4.3. Percentages in each age category of the overall MNI for each time period.

Time Period	Neonate	Infant	Child	Adoles.	Unaged Adult	Young Adult	Middle Adult	Old Adult
Hellenistic	0.0%	2.4%	7.1%	4.7%	20.0%	42.4%	20.0%	3.5%
Roman	4.2%	8.8%	16.0%	8.0%	22.7%	22.7%	13.4%	4.2%
Late Antique	3.5%	8.4%	18.5%	8.8%	21.1%	21.6%	15.9%	2.2%

Table 4.4. Percentages of each sub-adult age category out of the total number of sub-adults (n).

	n	Neonate %	Infant %	Child %	Adolescent %
Hellenistic	12	0	16.7	50	33.3
Roman	88	11.4	23.9	43.2	21.6
Late Antique	89	9	21.3	47.2	22.5

3.5% of the Hellenistic, which is meaningful considering the general inflation of the Hellenistic adult proportions. However, the Late Antique period has a larger proportion of individuals making it beyond Young adulthood, with a slightly larger (though negligible) proportion in the Middle and Old categories combined, at 18.1% compared to 17.6% in the Late Antique period. There are slightly more individuals reaching adulthood in the Roman period (61.9%) compared to the Late Antique period (60.1%) but the difference is again negligible and the age-at-death profiles for these two time periods are very similar.

Tables 4.3–4 and Figure 4.2 demonstrate that, for all three time periods, the child category is the best represented sub-adult group and the neonate category is the least well represented in every time period. The Hellenistic sub-adult sample is small (n=12) and therefore the numbers are not likely to be very meaningful as representative of the population. There are much larger proportions of adolescents (33.3% of sub-adults) and children (50%) in the Hellenistic than the equivalents for the Roman (Adolescent: 21.6%, Child: 43.2%) or Late Antique (Adolescent: 22.5%, Child: 47.2%) periods. The Hellenistic sample only had 16.7% of sub-adults in the infant category and no neonates, which suggests alternative burial treatment was particularly common amongst the youngest members of society, though excavation and preservation biases may also play a role in the absence of these individuals. Nevertheless, the difference between the sub-adult age categories for all three time periods was not statistically

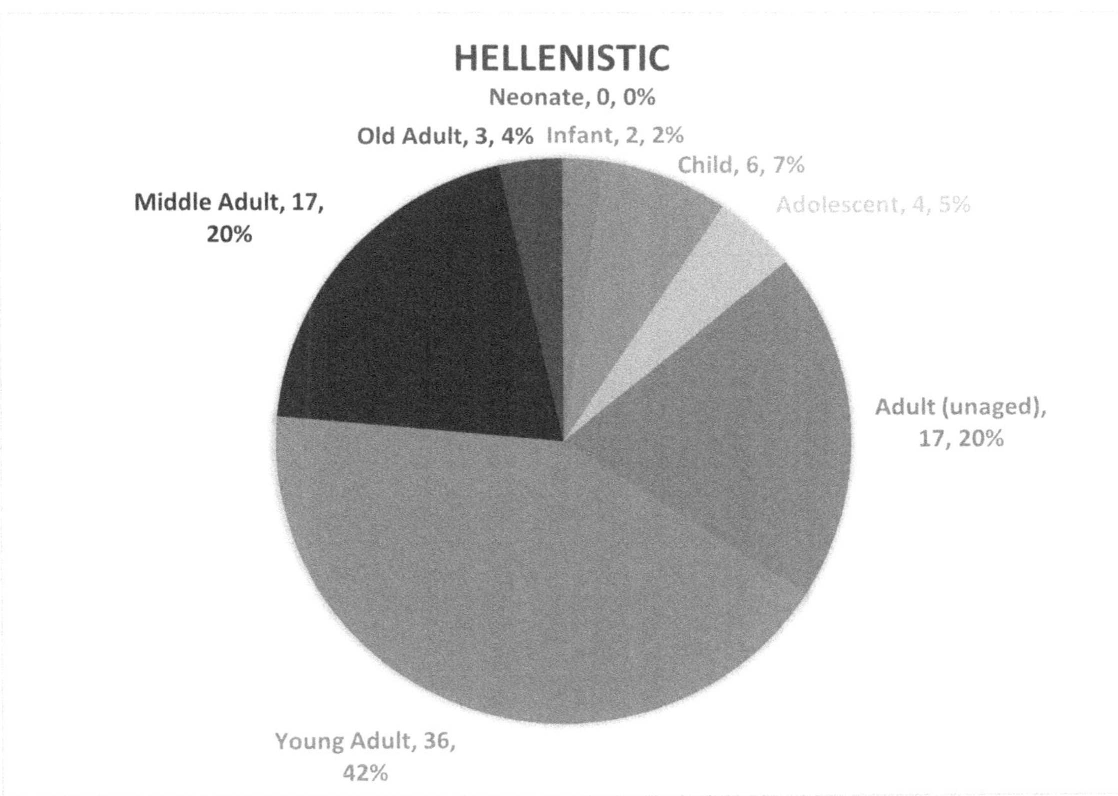

Figure 4.2. Pie chart showing MNI and proportions of individuals for each age category for the Hellenistic period.

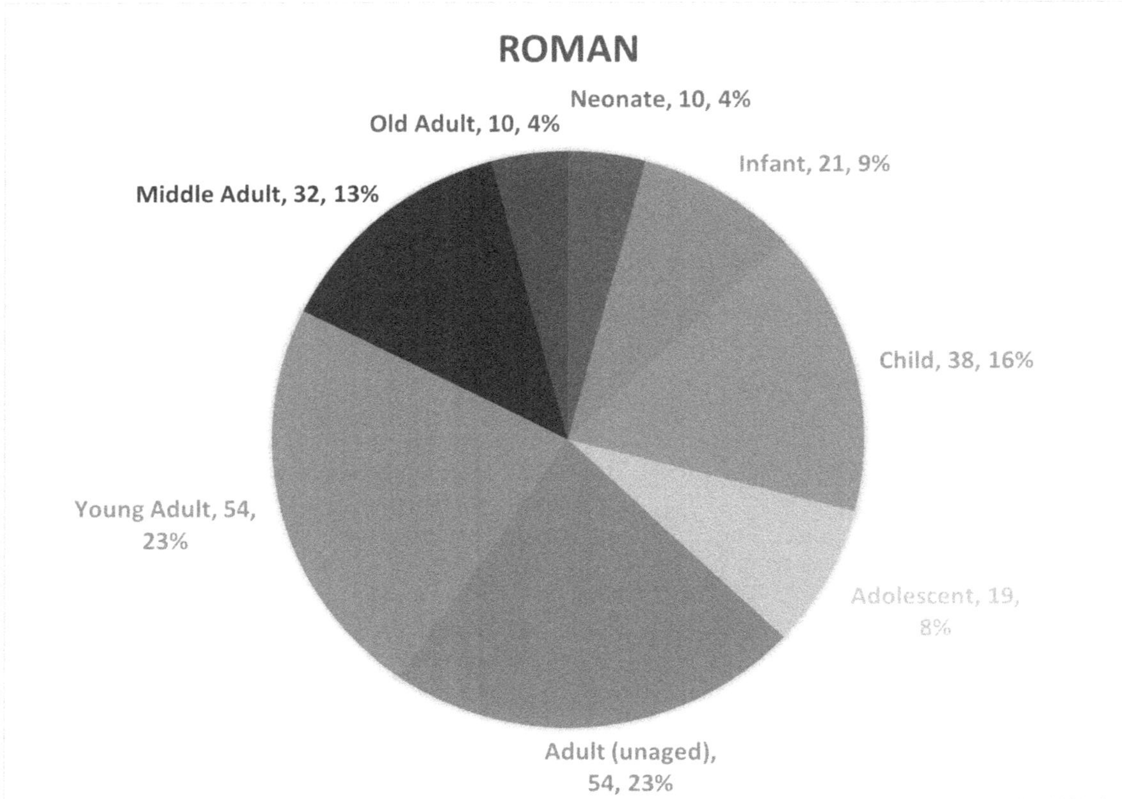

Figure 4.3. Pie chart showing MNI and proportions of individuals for each age category for the Roman period.

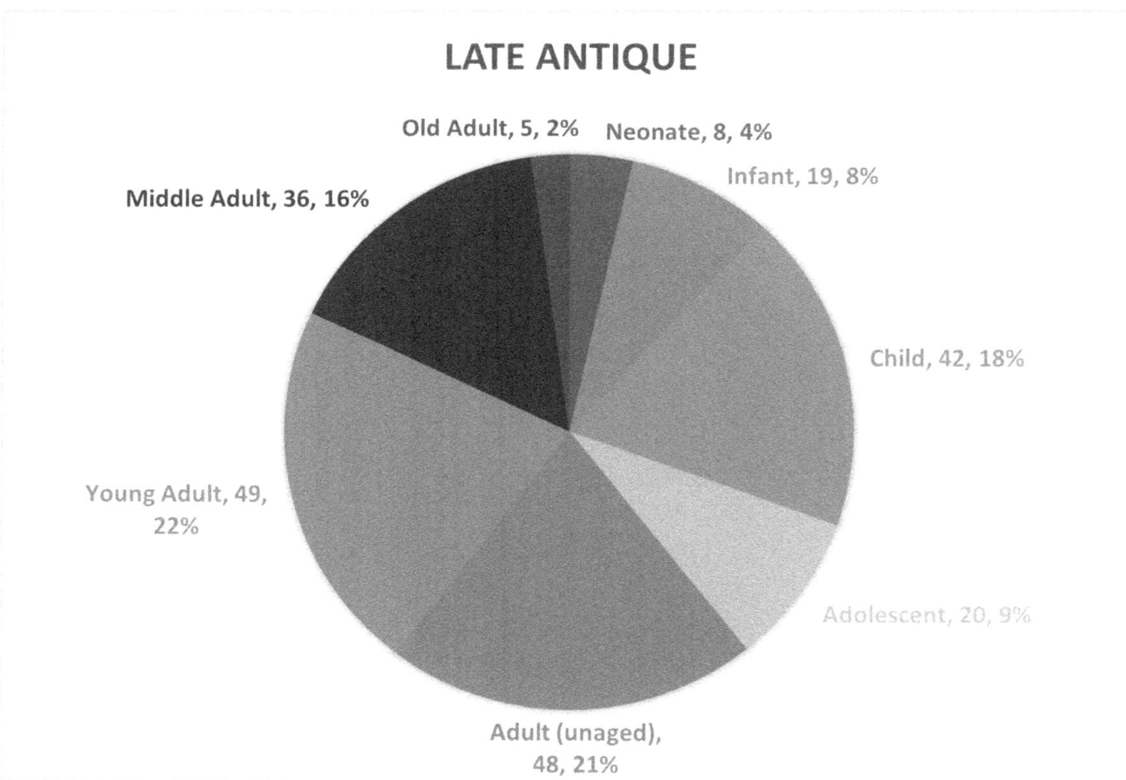

Figure 4.4. Pie chart showing MNI and proportions of individuals for each age category for the Late Antique period.

significant using a chi-square test (X^2=2.65, p=0.85). Just as the Roman and Late Antique adult samples were alike, the distribution amongst the sub-adult categories is also similar for the Roman and Late Antique periods. The older subadult categories have slightly larger proportions of individuals in the Late Antique period, with 69.7% of subadults in the adolescent and child categories combined, compared to 64.8% for the combined categories in the Roman period. Meanwhile, the infant and neonate groups have larger proportions in the Roman period with 35.3% for the combined categories, compared to 30.3% for the Late Antique infants and neonates combined. However, the difference between the older and younger sub-adult groupings for the Roman and Late Antique assemblages was not statistically significant using a chi-square test (X^2=0.48, p=0.49).

Figures 4.5–7 depict the proportions of adults in each of the Young, Middle and Old adult age categories for each time period. This avoids the skew that the different numbers of subadults for each time period can introduce into the comparison of the proportions of adults in each age group. This closer inspection of the adult categories (excluding the unaged adults) indicates that adult life expectancy is in fact lowest in the Hellenistic period, with relatively few individuals surviving into Middle or Old adulthood, compared to either the Roman or Late Antique time periods. All three time periods have the same pattern of the Young Adult category being the best represented, followed by Middle Adult, and lastly the Old Adult group, demonstrating life expectancy was not very high in any period. However, while the distribution of individuals is quite similar for the Roman and Late Antique periods, the Hellenistic assemblage is markedly different with a greater proportion of the population dying in early adulthood.

4.3.3. Sex

For the discussion of sexed individuals, the numbers refer to those identified in the MNI counts as opposed to isolated elements. The Hellenistic sample had 31 females (44.3%), 16 males (22.9%), and 23 of unknown sex (32.9%), giving a total of 67% of individuals being assigned a sex category (Figure 4.8). The Roman assemblage had 36 females (25.0%), 39 males (27.1%), and 69 of unknown sex (47.9%), meaning 52% of individuals were sexed (Figure 4.9). The Late Antique group had 36 females (27.1%), 41 males (30.8%), and 56 of unknown sex (42.1%), giving a result of 58% of individuals being sexed (Figure 4.10).

The sex distribution profiles for the Roman and Late Antique periods are very similar, with close to an equal distribution between the sexes, and marginally more males in each case. However, the Hellenistic distribution is markedly skewed, with two thirds of adults (of identified sex) being female, and the Hellenistic period has the highest proportion of adults of identifiable sex, with 67%. This, again, may indicate that the Hellenistic North Cemetery assemblage is not fully representative of the entire population and that a particular demographic or social sub-set of society was being buried in this cemetery. It is also possible that significant numbers of young adult males died away from the city, as soldiers, mercenaries,

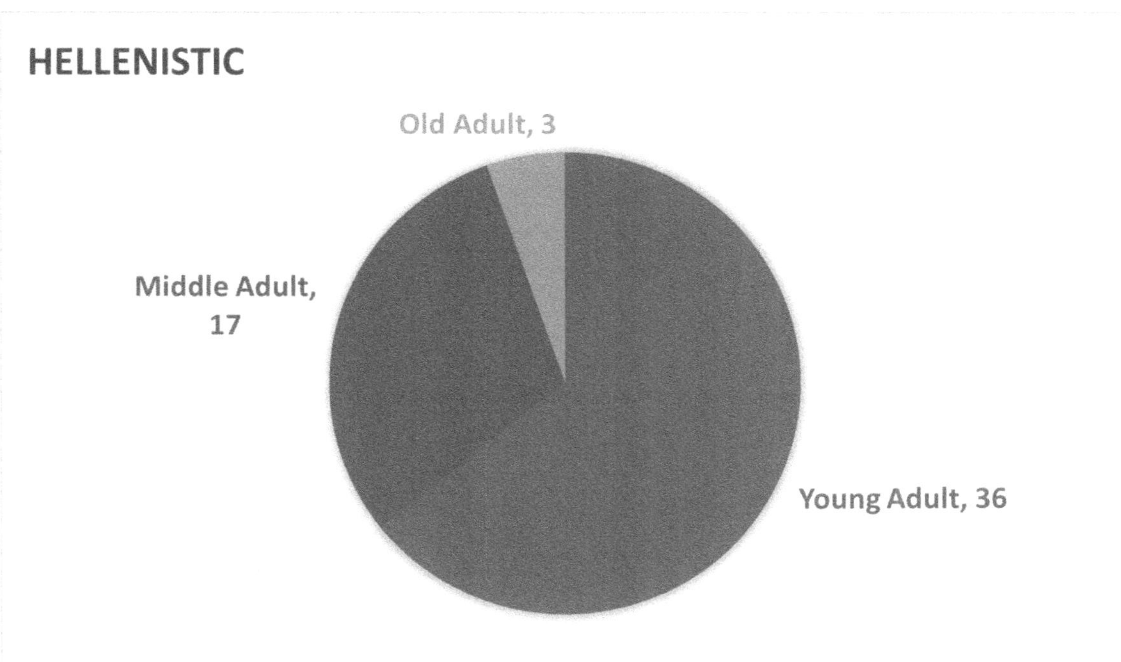

Figure 4.5. Proportions of each age category that compose the adult MNI in the Hellenistic period.

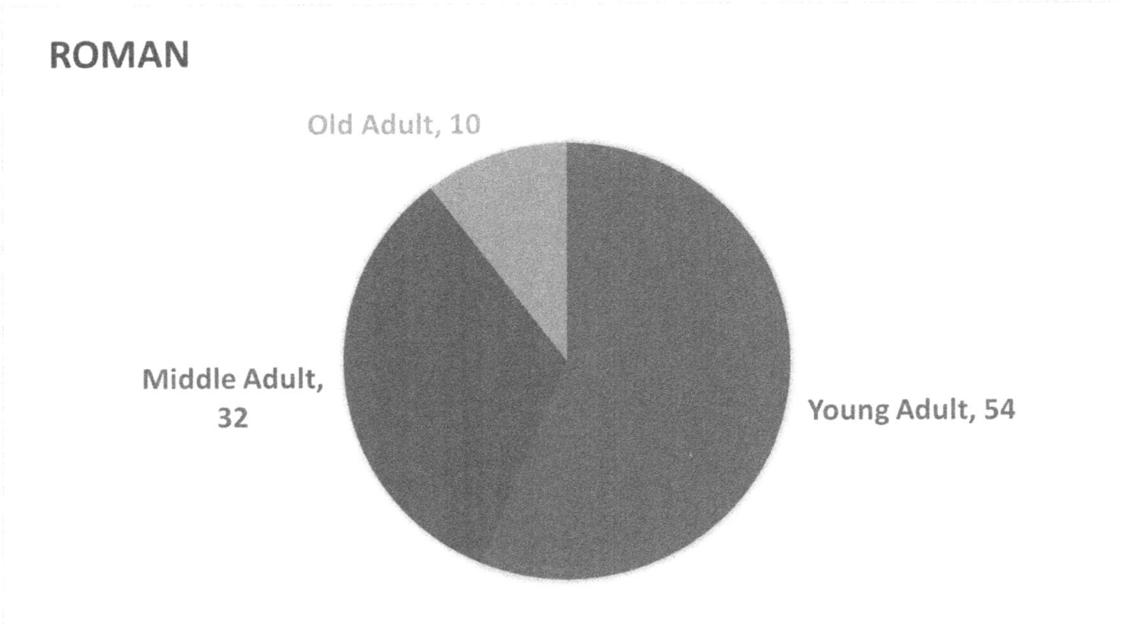

Figure 4.6. Proportions of each age category that compose the adult MNI in the Roman period.

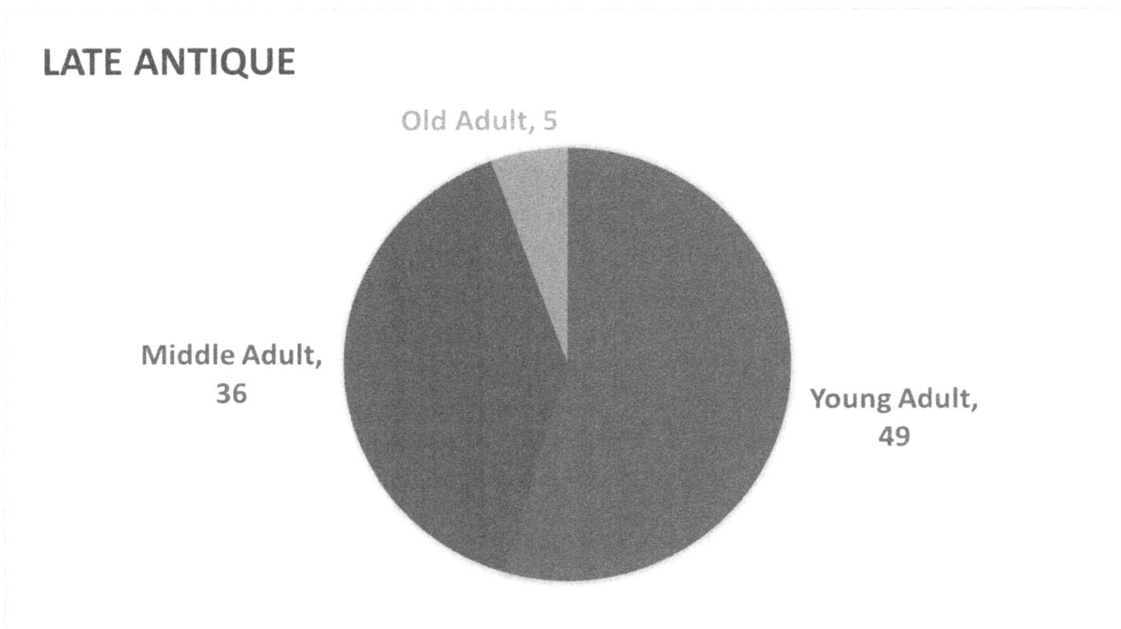

Figure 4.7. Proportions of each age category that compose the adult MNI in the Late Antique period.

merchants, emissaries, or ambassadors. This possibility is further discussed in Section 4.4.4.

4.4. Discussion

4.4.1. Population size and representativeness of the assemblage

It is important to consider the size of the assemblage and its social and demographic composition to understand the representativeness of the assemblage in relation to the once-buried population (i.e. the complete death assemblage). Making some gross assumptions of the size of the settlement, the population density, the length of a generation, and the proportion of adults in the population, Whitelaw (Whitelaw *et al.* 2017; 2018) has estimated population sizes based on the urban survey (KULP) evidence to set the size of this skeletal sample in perspective. The assumptions are that a generation lasts 25 years, adults make up 50% of the population, and that there was a middling population density of 100–150/ha. The extent of the settlement is estimated from the surface sherd distributions as 97–118.7 ha. for the Hellenistic period (323–67 BC), 89 ha. for the Early Roman period (67 BC- AD 100), 69.8 ha. for the Middle Roman period (2nd-3rd centuries AD), 49.7 ha. for the Late Roman period (4th-5th centuries AD), and 41.3 ha. for the Late Antique period (6th-7th centuries AD). As outlined in Table 4.5, this would mean a population density at any one time of 9705–17807 for the Hellenistic, 8896–13345 for the Early Roman period, 6975–10463 for the Middle Roman period, 4131–6197 for the Late Roman period, and 4968–74. The periods would span different numbers of generations with approximately 10 for the Hellenistic, 6.5 for the Early Roman, 8 for the Middle Roman, 8 for the Late Roman, and 8 for the Late Antique. Taking the mean population at any one time for each period and the assumption that adults are 50% of the population, the accumulated population across each phase would therefore be approximately 68780 for the Hellenistic period, 36142 for the Early Roman period, 34876 for the Middle Roman period, 24840 for the Late Roman period, and 20656 for the Late Antique period.

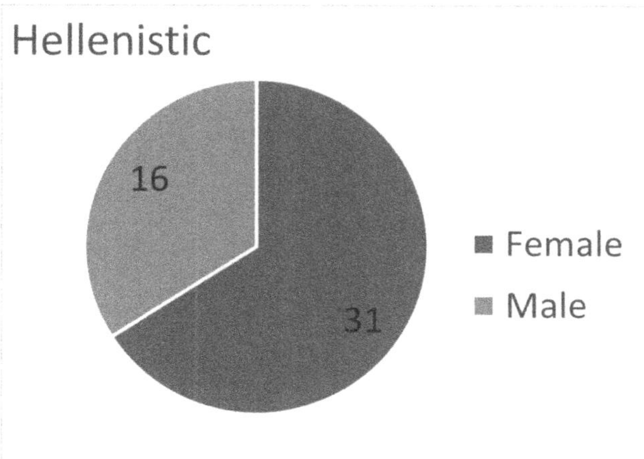

Figure 4.8. Proportions of females and males that compose the determinate-sex MNI in the Hellenistic period.

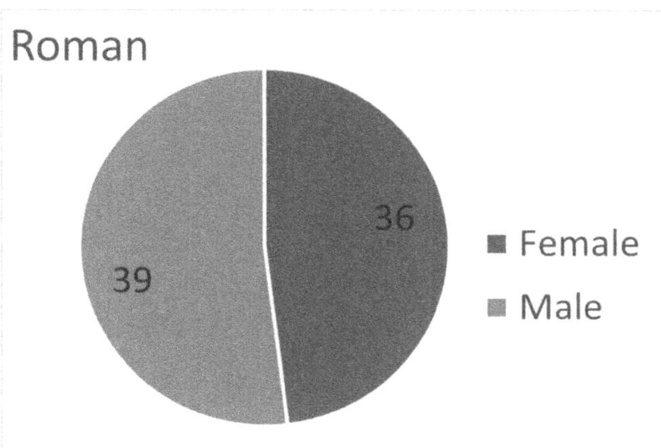

Figure 4.9. Proportions of females and males that compose the determinate-sex MNI in the Roman period.

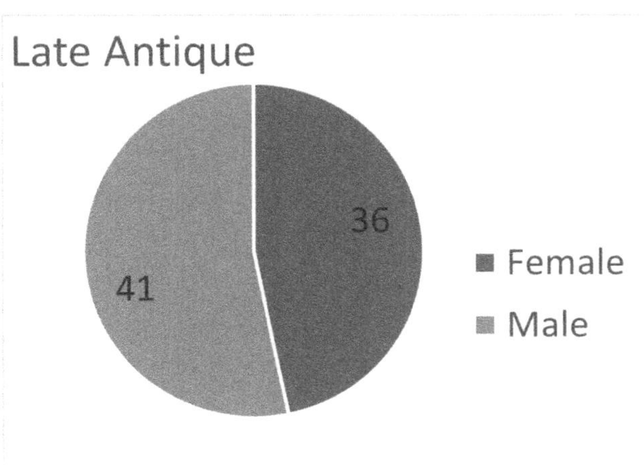

Figure 4.10. Proportions of females and males that compose the determinate-sex MNI in the Late Antique period.

This demonstrates the skeletal assemblage presented in this study is extremely small in comparison with the once-living (or once-buried) population, as almost inevitably are all archaeological skeletal assemblages for large urban sites. Therefore, it cannot be assumed that the assemblage is truly representative of the population. The investigation of the burial context (location, tomb form, burial goods) can give some indication of whether different social groups are present, and the presence of all age groups and both sexes would be expected to have a normal demographic distribution within the population. However, it is impossible to ascertain whether all sub-groups (social and demographic) of a population are represented, or whether the representation is proportionate. This is an inherent limitation of most archaeological skeletal assemblages (and other materials) and must simply be kept in mind for the interpretation of the results of any osteological analysis. The study of a sizeable sample has been achieved and, despite the aforementioned limitations, it can be taken as informative on aspects of past demography, society, and individual human lifeways.

4.4.2. Representation of society

The likelihood of an assemblage being representative of a cross-section of society in terms of social status can be assessed through the observation of how and where people were buried, the tomb form, burial goods, and a comparison of these factors with other sites in Crete. For the Hellenistic period there are only simple rock-cut pit and tile graves present in the sample and grave goods tend to be simple. Of all the Hellenistic graves known from Knossos, the only other tomb form attested was the cist grave type, of which there were examples mentioned, though not studied in detail, from the Fortetsa cemetery (Brock 1957), and one of possible Hellenistic date from north of the hospital site (*KS2*:44). There are a very small number of more elaborate grave goods from some of the KMF/78 tombs, including the gold earrings from Tomb 143 (Unit 31), a silver ring in Tomb 155 (Unit 37), a bronze pin from Tomb 37 (Unit 11) and the gold and silver coins from a number of tombs (T.70 [Unit20], T.143 [Unit 31],

Table 4.5. After Whitelaw *et al.* 2018 Figure 19, site size and population estimates for Knossos with 100–150/ha. being the most likely estimates in these time periods.

Time period	Extent	Area (ha.)	50/ha.	100/ha.	150/ha.	200/ha.
Hellenistic	Min.	97	4852	9705	14557	19410
Hellenistic	Max.	118.7	5936	11871	17807	23743
Early Roman		89	4448	8896	13345	17793
Middle Roman		69.8	3488	6975	10463	13950
Late Roman		49.7	2484	4968	7452	9935
Late Antique		41.3	2066	4131	6197	8262

Table 4.6. Population sizes at any one time and the accumulated total for each time period, calculated from Whitelaw *et al.* 2018 Figure 19.

	Population (at any one time)				Generations	Cumulative Total
	Min.	Max.	Mean	50%		
Hellenistic	9705	17807	13756	6878	10	68780
Early Roman	8896	13345	11121	5560.25	6.5	36142
Middle Roman	6975	10463	8719	4359.5	8	34876
Late Roman	4968	7452	6210	3105	8	24840
Late Antique	4131	6197	5164	2582	8	20656

T.150 [Unit 35], T.155 [Unit 37], T.167 [Unit 41], T.178 [Unit 43], T.215 [Unit 51], T.216 [Unit 52]).[18] The slight variation in accompanying grave goods – from none, to one or two unguentaria (the standard burial assemblage from the site), to a slightly larger number and selection of ceramic vessels, to the rarer inclusion of glass vessels, gold, silver and bronze coins, and other precious metal artefacts – may indicate individuals of different social standing. Pit, tile and cist graves are the most commonly attested tomb types throughout Crete in this time period, with a similar array of grave goods (Niniou-Kindeli *et al.* 1988; Pologiorgi 1991; Guyon 2008; Andreadaki-Vlazaki 2009; Sporn 2014). Therefore, it is possible that the upper echelons of society were not being buried in significantly more complex tomb forms. However, there are a small number of more elaborate tombs known from Chania, Aptera and Gortyn (Ioannidou-Karetsou 1974; Markoulaki and Niniou-Kindeli 1982; 2009; Tsigkou 2004;2009; di Vita 2010), including gold wreaths and jewellery like in the rich Hellenistic tombs of mainland Greece (e.g. Vergina: Andronikos 1984; Derveni: Themelis and Touratsoglou 1997; Pellas: Lilimbaki-Akamati and Akamatis 2014; Northern Peloponnese: Dimakis 2016). Some of these monumental Hellenistic tombs on Crete were reused into Roman times (Niniou-Kindeli 2005, 1026; 2009, 148). While it must be the case that there were as yet unexplored cemeteries further from the centre of Knossos, these examples of elaborate tombs at Chania and Gortyn are close to the settlement where they would have potentially been visible as a symbol of status or wealth. Considering the extent and intensity of excavations and survey in the Knossos area, it seems unlikely that any great number of such tombs could have existed. Concurrently, if such tombs existed at Chania and Gortyn, it seems surprising that Knossos, as one of the preeminent centres of Hellenistic Crete, would not have any more elaborate tombs. Without any cist graves (known to have existed at Knossos) or more elaborate tombs (for which there is no evidence at Knossos, but a small number may have existed) represented in the studied skeletal sample, it seems unlikely that a complete cross section of society is present in the Hellenistic assemblage and that the higher status individuals in particular may be missing.

The Roman period had a much wider range of tomb forms at Knossos, with pit, tile and cist graves, sculpted stone sarcophagi, rock-cut chamber tombs and various forms of built tombs or mausolea. There are only two Roman pit graves included in the sample due to the lack of available skeletal material from these tombs and the only cist or stone-lined tombs are from the later Roman period (4th century AD onwards). The bones from six tile graves were studied but as these tombs are generally single or

[18] These are examples of non-pottery grave goods associated with tombs from the studied skeletal assemblage. The full range of Hellenistic grave goods from Knossos is outlined in Chapters 2 and 3 (Sections 2.1.3 and 3.5).

double burials, this still represents a small sample size. The appearance of larger communal tombs, both rock-cut and built, demonstrates new preferences in burial practices around the time that Roman migrants and cultural elements were becoming increasingly evident at Knossos. The range of tomb forms present in this period represents greater differentiation between the societal strata in how they were able to or wished to present themselves and their kin in the burial sphere.

This increase in tomb diversity, size (and number of occupants), and monumentality is matched by other centres across Crete. At Kissamos in West Crete there excavated examples of pit, tile and cist graves, jar burials, rock-cut chamber tombs and various forms of monumental built tombs (Pologiorgi 1991; Niniou 1993; Paterakis 2011; Skordou 2016). The monumental built tomb from Kissamos presented by Skordou (2016), with the vaulted roof and subterranean chamber appears to be the same type as several known examples from Knossos, including the Topana tomb (Unit 104) and KMF Tomb 33 (Unit 68). Various forms of monumental built tombs or mausolea have been excavated at Chania, Aptera, Kissamos, Gortyn, Ierapetra, Elyros, Lasaia, Sougia, Lissos, and Matala. (Vasilakis 2004; Guyon 2008, 112–14; di Vita 2010; Apostolakou 2011; Paterakis 2011; Skordou 2016). Late Hellenistic and Roman rock-cut chamber tombs are also known from Kissamos, Polyrrenhia, Rhokka, Khandanos, Hyrtakina, Elyros, Chania, Aptera, Lappa, Pantomatrion, Allaria, Argyroupoli (Rethymnon), Eleutherna, Falagari and Faneromenis (Phaistos), Matala, Agios Thomas, Rhizenia, Heraklion, Pannona, Arkades, Praisos, and Prinias, while earlier examples of similar tombs are known from Alexandria in Egypt, Cyprus, Rhodes, Kos, Rinea (Cyclades) and Samos (Niniou-Kindeli *et al.* 1988; Hatzi-Vallianou 1995, 1019; Gavrilaki 2004; Niniou-Kindeli 2004, 327; 2009, 148; Guyon 2008, 107–9; Markoulaki 2009; Tzanakaki 2011; Skordou 2020). Over sixty sculpted stone sarcophagi, which were largely imported, are known from a number of sites on Crete, including Gortyn, Chersonesos, Malia, Aria and Ierapetra (Guyon 2008, 117–19; di Vita 2010, 350). Many pit, tile and cist graves have also been uncovered from this time period, including those at Chania, Agios Nikolaos, Gortyn, Axos, Ierapetra, Sfakaki Pangalochori, and Stavromenos (Catling 1984, 67; Davaras 1987; Andreadaki-Vlazaki 1992; Apostolakou 1995; 1997; Papadopoulou 1997; di Vita 2010, 347).[19] With relatively few tile and pit graves in the Knossos skeletal sample, and with these tombs having fewer occupants (and therefore fewer skeletal remains) than the large communal/family tombs, it is clear that this group (or these groups) of society are not well-represented.

There was less diversity in tomb forms in the Late Antique period with all the known tombs from Knossos being some form of masonry-built or stone-lined tomb. There is some variation in size and details, with some tombs being lined with large slabs, others built of smaller blocks or reused *spolia*, and with some having plastered walls, drainage holes, and other slight variations in features. Very few primary burials are known from this period, with the majority of the tombs being osteothekai or ossuaries. This prompts the question of what the primary burial customs were and whether the primary burials were in the same tomb. In the Fortetsa Fork tomb (Unit 4), some stacking of similar skeletal elements was observed during excavation and they do not appear to be designed with pits or niches for the clearing aside of earlier burials as has been observed in the Bronze Age chamber and tholos tombs of Crete (Branigan 1987; Triantaphyllou 2018). There were, however, some cases of articulated or partially articulated individuals in the upper levels of these tombs, demonstrating at least towards the end of their use, primary burials were interred in the osteothekai. At Late Antique Eleutherna and Corinth there are similar cases of tombs being used for large numbers of interments which appear to have been primary burials (Poulou-Papadimitriou *et al.* 2012, 388). The retrieval of small bones, such as carpals and phalanges, from many of the osteothekai at Knossos, supports the presence of at least some primary burials, as these bones are often left behind when the skeletal remains are moved to a secondary burial place.

Tile or *kalyvites* (tiles pitched like a tent) graves, various types of cist or stone-lined tombs and built or rock-cut vaulted tombs (or tombs using a combination of these features) are common throughout Greece in the Late Antique or Early Byzantine period (Poulou-Papadimitriou *et al.* 2012, 379). Like the osteothekai at Knossos, cists and built masonry tombs throughout Greece at this time employ a range of stone types and sizes, including *spolia* (Poulou-Papadimitriou *et al.* 2012, 388; Rife 2012, 175). A cemetery with a variety of stone-lined tombs is known from Kissamos. There is no skeletal report but it appears that these were primary interment graves, and the differences between the different tomb coverings and elements of construction appear to be chronological (Drosinou 1992; Diamantis 2004). There were also a number of inscriptions associated with these graves (Diamantis 1998), only two fragments of which are known from one of the Knossos graves (Tomb 244, Unit 84). Similar cist graves with individual single burials are known from Eleutherna (Stampolidis 2004b, 143), and this is the most common tomb form known from Greece in this time period – for example, they were predominant at Kenchreai (Rife *et al.* 2007), and common at Isthmia though tile and pit graves were also common (Rife 2012). In considering whether it is likely that the osteotheke burials represent a complete cross section of society, it is important to consider the likelihood that other tomb types existed at Knossos based on the comparative examples known from other sites on Crete. It seems likely that there will always be some simple pit graves, which are the most difficult to detect archaeologically, particularly for a time period that would have had few burial accoutrements.

[19] In Guyon's (2008) thesis, he lists over 400 pit graves known from Cretan sites in the Hellenistic and Roman periods (see p.99 for a complete list of sites and references to his catalogue), as well as almost 300 tile graves (p.100), and nearly 200 cist graves (p.102).

4.4.3. Age structure of the assemblage

As discussed in the introduction to this chapter (4.1), it is unrealistic to expect mortality rates and age structure to be reconstructed in any great detail from any skeletal assemblage and it was even more difficult with the fragmentation and commingling of much of the material studied here. It is important to recognise that certain knowledge can never be achieved from palaeodemographic data, even with the largest and best skeletal sample imaginable. The most that can be expected is a general age pattern of death for a past population, and simple methods and models that can achieve this are preferable to complicated life table models (Wood *et al.* 2002). Although even simple models cannot be used on very fragmentary material that is unable to provide ages-at-death for much of the assemblage or identify individuals within commingled material.

The ratio of adults to sub-adults was 100:17 for the Hellenistic period, 100:62 for the Roman period, and 100:66 for the Late Antique period. Expressed differently, this means that sub-adults made up 14.1% of the Hellenistic assemblage, 37.0% of the Roman assemblage and 39.2% of the Late Antique assemblage. Sub-adults are almost always underrepresented in archaeological assemblages due to a combination of different depositional rights for some sub-adults (particularly infants) and poorer preservation for smaller, more fragile bones with a lower mineral component. In a living population, sub-adults tend to make up half the population at any point in time (ratio of 1:1 for adults and sub-adults) (Kamp 2001; Margerison and Knüsel 2002). However, this will not be the same in a death assemblage as it is in the living population. The entire child population is not represented in the death assemblage as, although some children die, particularly with the high infant mortality rates in ancient populations, many children survive to adulthood (and are obviously represented as adults in the archaeological assemblage). It is, therefore, difficult to identify what a typical ratio of adults to sub-adults should be from a 'normal' ancient, attritional death assemblage, though sub-adults representing a little over a third of all individuals has been deemed normal for ancient archaeological assemblages (Fiorin *et al.* 2017). The study of a selection of early and middle Byzantine sites on Crete collectively produced a very similar ratio of adults to sub-adults to the Roman and Late Antique Knossos samples, with 100:64 (i.e. sub-adults are 39.1% of the total number of individuals) (Bourbou 2010, 106). These sites were not large, dense urban centres that are likely to have suffered greatly from population pressures and poor sanitation conditions that come with it, and from the burial types they are likely to be attritional death assemblages, rather than plague, natural disaster or war cemeteries that are likely to have atypical demographic profiles (Margerison and Knüsel 2002).

The lack of sub-adults in the Hellenistic assemblage, as previously mentioned (4.3.2), was likely due to a combination of differential burial practices for sub-adults and preservation and excavation biases. It is known that infant mortality was high in all pre-modern societies and there are no neonates and very few infants in the Hellenistic assemblage, which is likely to be a burial bias in the cemetery. There were no sub-adult individual burials, besides the burials of three adolescent individuals who would have been seen socially as adults, even if they were not biologically fully mature. All other sub-adults were interred with adults. This could indicate that sub-adults were generally buried in a different cemetery and were only present in the North Cemetery graves when interred with an adult. This was also found to be the case at Late Hellenistic-Early Roman Athens, where no infant or younger child burials were found in individual graves, but these remains were found in multiple burials alongside older sub-adults and adults (Lagia 2007, 306). The transition from childhood to adulthood seems to have occurred between the ages of twelve and twenty-one years, from the initiation of puberty to physical maturation (Grubbs and Parkin 2013, 6). This transition for females generally took the form of marriage, which under Roman law was legal from twelve years but was likely more common in the later teenage years on average (Alberici and Harlow 2007, 194). For males, there were rights of initiation, removing them from the female domestic sphere and bringing them into the citizen body, which marked their social role as an adult (Langdon 2007, 182). The age at which this occurred varied from fourteen in some Hellenistic Greek cities, to fifteen or sixteen at Rome, and seventeen or eighteen in Classical Athens (Garland 2013, 208).

However, it is important to consider the possibility that the lack of Hellenistic sub-adults is an excavation bias. Although the area was intensively excavated, there was a great deal of initial clearing of the Medical Faculty site (KMF North Cemetery) by JCB digger and element retrieval was poor for many of these simple pit graves which were presumably more easily missed initially and less well protected by architecture than the later built and stone-lined tombs in the same area. A group of Roman tile graves in the Staphylakis field (*KS2*:171, Monastiriako Kephali) were left unexcavated in 1975 due to the extent of the damage caused by a plough, demonstrating how close to the surface tombs of this date can be (Callaghan, Catling, *et al.* 1981). It is unlikely to be a preservation bias, as particularly child and adolescent bones are almost as likely to survive as adult ones, though it is possible this partially contributes to the issue, particularly in the case of infant and neonate bones (Bello and Andrews 2006). However, it is also common for neonates, infants and young children to be buried separately or to not be given a formal burial (Lagia 2007; Clement *et al.* 2009; Hillson *et al.* 2009; Bourbou and Themelis 2010; Liston and Rotroff 2012; Liston *et al.* 2018).

The child category is the best represented sub-adult category in each time period and neonates were the smallest category in each case. The small numbers of neonates can be attributed to poorer preservation, greater difficulty in recognising and retrieving small elements, as well as possible alternative burial practices and locations for the youngest members of society (Andrews and Bello 2006; Bello and Andrews 2006; Bello *et al.* 2006). The child category (c.3–12 years) is over-represented compared to the other sub-adult categories in each time period. This could be in part due to the inclusion of individuals of weaning age at the lower end of the age range, who would have been particularly vulnerable to infectious diseases. It may also be exaggerated by preservation bias against the more delicate infant remains, and by the underrepresentation of adolescents in a fragmentary assemblage due to ageing criteria. Adolescents at the upper end of the age range may be assigned as unaged adults if epiphyses have fused, which can occur early on in adolescence for some bones and for some individuals (Schaefer *et al.* 2009). If metric ageing methods were not possible, some adolescents at the younger end of the adolescent scale may also have been assigned to the child category.

The differences in proportions of individuals in each of the sub-adult categories for each time period was not statistically significant. However, in comparing the Roman and Late Antique distributions of individuals across these categories, the Late Antique older sub-adults (adolescents and children combined) had a slightly larger proportion of individuals than the Roman older sub-adults, while the combined infant and neonate groups had larger proportions in the Roman period compared to the Late Antique. A high infant mortality rate is expected in all ancient populations due to the difficulties of childbirth as well as environmental impacts. Death in later childhood and adolescence is more likely to be caused by unsanitary conditions and outbreaks of disease. This would be expected of the Hellenistic period when population pressure on the urban environment and on resources was likely to have been at its greatest as not only was the urban population at its largest since the Neopalatial period, but it was also largely a subsistence economy, dependent on local resources rather than imports. Although the Hellenistic results do support this theory, the sample size is too small for this to be taken as a reliable result. The Late Antique adolescent and child proportion of sub-adult deaths was greater than that of the Roman period, with the Roman period being better represented in the infant and neonate categories. The difference between the age categories was negligible and not statistically significant; therefore, it may be a case that conditions affecting sub-adult deaths were not substantially different between the Roman and Late Antique periods.

The most meaningful comparison of the age structure of the assemblage across the three time periods lies within the adult categories. The Hellenistic assemblage has a substantially larger proportion of individuals in the Young Adult category, with relatively few individuals surviving into Middle or Old adulthood (36% of adults). With 44% of Roman adults and 45% of Late Antique adults surviving beyond Young adulthood, this demonstrates a higher adult life expectancy in these times. This suggests that the increased prosperity and investment in public building works in the Roman period and the continued prosperity in the Late Antique period with some evidence for maintenance of infrastructure may have increased life expectancy and thus improved quality of life. This could have been by reducing conditions favourable to the proliferation of infectious diseases with improved sanitation conditions, or an improved diet. It is, however, surprising that there would not be a greater difference between the Roman and Late Antique assemblages' age-at-death structure. If there was a substantial improvement in sanitation conditions in the Roman city, then this may account for why the transition from the Roman to Late Antique periods did not affect death rates or life expectancy in the population as noticeably. Any improvement in sanitation could have been due to better infrastructure (aqueduct, baths, drains, sewers) or simply due to the decrease in population. While studies have indicated that Roman knowledge of and infrastructure relating to hygiene spread throughout the Empire (Hobson 2009; Yegül 2010; Jansen *et al.* 2011; Koloski-Ostrow 2015; Pitts and Versluys 2015b), recent parasitological studies have suggested that public sanitation measures were insufficient and there was no improvement to health due to such measures (Mitchell 2017; Ledger *et al.* 2018). The transition from the Roman to Late Antique periods would have been a very gradual transition in terms of settlement and population size. The settlement contraction in the Late Hellenistic period, followed shortly after by the Roman invasion, and then the establishment of the Roman colony represent a more dramatic and fast change to the population size and to the administrative workings of the settlement and its infrastructure. As an example of improved infrastructure, countless Roman drains have been identified during rescue excavations, particularly in the area of the modern upper village at Knossos (Sweetman and Grigoropoulos 2010), and one identified during the 1910 excavations (Benton 1937; *KS2*:132), and at some point in the Roman period, possibly beginning in the 2nd century AD, an aqueduct was constructed with evidence that rebuilding continued into the Late Antique period (Hood and Smyth 1981; Whitelaw *et al.* 2019).

4.4.4. Sex structure of the assemblage

A remarkably skewed ratio of females to males was observed in the Hellenistic period. There is some evidence to support the notion that significant numbers of prime age males died away from Knossos, such as the assumed mercenaries buried in the Hadra hydria at Alexandria in Egypt. The inscriptions on many of these cinerary urns indicate that they contained the remains of foreign officials, dignitaries, and mercenaries, and the cremation practice demonstrated a deviation from the accepted local customs (Landvatter 2013, 106). It is proposed that these hydria were manufactured in central Crete, at Knossos even, though they are found in many locations around the Eastern Mediterranean and beyond (Callaghan 1980; Callaghan and Jones 1985; Enklaar 1985; 1986; Chaniotis 1999). Cremation burials are not known from Knossos in this time period but it was an accepted, though minority, custom in the Hellenistic world and appeared to be the non-local custom at Alexandria (Landvatter 2013). Wars and territory disputes are reported to have been rife in Crete during the Hellenistic period, as well as Crete being renowned as a place that supplied the Hellenistic armies with mercenaries (Chaniotis 1999, 183). The discovery of a Hellenistic mass grave of young adult males at Chania (ancient Kydonia) suggests that due to these wars and disputes, warriors were at least sometimes buried in such communal graves rather than bodies being transported back to their home city for a family burial. The dating of this grave to the late 4th or early 3rd century BC may indicate that this mass burial was the result of a conflict stimulated by Knossos with Chania in 346 BC, though relatively few conflicts are specifically attested to in the written history (Bourbou and Niniou-Kindeli 2009).

The sex structure for the Roman and Late Antique assemblages was close to equal for each sex, with males representing marginally over half the sample of adults of identified sex in each case. This simply demonstrates that there were no significant exclusions or biases in burial location based on sex. These cemeteries were inclusive of all demographic groups and are likely to have been family tombs that included females and males of all age groups.

4.5. Conclusion

In this chapter, the representativeness – in terms of age, sex and social status – of the skeletal sample has been ascertained as well as can be achieved from the available evidence. An insight into the demographic structure of the assemblage and the shortcomings of its representativeness will aid in the interpretation of the analyses in the following chapters, across the time periods and demographic and social groups of the assemblage. This chapter enables an awareness of where there are likely or possible sample biases and also presents the important analysis (in itself) of the 'life expectancy' of the assemblage from the age-at-death categories. As broad age categories are employed, it is not a true calculation of life expectancy at birth (as would be calculated for modern demographic studies). The analysis presented here was lower resolution than could have been achieved from a more intact and less commingled assemblage. Considering the condition of the material, the use of wide age categories has at least enabled a broad picture to be created of the 'life expectancy' of the population.

5

Stable Isotope Analysis

5.1. Background

5.1.1. Isotopes and bone composition

Isotopes are atoms of the same element with different masses, meaning the same number of protons but different numbers of neutrons. They can be radioactive (unstable), like carbon-14 (^{14}C) which decays at a steady rate, or stable, like the carbon stable isotopes, ^{12}C and ^{13}C, which have atomic masses of 12 and 13 respectively, and the nitrogen stable isotopes, ^{14}N and ^{15}N, which have atomic masses of 14 and 15 respectively. In different parts of the natural environment and in different biological materials the isotopic ratios (i.e. ^{12}C:^{13}C or $\delta^{13}C$) will vary (Katzenberg 2008; Hoefs 2009). These variations are very small and therefore, rather than being expressed as a ratio of one isotope to another, the ratio is measured in comparison with the isotope ratios in an internationally recognised standard in per thousand or per mil (‰) (van der Merwe 1982). The standard for carbon isotopes is a fossil mineral Vienna PeeDee Belemnite (VPDB), which contains more ^{13}C than most biological materials, therefore $\delta^{13}C$ is usually a negative number (Long 1995; Hoefs 2009; Jochum and Enzweiler 2014). The standard for nitrogen isotopes is atmospheric nitrogen (AIR) and $\delta^{15}N$ is usually a number above zero due to most biological materials having more ^{15}N than the standard (DeNiro 1987, 182; Jochum and Enzweiler 2014, 62).

Bone is composed of an organic matrix of structural protein called collagen, which contains crystals of calcium phosphate, largely as hydroxyapatite. By weight, dry bone is approximately 30% organic (of which 85–90% is collagen, the remainder being made up of non-collagenous proteins, proteoglycans, and lipids) and 70% inorganic mineral (Katzenberg 2008). Collagen is made up of approximately 35% carbon and 11–16% nitrogen and is therefore the preferred material for carbon and nitrogen isotope analysis (van Klinken 1999). Bone carbonate (the inorganic hydroxyapatite) can also be analysed but is more susceptible to alteration in the burial environment (diagenesis) (Schoeninger and DeNiro 1982; Lee-Thorp *et al.* 1989, 586). The two materials can be analysed alongside each other to demonstrate different aspects of diet. Collagen carbon primarily represents dietary protein, whereas apatite carbon is more representative of the whole diet (Ambrose and Norr 1993; Keenleyside *et al.* 2006). Strontium and oxygen isotope analysis, used in both dietary and migration studies, can be done on the mineral component of the bone, but again, due to the high likelihood of diagenesis in bone, tooth enamel is a more common resource for these studies as it preserves the *in vivo* isotope signature (Price *et al.* 1994; Balasse *et al.* 2003; Evans *et al.* 2006).

5.1.2. Isotopes as dietary indicators

Different isotope masses mean that fractionation occurs with natural processes, such as photosynthesis and metabolism, as the heavier isotopes, such as ^{13}C, react more slowly than the lighter isotopes, such as ^{12}C. Fractionation affects the relative abundance of isotopes, which means that the ratios in the atmosphere and in plant tissues will be different due to this process. Different types of plants fix carbon by different photosynthetic pathways. Tropical plants, such as maize, millet, sorghum and sugarcane, fix carbon via the C_4 or 'Hatch-Slack' pathway, while most plants from temperate regions follow the C_3 or 'Calvin' pathway (van der Merwe 1982, 596–97; Katzenberg 2008, 423). Atmospheric CO_2 had an approximate $\delta^{13}C$ value of −7‰ prior to the industrial revolution and mass burning of fossil fuels (Katzenberg 2008, 425). With fractionation in the photosynthesis process C_4 plants tend to range from −9 to −14‰, while C_3 plants have a range from about −20 to −35‰ (Deines 1980; Katzenberg 2008, 423). When these plants are then eaten by humans or animals, there is further fractionation with the metabolic processes, but the different plant types and their values will be reflected in the tissues of the consumer. A small number of plants, including pineapples, follow the CAM photosynthetic pathway with intermediate values. The difference in $\delta^{13}C$ of the diet and that of the various body tissues is variable but it is estimated to increase by 1‰ in the whole body and by 3–5‰ in bone collagen at the first level of consumption (from plants to herbivores) but by 0–2‰ thereafter by trophic level (DeNiro and Epstein 1978; van der Merwe and Vogel 1978; Ambrose and Norr 1993; Bocherens and Drucker 2003; Katzenberg 2008). However, this fractionation level is more variable and unpredictable than the $\delta^{15}N$ fractionation between trophic levels (Schoeninger 1985; Perkins *et al.* 2014). Tests have been conducted to see if the trophic level effect on $\delta^{13}C$ varied between terrestrial, marine coastal and open ocean environments, and it was suggested by Van der Merwe (1982) that the trophic level effect for carbon occurred only at the step between plants and primary consumers (herbivores), but no consistent patterns have been observed (van der Merwe 1982; Rau *et al.* 1983; Schoeninger 1985). Atmospheric nitrogen (N_2), as the primary standard, has a value of 0‰. Legumes have $\delta^{15}N$ values very similar to the atmosphere, due to their symbiotic relationship with bacteria that live in their roots and can fix nitrogen, making it available to the plant (Brill 1977). Non-leguminous plants are more enriched in the heavier ^{15}N and therefore have elevated $\delta^{15}N$ values. Nitrogen isotopes vary depending on trophic level and $\delta^{15}N$ values increase by approximately 3–5‰ at each level of the food chain (Schoeninger and DeNiro

1984; Bocherens and Drucker 2003; Hedges and Reynard 2007), though recent work has demonstrated this should be closer to c.6‰ (O'Connell *et al.* 2012).

Marine and terrestrial based diets can also be distinguished from one another due the different carbon sources in the sea and the atmosphere. Carbon is available for marine organisms as dissolved carbonate, with a $\delta^{13}C$ value of 0‰, while atmospheric CO_2 is −7‰. Longer food chains in marine environments result in marine mammals at the top of the food chain also having elevated $\delta^{15}N$ values compared to most terrestrial carnivores (Schoeninger and DeNiro 1984; Lubell *et al.* 1994, 205). Therefore, there can also be a distinction between humans consuming shellfish and small fish compared to those eating larger fish further along the food chain. Freshwater resources have highly variable $\delta^{13}C$ values due to the range of sources the carbon can be obtained from, including atmospheric CO_2, CO_2 in the water, carbonate from rocks and soils, and decomposition products or waste from plants and animals living in the water (Zohary *et al.* 1994; Katzenberg 2008, 427) . There is variation in $\delta^{15}N$ of plants from inland versus coastal regions and arid versus wetter regions (Virginia and Delwiche 1982; Shearer *et al.* 1983; Heaton 1987; Sealy *et al.* 1987), and these signatures are passed up the food chain. $\delta^{15}N$ values are also elevated by breast feeding and at times of insufficient protein intake when the body has to reutilise the existing tissues in the body (Hobson *et al.* 1993; Katzenberg 2008, 428). Thus, stable carbon and nitrogen isotope analysis can be used in palaeodietary studies to determine these aspects of ancient diets and this provides the basis of the expression, 'you are what you eat.'

Just as the isotopic ratios between different tissues in the body are variable, there can also be a small amount of variation between collagen samples taken from different bones of the body, if there is a change in dietary habits over time, due to the different turn-over rates of bone in the different bones of the body. Studies on animals with controlled diets showed no isotopic difference between collagen of different bones when the diet remained constant (Deniro and Schoeniger 1983; Sealy *et al.* 1995). Bone is a living tissue, during an individual's lifetime, that is constantly being renewed through osteoblasts removing old bone cells and osteoclasts creating new ones. On average the turnover rate of bone in adults is 3.6% per year though this can be quite variable depending on various factors, including age, sex, environment, genetics, physical activity and disease (Hedges *et al.* 2007; Bronner 2008, 521). The turnover is faster in smaller bones with thin cortical bone and more cancellous bone, such as the ribs, and slower for a larger bone with thick cortical bone, such as the femur. Therefore, when sampling for stable isotope analysis, a rib sample might, for example, represent diet from the last 5 years, while a femur sample might represent diet from the last 20 years (Sealy *et al.* 1995; Cox and Sealy 1997; Bell *et al.* 2001; Hedges *et al.* 2007; Pollard *et al.* 2012). This will also vary between adults and sub-adults, with sub-adults having a faster bone turnover (more than twice the adult rate), and to a lesser extent between individuals, though decreases considerably with age, particularly in women (Cho *et al.* 2006).

5.1.3. Diet in the Graeco-Roman world

Most diets in Europe would have been based on C3 plants. The predominant crop in the Graeco-Roman world was wheat but a wide range of other C3 plants were consumed including other cereals (barley, oat, rye), legumes (lentils, beans, peas, chickpeas), fruits (grapes, figs, olives, dates, pears), vegetables (carrot, celery, leek, onion), nuts (almonds, chestnuts, hazelnuts), leaves (lettuce, cabbage, vine, wild greens), herbs (dill, mint, fennel, wild herbs), and spices (coriander, sesame, poppy, mustard) (Livarda 2014; Robinson and Rowan 2015; Margaritis 2015a; Rowan 2017; Erdkamp and Holleran 2018). The variety of plants available is known from both archaeobotanical remains and written sources. C4 plants come from tropical environments and most were not introduced into this part of the world until later in the medieval period. Millet was present in Greece as far back as the Neolithic period and was attested to throughout the Roman Empire, as animal feed particularly, but also as a porridge and in beer brewing, but it was never a popular or widespread crop. It is known from both ancient texts and the archaeological record as charred plant remains (Dalby 2003; Murphy 2016).

Meat, dairy products and eggs also featured in many diets as a supplement to the staples. Texts and art tend to represent the diets of the elite and banquets in particular, and therefore tend to overrepresent the importance of meat in the diet. Goat/sheep was the most important meat source at most Mediterranean sites, though pork became more prevalent in the Imperial Roman period, particularly in western central Italy (King 1999; 2001). Poultry and cattle bones also tend to be present in most animal bone assemblages, alongside a relatively insignificant proportion of various other species. Fish bones were often missed at sites in the past, prior to the systematic implementation of flotation during excavation, meaning that their inclusion in diets has often been overlooked. Accounts differ on the reception of seafood by past populations. Fish could, at certain times and places in the past, be an easily procured product and the staple diet of the fisherman, but could also be an exclusive, expensive luxury item. It is also sometimes seen as a moral taboo or something to be feared due to its provenance in the sea, which could be a dangerous and alien place (Purcell 1995).

Meat and fish would not have been staples in the diet, but rather supplements, and even in the more elite diets would not have been eaten on a daily basis. In most locations, meat would have been a more important resource than fish, as agriculture was a more important and reliable practice than fishing. The majority of fish consumed would have been small-fry, but the range of fish available could be expanded by salting or drying fish to extend their consumable life (Gallant 1985; Purcell 1995). In the Roman period particularly, fermented or salted fish pastes and sauces were traded extensively throughout the provinces (Garnsey 1999). Fresh fish was a desirable and exclusive product known from Classical and Roman literary works and was sold at fish markets, for example the one at Roman Corinth which is known from the inscriptions in both Greek and Latin which would have marked the entrance to the market (Williams 1993; Davidson 1997). It is possible that small dietary contributions from low trophic level fish might be difficult or impossible to detect isotopically. Coastal sites are likely to have a more substantial contribution from seafood in the diet as demonstrated by the Late Antique fish bone assemblage from Itanos in East Crete, though fish bones are also found at inland sites such as Eleutherna. A great number of fish species were present though the main ones were sea bream, parrot-fish, groupers/combers and picarels, as well as seashells, crustaceans and sea turtles (Mylona 2003b). In addition to the fish bone evidence, there are a number of (presumed-Roman) fish tanks along both the north and south coasts of Crete, which were rock-cut structures along the tide-line of the sea which would have kept a supply of live fish to overcome some of the problems of preservation (Mylona 2003b). The names of over 110 fish and around 30 other marine organisims are recorded in the Byzantine literature, demonstrating largely the same species were being eaten as had been attested to in the Roman period (Bourbou 2010, 129). While meat and other terrestrial animal products (dairy and eggs) would have been more commonly consumed than fish at most sites, livestock was a less economical use of land than arable farming, therefore plants would have made up the majority of people's diets.

The relative paucity of fish bone assemblages means that isotopic studies of fish bones are less common than for terrestrial animal bones as control samples for human dietary studies. Additionally, different types of fish have a wide range of values, therefore a small sample from a site may not represent the complete range of fish being consumed at the site. However, Table 5.1 displays results of isotopic studies of fish from Mediterranean regions and shows how wide-ranging the values are (including overlap with terrestrial values). This demonstrates that it cannot be determined conclusively that a diet did not contain fish from stable isotope analysis (Lightfoot, Šlaus, and O'Connell 2012; Vika and Theodoropoulou 2012). Studies conducted on Early-Middle Byzantine samples at Eleutherna and Stylos on Crete each had an outlier that indicated a more significant marine contribution in the diet than for any other individuals sampled (Bourbou 2010, 156; Bourbou *et al.* 2011). These were both inland sites and this is likely to simply demonstrate movement of people from coastal sites. Fish bones are, however, found at inland sites, including Knossos and Eleutherna and are a more common find at both coastal and inland sites in Crete than in other regions of Greece (Mylona 2003a, 193). It is, therefore, possible that the outlier diets of these individuals simply come down to personal preference.

The animal bones from Early Roman contexts (pre-2nd century AD) at the Unexplored Mansion site at Knossos indicate the main meat source was sheep/goat (55.5% of this assemblage), with substantial contributions from pig (26.2%) and cattle (15.8%), and a much smaller contribution from chicken (1.5%). There were four

Table 5.1. Stable isotope values of fish from the Mediterranean and neighbouring regions. [1]After Lightfoot *et al.* 2012 [2]Lakeside (freshwater) [3]Freshwater and marine.

Study	Age of samples	Material	*n*	Range in $\delta^{13}C$ (‰)	Range in $\delta^{15}N$ (‰)
Italy (Francalacci 1988)[1]	Epipalaeolithic to Middle Neolithic	Collagen	1 (C), 2 (N)	−10.6	9.8 to 11.4
Tunisia (Keenleyside *et al.* 2009)[1]	Roman/Late Roman	Collagen	2	c. −12 to −10.5	c. 8 to 10
Croatia (Lightfoot *et al.* 2011)[1]	Mesolithic and Neolithic	Collagen	9	−15.1 to −12.1	5.6 to 9.7
Sicily (Badalamenti *et al.* 2002)[1]	Modern	Muscle	No data	−18.8 to −16.9	9.4 to 11.2
Mallorca reefs (Jennings *et al.* 1997)[1]	Modern	Muscle	176	−19.2 to −16.1	8.4 to 13.8
Corsica (Pinnegar and Polunin 2000)[1]	Modern	Muscle	54	−19.6 to −16.3	4.6 to 9.8
Youra (Vika and Theodoropoulou 2012)	Mesolithic- Final Neolithic	Collagen	14	−19.2 to −9.3	3.6 to 9.2
Dispillio (Vika and Theodoropoulou 2012)[2]	Neolithic	Collagen	5	−19.8 to −11.9	4.9 to 9.5
Archontiko (Vika and Theodoropoulou 2012)[3]	Bronze Age	Collagen	5	−19.6 to −14.8	8.6 to 10.9
Toumba Thessaloniki (Vika and Theodoropoulou 2012)	Middle Bronze- Early Iron Age	Collagen	9	−12.2 to −7.6	5.8 to 12.1
Karabournaki (Vika and Theodoropoulou 2012)	Archaic-Classical	Collagen	9	−16.6 to −7.3	4.3 to 11.6
Velia (Craig *et al.* 2009)	Roman	Collagen	4	−14.9 to −12.6	9.1 to 12.1

examples of fish bones, representing 2 different species, and it is likely these are underrepresented due to poor retrieval of such tiny bones during excavation and deposits were not sieved. The bones from 2nd-3rd century levels in the same report are not taken to be representative of diet, as the large numbers of sawn-off bone terminals demonstrates a production area for bone tools, over representing the dense long bones of cattle and horses (Bedwin 1992). An animal bone assemblage studied from Eleutherna (1500 BC- 11th/12th century AD) indicates a similar pattern over a broad time period of sheep/goats being the main focus of animal husbandry, followed by pigs and with cattle more often being kept as draught animals. Wild animals, such as wild goats and hares, made up about 5% of the assemblage (Nobis 2003). Sheep/goats were the dominant species in animal bone assemblages (followed by pigs) across a broad time period for sites across Greece. Further examples include Neolithic and Bronze Age Knossos (Isaakidou 2004), Bronze Age Agia Triada (Wilkens 1996), Bronze Age, Classical and Roman Eleusis (Cosmopoulos *et al.* 2003), Hellenistic Halos (Prummel 2003), and Geometric and Byzantine Gortyn (Wilkens 1996).

A Protogeometric archaeobotanical assemblage excavated below the Roman Villa Dionysus, though of an earlier date than this study, demonstrates the variety of foodstuffs available at the site previously. Barley and glume wheats (predominantly emmer, with some einkorn) were the main cereals recovered, with only tentative suggestions of some free-threshing (common/durum) wheats. As a product of differential preservation, the cereal remains were outnumbered by fruits (olive, fig and grape predominantly), nuts (almonds), and wild species. Legumes were also present and included bitter vetch, celtic bean and pea. Small numbers of fish scales and urchin spines were also recovered from some flots. These soil samples taken from two sequential Protogeometric floor deposits were quite a homogenous fill and interpreted as largely domestic cooking and consumption debris (Livarda 2012). At three Hellenistic country houses in southern Macedonia, close to the Aegean coast, the study of plant remains demonstrated different agricultural practices and economic functions within a small region but many of the main foodstuffs were the same as those observed at Protogeometric Knossos, confirming this widespread (over space and time) core Mediterranean diet. At these sites glume wheats were less common than the free-threshing wheats but barley was also commonly found. Fruits (olives, grapes, figs, danewort, cornelian cherry), nuts (hazelnuts, walnuts, almonds), legumes (lentil, bitter vetch, pea, grass pea, celtic bean), wild species/weeds (lupine and medic), and some non-staple crops and plants for flavouring foods (sesame, pine) demonstrate both the core foodstuffs and the sort of variety that diets would have consisted of at this time (Margaritis 2015a; 2015b). Mineralized plant remains (as well as some fish bones, urchin spines, and splinters from larger mammal bones) from the Cardo V sewer at Herculaneum, for example, provide evidence for a diverse diet, with the major grain staples (various types of wheat, barley, and millet) supplemented by a wide variety of fruits, vegetables, legumes, herbs and spices (Robinson and Rowan 2015; Rowan 2017). Cereal grains, legumes, seeds and stones of fruits usually survive due to being carbonised but the highly perishable vegetable and tuber crops tend not to survive except in extreme dry conditions and the variety of such plants is better known from sites in Egypt (Zohary and Hopf 2000).

Despite texts expressing the strict dietary restrictions and fasting regimens, archaeobotanical evidence from the 5th–7th century Kom el-Nana monastery in Egypt demonstrates that the general diet at the site was high in variety and flavour (including onion, cumin, coriander, dill, fennel and juniper) (Harlow and Smith 2001; Luff 2007). The common staples of wheat, barley, grapes, olives, figs, nuts and lentils, were supplemented by dates, wild apples, beets, cucumber/melon, carrot, celery, pomegranate, peach and mulberry, amongst other things.

5.1.4. Isotopic evidence for Mediterranean diets

In Holocene Europe, typical $\delta^{13}C$ values for human C3 terrestrial consumers are around −20‰, though Table 5.12 suggests that for Mediterranean sites the average is more like −19‰, but this may be due to a marine component in the diet at a number of sites. Individuals consuming diets that consisted of protein derived exclusively from marine or C4 terrestrial sources have $\delta^{13}C$ values of approximately −12‰. Terrestrial diets that included meat generally have $\delta^{15}N$ values of around 8–10‰, while marine consumers can have values as high as 20‰ (Richards and Mellars 1998; Triantaphyllou *et al.* 2008; Stevens *et al.* 2010; Lightfoot *et al.* 2012). However, these can vary due to faunal isotope baselines varying due to local climate. Arid climates, such as those found at the Dakhleh Oasis in Egypt, can result in elevated $\delta^{15}N$ values of C3 plants but the $\delta^{13}C$ values for both the plants and their consumers remain in the typical C3 range (Dupras 1999; Dupras *et al.* 2001; Dupras and Tocheri 2007).

The majority of human dietary isotopic studies in Greece have been on Prehistoric populations. Post-Bronze Age exceptions include Triantaphyllou's investigations of a number of Early Iron Age sites in Northern Greece (Triantaphyllou 2001; 2015), Panagiotopoulou and Papathanasiou's (Papathanasiou *et al.* 2013; Panagiotopoulou and Papathanasiou 2015) study of a Geometric cemetery at Agios Demetrios, Vika's work at Classical and Hellenistic Thebes (Vika *et al.* 2009; Vika 2011), Lagia's study of Classical, Hellenistic and Imperial Roman Athens and Laurion (Lagia 2015), and another multi-period study for Hellenistic to Byzantine Helike in Achaea (McConnan Borstad *et al.* 2018). There are studies from Classical Greek colonies in (modern) Bulgaria at Apollonia Pontica (Keenleyside *et al.* 2006; Kwok and Keenleyside 2015) and Mesembria (Moles 2012; Bonsall *et al.* 2015), in Italy, at Metaponto (Henneberg *et al.* 1999; Henneberg and Henneberg 2003), and in Magna Graecia at Archaic Syracuse in Sicily (Tanasi *et al.* 2018).

Extending the review of dietary isotopic studies to assemblages in the Mediterranean Roman Empire, there have been studies conducted at various Imperial Roman period sites in Italy (Prowse 2001; Prowse *et al.* 2004; 2005; Craig *et al.* 2009; Crowe *et al.* 2010; Sperduti *et al.* 2012; Killgrove and Tykot 2013; 2018; Ricci *et al.* 2016), Leptiminus in Tunisia (Keenleyside *et al.* 2009), the Dakhleh Oasis in Egypt (Dupras 1999; Dupras *et al.* 2001; Dupras and Tocheri 2007), and in Asia Minor (Lösch *et al.* 2014; Propstmeier *et al.* 2017; Wong *et al.* 2017). For comparable Late Antique or Early Byzantine populations, there are studies from a variety of sites on Crete and mainland Greece (Bourbou and Richards 2007; Bourbou 2010; Bourbou *et al.* 2011; 2013; Bourbou and Garvie-Lok 2015; Kwok 2015) and for medieval Greece (Garvie-Lok 2001). There are also studies from Rome's catacombs (Rutgers *et al.* 2009), Roman and Late Antique sites in Dalmatia (Croatia) (Lightfoot *et al.* 2012). A summary of the results of these studies is outlined in Table 5.12.

Isotopic studies for Greek and Roman sites generally suggest a C3 diet with most individuals having some access to animal products and more occasionally with some individuals at some sites consuming fish. A general trend of increased protein consumption from prehistoric to historic times in Greece has been observed (Triantaphyllou 2001, 135; Vika 2011, 1161; Lagia 2015, 138). In prehistory there were a greater number of largely vegetarian diets and the inclusion of seafood in the diet was particularly rare, only being evident in Grave Circles A and B at Mycenae and at Neopalatial Knossos (Richards and Hedges 2008; Nafplioti 2016). Changes have been observed over time at some sites, particularly in terms of marine consumption. A marine component in the diet was identified in the Imperial Roman period at sites in Dalmatia which was not present in either the preceding Iron Age or succeeding Early Medieval period. Likely due to Christian fasting rules, a number of sites have identified an increase in marine consumption (or a noteworthy contribution from marine foods in this time period though there may not be site-specific data from the preceding period with which to compare it) in the Late Roman or Early Byzantine periods, though sometimes only for clergical sub-groups of the population (Garvie-Lok 2001; Bourbou and Richards 2007; Salamon *et al.* 2008; Bourbou *et al.* 2011; Moles 2012; Reitsema *et al.* 2016). Bourbou (2010, 158) compares the Byzantine results to prehistoric studies in Greece which showed no marine consumption, due to the lack of studies for intermediate time periods at the time, and with no earlier studies at these sites it is difficult to know whether the inclusion of marine foods in the diet is new in the Late Antique period. The level of elevation in the nitrogen values at Thebes, without a matching elevation in the carbon values to suggest marine consumption, is explained by the inclusion of freshwater fish in the diet, for which Vika (2009) draws a comparison with the written sources which attest to such foods being consumed. Despite the broader trend over time, from prehistoric to historic Hellenic Greece, of increasing protein consumption, the trend at Athens from Classical to Hellenistic and into Roman times was of decreasing protein levels in the diet (Lagia 2015). This suggestion of a deterioration in standards of living was supported by an increase in skeletal lesions indicative of periods of malnutrition or disease and demonstrates how large-scale urban changes and the pressures caused by a large population can impact individual lives and diets.

Differences between locations, namely nearby cemeteries, have also been investigated. While at Metaponto there was no significant difference in diets detected isotopically between the urban and rural cemeteries (Henneberg and Henneberg 2003), at Rome there was a difference between urban and suburban diets, with some C4 plant consumption in individuals from the suburban Castellaccio Europarco cemetery. There was also a greater amount of marine food in the diet of the sample from coastal Isola Sacra compared to the inland cemeteries at Rome (Killgrove and Tykot 2013, 34). There is often a subtle distinction between male and female diets but the difference is variable between different sites and often not statistically significant. At Metaponto, though the difference in protein intake between males and females was small, there was a greater difference between the sexes in the urban cemetery individuals compared to the rural cemetery (Henneberg and Henneberg 2003). The main age-related difference is in breastfeeding infants, who have elevated $\delta^{15}N$ values as they are a trophic level above their mothers (Dupras *et al.* 2001; Fuller *et al.* 2006; Dupras and Tocheri 2007; Keenleyside *et al.* 2009; Bourbou *et al.* 2013; Bourbou and Garvie-Lok 2015; Kwok and Keenleyside 2015; Reitsema *et al.* 2016). Other age-related differences, particularly among adult diets, are rarely observed. However, at Classical to Imperial Roman Athens, a significant difference was observed between Young Adults and both Middle and Old Adults (Lagia 2015, 133). This may indicate a greater level of social stratification or administrative control over food distribution at Athens compared to smaller centres and the importance of age in this setting.

Stable isotope analysis, though providing direct evidence of a specific individual's diet, only gives broad characteristics of certain food-types being consumed. Details of what these diets would have contained can be inferred from ancient texts and art, and archaeological remains, including animal bones, charred plant remains, residues, and coprolites. The importance of a holistic approach is evident from the fact that there are foods known from the archaeobotanical remains that are never mentioned in texts, as well as perishable foods, such as dairy produce, which generally do not leave a trace archaeologically but are known to have been part of the diet from the literary sources (Harlow and Smith 2001; Dalby 2003, 22). The core diet of the Greeks and the Romans is often described as the 'Mediterranean triad'. This consisted of bread, wine, and oil (or grain, grape and olive), and it was so deeply integrated into the diet and culture of the people of the region, as well as being central to Greek and Roman economy, that it continued into the Byzantine Empire (Wilkins and Nadeau 2015,

10). Texts and art often focus on feasting and ritualised meals, such as the symposium, though texts also include administrative records for taxation or supply purposes, accounts by doctors and travellers, references in plays and treatises, and dietary regimens at monasteries for the later Roman and Byzantine periods.

5.2. Method

5.2.1. Sampling

Bone samples for stable carbon and nitrogen isotope analysis were selected from across a range of contexts in order to represent the different time periods, burial locations, and tomb forms present at the site. Although the selection of samples had to be carried out prior to the full skeletal analysis of the assemblage, due to the long processing time for sample permits in Greece (13 months in this instance), they were also selected according to the amount of demographic information that could be obtained. This sometimes meant that samples had to be taken from the skull or pelvis, particularly for the commingled material. Having thick cortical bone often produces the best results as this is less prone to diagenesis; therefore, long bones are the preferred bone to sample, particularly the femur, tibia or humerus. Where it was possible, in the case of individual burials, a long bone sample was taken. Contextual information for each sample is outlined in Appendix C Table 1.[20]

The 93 bone samples were transported to the Wolfson Laboratories at UCL's Institute of Archaeology to be cleaned and prepared. The samples were cut to an appropriate size of c.0.5–1g using a cutting wheel attachment drill head and cleaned using a sandblaster to remove a layer from the external surface of the bone, then placed in labelled and weighed 12ml glass test tubes, and then the test tube was weighed again to obtain the sample weight. This part of the process took c.4 days, though the work had to be spread across 2 weeks due to equipment availability.

5.2.2. Collagen extraction

To carry out the isotopic analysis, the collagen component of the bone has to be isolated. The collagen extraction process was carried out following the method of Longin (1971) as adapted by Brown *et al.* (1988), which is considered to be the most rigorous extraction method, appropriate for extracting the maximum collagen yield from poorly preserved samples (Sealy *et al.* 2014). This process involves immersing the cleaned bone sample in 8ml of cold 0.5M HCl, covering the whole test tube rack with aluminium foil and leaving it in the fridge for several days, shaking once or twice daily. The acid was changed every 2–4 days ideally, until the inorganic component of the bone was demineralised. This step of the process can vary greatly between samples in how long it takes for the formation of bubbles (effervescence) to cease and the sample to become soft and translucent and float to the surface. It was also necessary to work this schedule of acid changes around weekends when there was no access to the lab for checking the samples, therefore it was generally ideal to change the acid on Mondays and then again on Wednesdays or Thursdays. Appendix C Table 1 demonstrates the number of days each sample spent in 0.5M HCl and the number of acid changes undergone for each sample prior to sufficient demineralisation.

A chunk of bone was used in preference to powdered bone as studies have shown that in poorly preserved bone this method produces more dependable results with acceptable C/N ratios (Schurr 1992; Garvie-Lok 2001). This stage is often followed by a NaOH treatment to remove humic contaminants; however, this process was omitted, which is a common methodological variation (e.g. Mays 1997; Richards and Hedges 1999; Lillie and Richards 2000), as it can result in a degree of sample loss due to the vulnerability of collagen to the chemical (Stafford *et al.* 1988; Mueller 1989; Katzenberg 1989; Bocherens *et al.* 1999). The demineralised bone sample was then filtered through an Ezee filter and rinsed three times with distilled water. The remaining sample was then gelatinised by being heated in pH 3.0 water (about 8ml) in the laboratory oven at 75°C for 48 hours. The solution was again put through an Ezee filter, into a pre-weighed and labelled test tube, and frozen for over 24 hours in the −20°C freezer before being transferred to the condenser chamber of the freeze-drier to chill the samples further, to below −31°C. The samples were then placed on the shelves in the vacuum jar over the condenser chamber and the vacuum pump was turned on to begin the freeze-drying process. It was left here for c.4 days until dry and then weighed to give the collagen yield. The collagen extraction process was done in two batches. Batch 1 (S1-S37) was 37 samples and took just over 4 weeks from going into the acid to going into the freezer, and a total of 6 weeks including the freeze-drying procedure. Batch 2 (S38-S93) was 56 samples and again took over 4 weeks for the collagen extraction and a total of 5 weeks including the freeze-drying (summarised in Table 5.2, with full results in Appendix C Table 1). Ideally the batches would have been equal sizes and the only reason for this not being the case was an electrical fault in the sandblaster after S37, with it remaining out of order for 2 weeks, and the need to get the first batch started. These processes, including weighing and labelling test tubes, acid changes and triple rinsing degraded samples using Ezee filters, testing the flexibility and firmness of the samples, and keeping a laboratory notebook to keep track of the progress of the samples and note any unusual developments, could be time consuming and took up to 3 hours per day for c.4 days per week for the duration of the collagen extraction process.

[20] Appendix C can be accessed at https://doi.org/10.30861/9781407360355-AppendixC

Table 5.2. Dates for collagen extraction processes for the two batches of bone samples.

	Batch 1	Batch 2
Into 0.5m HCl	23/01/17	09/02/17
Into oven	21/02/17	08/03/17
Out of oven	23/02/17	10/03/17
Into freezer	23/02/17	10/03/17
Into freeze drier	28/02/17	13/03/17
Out of freeze drier	06/03/17	16/03/17

5.2.3. Isotopic analysis

The extracted collagen was then transferred to the UCL Bloomsbury Environmental Isotope Facility (BEIF) in transport tubes, and here the samples were weighed, using a Mettler Toledo XP6 Microbalance, and sealed into 5x7mm tin capsules by being tightly folded and placed into wells in the capsule trays for analysis. The intricate weighing of small amounts of collagen and laboratory standards to within a narrow range is a delicate and time-consuming process and took 2 ½ days. The elemental analysis was done in three batches (of up to 27 samples per batch) and a further three repeat batches to replicate results (a further 2 ½ days of weighing samples into tin capsules), using a ThermoFisher Delta V Advantage stable isotope mass spectrometer attached to a Flash EA 1112 flash combustion elemental analyser. High precision stable isotope values of $\delta^{13}C$ and $\delta^{15}N$ are determined using a gas chromatographic separation column linked via a CONFLO IV interface to the mass spectrometer.

5.2.4. Indicators of diagenesis and contamination

Degradation of the bone collagen and the inclusion of contaminants in the sample are two distinct processes that can both affect the isotopic signatures needed for palaeodietary study. For results to be dependable, it is important to ensure that the collagen has not undergone any diagenetic degradation, which can commonly occur in archaeological bone samples and therefore studies have been carried out to develop means of assessing this diagenesis (DeNiro, 1985; Schoenenger *et al.* 1989; Van Klinken 1999). The indicators of diagenesis used for this study are collagen yield by weight, atomic C/N ratio, and carbon (%C) and nitrogen (%N) content. Collagen yield is useful as the smaller the amount recovered, the greater the chance that it has been degraded or contains other materials that can produce anomalous $\delta^{13}C$ and $\delta^{15}N$ values. Although opinion varies on selecting an appropriate cut-off point, below which the sample should be rejected, it is somewhat arbitrary as the degradation process is a gradual one (Garvie-Lok 2001). However, a 2% collagen yield cut-off is commonly recommended by other studies (De Niro and Weiner 1988; Ambrose 1990; Mays 1997). Atomic C/N ratio, measured by the elemental analyser, can indicate diagenesis on two levels. When collagen is broken down and lost, carbon and nitrogen can be differentially lost (Ambrose 1990). For this study anything below 1% collagen was treated with extreme caution, though samples were included and classified as borderline acceptable if the other measures indicated acceptable collagen preservation and the results were within a normal range. The most important indicator of acceptable collagen preservation is the atomic C:N ratio, which can be altered by the inclusion of carbon-rich contaminants, such as lipids (Garvie-Lok 2001). For this study a range of 2.9 to 3.6 for C:N ratios was used, as recommended by DeNiro (1985). The carbon (%C) and nitrogen (%N) content, also measured in the elemental analyser, demonstrate the concentration of these atoms in the sample. The accepted values fall within the ranges of 13%-47% for %C and 5%-17% for %N, as advocated by Ambrose (1990). When used together these assessments of diagenesis should enable any degraded samples to be identified and rejected.

Acceptable collagen preservation was present in 80% of samples (including the 10% of samples which were considered borderline acceptable). This was a far greater number of usable samples than was predicted for this region of the world, considering some comparable studies (for example, 13% [7/53] at Roman/Byzantine Hierapolis in Turkey (Wong *et al.* 2017)). Though preservation varies greatly within any region, with 80% (106/132) acceptable preservation found in sample from Roman and Byzantine Pergamon in Turkey (Propstmeier *et al.* 2017). The bone type used for each sample is listed in Appendix C Table 1. Interestingly, there does not appear to be a close relationship between the bone type sampled and collagen preservation, and the failed samples (those with poor or no collagen preservation) came from a variety of bone types. Figure 5.1 suggests that the pelvis samples had the greatest levels of acceptable preservation, although the fewest samples came from this group. Unacceptable preservation was most common among the skull samples though the levels of acceptable and unacceptable preservation were similar to the long bone samples.

5.2.5. Tests for diagenesis

Both the $\delta^{13}C$ and $\delta^{15}N$ values can be plotted against each of the preservation indicators to ensure that there is no correlation, and therefore no degradation or contamination of the samples due to factors that would affect these preservation indicators. The $\delta^{13}C$ and $\delta^{15}N$ values were plotted against the collagen yield, %C, %N and C:N values. No correlation was found as indicated in Figures 5.2–5.7. Additionally, Pearson's correlation coefficient tests were carried out to confirm this apparent lack of correlation and these demonstrate that no correlation was present. The results of these tests are set out in Table 5.3.

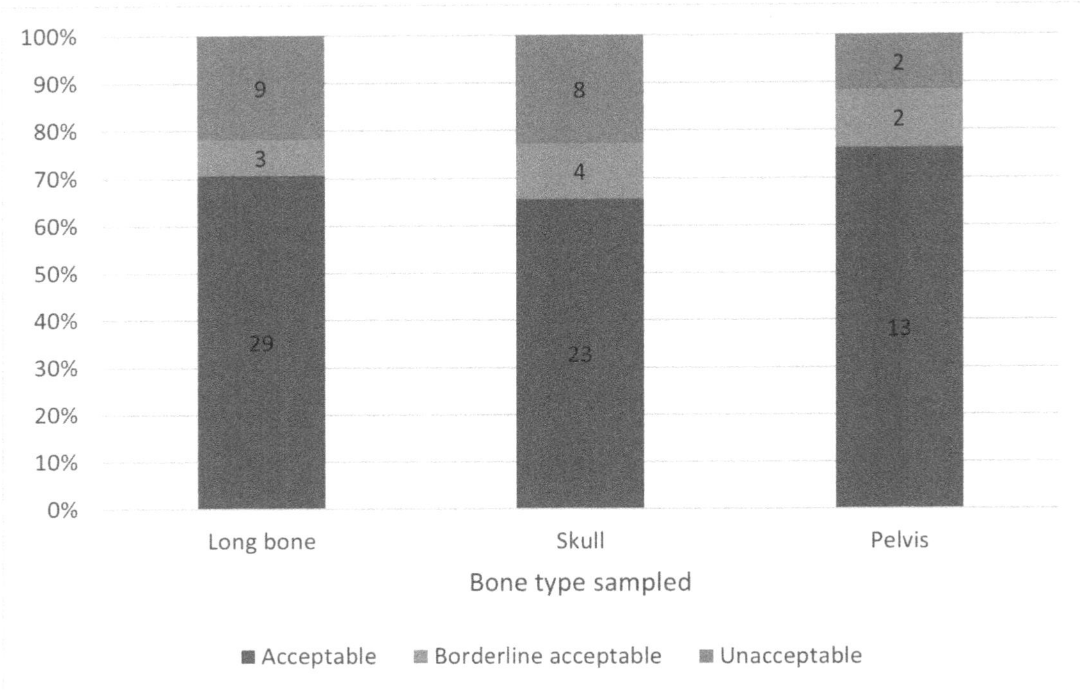

Figure 5.1. Stacked bar chart showing percentages of preservation levels for each bone type sampled with numbers of samples labelled on the bars.

5.3. Results

Though contemporary plant and animal bone control samples from Knossos were not available for analysis (Moles *et al.* 2022), there are isotopic studies of Neolithic and Bronze Age plants and faunal remains from Knossos, as well as a small number of Early-Middle Byzantine animal bone samples from elsewhere on Crete (Bourbou 2010; Nafplioti 2016; Nitsch *et al.* 2019; Issakidou *et al.* 2022). Though the Knossos samples are geographically appropriate and should control for the variation in isotope values affected by geology, climate and distance from the sea, they are temporally distant by thousands of years which could be problematic as they would

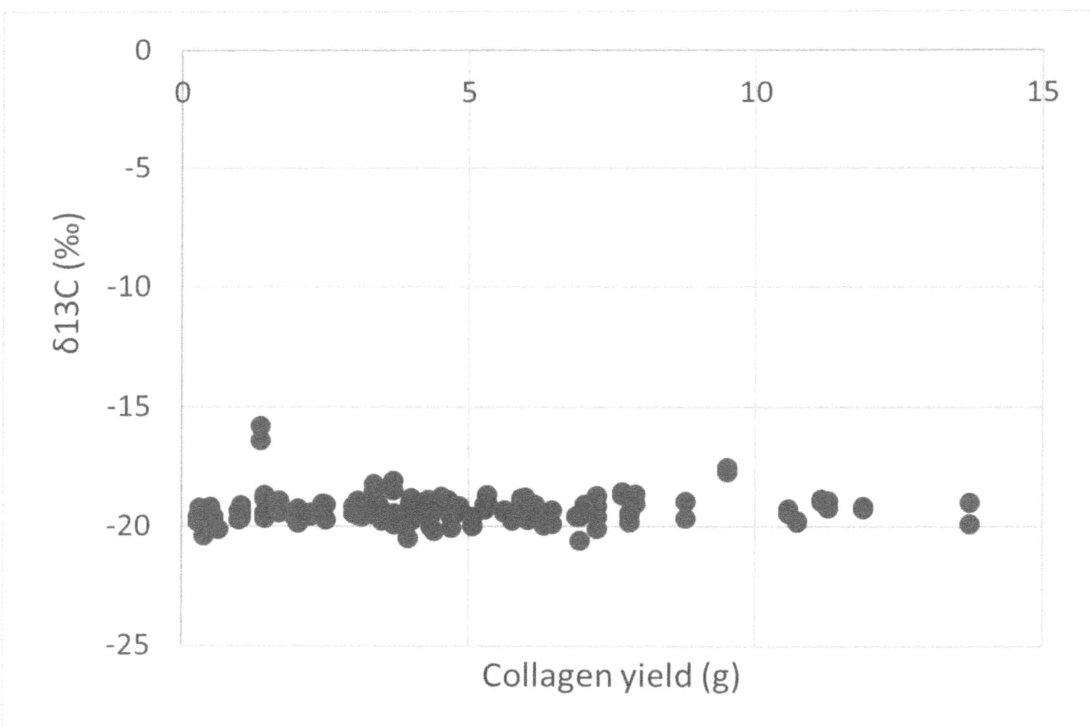

Figure 5.2. Scatter plot showing no correlation between δ^{13}C and collagen yield.

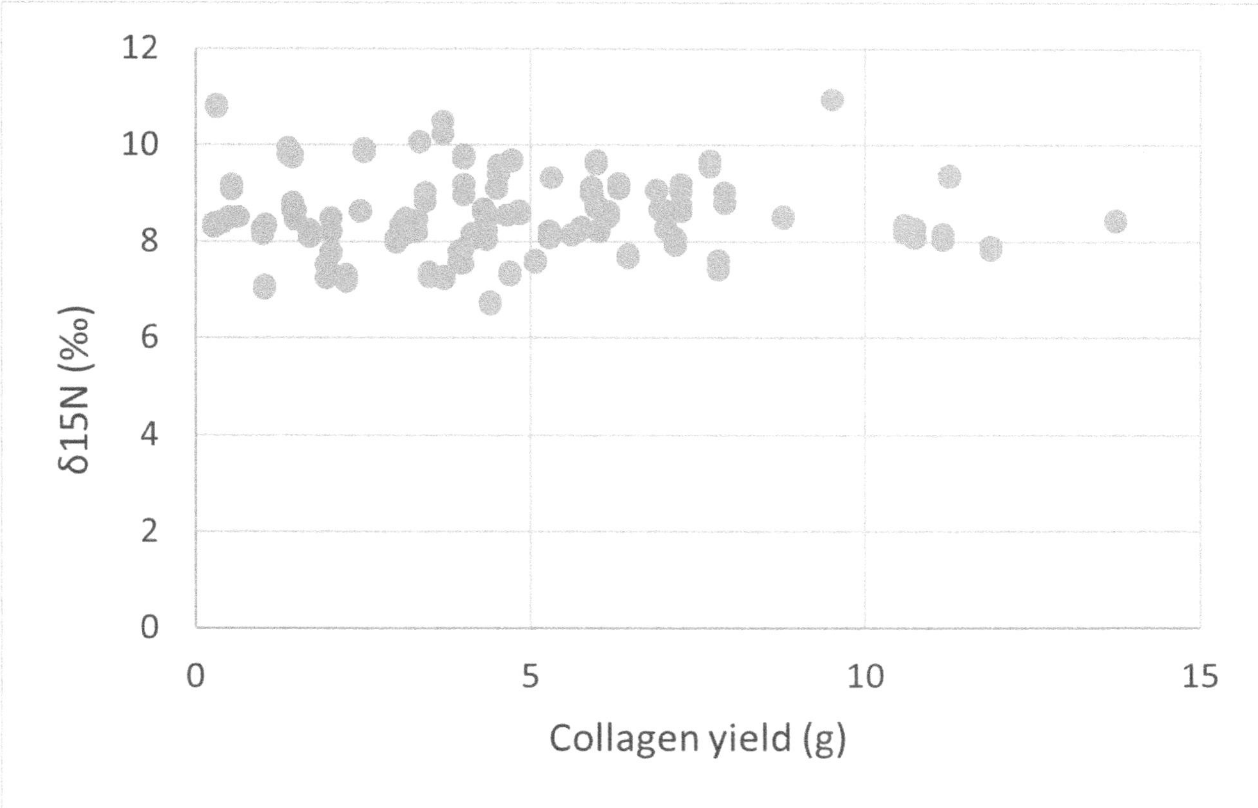

Figure 5.3. Scatter plot showing no correlation between $\delta^{15}N$ and collagen yield.

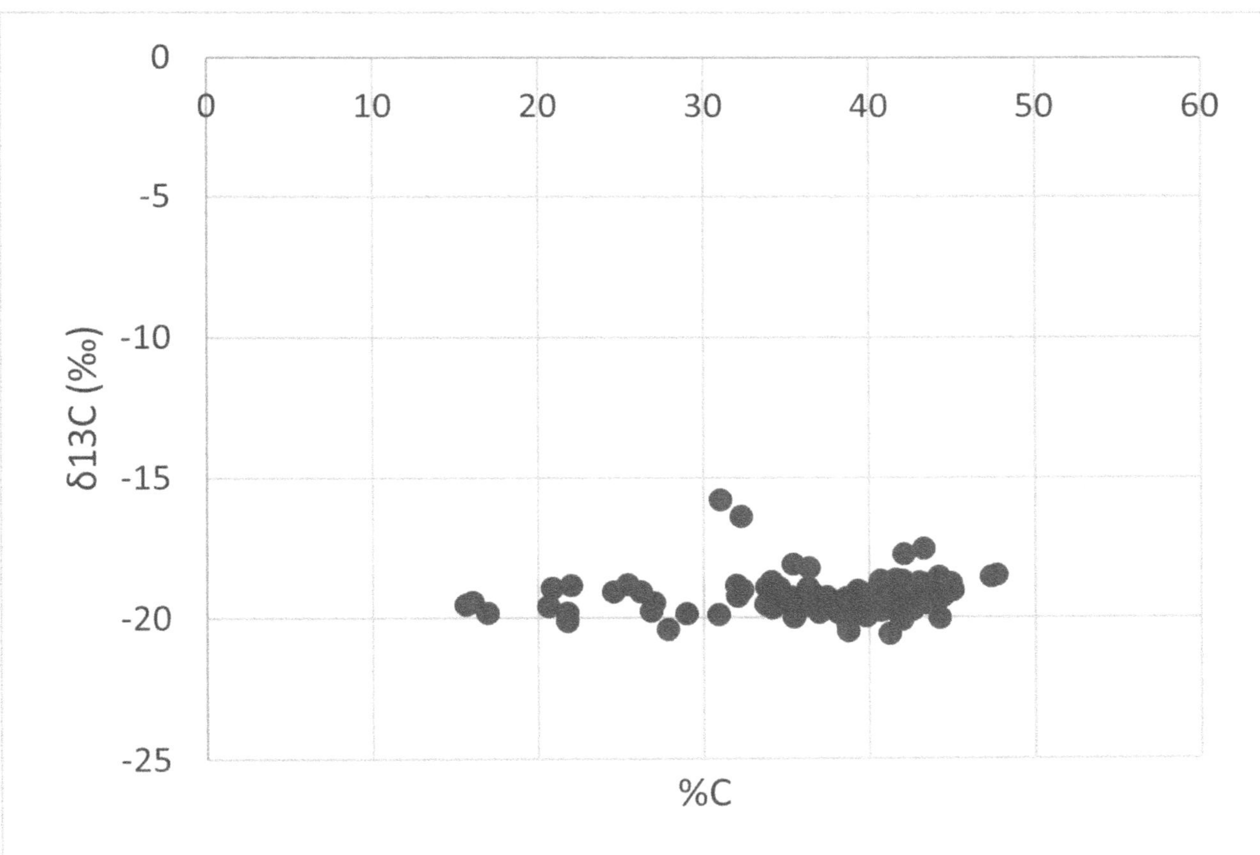

Figure 5.4. Scatter plot showing no correlation between $\delta^{13}C$ and %C.

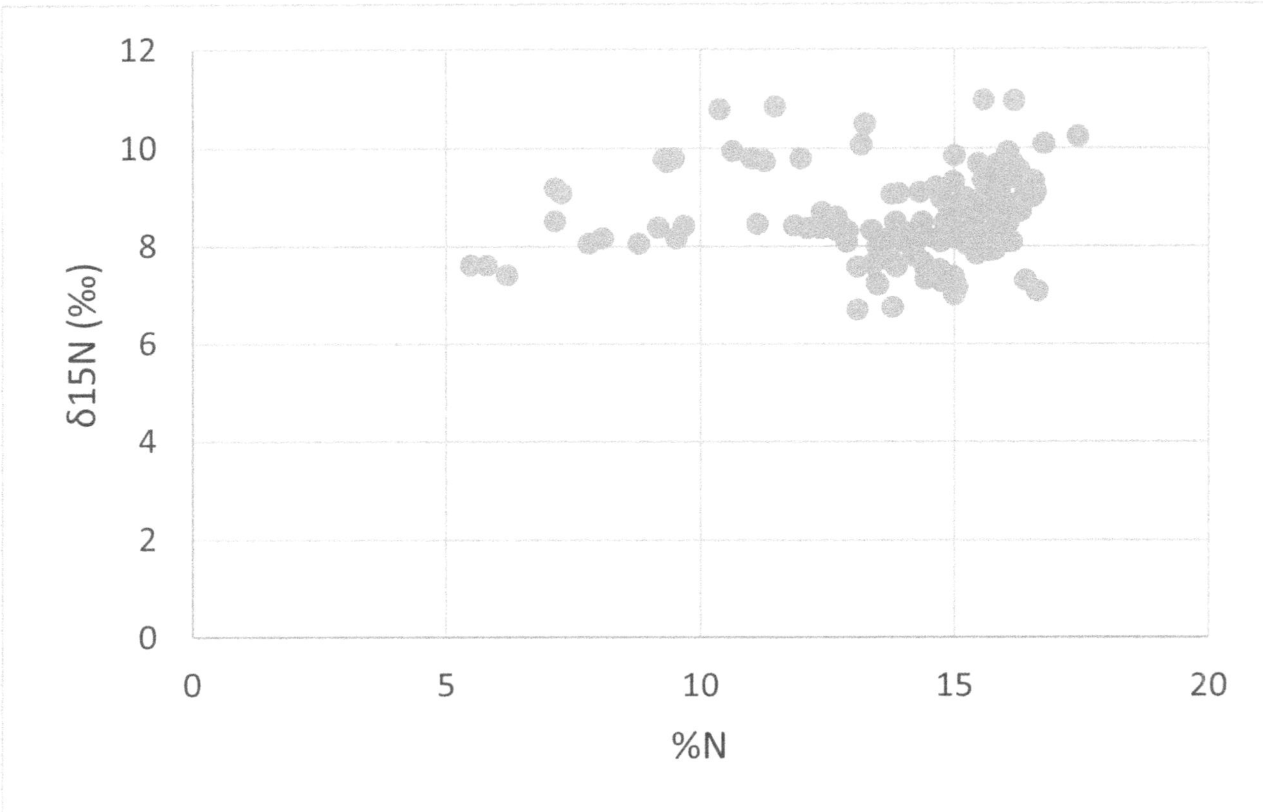

Figure 5.5. Scatter plot showing no correlation between δ^{15}N and %N.

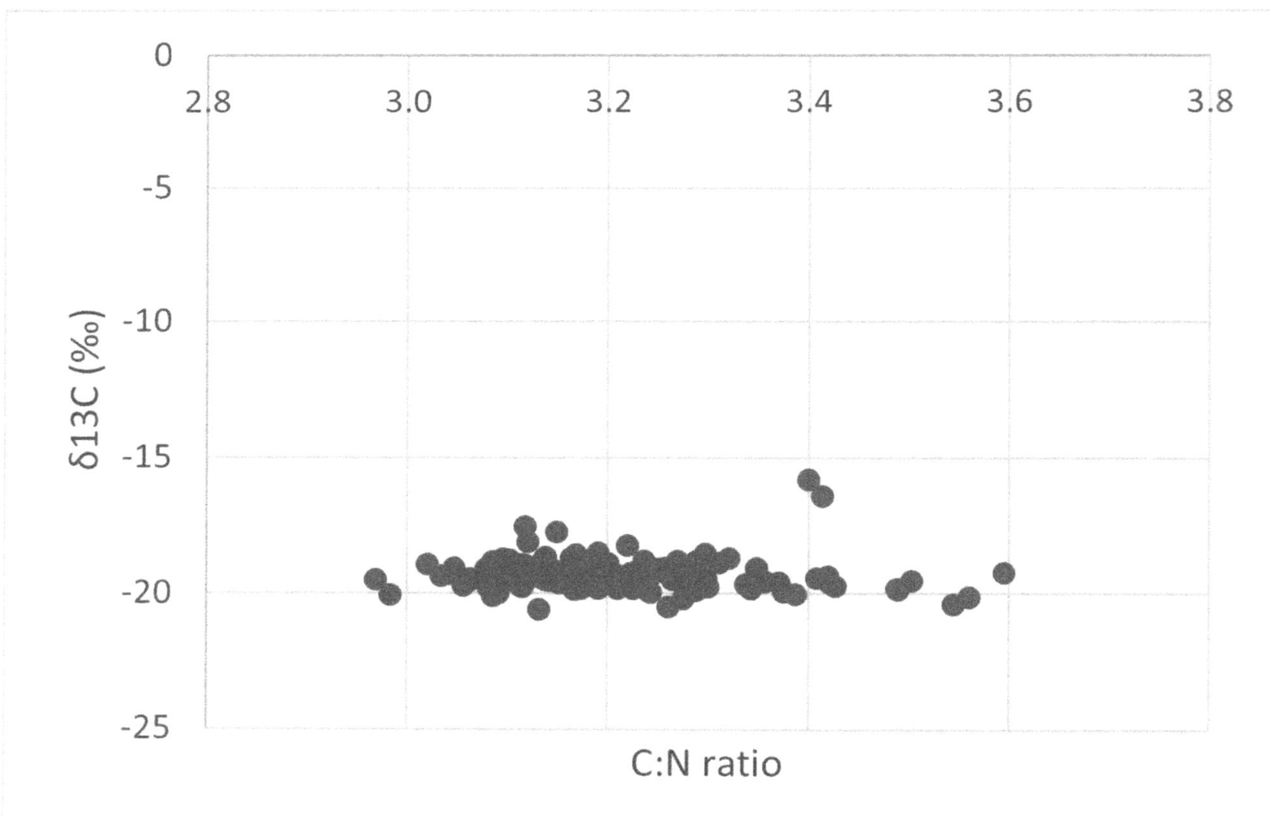

Figure 5.6. Scatter plot showing no correlation between δ^{13}C and C:N ratio.

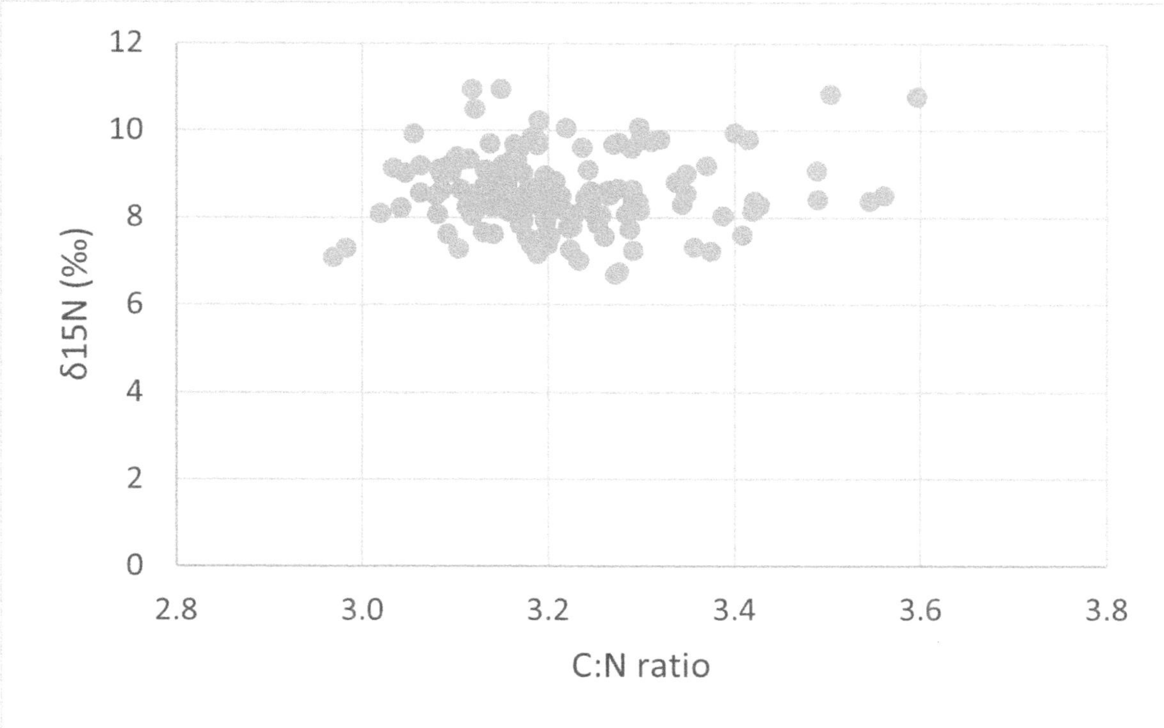

Figure 5.7. Scatter plot showing no correlation between $\delta^{15}N$ and C:N ratio.

Table 5.3. Results of Pearson's correlation coefficient tests with all values *p*>0.05 demonstrating no correlation between the isotopic signatures and the collagen preservation indicators.

	Collagen yield		%C		%N		C:N	
	r	*p*	r	*p*	r	*p*	r	*p*
$\delta^{13}C$	0.077	0.513	0.079	0.505	0.078	0.510	−0.065	0.585
$\delta^{15}N$	0.020	0.866	0.070	0.554	0.059	0.618	0.087	0.460

not account for different faming strategies or certain environmental changes in the Hellenistic, Roman and Late Antique periods. However, plotting these published control samples on the same graph as the present study's samples demonstrates a valid fractionation level between the animal control values and the human values. This suggests that factors, such as manuring crops, which can affect the nitrogen isotope values (Fraser *et al.* 2011; Bogaard *et al.* 2013), were not significantly different across time at the site. The results by Issakidou *et al.* (2022) were only published after the analysis for the present study had been conducted but demonstrate wide-ranging values within the faunal sample, suggesting a wide range of diets for animals in these time periods (Figure 5.8).

Moles *et al.* (2022) presented the human results analysed for this study alongside a variety of plant, terrestrial fauna and fish control samples and other human isotopic results from various periods at Knossos. Samples of human bone from two later Bronze Age cemeteries were analysed by Nafplioti (2015; 2016) and a Subminoan sample was analysed as part of the present study as an intermediate sample linking the earlier and later studies. It was not possible to sample the other intermediate time periods as all human remains from the Early Iron Age are cremations and no graves have been identified for the Archaic or Classical periods. The terrestrial plant and animal controls are outlined above. In the absence of isotopic analysis of fish remains from Knossos a selection of samples of Mediterranean fish of various time periods and locations were included, both modern and archaeological and including marine, euryhaline and freshwater species (Garvie-Lok 2001; Craig *et al.* 2009; Lightfoot *et al.* 2011; 2012; Vika and Theodoropoulou 2012). These fish values are outlined in Appendix C Table 3. Figure 5.9 summarises these results as mean values with standard deviations and Figure 5.10 displays these same summary values for only the human values. All the mean values (apart from for the Late Antique $\delta^{15}N$) are intermediate between the two Bronze Age sample sets, demonstrating that diet was much more variable in the Bronze Age samples compared to the historic periods. The Late Antique mean $\delta^{15}N$ is the most elevated value demonstrating the greatest access in this time period to high trophic level protein.

The high $\delta^{15}N$ values of the Neolithic free-threshing wheat samples demonstrate intensive manuring in this period. The Bronze Age $\delta^{15}N$ cereal values demonstrate more moderate manuring than in the Neolithic but with the $\delta^{15}C$ values suggesting a more intensive water management strategy. The legumes have lower $\delta^{15}N$ values, typical of nitrogen fixers, but with values about 0‰, these results are also consistent with manuring (Nitsch *et al.* 2019). If this level of intensive cultivation strategy involving manuring continued into the Hellenistic, Roman and Late Antique periods, some of the samples with lower $\delta^{15}N$ values may indicate individuals with relatively little animal protein in their diets. Some of the terrestrial fauna values have a lower mean $\delta^{15}N$ value than the contemporary cereals, indicating that this sample of livestock were not raised on manured cereals. If the Hellenistic, Roman and Late Antique livestock values were similar to these, the present sample human values would indicate that most individuals had some terrestrial animal foods in their diets.

5.3.1. Time period

Figure 5.11 plots $\delta^{13}C$ against $\delta^{15}N$ to show the values for each individual sampled for the different time periods. It also shows that the human values are more elevated than the control sample of local animal values. Most of the human samples likely demonstrate some meat consumption and the higher level of elevation in some isotopic values may indicate some marine food consumption. However, the wide-ranging terrestrial animal values may indicate that some individuals in the Hellenistic and Roman periods with $\delta^{15}N$ values similar to some of the herbivorous fauna

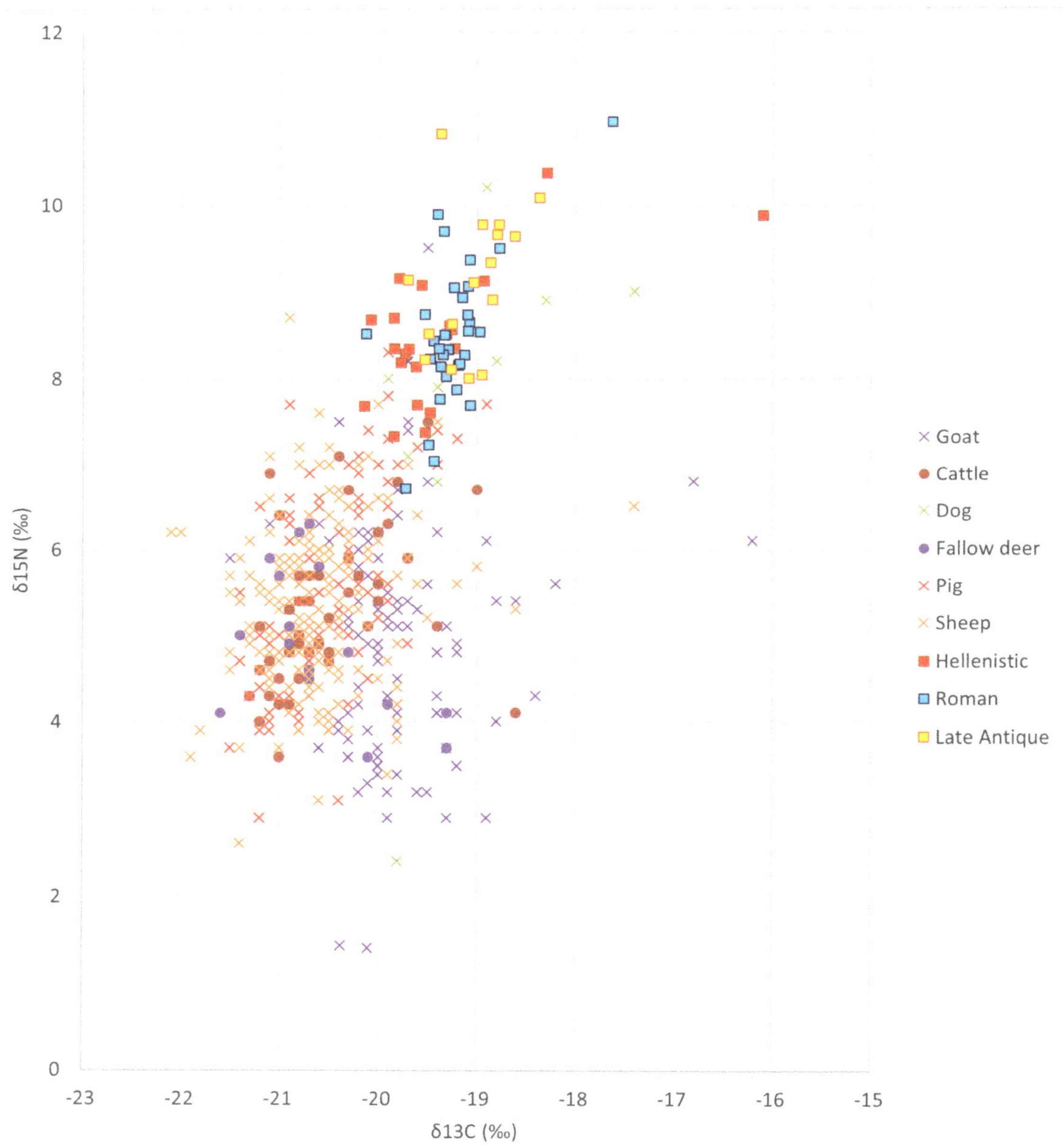

Figure 5.8. Scatter plot displaying stable carbon and nitrogen isotope values for the humans (squares) plotted by time period, using Neolithic and Bronze Age terrestrial fauna (Issakidou *et al.* 2022) as a control sample.

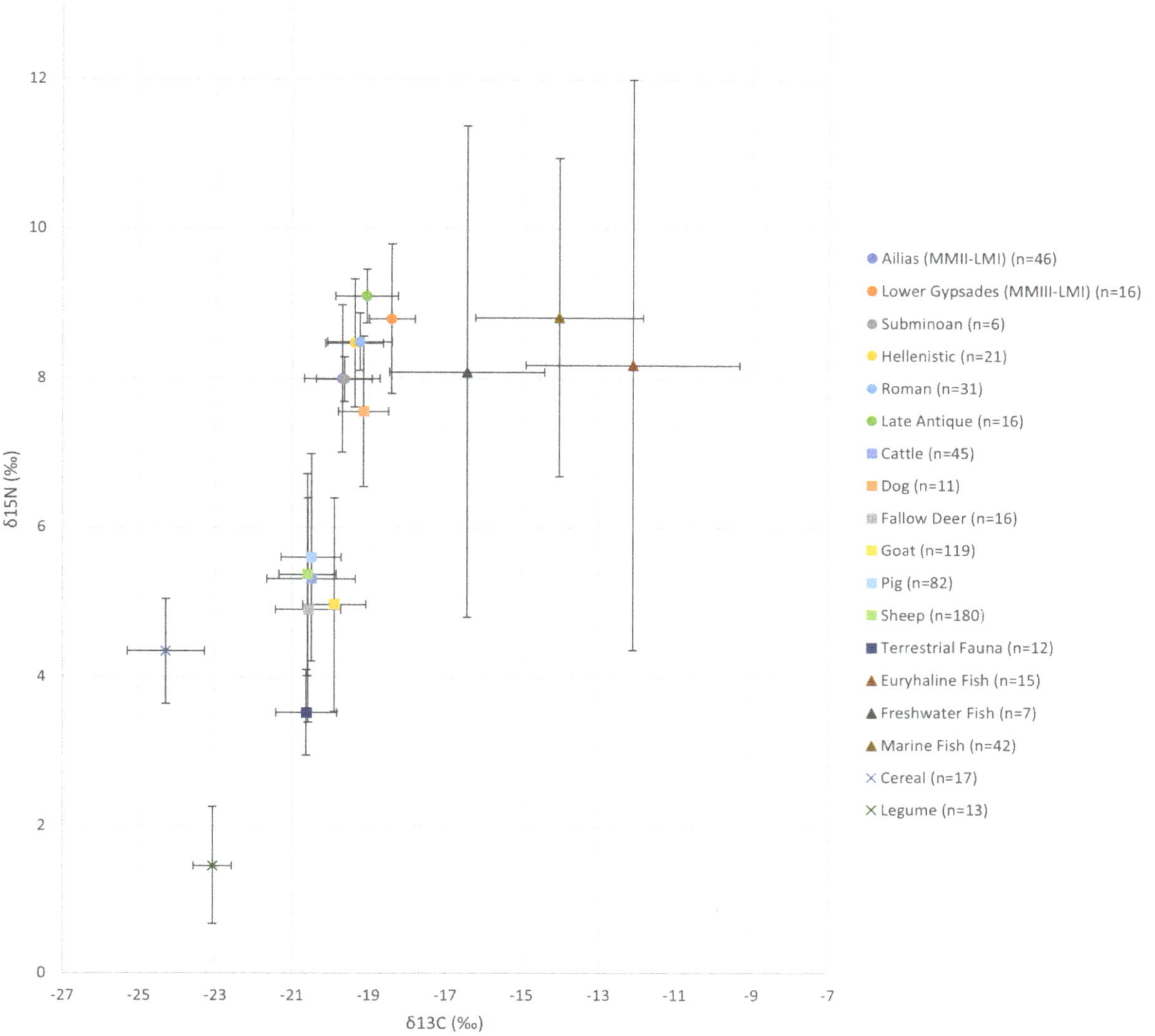

Figure 5.9. Scatter plot of mean isotope values with standard deviation bars for humans (circles) from different time periods at Knossos, terrestrial livestock (squares) of various species from Neolithic and Bronze Age Knossos (Issakidou *et al* 2022) and the 12 control samples originally used for comparison from Bronze Age Knossos (Nafplioti 2016), charred plants largely from Bronze Age Knossos but including four Neolithic samples (Nitsch *et al.* 2019), and a selection of Mediterranean fish values: the same as those displayed in Moles *et al.* (2022) and outlined in Appendix C Table 3.

may have had largely plant based diets (Figure 5.8). The results by time period are summarised in Table 5.4.

The animal samples have a wide range of variation, with some extremely low values (e.g. a sheep/goat with $\delta^{15}N$ 2‰), possibly suggesting the inclusion of legumes in some fodder. The wide-ranging values of the sheep and goat samples in particular may be due to a greater variability in diet due to a wider geographical range for these animals. The pig diets may reflect a mixture of some herbivorous and some omnivorous diets. The Unexplored Mansion Roman animal bone assemblage indicates sheep/goat was the main meat source, therefore this can account for some of the variability in the human values. Archaic law inscriptions

Table 5.4. Summary of isotopic values for each time period.

	n	Mean $\delta^{13}C$ (‰)	Lowest $\delta^{13}C$ (‰)	Highest $\delta^{13}C$ (‰)	$\delta^{13}C$ SD	Mean $\delta^{15}N$ (‰)	Lowest $\delta^{15}N$ (‰)	Highest $\delta^{15}N$ (‰)	$\delta^{15}N$ SD
Hellenistic	21	−19.4	−20.1	−16.1	±0.9	8.5	7.3	10.4	±0.8
Roman	31	−19.2	−20.1	−17.6	±0.4	8.5	6.7	11.0	±0.8
Late Antique	16	−19.1	−19.7	−18.4	±0.4	9.1	8.0	10.8	±0.8

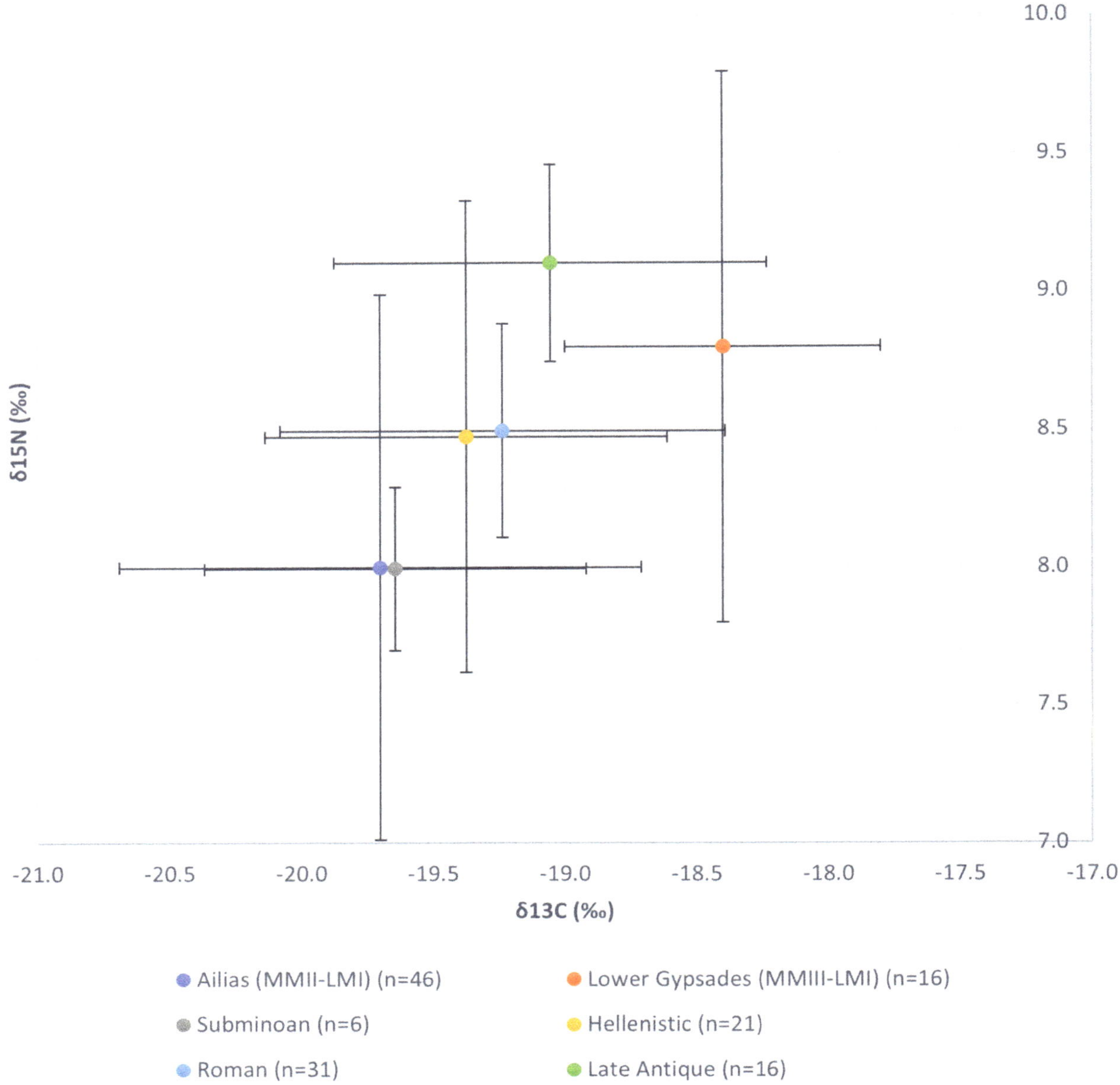

Figure 5.10. Scatter plot of mean human isotope values with standard deviation bars for different time periods at Knossos.

from Crete indicate widespread grazing with treaties between city-states for access to upland grazing, which could account for varied diets amongst livestock (Chaniotis 1999, 192–97; Gagarin and Perlman 2016, 42, 104).

The picture is generally one of increasing values over time for both $\delta^{13}C$ and $\delta^{15}N$, though the overlapping confidence intervals in Figures 5.12–13 illustrate no significant difference between the mean values. The Roman sample has more extreme lowest and highest $\delta^{15}N$ values, demonstrating a wider range of values than in the Hellenistic period. The difference between the median $\delta^{13}C$ values for the three time periods was highly significant (Kruskal-Wallis: $H=13.51$, $p=0.001$). Using the same test for the three sets of $\delta^{15}N$ values, the difference between the medians was not significant ($H=5.39$, $p=0.068$). However, the Late Antique mean $\delta^{15}N$ is substantially (0.6‰) higher and this proved to be highly significant using a t-test of equal means, compared to the earlier periods combined ($t=2.67$, $p=0.009$). Additionally, a Mann-Whitney pairwise test demonstrated significant differences between Hellenistic and Late Antique ($p=0.043$) and between Roman and Late Antique ($p=0.036$) $\delta^{15}N$ values. This sort of margin can be regarded as substantial considering the generally limited variation, with almost all values within a range that suggests a C3 terrestrial diet, largely with adequate access to animal products. Some of the lowest values, particularly for $\delta^{15}N$, may represent diets less rich in meat and, for these individuals, dietary protein may occasionally have been obtained from plant sources.

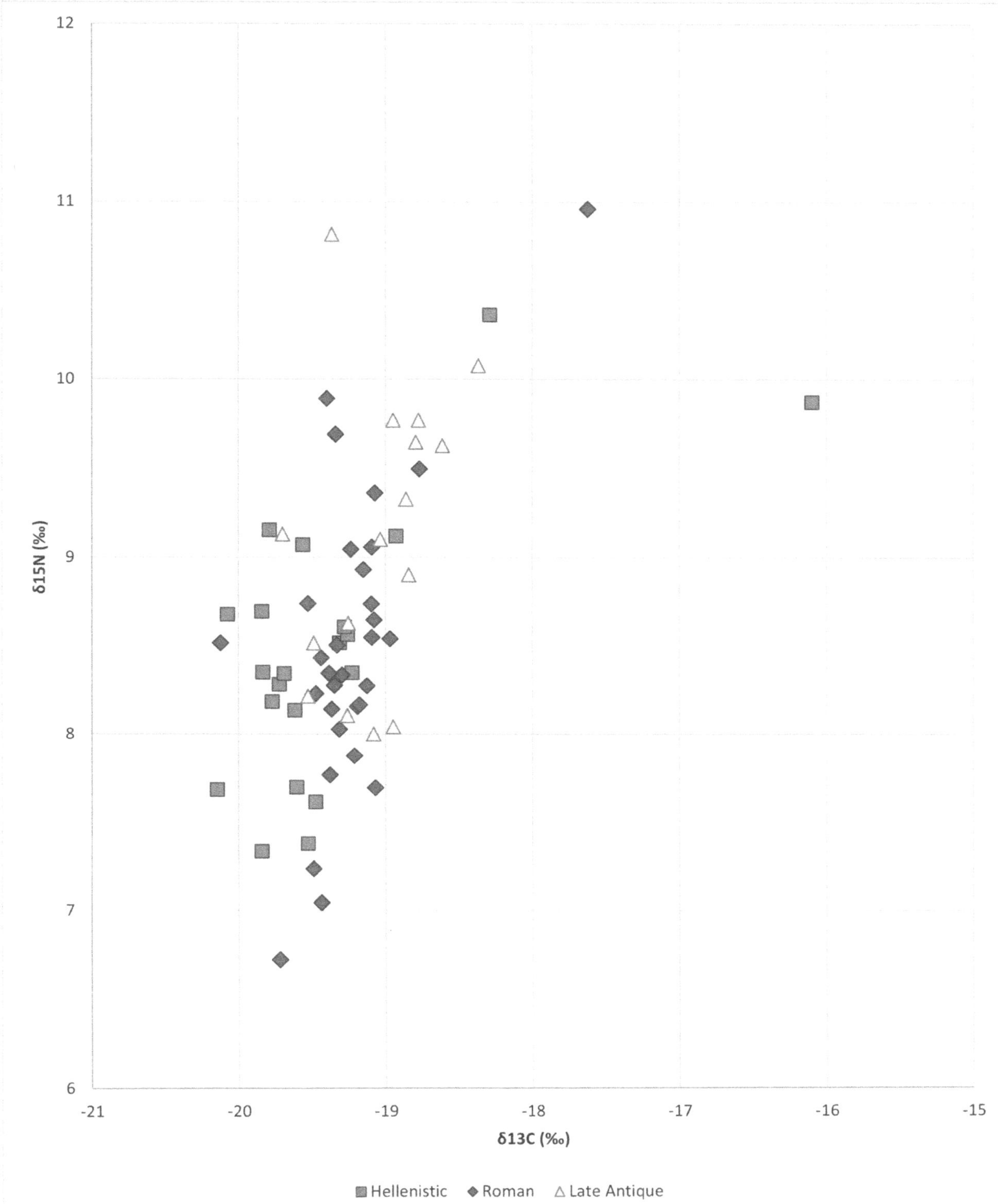

Figure 5.11. Scatter plot of isotope values for each time period.

There are only two Hellenistic samples with $\delta^{15}N$ values over 9.2‰. The Roman samples are not significantly different from the Hellenistic samples in terms of $\delta^{15}N$ values ($t=0.096$, $p=0.92$), with the majority lying between 8–9‰ but with six less elevated values and seven more elevated values. However, in terms of $\delta^{13}C$ values, the Roman samples are consistently slightly more positive. This was not statistically significant for a test of equal means, probably due to outlier Hellenistic values with higher carbon isotope values, but when tests for equal medians and variances were run the difference in $\delta^{13}C$ values between the Hellenistic and Roman groups proved to be statistically highly significant (Mann-Whitney test for equal medians: $U=176.5$, $p=0.006$; F-test for equal

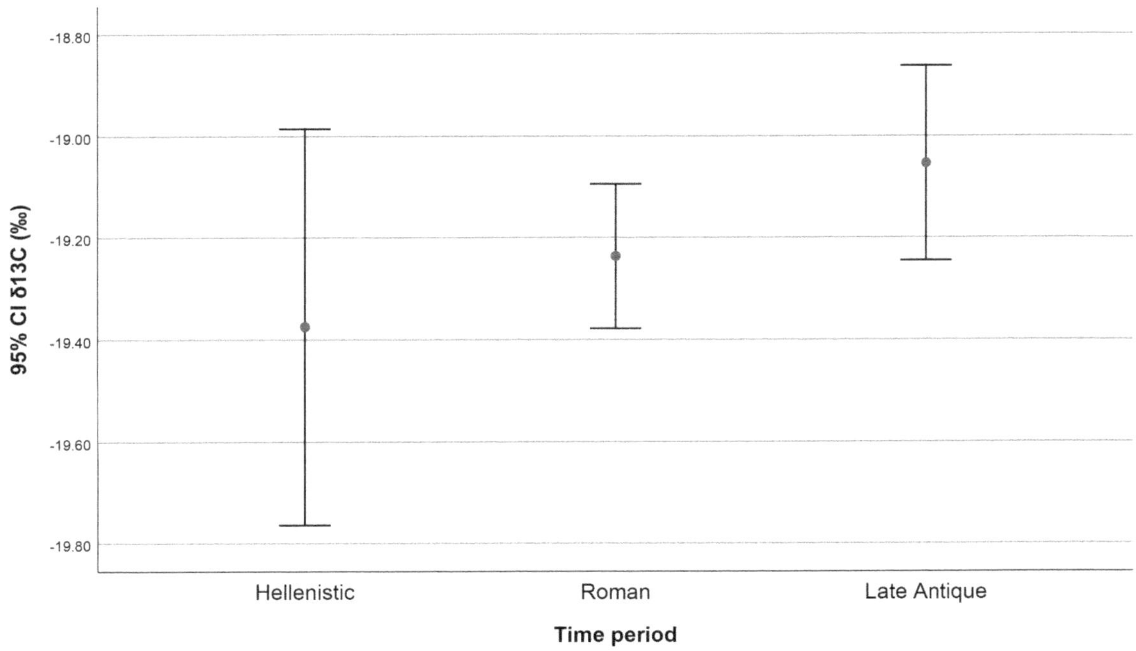

Figure 5.12. Error bar plot demonstrating mean $\delta^{13}C$ values with 95% confidence intervals for each time period.

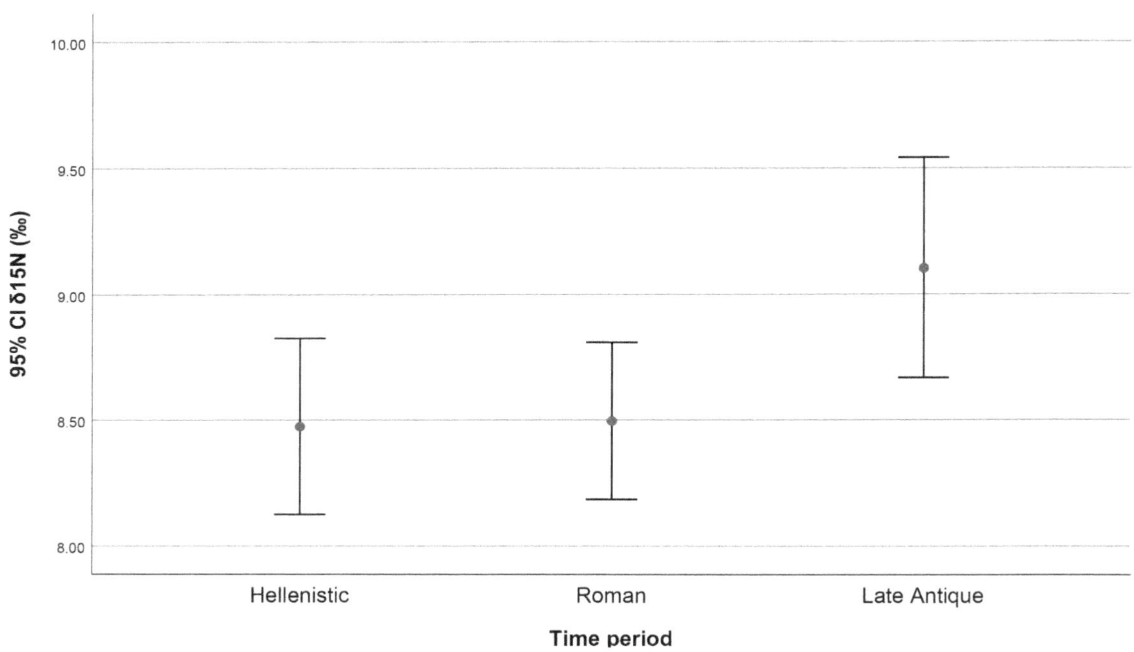

Figure 5.13. Error bar plot demonstrating mean $\delta^{15}N$ values with 95% confidence intervals for each time period.

variances: F=4.89, p=0.000). This elevation in $\delta^{13}C$ values could be due to a small amount of C4 crops being introduced into either animal or human diets, low trophic level fish or small amounts of fish consumption, or could be a variation in the type of meat being consumed or type of feed the livestock are getting. The Late Antique samples are more elevated in both $\delta^{13}C$ and $\delta^{15}N$ compared to both the Hellenistic and Roman samples. None of the Late Antique samples have $\delta^{15}N$ values lower than 8‰ and over half the values are higher than 9‰. Only four samples overall had $\delta^{15}N$ values over 10‰ and two of these were from the Late Antique period. This suggests that all the individuals in the Late Antique sample had ample quantities of meat or animal products to satisfy the body's protein requirements and some were also consuming fish.

There are two outliers that appear to have had a sizable fish component in their diets. The individual with the most elevated carbon signal (S22: −16.09, 9.87), was a Young Adult of Unknown sex, buried in a Late Hellenistic tile grave in the area of the North Cemetery excavated in 1976 as part of the Venezelion North Perimeter (VNP/76) excavations. Unfortunately, the other sample taken from the neighbouring tile grave to this one did not have sufficient collagen preservation for the result to be viable. These tombs were thought to have been Roman at the time of excavation but a more recent examination of the pottery reveals nothing convincingly Roman, therefore it is likely to have been a Late Hellenistic burial (Trainor, personal communication).

The other outlier who was consuming a significant amount of fish (S31: −17.62, 10.96), was a Young Adult Female, buried in a Roman rock-cut chamber tomb excavated next to the Sanatorium Basilica by Mervyn Popham in 1961 (KSM/61). Four other samples were taken from individuals in the same tomb, who all have remarkably similar isotope values to each other, but dramatically different to this outlier, implying C3 terrestrial diets that included meat consumption but with no significant contribution from marine resources. The fact that only one out of five analysed individuals, buried in the KSM/61 Roman rock-cut chamber tomb, had fish in her diet, suggests that it was unlikely to be social status that allowed her access to seafood, or at least not solely so. For both these outliers, it may have been personal preference that resulted in seafood consumption, or that they were relatively recent incomers to Knossos, having come from somewhere where seafood played a greater role in the general diet. The latter theory could be tested using other isotopic methods, such as strontium and oxygen isotope analysis.

Often there exists no further dating information for particular tombs beyond the general time period. However, where closer dating was available, these tombs have been assigned to narrower time periods and plotted on the following graphs in various combinations to try and see if the general pattern of more elevated values (and potentially increased meat and fish consumption) over time holds up when explored in more detail.

There are only 3 samples in the Hellenistic group that could be more closely dated and these were all Late Hellenistic. Therefore, unfortunately, no comparison over time within the Hellenistic period was possible. Comparing the Late Hellenistic to the Early Roman and subsequent time periods may also be fruitless due to the small sample size and the one (fish-eating) outlier elevating the mean values. There was no significant difference between the Hellenistic (as a whole) and Early Roman mean $\delta^{13}C$ values (Mann-Whitney: U=104.5, p=0.09). However, the difference between the Hellenistic (9.1‰) and Early Roman (8.3‰) $\delta^{15}N$ means was statistically significant (t-test: t=2.49, p=0.02), demonstrating that the elevated Late Roman values had cancelled out the more depleted Early Roman. This shows a pattern opposite to what was observed for the broader time periods of a general elevation in values and demonstrates less protein consumption in the Early Roman period compared to the Hellenistic period. These narrower time periods are defined as follows:

Early Hellenistic:	Late 4th-3rd century BC
Late Hellenistic:	2nd-1st century BC
Early Roman:	1st- 2nd century AD
Late Roman:	3rd-4th century AD
Late Antique (Early):	5th-early 6th century AD
Late Antique (Late):	Late 6th-7th century AD

The mean carbon and nitrogen values for the narrower time periods (Table 5.5 and Figures 5.14–17) support the trend of values becoming more elevated over time. An exception to the trend is the difference in mean $\delta^{13}C$ values between the Late Roman and Late Antique (Early) but this is a negligible difference of 0.1‰ and generally the $\delta^{13}C$ values are very similar. The trend is more noticeable in the mean nitrogen isotope values rising from 8.3‰ in the Early Roman to 9.1‰ in the Late Antique (Late). Figure 5.17 (which removes the 'noise' created by the samples with only more general time period in Figure 5.14 does not show any clear trend of elevation of values over time. The Early Roman samples are the most scattered and are particularly wide ranging in their nitrogen values. The Early Roman carbon values are all on the lower end of the scale, although when compared with the Hellenistic values, seen most clearly on the Hellenistic-Roman scatter graph (Figure 5.15), they are not quite so depleted in $\delta^{13}C$, demonstrating that this shift occurs between the Hellenistic and Early Roman phases (potentially in the Late Hellenistic or Early Roman periods).

The Late Roman samples have some overlap with the Early Roman samples, but generally demonstrate a trend of elevation in both carbon and nitrogen from the Early to Late Roman periods. This is supported by elevation in the mean $\delta^{13}C$ and $\delta^{15}N$ values, which are −19.2‰ and 8.8‰ for the Late Roman samples, though the difference was not statistically significant as indicated by t-tests

Table 5.5. Descriptive statistics for $\delta^{13}C$ and $\delta^{15}N$ values for each narrowly defined time period.

Time period	*n*	Mean $\delta^{13}C$ ‰	Lowest $\delta^{13}C$ ‰	Highest $\delta^{13}C$ ‰	$\delta^{13}C$ s.d.	Mean $\delta^{15}N$ ‰	Lowest $\delta^{15}N$ ‰	Highest $\delta^{15}N$ ‰	$\delta^{15}N$ s.d.
Late Hellenistic	3	−18.2	−19.3	−16.1	±1.8	9.0	8.5	9.9	±0.8
Early Roman	15	−19.4	−20.1	−19.0	±0.3	8.3	6.7	9.9	±0.9
Late Roman	8	−19.2	−19.4	−18.8	±0.2	8.7	8.3	9.5	±0.5
Late Antique (Early)	5	−19.3	−19.7	−18.8	±0.4	9.0	8.0	10.8	±1.1
Late Antique (Late)	7	−19.0	−19.5	−18.6	±0.3	9.1	8.1	9.8	±0.7

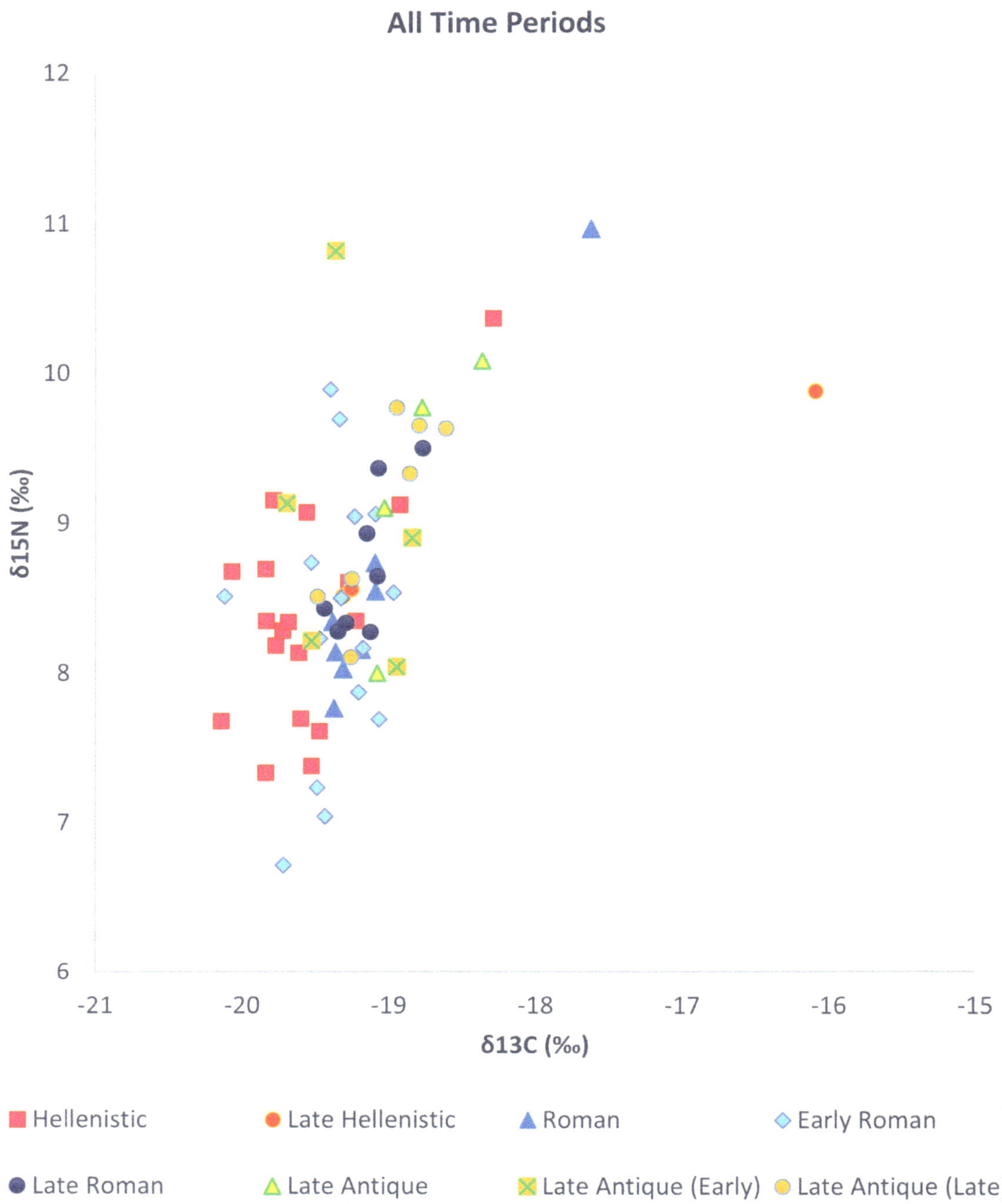

Figure 5.14. Scatter plot of isotope values for each time period, including the more narrowly defined periods where more specific dating was possible.

($\delta^{13}C$: t=−1.68, p=0.11; $\delta^{15}N$: t=−1.15, p=0.26) and the overlapping confidence intervals in Figure 5.18 and Figure 5.19. There does not appear to be a clear pattern of attributes for which Early Roman samples are most elevated. Taking the nine Early Roman samples with both $\delta^{13}C$ values over −19.5‰ and $\delta^{15}N$ over 8‰, both male and females represented and both chamber tombs and built tombs (the only two tomb types represented in the Early Roman sample) from locations north and south of the valley (North Cemetery, Topana, Monastiriako Kephali and Spilia) and there were other samples from these same tombs and same cemeteries with less elevated values. The four of these Early Roman samples with $\delta^{15}N$ values over 9‰, similarly come from a range of tomb types and locations, and males and females are equally represented.

There is a less significant difference for the Late Roman to Late Antique (Early), with a slight decrease in the $\delta^{13}C$ value to 19.3‰ but an elevation in the $\delta^{15}N$ to 8‰. The decrease in carbon values can be explained by two 'outliers' on the Late Roman-Late Antique scatter plot (Figure 5.16). It is always necessary to bear in mind that

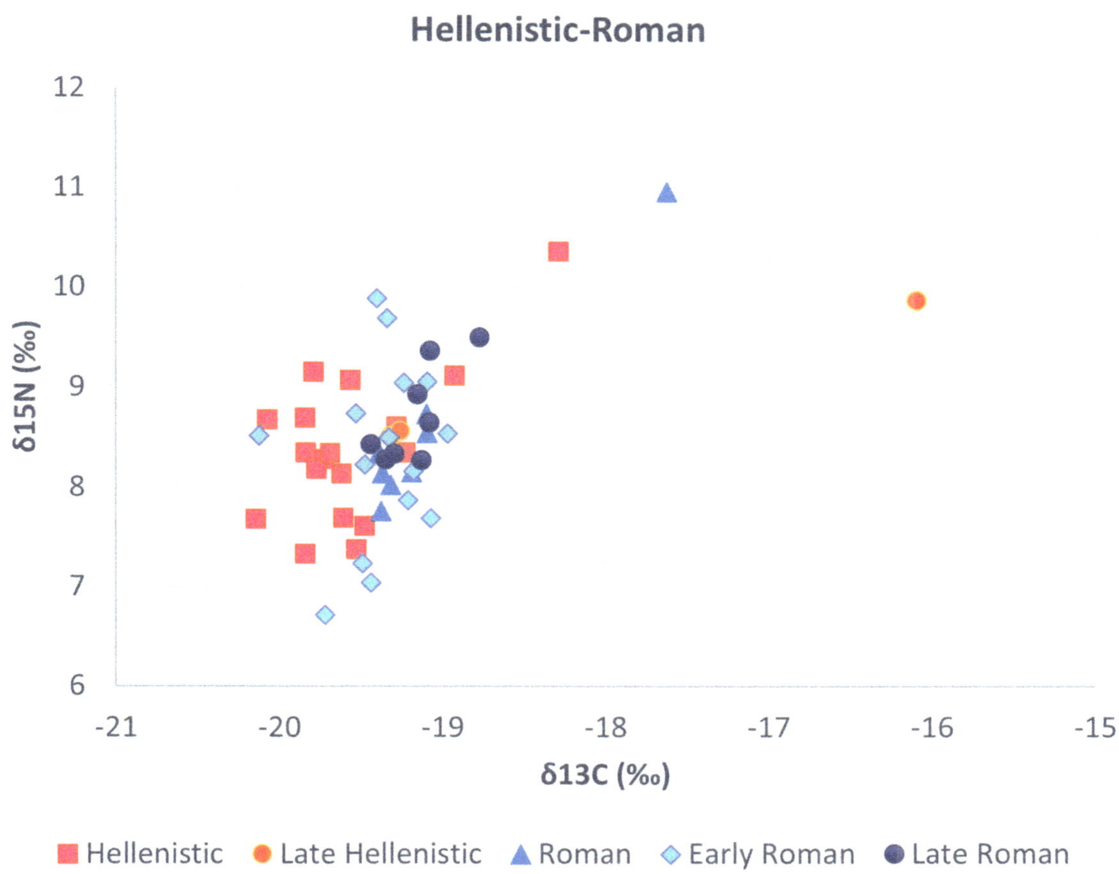

Figure 5.15. Scatter plot of isotope values for the Hellenistic and Roman time periods.

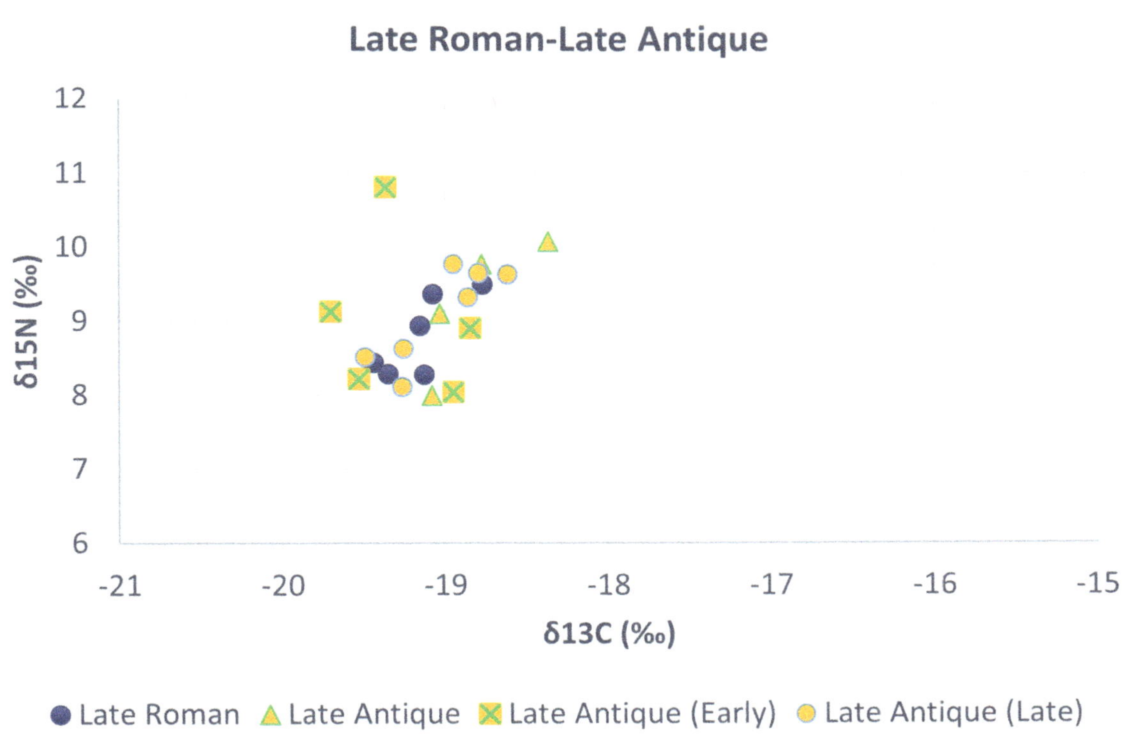

Figure 5.16. Scatter plot of isotope values for the Late Roman and Late Antique time periods.

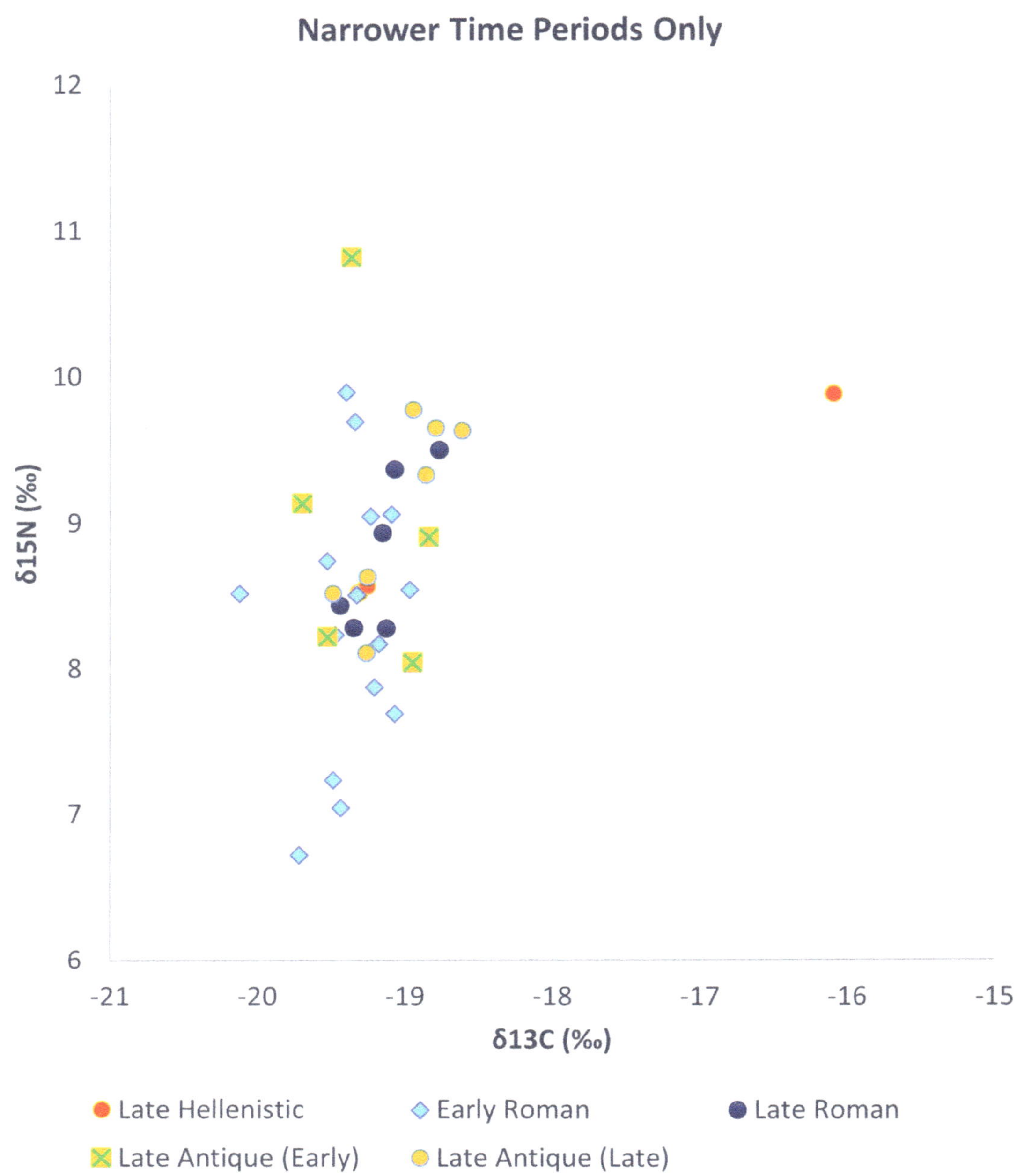

Figure 5.17. Scatter plot of isotope values for only the more narrowly defined time periods.

these could be skewed values as both these samples had poor structural integrity during collagen extraction while in acid and low collagen yields, though both were deemed to have acceptable preservation levels by all other indicators. Additionally, these are not truly outliers when looked at with all the results present, as there are many Hellenistic and Early Roman values that are similar. This is particularly true for S84 ($\delta^{13}C$ −19.7‰, $\delta^{15}N$ 9.1‰); whereas S78 ($\delta^{13}C$ −19.4‰, $\delta^{15}N$ 10.8‰) has a markedly high nitrogen value without a high carbon value that might be expected from the general correlation and is a more distinctive value. The general trend from Late Roman to Late Antique (Early, Late and unspecified), as observed from Figure 5.16, is that values again are increasingly elevated with relatively more values above the −19‰ line for $\delta^{13}C$ and the 9‰ line for $\delta^{15}N$. The mean values continue to demonstrate a trend of elevation from the Late Antique (Early) to Late Antique (Late) with the mean $\delta^{13}C$ at −19‰ and the mean $\delta^{15}N$ at 9.1‰. This was not statistically significant ($\delta^{13}C$: t=−1.25, p=0.24; $\delta^{15}N$: t=−0.14, p=0.89), which may be because the sample size was small.

Therefore, this more detailed analysis of the trend over time, using narrower time periods, supports the more general picture observed from the analysis using the broader time periods of a gradual elevation of both carbon

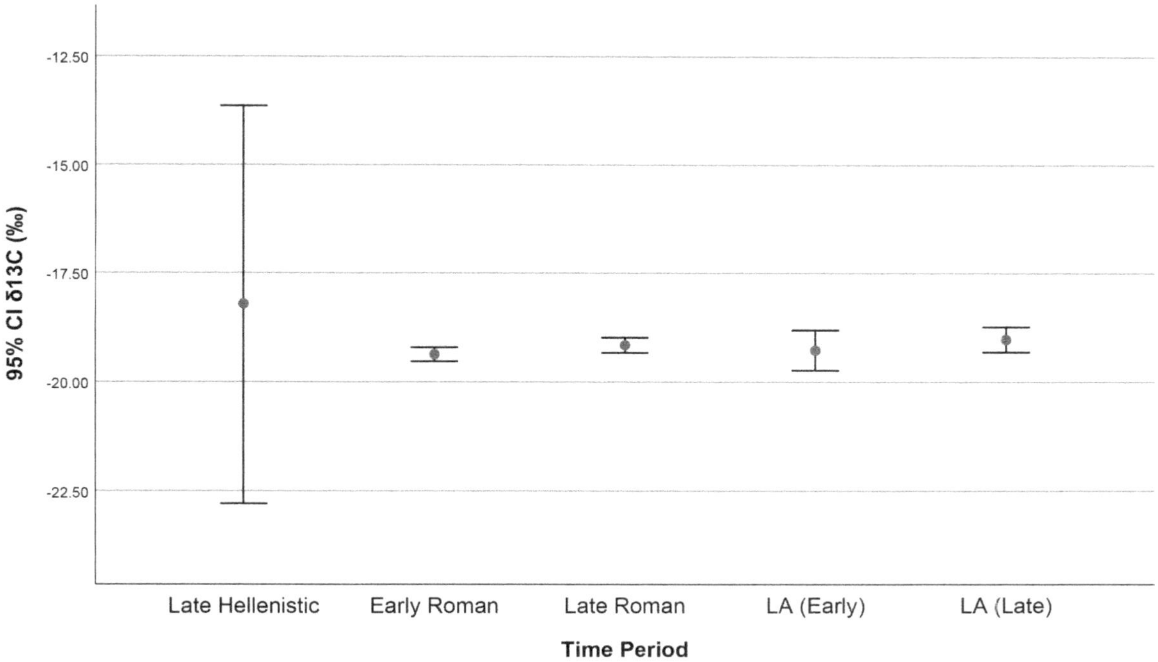

Figure 5.18. Error bar plot demonstrating mean $\delta^{13}C$ values with 95% confidence intervals for each narrowly defined time period.

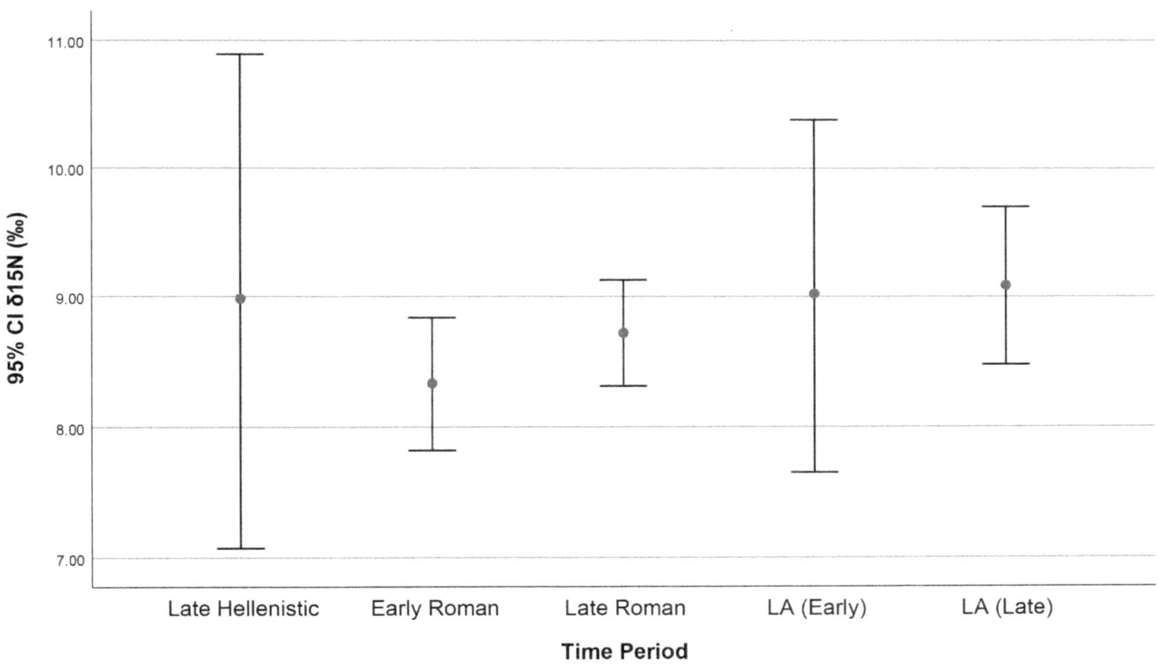

Figure 5.19. Error bar plot demonstrating mean $\delta^{15}N$ values with 95% confidence intervals for each narrowly defined time period.

and nitrogen values over time. This suggests that with the progressive reduction in settlement and population size, and potentially the coincident reduction of urban pressures on resources and distribution of food, there was an increase in meat or other animal products in people's diets.

5.3.2. Sex

Summary $\delta^{13}C$ and $\delta^{15}N$ values are laid out in Table 5.6 for females and males, which demonstrate that the mean $\delta^{13}C$ and $\delta^{15}N$ values are almost identical. The female samples have a much broader range of values for both carbon and nitrogen isotopes, demonstrating that across the sample, female diets were more variable, though tests for equal variances were not statistically significant ($\delta^{13}C$: F=1.68, p=0.15; $\delta^{15}N$: F=1.8, p=0.1). There are twice the number of females (n=8) as there are males (n=4) with $\delta^{15}N$ values below 8.0‰. This demonstrates fewer male diets with these low nitrogen values that may suggest lower levels of animal products in these diets. There are also more

Table 5.6. Descriptive statistics for $\delta^{13}C$ and $\delta^{15}N$ values for females and males.

	n	Mean $\delta^{13}C$ (‰)	Lowest $\delta^{13}C$ ‰	Highest $\delta^{13}C$ ‰	$\delta^{13}C$ St.Dev.	Mean $\delta^{15}N$ ‰	Lowest $\delta^{15}N$ ‰	Highest $\delta^{15}N$ ‰	$\delta^{15}N$ St.Dev
Female	35	−19.3	−20.1	−17.6	±0.5	8.6	6.7	11.0	±1.0
Male	31	−19.3	−19.8	−18.3	±0.4	8.6	7.2	10.4	±0.7

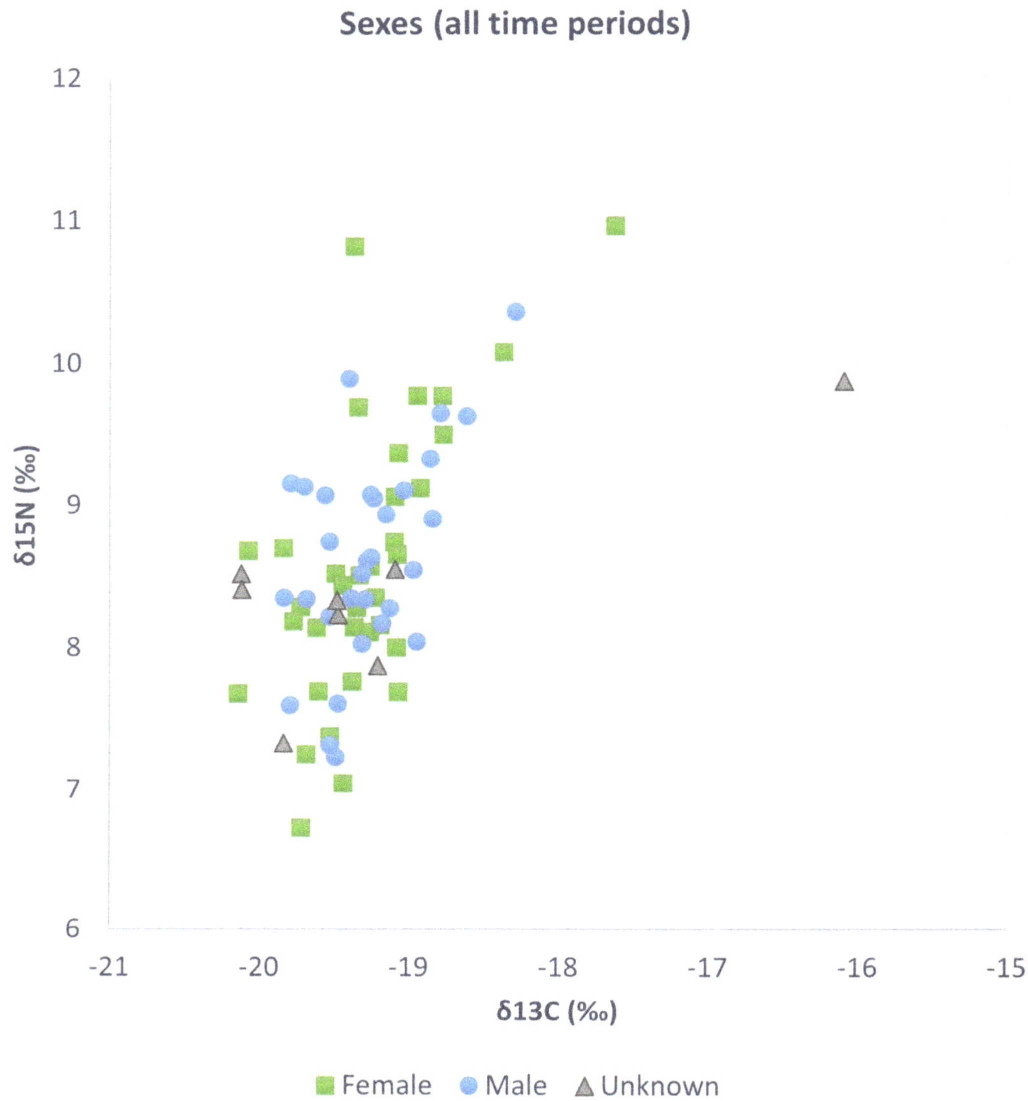

Figure 5.20: Scatter plot of isotope values for the sexes.

Table 5.7. Descriptive statistics for $\delta^{13}C$ and $\delta^{15}N$ values for females and males within each time period.

	n	Mean $\delta^{13}C$ ‰	Lowest $\delta^{13}C$ ‰	Highest $\delta^{13}C$ ‰	$\delta^{13}C$ s.d.	Mean $\delta^{15}N$ ‰	Lowest $\delta^{15}N$ ‰	Highest $\delta^{15}N$ ‰	$\delta^{15}N$ s.d.
Hellenistic Females	11	−19.6	−20.1	−18.9	±0.4	8.3	7.4	9.1	±0.5
Hellenistic Males	8	−19.4	−19.8	−18.3	±0.5	8.8	7.6	10.4	±0.8
Roman Females	16	−19.1	−19.7	−17.6	±0.5	8.5	6.7	11.0	±1.0
Roman Males	11	−19.3	−19.5	−19.0	±0.2	8.5	7.2	9.9	±0.7
Late Antique Females	7	−19.0	−19.5	−18.4	±0.4	9.3	8.0	10.8	±1.1
Late Antique Males	9	−19.1	−19.7	−18.6	±0.4	9.0	8.0	9.6	±0.6

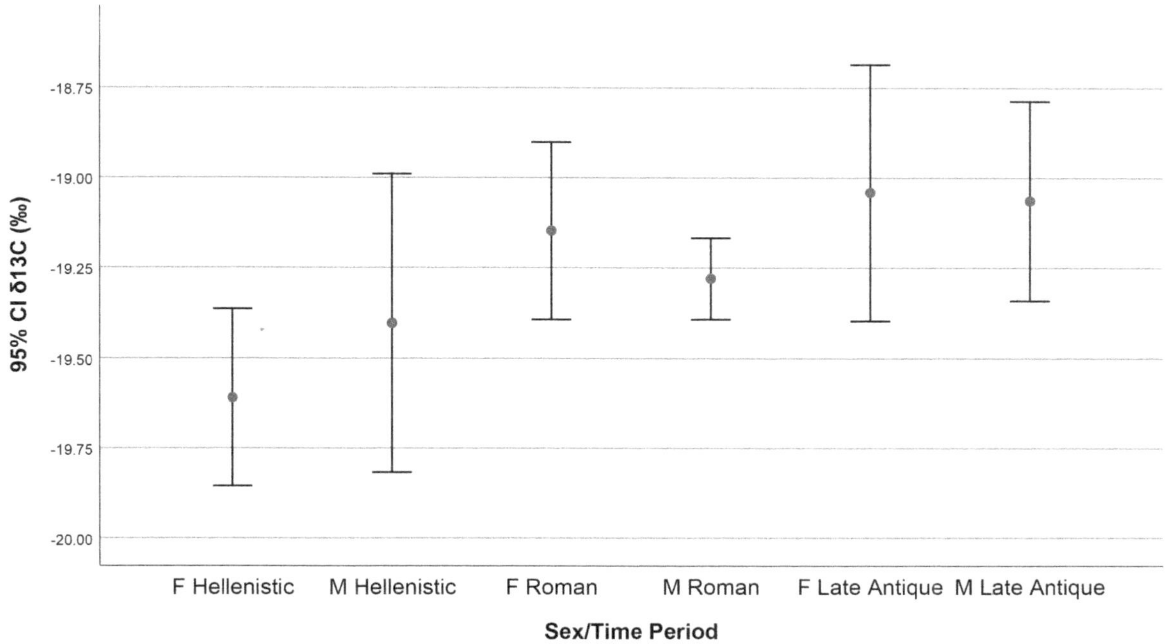

Figure 5.21. Error bar plot showing mean δ^{13}C values and 95% confidence intervals for females and males in each time period.

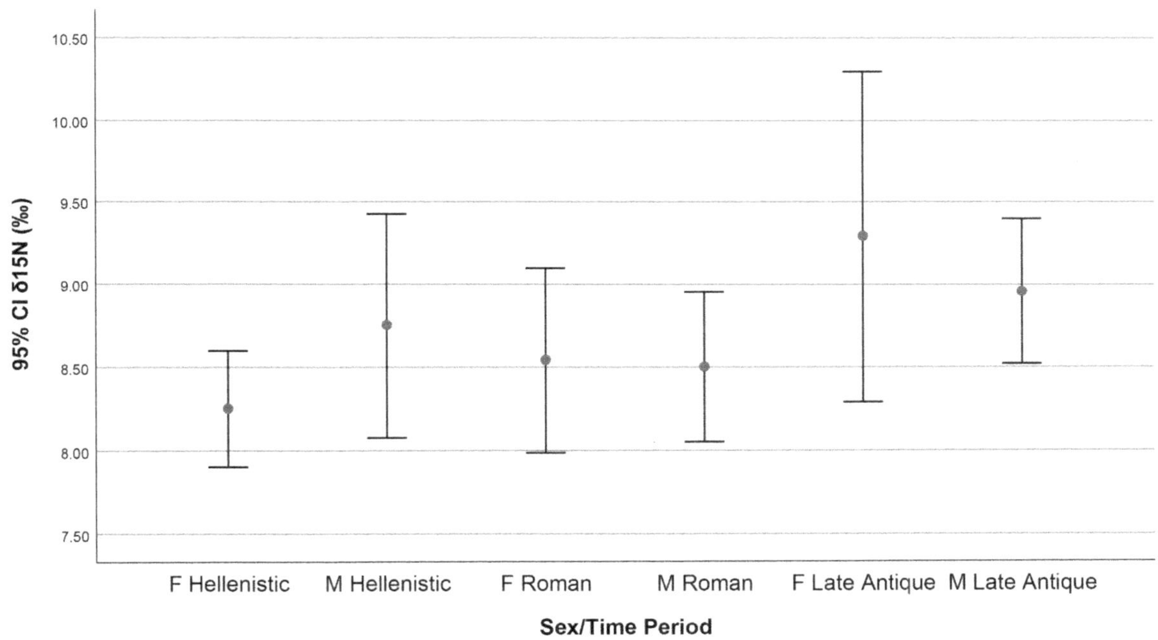

Figure 5.22. Error bar plot showing mean δ^{15}N values and 95% confidence intervals for females and males in each time period.

females represented in those samples with δ^{15}N values over 10.0‰, supporting more variation between different female diets.

Looking at sex-specific change over time, the same pattern of slight elevation of carbon mean values can be observed across the time periods from Hellenistic to Late Antique, though there is substantial overlap of confidence intervals (Figure 5.21). A three-sample test for equal medians showed the difference in female δ^{13}C values was statistically highly significant (Kruskal-Wallis: H=9.71, p=0.0077). Unlike for the female groups, the difference between the male values for δ^{13}C were not significant (Kruskal-Wallis (medians): H=5.58, p=0.06; one-way ANOVA (means): F=2.13, p=0.14). There was an increase in female δ^{15}N values for each time period but the male Roman mean δ^{15}N was lower than for the Hellenistic period and substantial overlap of confidence intervals indicates no significant differences (Figure 5.22).

Looking at time-period-specific differences between the sexes, in each instance the male δ^{13}C values are slightly

Table 5.8. Results from statistical tests comparing isotope values for females and males within each time period.

Female vs. Male						
	$\delta^{13}C$			$\delta^{15}N$		
	T-test (means)	Mann-Whitney (medians)	F-test (variances)	T-test (means)	Mann-Whitney (medians)	F-test (variances)
Hellenistic	t=−1.04 *p*=0.31	U=35.5 *p*=0.51	F=1.85 *p*=0.37	t=−1.65 *p*=0.12	U=27.5 *p*=0.19	F=2.45 *p*=0.19
Roman	t=0.91 *p*=0.37	U=73.5 *p*=0.49	F=7.65 *p*=0.00	t=0.11 *p*=0.91	U=87.5 *p*=1.00	F=2.41 *p*=0.16
Late Antique	t=0.11 *p*=0.91	U=30.5 *p*=0.96	F=1.12 *p*=0.85	t=0.80 *p*=0.44	U=24.0 *p*=0.46	F=3.50 *p*=0.10

higher than the female ones (Figures 5.23–25). More notably, the Hellenistic male mean $\delta^{15}N$ value is 0.5‰ higher than the female mean $\delta^{15}N$ value. The Roman male and female $\delta^{15}N$ mean values are the same, but the Late Antique female $\delta^{15}N$ mean value is 0.3‰ higher than the male mean. These are mostly quite small differences and statistically insignificant (Table 5.8). The difference in mean nitrogen values between Hellenistic males and females is quite sizeable and may indicate that during this time period males often had preferential access to animal products in their diets. However, it is not a statistically significant difference. The only test that showed a significant difference between sex/time period groups was for $\delta^{13}C$ variances between the Roman male and females (shaded in Table 5.8), which was highly significant ($p<0.01$). The Roman female $\delta^{13}C$ mean was higher (−19.1‰) with a larger range (1.7‰) and standard deviation (±0.5‰) than the male equivalents (mean: −19.3‰, range: 0.5‰, standard deviation: ±0.2‰).

5.3.3. Age group

The majority of individuals assigned to specific age groups (as opposed to the general 'Adult' group) are in the Young

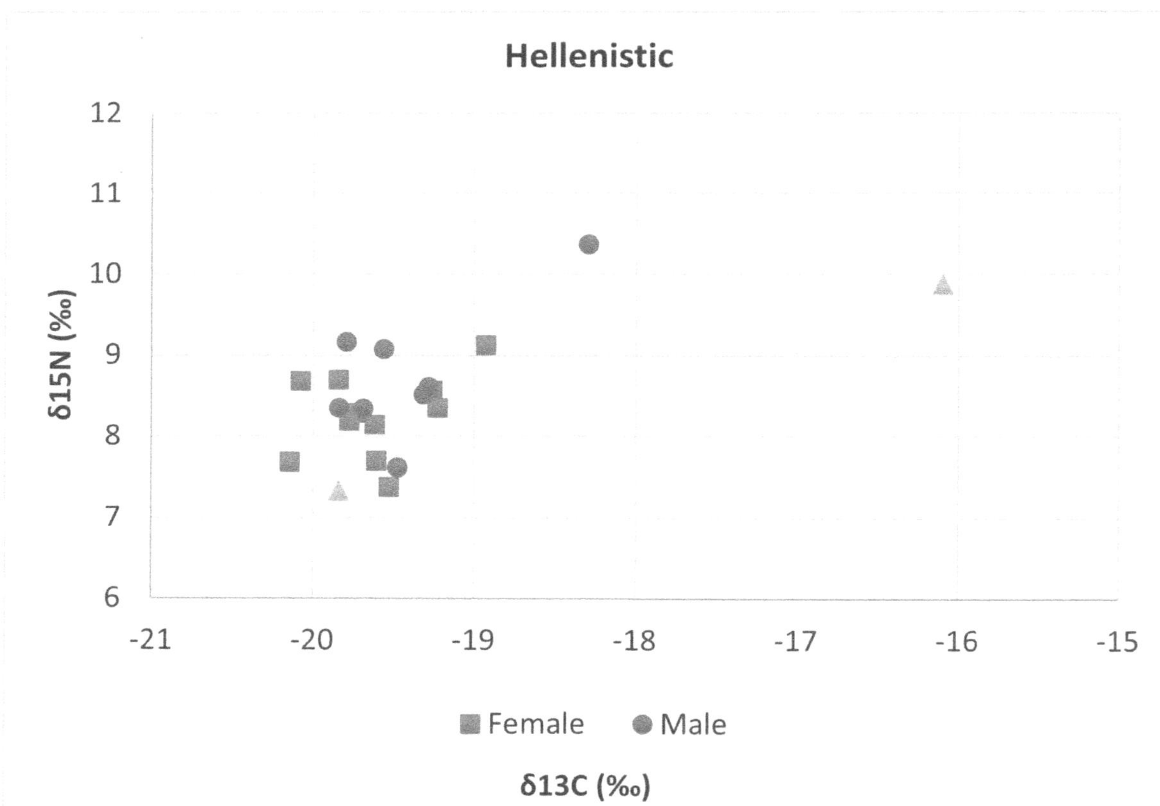

Figure 5.23. Scatter plot of isotope values for the sexes from the Hellenistic period.

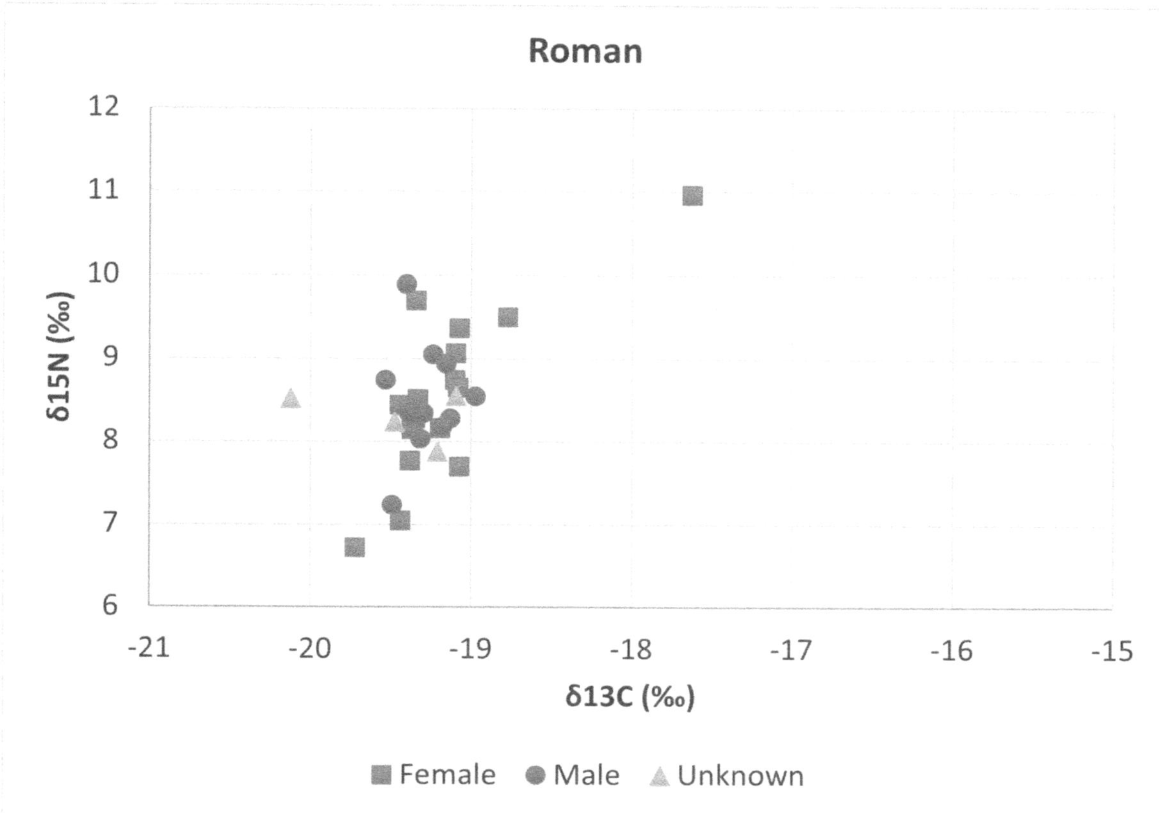

Figure 5.24. Scatter plot of isotope values for the sexes from the Roman period.

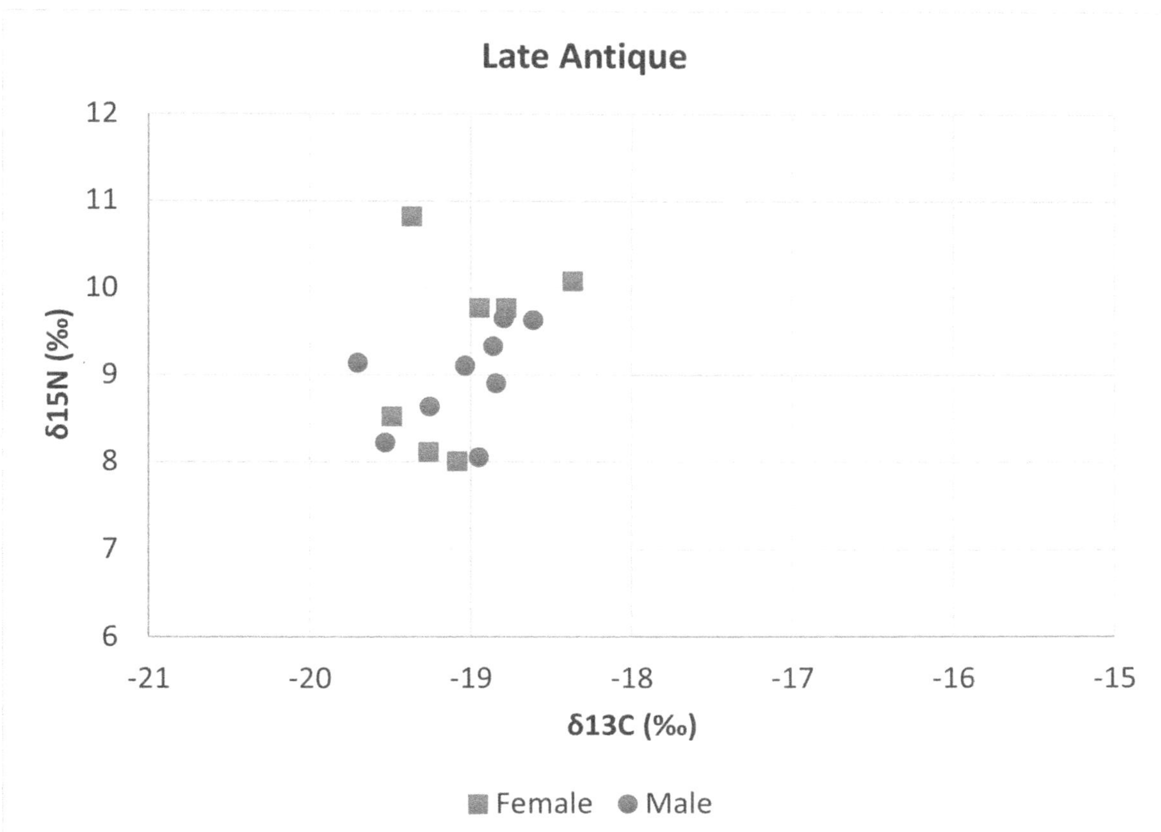

Figure 5.25. Scatter plot of isotope values for the sexes from the Late Antique period.

Table 5.9. Descriptive statistics for $\delta^{13}C$ and $\delta^{15}N$ values for each age group.

Age Group	*n*	Mean $\delta^{13}C$ ‰	Lowest $\delta^{13}C$ ‰	Highest $\delta^{13}C$ ‰	$\delta^{13}C$ SD	Mean $\delta^{15}N$ ‰	Lowest $\delta^{15}N$ ‰	Highest $\delta^{15}N$ ‰	$\delta^{15}N$ SD
Adolescent	5	−19.2	−19.5	−18.9	±0.2	8.3	7.4	9.8	±1.0
Young Adult	20	−19.2	−20.1	−16.1	±0.9	8.7	7.3	11.0	±0.8
Middle Adult	19	−19.2	−19.8	−18.6	±0.3	8.7	7.0	9.9	±0.7
Old Adult	1	−18.9	−18.9	−18.9		9.1	9.1	9.1	

Adult and Middle Adult categories, with only five samples representing the Adolescent group and a single example for the Old Adult group. Sub-adults were generally avoided during the sampling process as this would have introduced an additional variable which could have complicated the interpretation of the other variables present and, additionally, only a very small sample would have been available for each subadult category. Therefore, not only would it have been hard to identify any dietary trends for a large number of age categories with a small sample size in each, but the adult sample would have had to be reduced in size to allow for sub-adult samples to be included in the finite number of samples. However, some older adolescents were included, as it is likely that these individuals would have socially been considered to be adults.

The mean carbon values are extremely similar for all age categories and there is no substantial difference in the nitrogen values (Table 5.9). The Adolescent group, with the lower 8.3‰ mean $\delta^{15}N$ value, was not significantly different when compared with the Young Adult group (Two sample T-test for equal means: $t=-0.9$, $p=0.38$; Mann Whitney U test for equal medians: $U=37.5$, $p=0.41$). No patterns of different isotopic signatures for the different age groups or trends with the progression of age can be identified from the scatter graph (Figure 5.26) either.

5.3.4. Tomb type

Tomb type is used as an indicator of social status and, therefore, situating the tomb type within its time-period

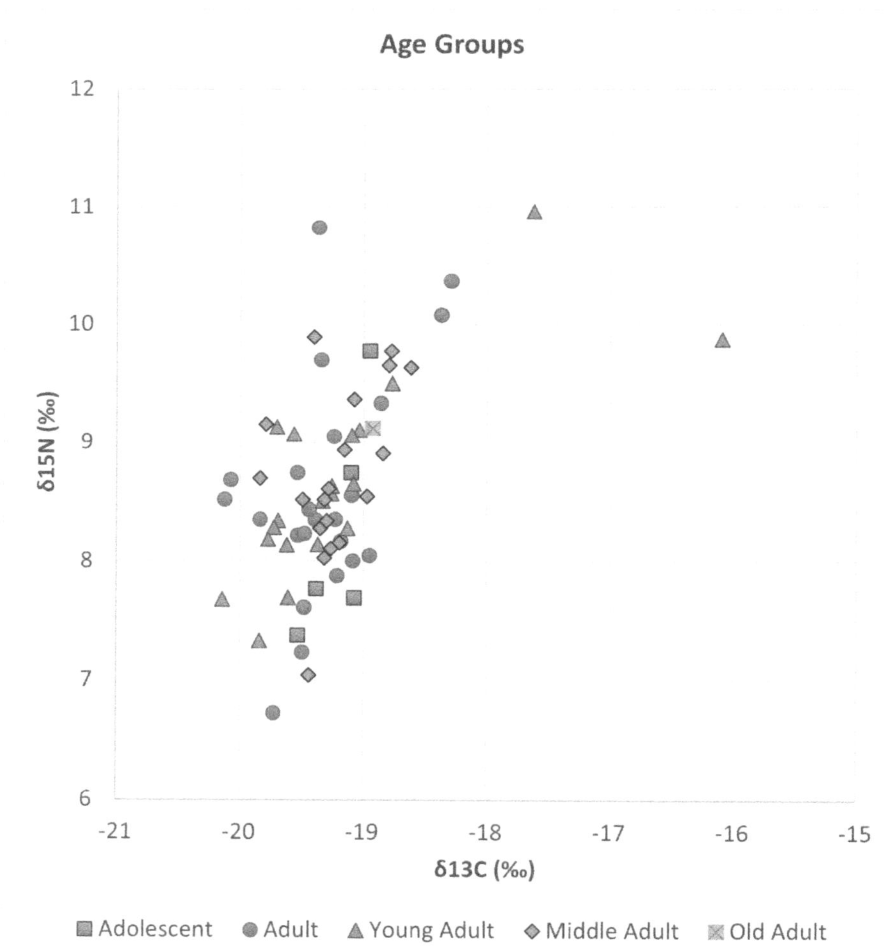

Figure 5.26. Scatter plot of isotope values for the age groups for all time periods.

context is important. Although similar tomb types can exist at different times their context, significance and use may be different. All tomb types for all time periods are plotted together on Figure 5.27 to situate each tomb type within the context of the whole sample. However, the time-period-specific scatter graphs (Figures 5.28–30) are more informative due to this contextualisation within a time period. Unfortunately, the Roman period is the only time period with a great deal of diversity in tomb types for the present assemblage. The Hellenistic graves are almost all pit graves, with a small number of tile graves (n=3). There are not enough tile graves for any pattern to be determined and the pit graves have a wide range of values. However, as was observed in general for the Hellenistic period, this group generally has more samples with the most depleted isotopic values, particularly in $\delta^{13}C$.

The Late Antique tombs are all varieties of stone-lined tombs, either the larger osteothekai or slightly smaller cist or stone-lined tombs (the terminology for these tombs has been discussed previously in Section 3.4), as well as one stone sarcophagus. The 'other stone-lined' tombs show no trend and there is no clear pattern of difference between the osteothekai and 'other stone-lined' tombs. However, with the Late Antique samples plotted on their own two slight groups can be identified in the osteotheke sample (Figure 5.30). This may be an artificial or arbitrary divide in the linear trend but there does seem to be one cluster in the $\delta^{13}C$ −19‰ to −18.5‰ and $\delta^{15}N$ 9‰ to 10‰ region and another cluster with values around $\delta^{13}C$ −19.5‰ to −19‰ and $\delta^{15}N$ 8‰ to 9‰. None of the variables explored in this study (tomb type, sex, age) appear to account for the divide which differentiates individuals with more and less animal and/or marine products in their diets.

The Roman period has the greatest diversity of tomb forms but the majority of tombs for the studied assemblage were the more elaborate rock-cut chamber and built tombs. For the Roman isotope sample there were 15 rock-cut chamber tombs, seven built masonry tombs, three stone-lined tombs, three tile graves, two cist graves and one pit grave. The built tombs, which architecturally indicate a higher social status (monumental structures of built masonry, often with barrel-vaulted roofs), are not particularly distinguished by their inhabitants' dietary status, as these isotope values are generally found quite centrally within the main cluster (Figure 5.27). Although Figure 5.29 (the Roman tomb types plot) shows that the built tomb values generally lie towards the upper end of the main cluster, there are no individuals with $\delta^{15}N$ values higher than 9‰ and the $\delta^{13}C$ and $\delta^{15}N$ mean values are quite middling compared to the other Roman tomb type averages (Table 5.10). This clustering of the built tomb results is also evident from the range ($\delta^{13}C$ 0.4‰, $\delta^{15}N$ 2‰) and standard deviation ($\delta^{13}C$ ±0.2, $\delta^{15}N$ ±0.6) values, even with one slightly lower value (S89: $\delta^{13}C$ −19.4‰, $\delta^{15}N$ 7.0‰).

The chamber tomb results are very variable, with outliers above and below the cluster, as demonstrated by the much larger range ($\delta^{13}C$ 3.7‰, $\delta^{15}N$ 4.3‰) and standard deviation ($\delta^{13}C$ ±0.5, $\delta^{15}N$ ±1.1) values compared to the built tomb samples. The difference in $\delta^{13}C$ variances between the built and chamber tombs was highly significant ($F=11.47$, $p=0.01$), but not significant for $\delta^{15}N$ ($F=3.03$, $p=0.18$). Other than for the built and chamber tombs, these samples are all too small for their mean values to be very reliable or for any further statistical testing to be attempted. There was no significant difference between the built and chamber tomb samples for either carbon or nitrogen mean or median values ($\delta^{13}C$: $t=0.14$, $p=0.89$; $U=42$, $p=0.48$; $\delta^{15}N$: $t=-0.66$, $p=0.52$; $U=44$, $p=0.57$). The chamber tomb nitrogen mean value was 0.3‰ higher than that of the built tombs due to the outlier (S31) with a $\delta^{15}N$ value of 11‰. Compared to the tight clustering of the built tomb samples, there is a lot more variety in the chamber tomb values.

Despite only having three samples, the Roman stone-lined tomb samples have noticeably elevated mean isotope values, particularly for $\delta^{15}N$ at 9‰ (a whole 1‰ higher than the tile grave mean). A pairwise Mann-Whitney test comparing the Built, Chamber, Tile and Stone-lined/Cist (grouped to give a large enough sample size) demonstrated the only significant difference between any of the pairs of tomb groups was in $\delta^{15}N$ for the Tile and Stone-lined/Cist groups ($U=0$, $p=0.037$). S25 (female, adult, KSM T.21, Unit 100), S26 (female, young adult, KSM T.18, Unit 97) and S27 (male, middle adult, KSM T.18, Unit 97) all come from the Sanatorium Basilica (KSM) cemetery, are of Middle/Late Roman date (3rd-4th century AD) and these individuals are likely to have been early Christians. As was observed from the study of the narrower time periods, these Late Roman samples have more elevated values

Table 5.10. Descriptive statistics for $\delta^{13}C$ and $\delta^{15}N$ values for each Roman tomb type.

Roman Tomb Type	n	Mean $\delta^{13}C$ ‰	Lowest $\delta^{13}C$ ‰	Highest $\delta^{13}C$ ‰	$\delta^{13}C$ SD	Mean $\delta^{15}N$ ‰	Lowest $\delta^{15}N$ ‰	Highest $\delta^{15}N$ ‰	$\delta^{15}N$ SD
Built	7	−19.2	−19.4	−19.0	±0.2	8.3	7.0	9.0	±0.6
Chamber	15	−19.3	−20.1	−17.6	±0.5	8.6	6.7	11.0	±1.1
Stone-lined	3	−19.1	−19.4	−18.8	±0.3	9.0	8.4	9.5	±0.5
Cist	2	−19.2	−19.3	−19.1	±0.2	8.5	8.3	8.6	±0.2
Tile	3	−19.3	−19.4	−19.2	±0.1	8.0	7.8	8.2	±0.2
Pit	1	−19.1	−19.1	−19.1		9.4	9.4	9.4	

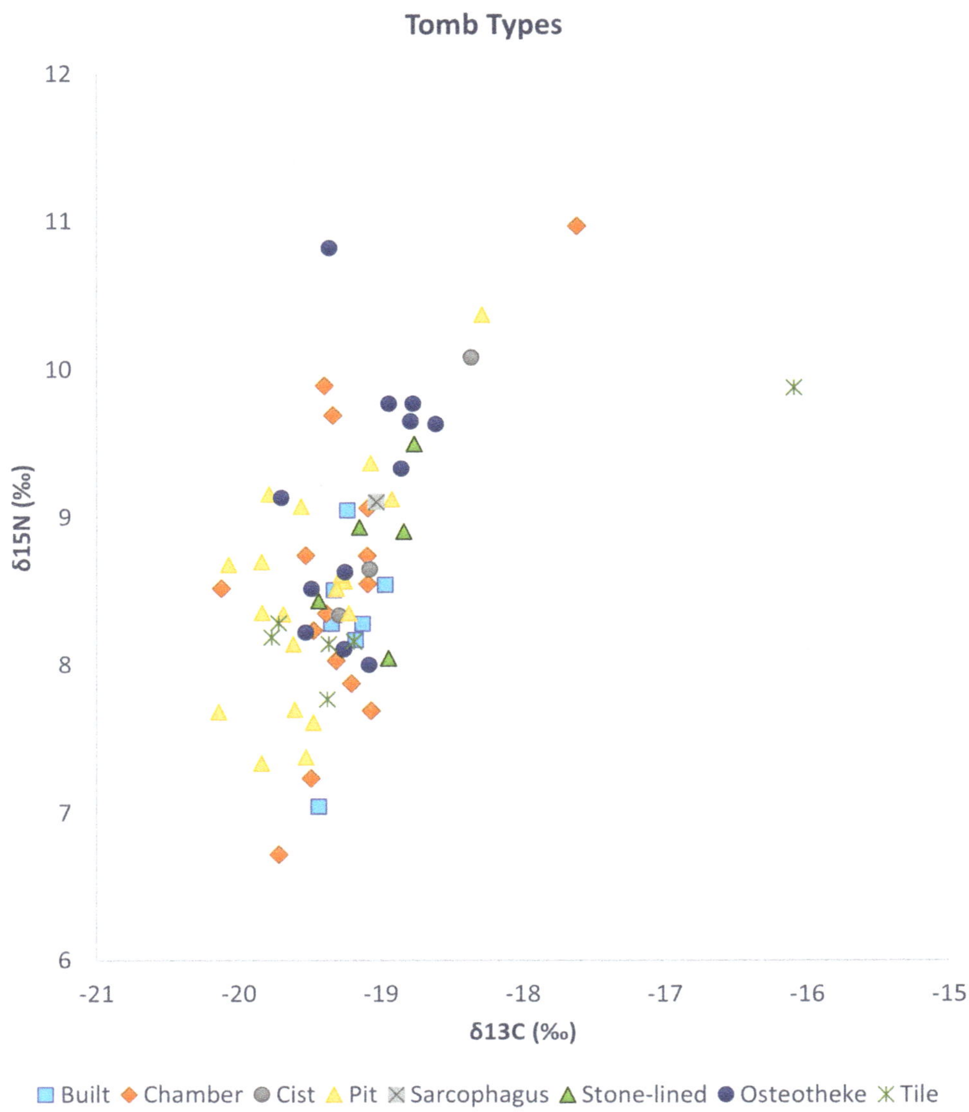

Figure 5.27. Scatter plot of isotope values for the tomb types for all time periods.

than the earlier Roman examples represented by the other tomb forms. Therefore, despite being more elaborate tomb forms (in the case of the 1st-2nd century, built and rock-cut chamber tombs), and the inhabitants potentially being of the highest social status for the time, conditions in the Late Roman and Late Antique periods were more conducive to this diet that likely involved more meat and in some cases more fish.

5.3.5. Cemetery (location)

All of the Hellenistic and Late Antique samples come from tombs in the North Cemetery, therefore, for these time periods there can be no comparisons made between the different cemeteries or regions of the Knossos valley. Just as there was the greatest diversity of tomb forms for the Roman period, this is also the time period for which we have material from a wide range of different cemeteries. The choice of burial ground may represent different social subsets of society. The mean, lowest, highest and standard deviation values for each cemetery are displayed in Table 5.11, and all the sample values are displayed in Figure 5.31.

There are four North Cemetery samples representing four different tombs. Three of these are tile graves (S65, S67, S68, all with $\delta^{13}C$ values just below −19‰ and $\delta^{15}N$ values close to 8‰) and one was a built tomb with a markedly more elevated nitrogen isotope value (KMF T.124, S66, $\delta^{13}C$ −19.2‰, $\delta^{15}N$ 9.1‰). This suggests, at least for the North Cemetery, that tomb type is a more important factor than cemetery for distinguishing dietary differences (and potentially social status as inferred both from the difference in tomb form and in diet). Though the sample size is very small, the built tomb sample having a markedly elevated $\delta^{15}N$ value compared to those from the tile graves, indicates that people of different social (and dietary) status were being buried in the North Cemetery but in different tomb forms.

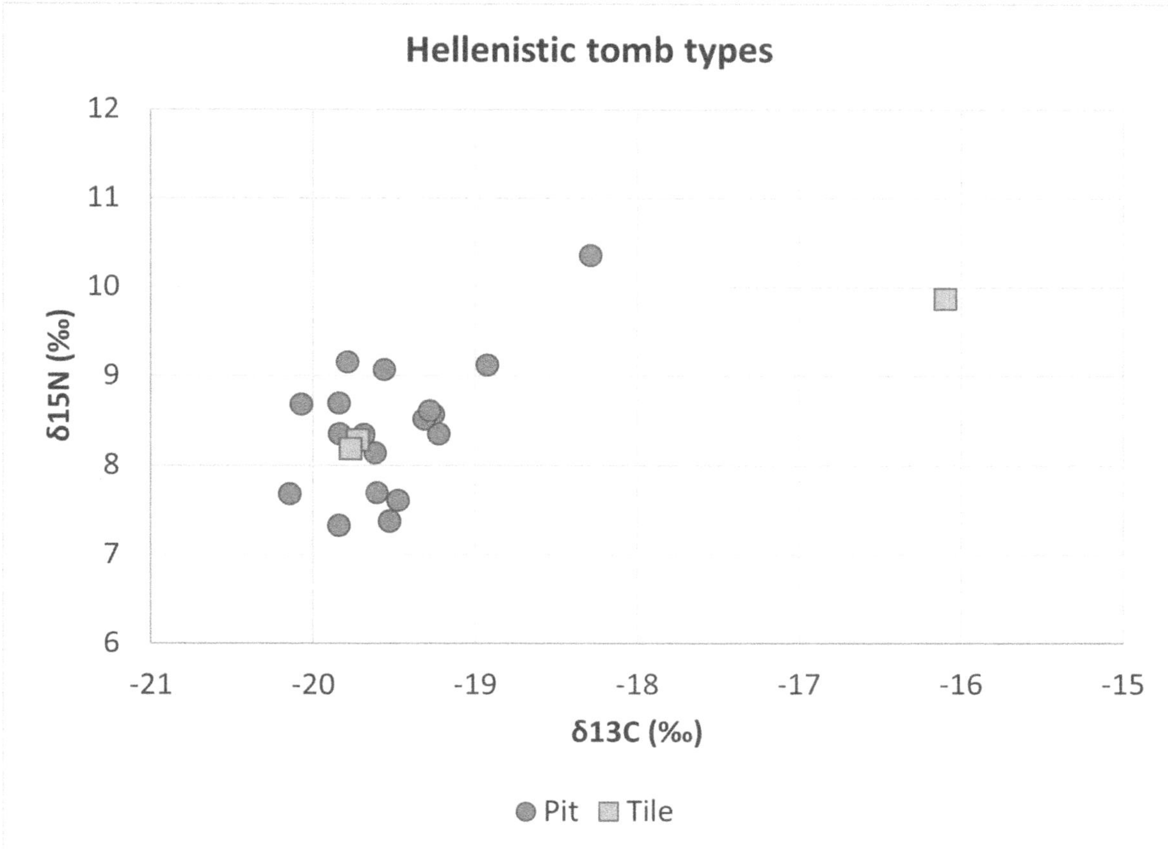

Figure 5.28. Scatter plot of isotope values for the Hellenistic tomb types.

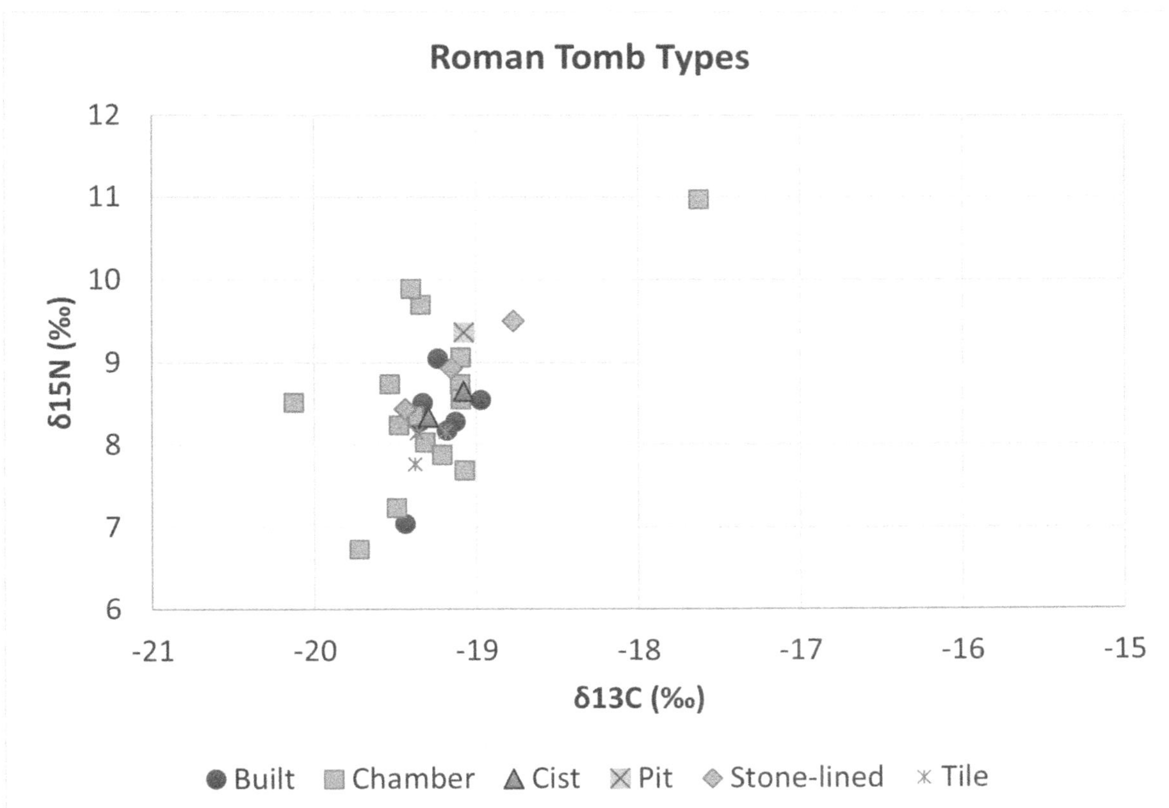

Figure 5.29. Scatter plot of isotope values for the Roman tomb types.

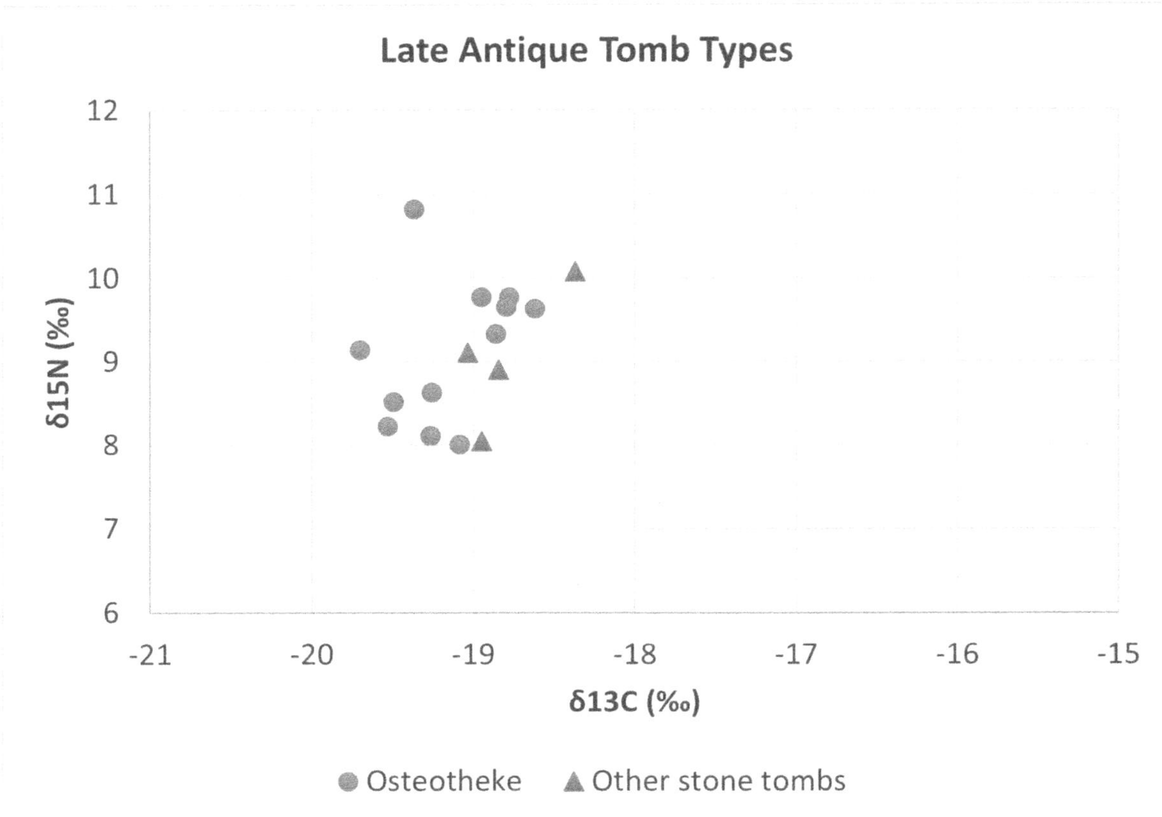

Figure 5.30. Scatter plot of isotope values for the Late Antique tomb types.

Table 5.11. Descriptive statistics for $\delta^{13}C$ and $\delta^{15}N$ values for the Roman cemeteries.

Roman Cemetery	*n*	Mean $\delta^{13}C$ ‰	Min. $\delta^{13}C$ ‰	Max. $\delta^{13}C$ ‰	$\delta^{13}C$ SD	Mean $\delta^{15}N$ ‰	Min. $\delta^{15}N$ ‰	Max. $\delta^{15}N$ ‰	$\delta^{15}N$ SD
Monastiriako Kephali	8	−19.5	−20.1	−19.1	0.3	8.4	6.7	9.9	1.1
Krevatina	2	−19.2	−19.3	−19.1		8.5	8.3	8.6	
North Cemetery	4	−19.3	−19.4	−19.2	0.1	8.3	7.8	9.0	0.5
Sanatorium	11	−19.0	−19.4	−17.6	0.5	8.9	8.0	11.0	0.8
Spilia	2	−19.3	−19.5	−19.2		8.1	7.9	8.2	
Topana	4	−19.2	−19.4	−19.0	0.2	8.1	7.0	8.5	0.7

The cemeteries at Spilia, Topana and near the palace entrance are represented by only a single tomb each. Three of the Topana barrel-vaulted built tomb (Unit 104) samples (S85, S96, S90) are clustered quite close together, with quite middling values within the whole sample. However, the fourth Topana tomb sample (S89) has significantly depleted values, particularly in $\delta^{15}N$ (7‰). This level of variation within a single tomb (also noted in other tombs, e.g. Units 1, 3, 5 and 93) demonstrates that making assumptions about social differences or changes over time from a small sample can result in false patterns being identified and such interpretations (such as that made from the four North Cemetery samples above) should be considered cautiously. The two samples (S18 and S20) from the cist tomb at Krevatina (Unit 105), excavated by Hutchinson in 1936, have quite similar isotope values and the $\delta^{15}N$ mean value is the second highest after the Sanatorium Cemetery mean.

The two Spilia chamber tomb (Unit 109) samples are close together in values, which in both carbon and nitrogen are below average in relation to the whole group. If these are compared to the acropolis rock-cut tombs (as part of a continuum of cemeteries cut into the hillsides to the south of the settlement of rock-cut chamber tombs with arcosolia and niches), the values are very scattered. Unusually, all the acropolis samples lie outside of the central cluster, both above and below, with three having very low $\delta^{15}N$ values (S9: 6.7‰, S10: 7.2‰, and S41: 7.7‰), one having a particularly low $\delta^{13}C$ value (S93: −20.1‰) and four samples with more elevated $\delta^{15}N$ values (S8: 8.7‰, S11: 9.7‰, S42: 9.9‰, and S43: 9.1‰).

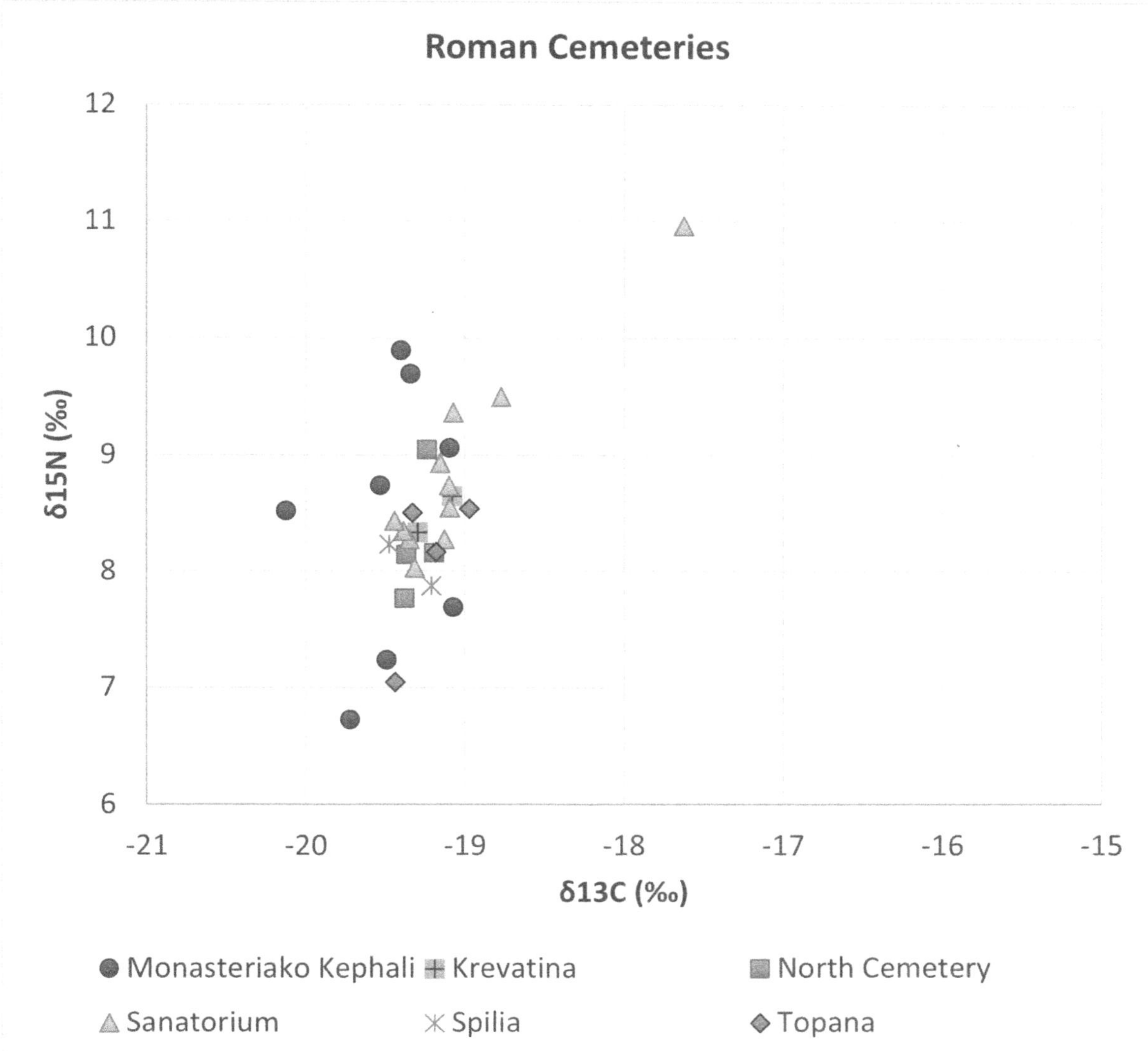

Figure 5.31. Scatter plot of isotope values for the Roman cemeteries.

The Sanatorium cemetery has the most elevated mean values for both carbon and nitrogen ($\delta^{13}C$ −19‰, $\delta^{15}N$ 8.9‰). The degree of elevation is partially due to the outlier values of S31 ($\delta^{13}C$ −17.6‰, $\delta^{15}N$ 11‰) but generally the samples from this cemetery are amongst the most elevated, with none lying below −19.4‰ or 8‰ for $\delta^{13}C$ and $\delta^{15}N$ respectively. As the Sanatorium Cemetery contained a large enough sample to represent a range of tomb types, sexes and age groups, it was possible to investigate these within the context of the cemetery. Five samples were from a single chamber tomb (Unit 93), two from a built tomb (Unit 94), one from a grave of unknown structure, termed a pit (Unit 99), and three from stone-lined tombs (two from Unit 97 and one from Unit 100). No clear pattern emerges for the different tomb types within the Sanatorium cemetery (Figure 5.32), nor is there any trend for the different age groups (Figure 5.34). However, Figure 5.33 shows these samples for the different sexes and indicates that females generally had higher carbon and nitrogen isotope values than the males. This was not statistically significant (Mann-Whitney: $\delta^{13}C$: $U=7$, $p=0.34$; $\delta^{15}N$: $U=4$, $p=0.11$) and it is a small sample (6 females, 4 males). The difference in the $\delta^{13}C$ variances for males and females were, however, statistically significant ($F=28.87$, $p=0.019$), as can be seen from the much broader range of female values compared to the clustering of male values.

All the Roman samples were also tested for differences by the region of the valley from which they came. This meant grouping the northern cemeteries (North, Sanatorium, Topana) and the southern cemeteries (Monastiriako Kephali, Spilia and Krevatina). The northern side of the city has generally been observed to be the 'wealthier' side of town with the widespread distribution of mosaics, while the industrial quarters were located to the south. That does not mean that the same pattern should be seen in the burial record and certainly the diversity of tomb forms in the North Cemetery suggests a mixed demographic in a single cemetery. Additionally, the rock-cut chamber tombs were largely to the south of the city and these are unlikely to represent individuals of low social status due to their complexity, elaboration, energy investment and visibility. The mean values for the

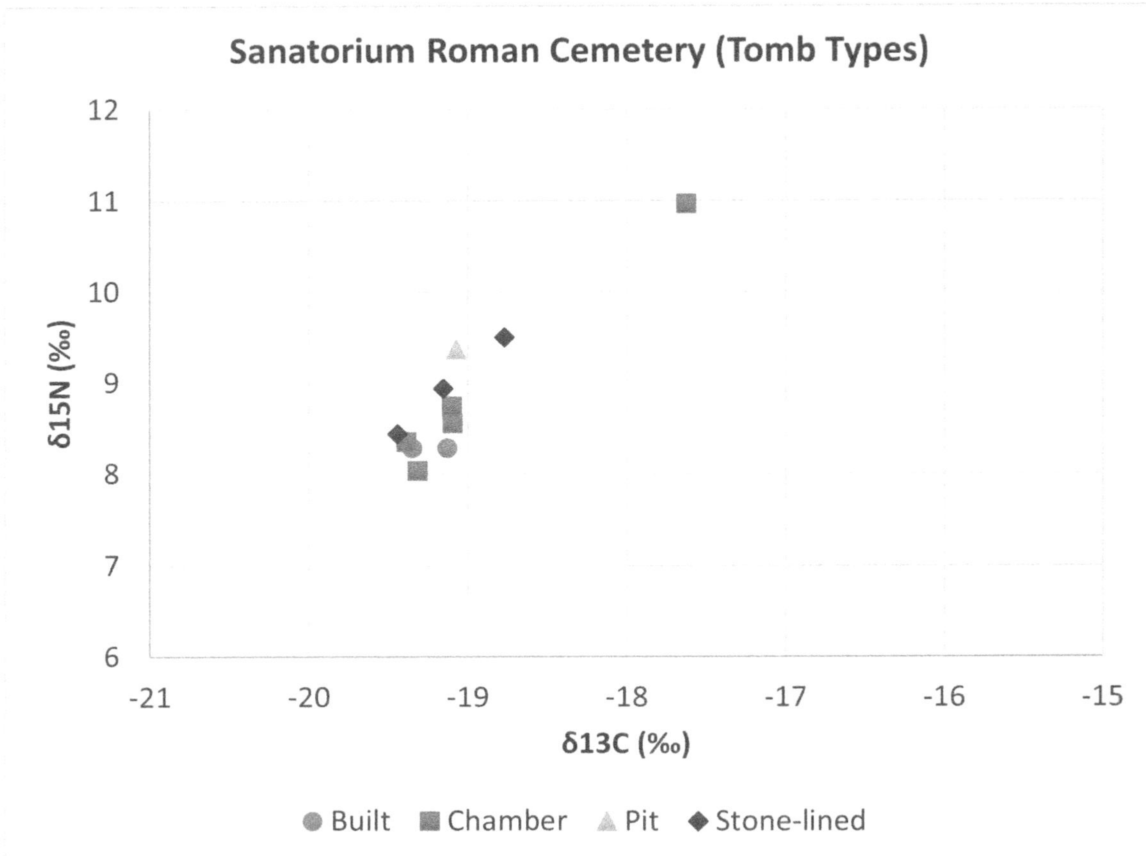

Figure 5.32. Scatter plot of isotope values for the Sanatorium Roman tombs by tomb type.

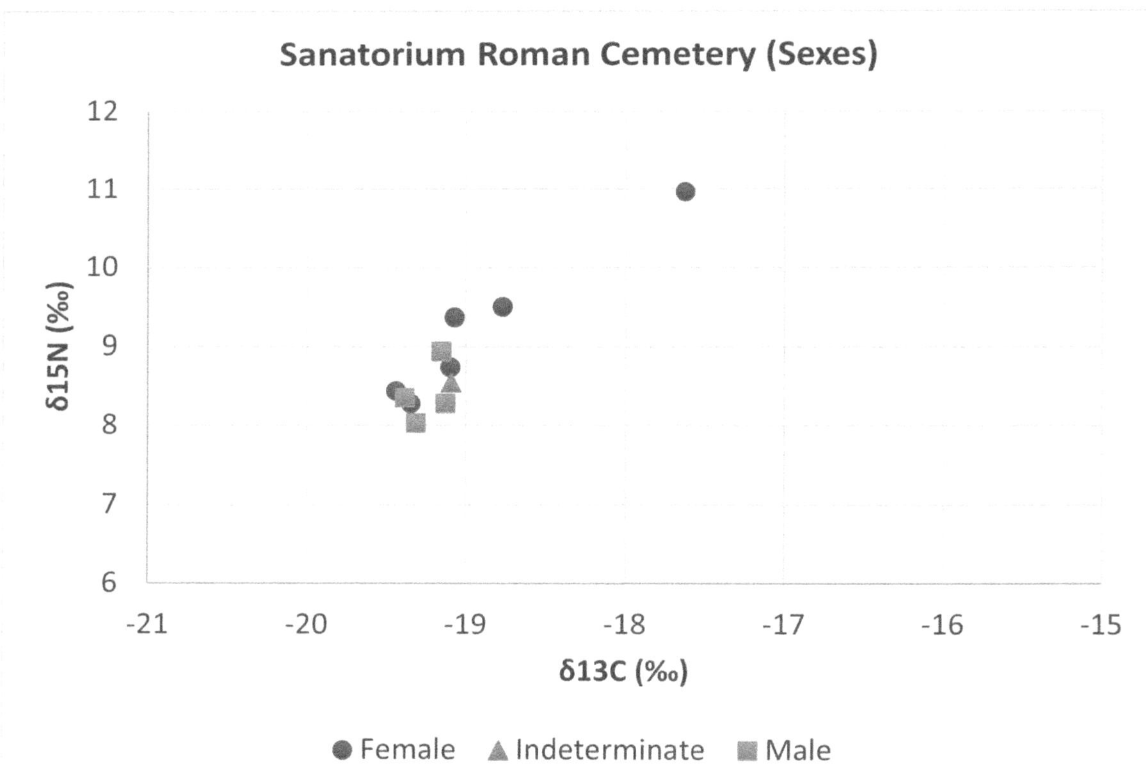

Figure 5.33. Scatter plot of isotope values for the Sanatorium Roman tombs by sex.

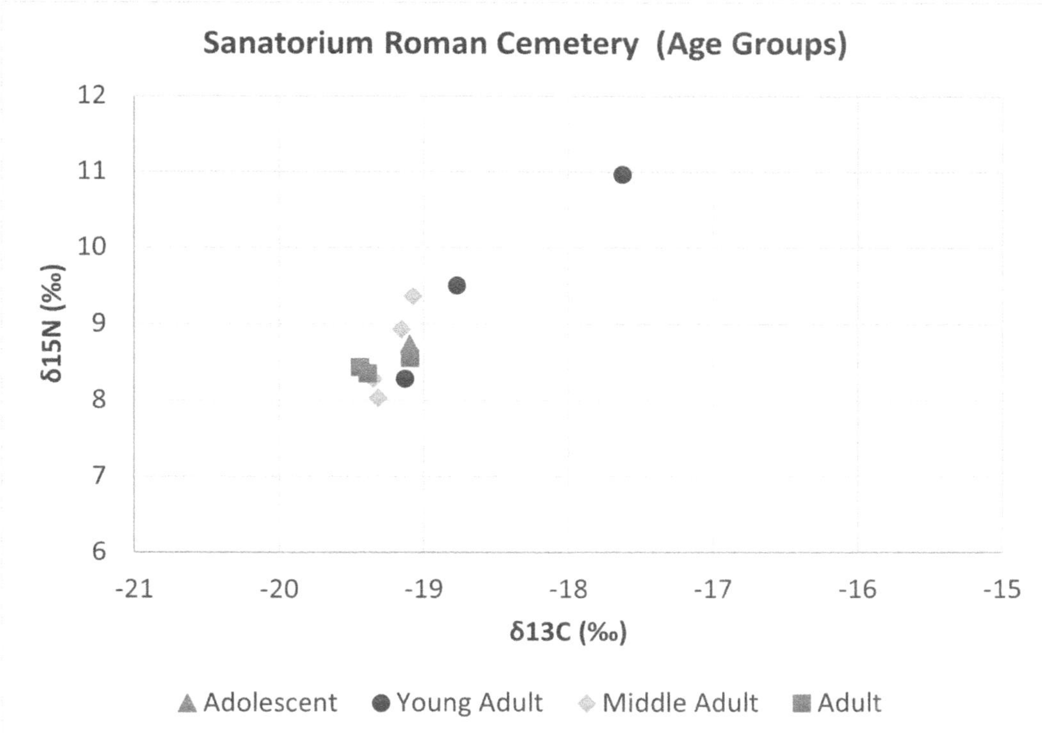

Figure 5.34. Scatter plot of isotope values for the Sanatorium Roman tombs by age group.

North group were −19.1‰ (n=19, s.d.=0.4) and 8.6‰ (n=19, s.d.=0.8) and for the South group were −19.4‰ (n=12, s.d.=0.3) and 8.4‰ (n=12, s.d.=0.9) for $\delta^{13}C$ and $\delta^{15}N$ respectively. The lack of a significant difference between the mean values is supported by the lack of any observable patterns in Figure 5.35, though the difference in $\delta^{13}C$ values was not far from the $p<0.05$ significance level (U=352.5, $p=0.057$), and the difference in $\delta^{13}C$ variances was statistically highly significant (F=3.78, $p=0.004$).

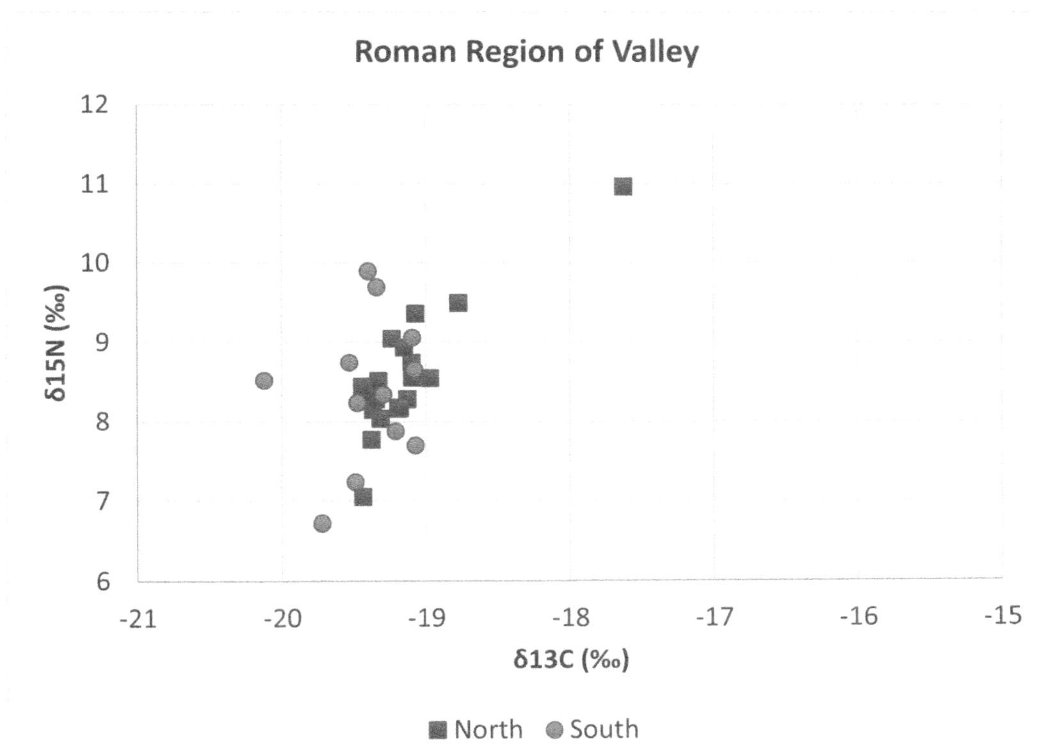

Figure 5.35. Scatter plot of isotope values for the northern and southern cemeteries within the Knossos valley.

5.4. Discussion

The diets of the majority of studied individuals were C3 terrestrial diets with the inclusion of terrestrial animal products. The isotopic signatures for most individuals indicate that there was meat or secondary animal products in their diets to satisfy their dietary protein requirements. A small number with the lowest $\delta^{15}N$ values still had occasional access to animal products but are likely to have subsisted off a largely vegetarian diet much of the time. Even these lowest values, however, demonstrate that animal products were not a very rare feature in any diet within the sample, as even the lowest human value ($\delta^{15}N$ 6.7‰) is over 2‰ higher than the highest faunal $\delta^{15}N$ value and almost 5‰ above the lowest faunal $\delta^{15}N$ value. The amount of animal products would nevertheless have been fairly modest in all diets (compared to modern Western expectations of meat consumption, which are unprecedented and unsustainable) and staple crops would have provided the bulk of the diet. The Recommended Dietary Allowance of protein for a healthy adult with minimal physical activity is currently 0.8 g protein per kilogram body weight per day (Food and Nutrition Board of the Institute of Medicine 2005, 589), which would be 40g for a 50kg individual or 64g for an 80kg individual per day. Animal husbandry is an extremely expensive use of land for food production compared to growing crops, and although intensive dairying supported livestock farming, meat remained a prestigious product (Sallares 1991). This is a common pattern throughout prehistory and history in Greece, where mixed farming has been common since the Neolithic and provided a more secure and less labour-intensive subsistence model than arable farming alone (Halstead 2008, 244; Papathanasiou and Richards 2015, 200).

Some values indicate that marine foods were included in some diets. In particular the two outlier values S22 and S31 (discussed in Section 5.3.4), but some of the other values at the upper end of the spectrum (those above $\delta^{13}C$ −19‰ and $\delta^{15}N$ 9.5‰) also likely indicate some fish consumption considering the level of elevation over the terrestrial faunal values. None of the isotope values in the present study reach the 11.5‰ $\delta^{15}N$ marine-terrestrial boundary recommended by Salamon *et al.* (2008) but other studies have discussed the wide range of marine organism values and the difficulty in detecting low trophic level fish in the diet (Lightfoot *et al.* 2012; Vika and Theodoropoulou 2012). Additionally, 10‰ is the cut-off that Papathanasiou and Richards (2015) have used for identifying a significant marine component in the diet. This indicates the importance of having local faunal values as a site-specific indicator of where terrestrial human values would be expected to lie.

5.4.1. *Time period*

Across the three time periods, Hellenistic, Roman and Late Antique, carbon and nitrogen isotope values increase slightly, though generally insignificantly (and there is a negligible difference in $\delta^{15}N$ means between the Hellenistic and Roman periods). The analysis of change over time using the narrower time periods indicates that a change in diet occurred in the Late Hellenistic or Early Roman periods which involved an elevation in the $\delta^{13}C$ values but a depletion in $\delta^{15}N$ values. This suggests that the change must have been caused by either the inclusion of a small amount of C4 plant (likely millet), a small amount of marine food or very low trophic level marine foods in the Roman diets, alongside less terrestrial meat consumption.

The Late Antique samples are significantly higher in both $\delta^{13}C$ and $\delta^{15}N$, though not by a very large margin in terms of absolute values, which suggests a small but consistent (across the sample) change in diets. This indicates a greater protein component in the diet and it is likely that this involved an increased (though still modest) amount of seafood. The investigation of the isotopic results for the narrower time periods suggests that this elevation in values was a gradual process starting in the 3rd or 4th century AD. This suggests that the shift in dietary habits may have been influenced by Christian asceticism. The later Roman and Late Antique graves are largely considered to be Christian graves due to either their association with a basilica church or their orientation, treatment of the body, grave architecture and lack of grave goods (Frend and Johnston 1962; Sweetman and Becker 2005). Although there are other possible reasons for increased fish consumption such as developments in fish preservation techniques, changes in attitudes towards the sea and sea life, or new trading partners or networks, the widespread adoption of Christianity and its fasting calendar coincides with the phenomenon at a number of sites in Crete, around the Mediterranean and across Europe (Garvie-Lok 2001; Polet and Katzenberg 2003; Bourbou and Richards 2007; Rutgers *et al.* 2009; Bourbou 2010; Bourbou *et al.* 2011; Reitsema *et al.* 2016). At the site of Helike in Achaia, the study of stable carbon and nitrogen isotopes for the Hellenistic, Roman and Byzantine periods should be directly comparable to the present study, but unusually fish consumption was found to be at its highest in the Hellenistic period. This was explained, however, by the seismic activity which had created a lagoon that may have enabled greater and more diverse access to fish and highlights the importance of site specific knowledge, including such unusual environmental circumstances (McConnan Borstad *et al.* 2018).

The isotopic study of diet at Classical, Hellenistic and Imperial Roman Athens is closely comparable to the present study due to its status as a large urban centre that was well-connected within Mediterranean networks (Lagia 2015). As at Knossos, the results indicated a changing diet across the three time periods. However, the trend was largely the opposite of that observed at Knossos as there was a decrease in $\delta^{15}N$ values over time (though it is not directly comparable as it is generally an earlier – and importantly, pre-Christian – time period being studied). However, at the transition from the Hellenistic to Roman periods, individuals at both sites experienced a fall in protein consumption demonstrated by the depletion of nitrogen isotopic values. While at Athens, this is a continuing downward trend, at Knossos there is a significant increase in carbon and nitrogen isotope values from the Late Roman period onwards. Therefore, Knossos does not really fit the trend of having increased protein consumption in times of economic and cultural growth and prosperity, which are likely in decline throughout the Late Roman and Late Antique periods, as indicated by the reduction of population, lack of building projects and relative lack and diversity of artefacts. At Athens there were no significant differences between the different cemeteries, tomb types, or between the sexes, which is generally a pattern matched at Knossos, though some subtle differences were observed.

5.4.2. Sex

As observed above there was no isotopic difference between male and female diets for the whole sample from Knossos. This is frequently the case at comparable sites (Keenleyside *et al.* 2009; Lagia 2015). However, this does not mean that differences did not exist as the isotopic results could not detect a difference between different cuts of meat or between meat and other animal products. Some difference was observed in the distribution of results that indicated more varied female results and more clustered male results. Although there were more female $\delta^{15}N$ values both below 8‰ and above 10‰, a test for different variances was not statistically significant. Nevertheless, with fewer males in the region below 8‰ and the greater clustering of male values there is some suggestion that male diets generally, and more consistently than female diets, contained animal protein. At a number of temporally comparable sites small but consistent differences have been observed between the sexes, which also show that males often have slightly more elevated isotopic values (Henneberg and Henneberg 2003; Prowse *et al.* 2005), which supports the indication that there could be discrepancies between the diets of males and females.

Within each time period, the picture was generally the same, with very little difference being detected between male and female diets. Although it was not a statistically significant difference, Hellenistic male $\delta^{15}N$ mean value was 0.5‰ more elevated than the female value, which may indicate more protein in Hellenistic male diets. However, a larger sample would be needed to confirm or refute this suggestion. The only difference that was deemed statistically significant in the comparison of male and female diets was in the Roman $\delta^{13}C$ variances, indicating that Roman female diets were more varied and supported by the greater range and standard deviation of female values.

5.4.3. Age group

No differences were isotopically detectable between the diets of individuals from different age groups. Adolescents were included in the study, due to the likelihood that they were socially considered to be adults. However, younger sub-adults were excluded to avoid additional confounding factors introduced by additional variables and because it is usual for infants and young children to have elevated $\delta^{15}N$ values. This is caused by breastfeeding, which results in the isotope values of the infant reflecting a trophic level above that of the mother. For this reason, in Table 5.12 which sets out the data for comparable studies, infants and young children's values were also removed where possible (if a full list of data was published).

Unfortunately, very few Old Adults were included in the sample. However, it is very unusual for significant differences to be detected between adults of different ages. At Athens a difference between the Young Adults and both the Middle and Old Adults was found to be significant for the $\delta^{15}N$ results, and therefore in the quantities and types of protein in the diet (Lagia 2015). At Isola Sacra a similar trend was found with the older adults having more elevated $\delta^{15}N$, although in the Athens study the Middle Adults had slightly higher values than the Old Adults (Prowse *et al.* 2005; Lagia 2015). Such differences between adult age categories are not very common.

5.4.4. Tomb type

The lack of diversity in the Hellenistic and Late Antique tomb forms meant that no analysis of differences between tomb types could be conducted for these time periods. The Hellenistic graves were all pits, with the exception of three tile graves and the Late Antique samples all came from stone-lined tombs (the majority of which were defined as osteothekai). However, the Roman samples came from a broad range of tomb types, with this being the time period that had the greatest diversity in tomb forms.

The Roman samples that came from the more elaborate built and rock-cut chamber tombs did not portray individuals with superior diets in the form of greater access to protein or with the inclusion of fish. The results from the rock-cut chamber tomb samples were very varied, while most of the built tomb samples were very closely clustered. Although there was a highly significant difference in $\delta^{13}C$ variances between these tomb types, there was no significant difference between their mean values.

The stone-lined tombs had the samples with the most elevated values, particularly for $\delta^{15}N$ with a mean of 9‰. This was a whole 1‰ more elevated than the tile grave mean value, which was the lowest mean value for all the tomb forms and was a statistically significant difference. However, these samples (S25, S26, and S27) were all later Roman (3rd-4th century) tombs from the Sanatorium Basilica cemetery. This cemetery, though it predated the basilica, was judged to have been an early Christian cemetery due to the deliberate positioning and alignment of the basilica with the tombs and the incorporation of Tomb 8 into the nave (Frend and Johnston 1962, 188). Therefore, this observed difference for the stone-lined tombs having higher carbon and nitrogen isotope values (likely indicative of a small increase in marine food in

Table 5.12. Stable carbon and nitrogen isotope values from comparable sites throughout Crete, Greece, the Mediterranean and neighbouring regions.

Site	Region	Location	Time period	*n*	Mean $\delta^{13}C$ ‰	Lowest $\delta^{13}C$ ‰	Highest $\delta^{13}C$ ‰	$\delta^{13}C$ SD ‰	Mean $\delta^{15}N$ ‰	Lowest $\delta^{15}N$ ‰	Highest $\delta^{15}N$ ‰	$\delta^{15}N$ SD ‰	Reference
Knossos (Gypsades)	Crete	Inland	Neopalatial (MMIII-LMI)	16	-18.4	-20.3	-17.4	1.0	8.8	7.3	9.8	0.6	Nafplioti 2016
Knossos (Ailias)	Crete	Inland	Neopalatial (MMII-LMI)	46	-19.7	-21.4	-17.4	1.0	8.0	6.2	9.8	1.0	Nafplioti 2016
Knossos	Crete	Inland	Subminoan	6	-19.6	-20.1	-19.3	0.3	8.0	7.2	9.1	0.7	Present study
Thebes	Boeotia	Inland	Classical	30	-19.2	-20.2	-18.1	0.5	10.6	8.9	14.5	1.1	Vika 2011
Apollonia	Black Sea (Bulgaria)	Coastal	Classical	54	-18.5	-19.5	-17.8	0.5	10.1	8.5	12.2	0.8	Keenleyside, Schwarz and Panayotova 2006
Mesembria	Black Sea (Bulgaria)	Coastal	Classical-Hellenistic	9	-18.9	-19.3	-18.5	0.2	10.1	9.4	11.2	0.6	Moles 2012
Knossos	Crete	Inland	Hellenistic	21	-19.4	-20.1	-16.1	0.9	8.5	7.3	10.4	0.8	Present study
Thebes	Boeotia	Inland	Hellenistic	44	-19.2	-19.8	-15.9	0.6	9.6	8.2	10.9	0.7	Vika 2011
Athens	Attica	Inland	Hellenistic	20	-19.0	-19.7	-17.6	0.6	9.9	8.5	11.3	0.8	Lagia 2015
Helike	Achaea, Peloponnese	Coastal	Hellenistic	6	-17.7	-18.5	-16.9	0.7	9.3	8.8	9.8	0.4	Borstad, Garvie-Lok and Katsonopoulou 2018
Athens	Attica	Inland	Imperial Roman	14	-19.1	-19.8	-18.7	0.3	9.7	8.8	10.7	1.7	Lagia 2015
Gabii (near Rome)	Italy	Inland	Imperial Roman	18	-18.8	-19.3	-15.8	0.8	10.7	8.5	11.5	0.9	Killgrove and Tykot 2018 (in press)
Casal Bertone (Rome)	Italy	Inland	Imperial Roman	26	-17.8	-19.5	-16.8	0.6	10.1	7.0	11.8	1.4	Killgrove and Tykot 2013
Castellaccio Europarco (Rome)	Italy	Inland	Imperial Roman	8	-17.8	-19.5	-12.5	2.2	9.3	7.8	11.5	1.3	Killgrove and Tykot 2013
Isola Sacra (Rome)	Italy	Coastal	Imperial Roman	102	-18.8	-17.8	-19.7	0.3	10.8	7.5	14.4	1.2	Prowse *et al.* 2004, Crowe *et al.* 2010
ANAS (Rome)	Italy	Inland	Imperial Roman	14	-19.4	-20.0	-18.9	0.4	9.5	6.9	11.3	1.8	Prowse *et al.* 2004
Velia	Italy	Coastal	Imperial Roman	117	-19.4	-20.0	-18.7	0.3	8.6	6.4	14.1	1.3	Craig *et al.* 2009, Crowe *et al.* 2010

Herculaneum	Italy	Coastal	Imperial Roman	75	-19.2	-20.2	-18.2	0.4	10.1	8.2	11.7	0.8	Craig *et al.* 2013, Martyn *et al.* 2018 (in press)
Paestum	Italy	Coastal	Imperial Roman	22	-19.5	-20.9	-18.5	0.7	8.1	7.5	9.4	0.5	Ricci *et al.* 2016
Ephesus	Asia Minor (Turkey)	Coastal	Imperial Roman	42	-18.9	-19.7	-17.8	0.4	9.2	4.8	11.2	1.1	Lösch *et al.* 2014
Knossos	Crete	Inland	Roman	31	-19.2	-20.1	-17.6	0.4	8.5	6.7	11.0	0.8	Present study
Helike	Achaea, Peloponnese	Coastal	Roman	10	-19.3	-19.9	-17.1	0.8	8.5	7.1	9.0	0.6	Borstad, Garvie-Lok and Katsonopoulou 2018
Zadar-Relje	Dalmatia (Croatia)	Coastal	Roman	51	-18.9	-19.6	17.8	0.4	10.0	9.0	12.9	0.7	Lightfoot, Šlaus and O'Connell 2012
Vis-Bandirica	Dalmatia (Croatia)	Coastal	Roman	14	-18.9	-19.4	-18.5	0.3	9.7	8.5	10.5	0.7	Lightfoot, Šlaus and O'Connell 2012
Kellis 2, Dakhleh Oasis	Egypt	Inland	Roman	63	-18.9			0.2	17.9			0.7	Dupras 1999
Pergamon	Asia Minor (Turkey)	Inland	Roman	75	-18.7			0.5	9.9			0.9	Propstmeier 2017
Rome catacombs	Italy	Inland	Late Roman	22	-19.8	-20.8	-18.9	0.4	10.6	9.7	11.9	0.8	Rutgers *et al.* 2009
Leptiminus	Tunisia	Coastal	Roman-Late Antique	58	-17.8	-19.0	-16.5	0.6	12.8	10.0	15.7	1.3	Keenleyside *et al.* 2009
Hierapolis	Asia Minor (Turkey)	Inland	Roman-Middle Byzantine	7	-19.3	-20.5	-18.9	0.5	9.8	8.9	11.1	0.8	Wong *et al.* 2017
Knossos	Crete	Inland	Late Antique	16	-19.1	-19.7	-18.4	0.4	9.1	8.0	10.8	0.8	Present study
Eleutherna	Crete	Inland	Late Antique	27	-18.9	-19.6	-16.9	0.6	8.2	5.6	11.5	1.4	Bourbou, Fuller and Richards 2008, Bourbou 2010, Bourbou *et al.* 2011
Messene	Messenia, Peloponnese	Inland	Late Antique	21	-19.2	-20.0	-18.7	0.3	8.7	7.3	11.7	0.9	Bourbou, Fuller and Richards 2008, Bourbou 2010, Bourbou *et al.* 2011
Sourtara	Macedonia	Inland	Late Antique	27	-18.2	-18.8	-17.8	0.3	9.5	9.1	10.1	0.3	Bourbou, Fuller and Richards 2008, Bourbou 2010, Bourbou *et al.* 2011
Podvršje	Dalmatia (Croatia)	Coastal	Late Antique	11	-18.5	-18.9	-17.7	0.3	10.9	9.8	12.1	0.9	Lightfoot, Šlaus and O'Connell 2012
Nemea	Argolid, Peloponnese	Inland	Late Antique	17	-19.4	-19.1	-19.7	0.2	8.6	7.2	9.6	0.7	Kwok 2015

(Continued)

Table 5.12. (*Continued*)

Site	Region	Location	Time period	*n*	Mean $\delta^{13}C$ ‰	Lowest $\delta^{13}C$ ‰	Highest $\delta^{13}C$ ‰	$\delta^{13}C$ SD ‰	Mean $\delta^{15}N$ ‰	Lowest $\delta^{15}N$ ‰	Highest $\delta^{15}N$ ‰	$\delta^{15}N$ SD ‰	Reference
Abdera	Macedonia	Coastal	Late Antique-Middle Byzantine	4 (?)	-18.8			0.4	9.5			1.1	Agelarakis in Bourbou 2010
Mesembria	Black Sea (Bulgaria)	Coastal	Early-Late Byzantine	12	-18.6	-19.5	-16.8	0.7	10.3	7.6	11.9	1.1	Moles 2012
Helike	Achaea, Peloponnese	Coastal	Byzantine	8	-18.7	-19.6	-17.5	0.8	9.2	8.5	10.2	0.7	Borstad, Garvie-Lok and Katsonopoulou 2018
Kastella	Crete	Coastal	Middle Byzantine	19	-18.8	-19.4	-18.2	0.3	9.1	7.8	10.9	1.2	Bourbou and Richards 2007, Bourbou 2010, Bourbou *et al.* 2011
Nemea	Argolid, Peloponnese	Inland	Middle Byzantine	18	-19.0	-19.8	-16.0	0.8	8.6	7.6	9.8	0.6	Garvie-Lok 2001, Bourbou 2010, Bourbou *et al.* 2011
Petras	Crete	Coastal	Middle Byzantine	12	-19.2	-20.2	-18.6	0.3	9.4	8.5	10.8	0.7	Garvie-Lok 2001, Bourbou 2010, Bourbou *et al.* 2011
Stylos	Crete	Inland	Middle Byzantine	10	-18.8	-20.0	-17.6	0.7	9.4	7.5	13.2	1.7	Bourbou, Fuller and Richards 2008, Bourbou 2010, Bourbou *et al.* 2011
Servia	Macedonia	Inland	Middle-Late Byzantine	13	-18.7	-19.2	-17.6	0.3	8.7	8.2	9.7	0.5	Garvie-Lok 2001, Bourbou 2010, Bourbou *et al.* 2011

the diet) is actually due to the time period and associated social changes, rather than being linked inherently to the tomb type and the inhabitant's social status.

The introduction of Christianity and the dietary rules that came with it is not the only social change that might have affected individuals' diets. There may have been improvements in preservation techniques for keeping fish longer. This varied regionally and over time, as although the decline of the Roman Empire resulted in the established networks for moving salted fish breaking down, the opening up of the Atlantic for fishing in the Medieval period resulted in new preservation techniques being employed and new networks linking the Atlantic and Mediterranean being developed (McCormick 2001; Van Neer and Ervynck 2004; Salamon *et al.* 2008). Changes in diet at this time could also have been due to the easing of pressure on resources or on the administration and distribution of food due to the reduction in settlement and population size. It may represent a return to a more personal or family level of food production, with the reduction in population, rather than a state administered food distribution system which may have been more necessary for the population size during the Hellenistic and Roman periods.

In the Hellenistic period, the *syssitia* communal meals for citizen males would have meant a degree of community-organised food distribution based on a subsistence economy (Chaniotis 1999, 182). A passage from Aristotle's *Politica* suggests that this was not only for men but that all women and children were also maintained on public funds (Viviers 1999, 227). This is not thought to have continued into the Roman period when elite competition for social and political status often overcame Greek ideologies of equality and participation (Donahue 2018). However, sacrifice and communal feasting would have been a regular feature of both Greek and Roman religion, which may also have controlled and regulated consumption (Ekroth 2007; Hitch 2015). Supply and distribution systems were required for large urban communities to function, as a large proportion of the population needed to be relieved of agricultural duties in order to carry out urban building labour or administrative tasks (Bernard 2016). During the Roman period, the economy on Crete changes as it becomes integral within Mediterranean networks with a particular focus on the mass export of wine and increased reliance on imported food (Chaniotis 1999, 211). However, an urban population dependent on this system was a high-risk enterprise due to problems that could occur with failed yields and grain transportation (Garnsey 1988; Morley 1996, 55–56). A return to small-scale subsistence farming reduced vulnerability to these problems, as individuals could choose to disperse landholdings, diversify produce and store surplus to secure a food supply (Garnsey 1988, 48). However, if the decreased population at Knossos was compensated for by the growth of the settlement at Heraklion production strategies may have continued on a similar scale to the previous periods for the wider region but may have returned to subsistence as opposed to being more dependent on imports.

5.4.5. Cemetery (location)

As the Hellenistic and Late Antique samples all came from tombs in the North Cemetery, the discussion of dietary differences between individuals buried in different cemeteries or locations is again restricted to the Roman period. Just as for the different tomb types, the burial location could potentially represent different social groups. Although the North Cemetery contained many of the monumental built tombs and these tombs would have been a display of social standing along the main route into the city from the north and from the coast, there was also a diverse range of tomb types here, suggesting a lack of exclusivity in the burial area as a whole. The Roman North Cemetery samples come from four different tomb types and therefore are likely to represent individuals of different social status. In this case, tomb type was more important than cemetery choice as a public display of status. Although it was observed that the built tomb individual had a much higher $\delta^{15}N$ value than the tile grave individual, indicating a diet with a greater protein component in the former, to extend this interpretation to an assessment of individuals buried in these tomb types in general is not possible. The example of the high degree of variation between two individuals' isotopic signatures within a single tomb, such as S86 and S89 in the Topana tomb, demonstrates how caution must be exercised when using small sample sizes and generalisations should not be inferred from a single individual's diet.

The Sanatorium cemetery had the highest $\delta^{15}N$ values, followed by the individuals from the Krevatina cist grave. These are Late Roman burials in stone-lined graves and as discussed for the tomb types (Section 5.4.4) it seems likely that the significant factor was the social change occurring in the later Roman period. The transition to Christianity may also have been the impetus for the initiation of a new cemetery on this site in the 3rd century AD. Within the Sanatorium cemetery sample, the results were investigated for difference by tomb type, sex and age. No patterns or significant differences were identified between the tomb types or age groups. This suggests that the different tomb forms did not have individuals of significantly different social status, or at least no difference that was isotopically detectable between their diets. While a slight difference was suggested between male and female diets, with the female isotopic mean value slightly higher and a statistically significant difference between the $\delta^{13}C$ variances, there was no significant difference in the mean values and the sample was small. The main difference, as was observed for the entire sample for all time periods, was that the female values were more variable and the male values were closely clustered together.

With cemeteries lying to the north and south of the settlement and differences observed for the settlement itself in terms of finds and building types between the northern and southern regions of the city, the differences between these two broad regions (North and South) were investigated. The northern side of the settlement had a widespread distribution of mosaics, as well as most of the public buildings such as the civic basilica and bath houses, though many of these were not constructed until the 2nd and 3rd centuries. In the southern part of the settlement residential and industrial areas have been identified, with kilns for pottery production and a dump site of Knossian and Cretan amphorae suggestive of an Early Roman warehouse or distribution centre (Whitelaw *et al.* 2016; 2017). The North mean values ($\delta^{13}C$ and $\delta^{15}N$) were only very slightly (and insignificantly) higher than the South ones. The South values were slightly lower and slightly more variable but there does not appear to be a meaningful difference between diets of individuals interred in cemeteries to the north or south of the settlement. Though, as mentioned in the Section 5.3.5, the pattern observed within the settlement (between the finds and architecture in the north and south) need not be extended to the consideration of where these different subsets of society were burying their dead. The existence of many built tombs to the north is an indicator that the burial record might also place the upper echelons of society to the north of the valley. However, relatively little material for sampling was available from most of the built tombs, therefore a mixed demographic appears to be represented. Additionally, the southern tomb forms are also quite elaborate, being largely represented by the rock-cut chamber tombs in this sample, therefore these samples are unlikely to represent the lower echelons of society. Large Late Roman built tombs are also known from the excavations at the Sanctuary of Demeter and Hogarth's Houses on Lower Gypsades though these were poorly preserved and there is no skeletal material for these tombs.

5.5. Conclusion

The Knossian diet in all time periods was one based on C3 plants and usually including some C3 animal products as well, and for some individuals some fish. Fish consumption was limited in most diets but there was a slight increase in marine organism consumption in the Late Antique period. The most significant differences in diets at Knossos are between the different time periods due to the social changes that were occurring. Diets were not as variable as they had been in the later Bronze Age, nor was the same level of intrapopulation variation observed within any single period between those of different social status or by demographic characteristics. This indicates less social differentiation or hierarchy within each of the Hellenistic, Roman and Late Antique periods, or that the excavated skeletal remains (and therefore the sample) only represents a fairly homogeneous social group for each time period. While the latter is possible for the spatially-limited Hellenistic and Late Antique samples, it seems highly unlikely for the Roman sample which represents a wide range of tomb types and burial locations around the city. This suggests that there were not dramatic differences in diet between different social groups or that the differences were not isotopically detectable. Even the individuals of low social standing had some animal products in their diet, and these individuals would not be detectably different from individuals eating dramatically larger quantities of these foods. $\delta^{15}N$ values are not elevated by excess quantities of protein as excess protein cannot be absorbed and passes out of the system in urine, leaving no trace. The difference between protein intake from dairy or from meat would also not be distinguishable as all animal products have similar isotopic values.

A tentative pattern is suggested by Papathanasiou and Richards (2015, 201) in their concluding chapter for *Archaeodiet in the Greek World* of higher animal protein consumption in times of economic and cultural growth and prosperity, such as for the elite classes of the Mycenaean civilisation and at Classical Athens. Though they concede that a great deal more data are needed to support this assertion. The Knossos data do not fit with this pattern. It is most likely that the Roman period was the period of greatest economic and cultural growth and prosperity, as reflected in the greater monumentality and abundance of building projects as well as conspicuous displays of wealth and status in both the private and burial spheres, though this is not apparent until the 2nd and 3rd centuries. Less is known about the Hellenistic city and it is likely that in developing the Roman city evidence of its predecessor was removed. It was, however, more extensive than the Roman city and considered to be politically successful as one of the foremost centres in Crete. Despite accounts of mercenaries, pirates, wars and unrest, Hellenistic Knossos was also an economically thriving and culturally prominent city. Although there was a steady demographic decline throughout the Roman period, this was independent of prosperity. The basilica churches and their elaborate mosaics indicate a prosperous community at Late Antique Knossos and it was the Late Antique sample that had the individuals with the most isotopically elevated dietary signatures, indicating the consumption of higher trophic level proteins. This most likely took the form of a small (but increased) amount of fish in the diet.

6

Dental Disease

The study of dental disease can be extremely informative for aspects of ancient diets. Everything that is eaten comes into contact with the teeth. Although a series of endogenous, pathogenic and environmental processes influence the manifestation of dental diseases, diet is the primary influencer. The most common dental diseases occur due to the build-up of plaque that occurs on the surfaces of the teeth and the cumulative effect of pH environment of that plaque (Hillson 1996; 2008a; 2008b). This dense accumulation of bacterial micro-organisms can result in dental caries (teeth), gingivitis (soft tissue), periodontal disease (alveolar bone), granulomata and abscesses (periapical bone), and can mineralise to form dental calculus (tooth surfaces), which can often lead to tooth loss or extraction. Gingivitis, of course, cannot be observed in skeletal material but periodontal disease and periapical lesions have also been excluded from a systematic study of dental disease for the Knossos assemblage due to the high levels of fragmentation, with many cases of partial or complete destruction of the alveolar process, or the bone being entirely absent with many teeth being recorded loose.

Dental caries is a disease process characterised by the focal demineralisation of dental hard tissues by organic acids produced by bacterial fermentation of carbohydrates in the diet (Larsen 2015, 67; Temple 2015, 434). It manifests itself variously as it progresses from slight enamel opacities to extensive cavities involving the partial or complete destruction of the crown and roots of teeth (Hillson 2008b). It is primarily indicative of a high carbohydrate diet. As such it has proved particularly useful in the study of major changes in subsistence patterns, for example at the transition from hunter-gatherer groups to more sedentary farming settlements (Lillie 1996; Lukacs 1996; Lillie and Richards 2000; Eshed *et al.* 2006; Temple and Larsen 2007; Lanfranco and Eggers 2010; Karsten *et al.* 2015). However, it has also proved useful for more subtle changes and differences in diets over time, between different populations or among different sub-groups of a population (Swärdstedt 1966; Girotti and Doro Garetto 1999; Bonfiglioli *et al.* 2003; Lukacs 2011; Šlaus *et al.* 2011; Tomczyk *et al.* 2013; Bonsall 2014). Periapical lesions are caused due to inflammation of the pulp chamber, when bacteria have access to it due to caries, attrition or fracture. These toxins can then pass through the apical foramen of the tooth to trigger inflammation in the periodontal tissues, causing the resorption of the bone to form a periapical granuloma, which can accumulate pus to become an abscess (Hillson 1996, 284–85).

Calculus is mineralised dental plaque that has adhered to the tooth surface, either as supra-gingival or sub-gingival calculus. Calculus can contribute to the occurrence of periodontal disease. Sub-gingival calculus forms within the periodontal pocket and its presence is associated with long-standing plaque deposits (Powell and Garnick 1978; Hillson 2008a, 312). As such it can be used to infer the presence and degree of periodontal disease (Brothwell 1981, 154; Ortner and Putschar 1981, 442; Lieverse 1999, 219). Its aetiology is little understood but it is known that an alkaline environment in the mouth is conducive to its formation. Diet is known to play a role but the other factors contributing to its formation are often overlooked (Lieverse 1999). High protein diets are thought to increase the alkalinity of the oral environment but this factor has been over-used in the interpretation of calculus. A high alkaline environment can be caused by the loss of carbon dioxide following saliva secretion and the production of ammonia from the metabolism of amino acids and urea (Hodge and Leung 1950; Mandel and Thompson 1967; Schroeder 1969; Mandel 1990; Margolis 1990). Caries, requiring an acidic environment, and calculus, requiring an alkaline environment, are often found on the same tooth (Hillson 1996, 260). Therefore, it is an oversimplification to interpret calculus as representing a high protein diet without any other factors being considered (Lieverse 1999). These other factors include the general chemical composition of oral fluids, biological processes, and cultural factors affecting the oral environment. Although it is known that the amount of calcium and phosphorus in the oral environment affect the weight of calculus deposit, there are still confounding factors in understanding what factors affect the presence of amounts of these minerals (Mandel 1974; Lieverse 1999).

Antemortem tooth loss is not technically a disease but is caused by different dental diseases, including caries and periodontal disease. Antemortem tooth loss is represented by remodelling sockets or remodelled spaces where a tooth has been lost prior to death. The alveolar process (the bone around the teeth forming the sockets) is a site of active remodelling at all ages for the development of teeth and in response to occlusion and wear processes (Hillson 2008a, 319). Inflammation of the supporting (periodontal) tissues can also cause alveolar bone loss. This is in relation to periodontal disease which also involves inflammation of the gums. It can result in tooth loss as a 'moat' is formed between the tooth and the bone by the receding alveolar margin and widening tooth socket, until eventually the periodontal ligament attachment for the tooth is lost (Hillson 1996, 266–67).

Some studies score dental diseases by individual which is problematic, particularly for caries, as it does not distinguish between an individual with a single mild lesion and one with many severe lesions. Scoring by tooth gives a more representative picture of caries prevalence across an assemblage (Steckel *et al.* 2002, 70). However, statistical evaluation of caries rates for epidemiological purposes is problematic in fragmented archaeological material. The DMF index records the number of decayed, missing or filled teeth for each individual to express the mean per individual across the assemblage. This does not account for having more than one lesion per tooth or for teeth lost by periodontal disease or post-mortem (Hillson 1996, 279–80; Temple 2015, 443). Scoring by tooth with highly fragmented material (often with poor retrieval of elements) can result in overrepresenting better preserved individuals while other individuals may be represented by a single tooth. Molars are more prone to caries than anterior teeth, and molars are less likely to be lost post-mortem, so assemblages with poor anterior tooth preservation will have artificially inflated caries rates (Hillson 1996, 280). Scoring each site of the tooth and considering the severity of lesions can help circumvent this to a certain extent, but when it comes to comparing different assemblages there is little that can be done to overcome the shortcomings of poor preservation, such as a lack of representation for anterior teeth.

6.1. Methods

6.1.1. Caries

Caries was scored using the Hillson (2001) method of scoring each surface of the crown and root on an 8-point scale of caries progression. Dental caries can be easily scored on both loose teeth and those in situ in the bone. This method enables the complete range of caries with different forms and aetiologies to be recorded for the assessment of the progressive nature of the disease. This allows for better interpretation of the disease than less comprehensive scoring systems. While the manifestation of caries can be affected by endogenous, pathogenic or environmental factors, it is primarily indicative of a predominantly carbohydrate diet, namely, a crop-based diet.

Coronal and root surface caries are both scored for a variety of sides and facets of both the crown and root respectively and this is done separately for different tooth types. The sites recorded and a brief description of the site where carious lesions can be initiated are outlined in Table 6.1. Root surface and attrition facet caries only develop later in life when the gingival margin has receded or occlusal enamel worn down respectively. Coronal caries can be initiated anywhere in the enamel of the crown, but the most common location is at the contact point or approximal surface between the teeth.

Most of the enamel caries types are scored on a scale of 0–8, with 0 meaning there is no lesion, 1 being the initial signs of a lesion (in the form of an opaque or stained patch on the crown surface) and 8 being the most severe lesion (gross coronal caries, involving the occlusal crown surface and contact area or pit, within the floor of which is the open pulp chamber, or open root canals). The root surface caries is scored in a similar way but with fewer stages and gaps in the numbering system to match the numbering of the other categories (scores 2-4 are missing as there are no equivalent stages identified for this type of caries). Each tooth is also scored for presence/absence, which includes additional nuanced options including 'partially erupted' and 'present with

Table 6.1. Descriptions for sites of the tooth where caries is scored.

Occlusal surface	Fissures, fossae, grooves, and sloping cusp sides that mark the occlusal surfaces of molar and premolar crowns.
Pit	Buccal pits at the end of fissures on the molar crown sides, or in the pits which sometimes mark the lingual surfaces of upper incisors.
Attrition facet	Facets created by attrition/wear exposing dentine.
Edge chipping	Antemortem chipped enamel at the edges of attrition facets.
Buccal enamel	Smooth surface on the labial/buccal crown, most commonly along the cervix of the crown just above the line of the gingivae.
Buccal root	Root surface either along the buccal cement-enamel junction or further down the root when this is exposed above the margin of the gingivae.
Distal contact	Contact point or approximal smooth surface on the distal crown side, just below the contact point between neighbouring teeth.
Distal root	Root surface either along the distal cement-enamel junction or further down the root when this is exposed above the margin of the gingivae.
Lingual enamel	Smooth surface on the lingual crown, most commonly along the cervix of the crown just above the line of the gingivae.
Lingual root	Root surface either along the lingual cement-enamel junction or further down the root when this is exposed above the margin of the gingivae.
Mesial contact	Contact point or approximal smooth surface on the mesial crown side, just below the contact point between neighbouring teeth.
Mesial root	Root surface either along the mesial cement-enamel junction or further down the root when this is exposed above the margin of the gingivae.

gross gross caries' (where the site of initiation is unknown as the lesion takes over much of the tooth). Appendix A in Hillson's (2001) paper provides comprehensive guidelines for this recording system. The recording was done in the Access skeletal database with dropdown options, including descriptions, to avoid any errors in misnumbering categories.

6.1.2. Calculus

Calculus is mineralised bacterial plaque which adheres to the surface of the tooth. Similar to caries, it is a result of conditions in the mouth and is primarily dependent on the diet, though it can be affected by a variety of factors. It is most commonly found close to salivary ducts, on the lingual surfaces of the anterior teeth and the buccal surfaces of the molars (Hillson 1996, 255). The exact aetiology of calculus is complex and its relationship to diet is little understood. It is known to derive from saliva and saliva content and is dependent on interactions between food and the bacterial environment surrounding the teeth. In the past it has been frequently misinterpreted, based on no clinical evidence, as being indicative of a high protein diet (Baer *et al.* 1961; Mandel 1974; Lieverse 1999). Meanwhile, caries was conversely interpreted as indicative of a high carbohydrate diet, but as both often occur in a single tooth, this interpretation has no merit. Calculus requires plaque deposits, therefore factors that result in an increased accumulation of plaque, such as poor oral hygiene and carbohydrate consumption, are likely contributing factors. However, heavy plaque deposits do not necessarily lead to large calculus deposits, therefore there are further factors to be considered in the initiation of mineralisation (Hillson 1996, 259). Genetic factors also contribute to its manifestation.

These difficulties in understanding calculus aetiology make the interpretation of its occurrence and changes and differences in its prevalence difficult to interpret. However, significant differences can be used alongside the evidence for caries and antemortem tooth loss to identify changes and differences in diet, even if their exact nature is unclear. Another problem with recording calculus is that it can be easily chipped off. With the poor storage conditions of many of the teeth in this assemblage it is likely that some calculus deposits will have been lost and whether this significantly affects the representativeness of the results cannot easily be ascertained. Often a small remnant of a calculus deposit was still visible on the tooth which indicated a larger deposit had once been there. This likely results in the over-scoring of slight deposits (Score 1) compared to the heavier deposits (Scores 2 and 3).

Calculus is scored using the Brothwell (1981) method which simply describes the calculus deposit, if present, on a scale of 0-3: 0 (absent), 1 (small amount, 'light' or 'slight'), 2 (medium amount, 'medium'), or 3 (large amount, 'considerable' or 'heavy'). The descriptions for the three categories for the presence of calculus also considers whether it is only on the crown surface, touching the root or overhanging the root respectively. While calculus is difficult to interpret, it is extremely simple and quick to record, therefore, it is hoped that when used in conjunction with caries patterns may occur, and though the nature of the difference between different diets may not be easily identified, the fact that there is a difference or a change is inherently interesting.

6.1.3. Antemortem tooth loss

Antemortem (or *intra vitam*) tooth loss is usually caused by plaque related diseases, namely periodontal disease and caries, though can also be caused by other factors, such as trauma (Niessen and Weyant 1989; Phipps and Stevens 1995; Hawkins *et al.* 1997; Stabholz *et al.* 1997; Oginni 2005; Lukacs 2007; Wasterlain *et al.* 2009). Antemortem tooth loss (AMTL) was recorded by counting remodelling sockets or fully remodelled gaps out of all the available teeth or empty sockets due to post mortem loss of teeth. This is integrated with the caries scoring system with scores 11 and 12 in the presence/absence category (Table 6.2) representing the three types of antemortem tooth loss recorded. As with the various different forms of caries,

Table 6.2. Caries scoring system with descriptions for each numbered category (after Hillson 2001).

[BLANK]	missing post-mortem and jaw with socket missing too.
0	tooth present, without gross gross caries.
7	gross gross carious cavity, involving the loss of so much of the tooth that it is not possible to determine whether the lesion was initiated in the crown or root.
8	gross gross carious cavity, involving the loss of so much of the tooth that it is not possible to determine whether the lesion was initiated in the crown or root, and there is a clear opening into an exposed pulp chamber or root canal.
10	tooth missing, leaving an empty socket in the jaw without any sign of remodelling.
11	tooth missing, leaving an empty cavity in which there are signs of remodelling, but the bone is not fully remodelled to a level contour.
12	tooth missing, with full remodelling of the jaw to leave a level contour.
13	no evidence that the tooth has ever erupted (as a result of young age, impaction or agenesis).
14	tooth partly erupted (crypt communicating with crest of alveolar process, or tooth not yet in wear).
15	anomalous eruption, so that the tooth has not reached its normal position in the tooth row.

there are intentional gaps in the scoring system to match the numberings of other categories.

6.2. Results

6.2.1. Caries

Results are presented by tooth, observing firstly whether caries of any degree is present or absent. Secondly, caries in the form of a cavity is presented, excluding the early signs of the presence of caries represented by the first two stages in the Hillson method, to make the results comparable with other assemblages using different caries scoring methods (generally as present or absent by tooth or by individual with the formation of a cavity). Finally, a cumulative score is presented which is the sum of the progression stage of each lesion on each site of a tooth, which is then totalled for all the teeth in any group and divided by the number of carious teeth in that group to give an average caries score per tooth which represents the mean severity of carious lesions. As well as presenting raw numbers of carious teeth (generally in parentheses expressed as a fraction of the total scorable teeth), the results are presented as percentages of the total number of scorable teeth, in order to make the results comparable across different time periods, tomb types, cemeteries or between the sexes. Results are not presented by individual due to the commingled nature of much of the material and the fact that many teeth had to be scored as individual, loose teeth rather than in the maxilla or mandible of an identifiable individual, and even when teeth where found in the dental arcade, or a fragment of it, often the mandible and maxilla could not be paired or one might exist without the other.

For all time periods combined, a total of 1572 teeth were recorded (Table 6.7). There was a total of 274 (17.4%) carious teeth and a total of 151 (9.6%) teeth with cavities (i.e. caries score 3 and above). The average cumulative caries score for all teeth was 1 (i.e. including teeth with a caries score of 0), and the average cumulative score for carious teeth was 6 (i.e. counting teeth with a caries score of at least 1). Caries is more common in certain tooth types, zones of the teeth and in older individuals. Therefore, before considering the main variables of the study it is important to consider the tooth types, tooth zones and age distribution of the assemblage.

6.2.1.1. Tooth type

Table 6.3 and Figure 6.1 demonstrate that caries is most common in the molars, followed by the premolars, as

Table 6.3. Caries counts and scores by tooth for each tooth type.

	Teeth with caries	Teeth with cavities	Average Score (per carious tooth – for all teeth)
Incisors	6.1% (20/326)	3.7% (12/326)	4.3 – 0.3
Canines	8.8% (15/171)	5.3% (9/171)	6.1 – 0.5
Premolars	18.1% (69/382)	7.1% (27/382)	6.4 – 1.2
Molars	24.5% (172/702)	15.0% (105/702)	6.1 – 1.5

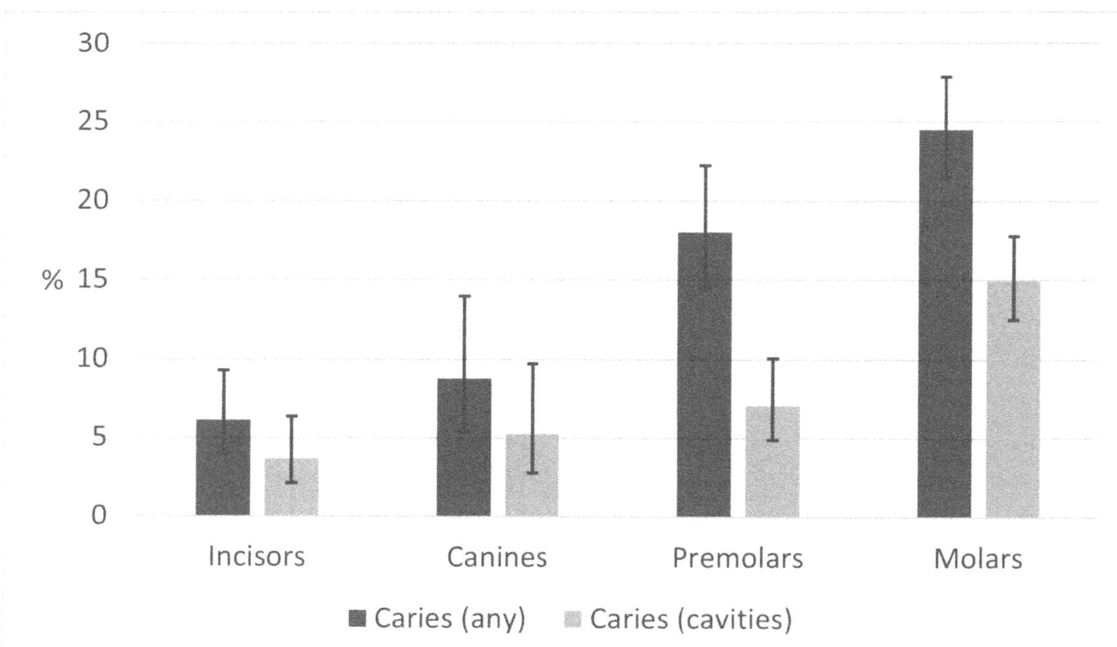

Figure 6.1. Prevalence of caries and cavities by tooth for each tooth type with 95% confidence interval error bars.

was expected due to the fissure systems on their occlusal surfaces (Hillson 2008b, 117). Both had significantly higher caries levels than the canines and incisors (see non-overlapping confidence intervals for caries prevalence in Figure 6.1). As the variables for which caries prevalence is being considered are unlikely to be evenly represented by all tooth types it is important to consider that the varying proportions of tooth types could be the cause of a significant difference between two variables. Figure 6.2 demonstrates the expected (or ideal) proportions of each tooth type based on a complete, normal dentition, including the third molars, and the proportions of each tooth type for each of the time periods. Table 6.4 displays the numbers and proportions of each tooth type for all of the main variables being studied in the chapter to provide a control for the following results. The most commonly underrepresented tooth type is the incisor, followed by the canine. Molars are nearly always overrepresented due to more often being preserved within the jaws, and potentially due to their being larger and therefore more visible even when loose for collection during excavation. However, if these under- and over-representations are similar for each of the variables being compared then it will not bias the comparison. Considering the time periods, for example, the molars and premolars are over-represented in each case, and the incisors and canines are under-represented (Figure 6.2). The Roman and Late Antique distributions are very similar, while the Hellenistic distribution is closer to the 'expected' proportions but this is unlikely to be a significant enough difference to bias the results.

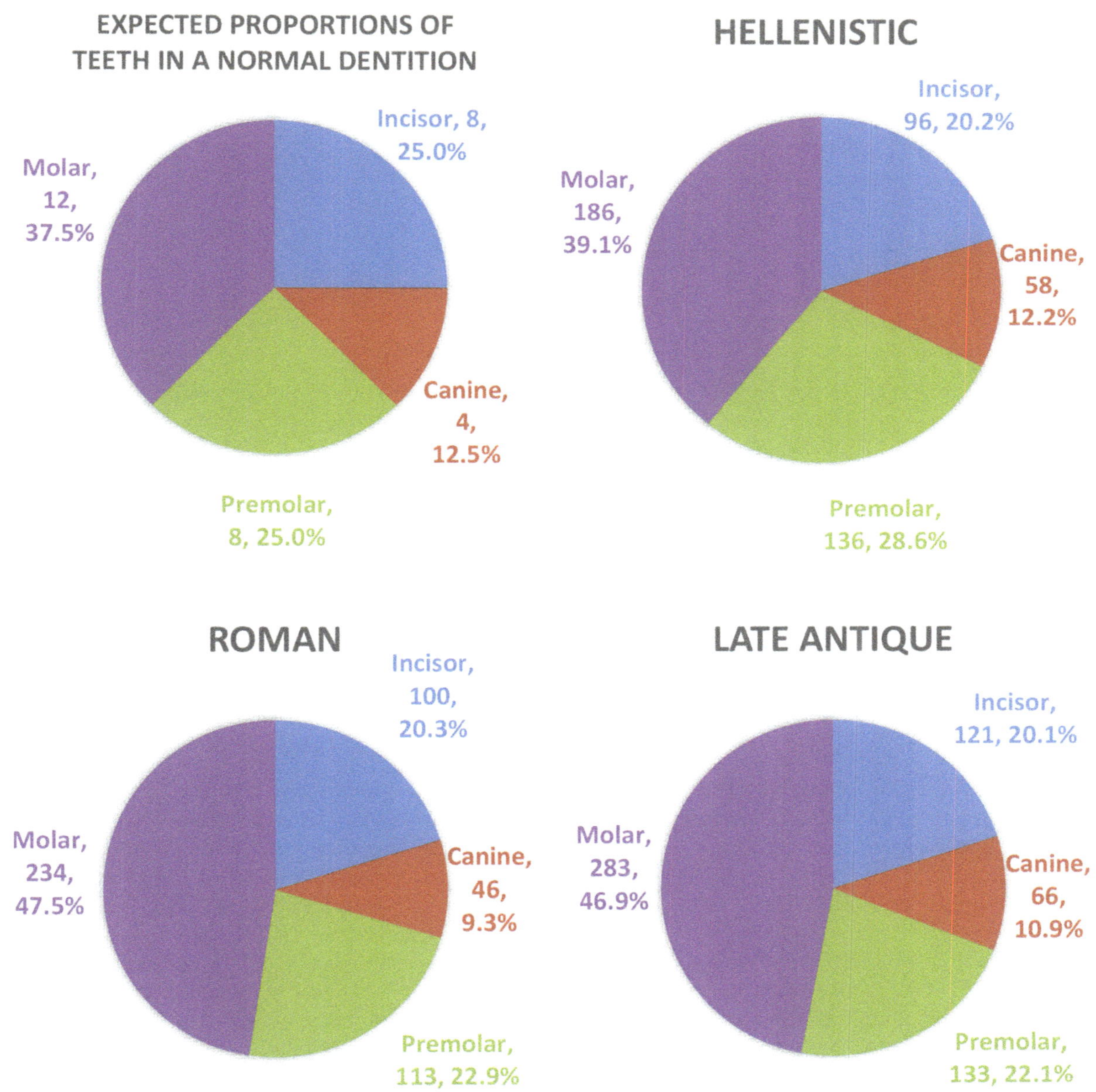

Figure 6.2. Pie charts demonstrating expected proportions of each tooth type in a normal dentition (assuming third molars are present) and the proportions of each tooth type present in the assemblage for each time period.

Table 6.4. Proportions and numbers of each tooth type for each of the main variables within the main categories under study.

	Incisor	Canine	Premolar	Molar
Expected Values	**25.0% (8)**	**12.5% (4)**	**25.0% (8)**	**37.5% (12)**
Time Periods				
Hellenistic	20.2% (96)	12.2% (58)	28.6% (136)	39.1% (186)
Roman	20.3% (100)	9.3% (46)	22.9% (113)	47.5% (234)
Late Antique	20.1% (121)	10.9% (66)	22.1% (133)	46.9% (283)
Sexes				
Female	21.4% (134)	12.0% (75)	26.2% (164)	40.4% (253)
Male	22.7% (100)	12.0% (53)	26.1% (115)	39.2% (173)
Age Groups				
Child	27.9% (24)	8.1% (7)	9.3% (8)	54.7% (47)
Adolescent	21.5% (29)	11.9% (16)	26.7% (36)	40.0% (54)
Young Adult	21.3% (211)	10.4% (103)	25.0% (248)	43.3% (429)
Middle Adult	17.3% (56)	12.4% (40)	23.8% (77)	46.4% (150)
Old Adult	9.8% (4)	9.8% (4)	31.7% (13)	48.8% (20)
Tomb Types				
Built	13.4% (13)	3.1% (3)	21.6% (21)	61.9% (60)
Chamber	22.0% (48)	7.8% (17)	21.1% (46)	49.1% (107)
Osteotheke	20.1% (100)	10.9% (54)	21.3% (106)	47.7% (237)
Stone-lined	23.0% (26)	10.6% (12)	23.0% (26)	43.4% (49)
Cist	20.4% (20)	13.3% (13)	24.5% (24)	41.8% (41)
Tile	18.8% (18)	14.6% (14)	27.1% (26)	39.6% (38)
Pit	20.7% (92)	12.8% (57)	28.3% (126)	38.2% (170)
Cemeteries				
Monastiriako Kephali	22.7% (29)	8.6% (11)	21.9% (28)	46.9% (60)
Krevatina	22.2% (4)	22.2% (4)	22.2% (4)	33.3% (6)
North Cemetery (Hellenistic)	21.7% (105)	12.0% (58)	28.1% (136)	38.2% (185)
North Cemetery (Roman)	19.4% (18)	12.9% (12)	21.5% (20)	46.2% (43)
North Cemetery (Late Antique)	20.4% (120)	9.0% (53)	22.4% (132)	48.1% (283)
Sanatorium	19.7% (30)	9.9% (15)	26.3% (40)	44.1% (67)
Spilia	21.2% (11)	9.6% (5)	21.2% (11)	48.1% (25)
Topana	10.4% (5)	4.2% (2)	22.9% (11)	62.5% (30)

No significant different in caries prevalence was noted between the maxillary (19.2% of 667 teeth) and mandibular (16.1% of 905 teeth) teeth (Moles 2023).

6.2.1.2. Tooth zone

Caries was scored by the sites or zones of the tooth as outlined in Table 6.1, with the results presented by tooth type and for all the teeth combined in Table 6.5. Figure 6.3 depicts these results as a bar chart for each tooth type, while Figure 6.4 shows the results for all tooth types combined. Figure 6.5 groups the tooth zones together into similar types to get a better overall picture of the zones of the teeth most affected by caries.

The most common sites for caries on the molars and premolars were the mesial and distal contact areas and the occlusal surfaces (fissures). Caries was less common in the incisors and canines but was most common in the attrition facets (where wear had exposed dentine on the occlusal surface) and on the buccal enamel and root surface/cemento-enamel junction (CEJ). The tendency of attrition facets and root surfaces to be the most common sites for caries has been found to be a familiar pattern amongst archaeological agriculturalist groups that were typified by high attrition rates alongside a high starch, low sugar diet (Hillson 2008b, 125). The high wear rates (and the resultant continued eruption) cause the more vulnerable surfaces at the CEJ and enamel-dentine junction (EDJ) to be exposed.

Table 6.5. Numbers of caries, counts of zones scored, and percentage of caries for each tooth zone, presented for each tooth type and for all the teeth combined.

	Edge chip.	Attrit. facet	Buccal enamel	Bucc. root	Distal contact	Dist. root	Lingual enamel	Ling. root	Mesial contact	Mes. root	Occlus. surface	Pit
Incisor Caries	0	5	7	7	3	1	1	1	2	5	0	1
Zones scored	290	293	326	316	314	315	322	316	318	316	0	129
% caries	0.0	1.7	2.1	2.2	1.0	0.3	0.3	0.3	0.6	1.6		0.8
Canine caries	0	3	3	3	3	4	2	2	2	0	0	0
Zones scored	156	156	169	163	166	164	167	162	162	164	0	0
% caries	0.0	1.9	1.8	1.8	1.8	2.4	1.2	1.2	1.2	0.0		
Premolar caries	0	5	6	11	20	12	0	5	19	4	13	0
Zones scored	242	250	330	368	367	354	374	371	366	372	367	0
% caries	0.0	2.0	1.8	3.0	5.4	3.4	0.0	1.3	5.2	1.1	3.5	
Molar caries	1	14	15	21	45	23	7	13	67	31	52	10
Zones scored	467	462	687	675	668	667	683	670	672	662	689	661
% caries	0.2	3.0	2.2	3.1	6.7	3.4	1.0	1.9	10.0	4.7	7.5	1.5
Total caries	1	27	31	42	71	40	10	21	90	40	65	11
Zones scored	1155	1161	1512	1522	1515	1500	1546	1519	1518	1514	1056	790
% caries	0.1	2.3	2.1	2.8	4.7	2.7	0.6	1.4	5.9	2.6	6.2	1.4

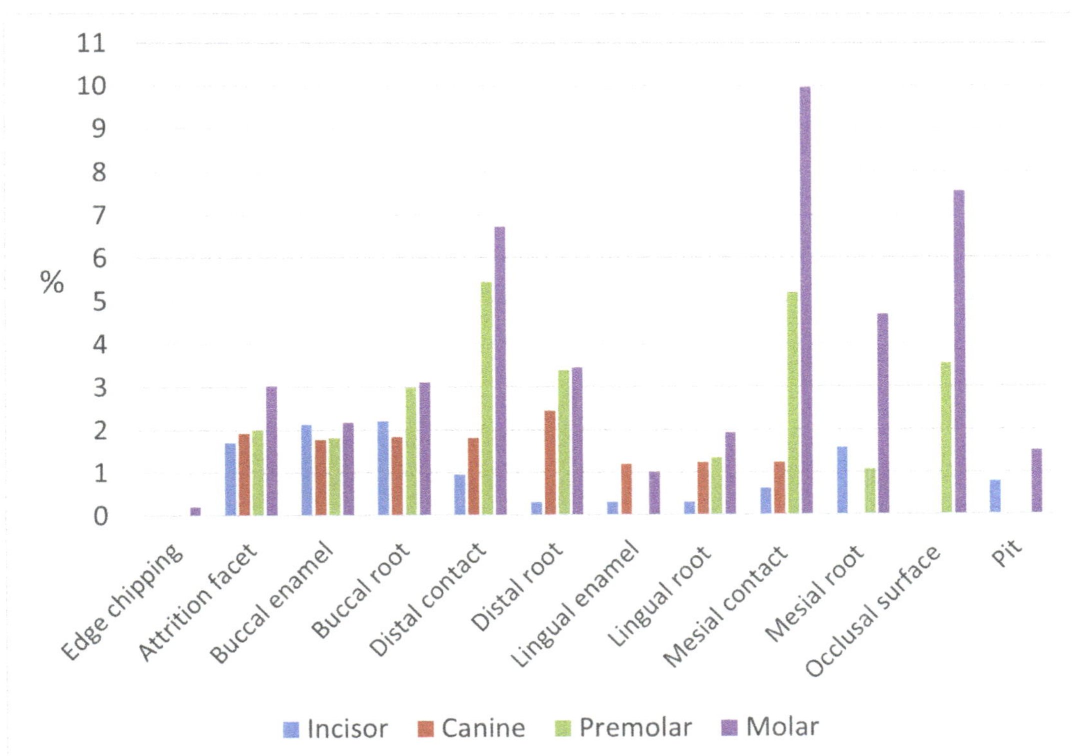

Figure 6.3. Caries prevalence for each zone scored on the teeth by tooth type.

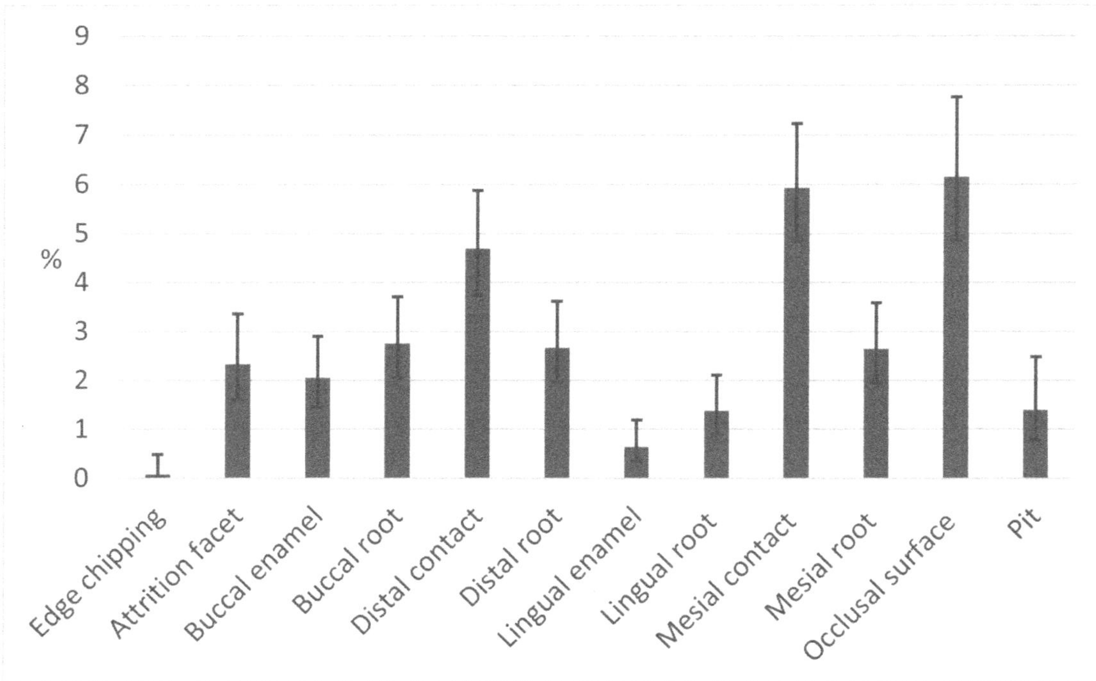

Figure 6.4. Caries prevalence for each zone scored on the teeth for all teeth (tooth types combined) with 95% confidence interval error bars.

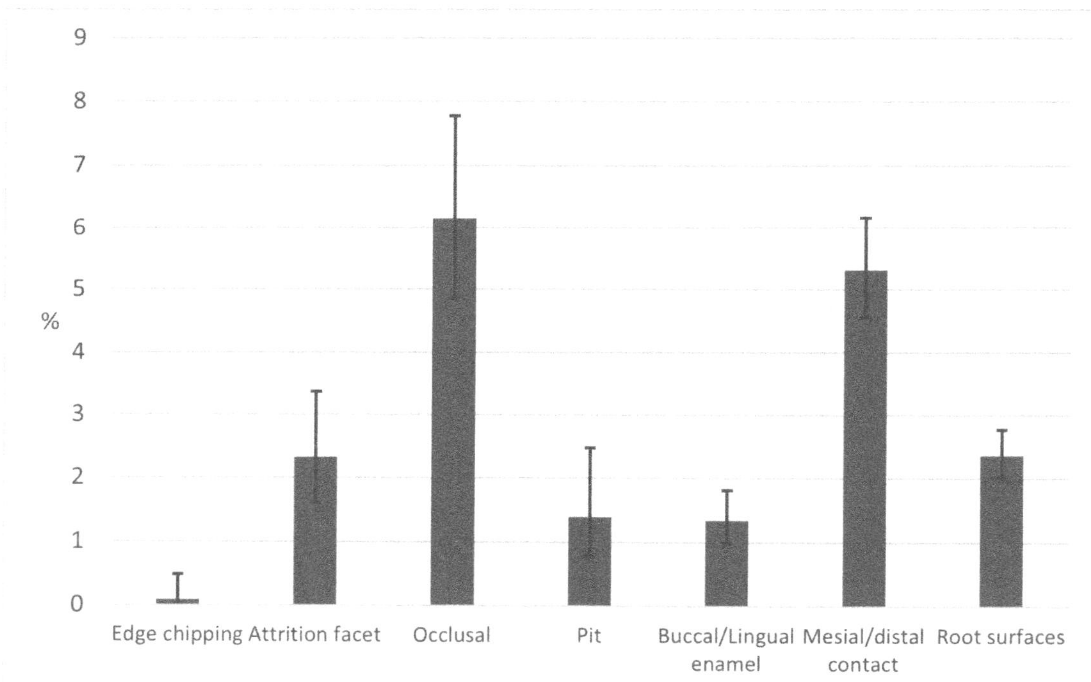

Figure 6.5. Caries prevalence for the tooth zones grouped into similar types for all teeth with 95% confidence interval error bars.

However, with caries being more common in the molars and premolars, the overall pattern has the highest caries rates in the occlusal surfaces and mesial/distal (interproximal) contact areas and these were significantly higher rates than for the attrition facets or roots surfaces, as demonstrated by the non-overlapping confidence intervals (Figure 6.5). This could be due to the low wear rates or young ages-at-death (most ages were determined by dental wear) not exposing the CEJ or EDJ for as long or in as many teeth as in other agricultural communities with starch staples in their diets. Although the prevalence of caries is much lower, the pattern of higher caries on the occlusal and interproximal surfaces is more comparable to modern western caries patterns which have been attributed to the high sugar and starch diets and high frequency of snacking during childhood (Hillson 2008b, 120). This could be indicative of a higher sugar content in the diets at Knossos than was customary in agricultural populations, meaning that caries often occurred in a tooth prior to the exposure of dentine from wear, or the CEJ from continual eruption.

6.2.1.3. Age group

Caries should be highly age progressive, though factors such as antemortem tooth loss and wear can mask this to a degree in the results (Hillson 1996, 284). Additionally, small sample sizes, particularly in the Old Adult category, may produce unrepresentative results. The results are displayed in Table 6.6 and Figures 6.6–7. The overall trend for caries (any, i.e. including early stage and cavitous caries), was that it became more common with increasing age, other than the Adolescent result being slightly elevated above the Young Adult one. Both the cavities results and the average caries scores show a trend of progression with age from childhood through to middle-adulthood though there is overlap of confidence intervals which could be due to the small sample sizes for some groups or a lack of significant differences. Notably, the confidence intervals for Young and Middle Adult (the two largest sample size groups) cavities do not overlap indicating a significant difference. The Old Adult caries prevalence is likely lower due to the aforementioned issues of tooth loss, wear and sample size. Figure 6.7 demonstrates relatively low levels of early-stage caries for the Young and Middle Adult categories. Early-stage caries is most commonly observed on the interproximal attrition facets (between the teeth). For complete mandibles and maxillae with closely packed teeth prohibiting a view of these facets of the teeth firmly fixed within the jaws (which are most common for the Young and Middle Adult categories) these facets often could not be scored. This may have resulted in the underscoring of early-stage caries for some teeth.

Table 6.6. Prevalence of caries, cavities and carious scores for the age groups.

	Teeth with caries	Teeth with cavities	Average Score (per carious tooth – for all teeth)
Child	8.1% (7/86)	1.2% (1/86)	2.3 – 0.2
Adolescent	17.8% (24/135)	6.7% (9/135)	2.8 – 0.5
Young Adult	16.8% (166/991)	8.9% (88/991)	5.5 – 0.9
Middle Adult	20.7% (67/323)	15.2% (49/323)	9.0 – 1.9
Old Adult	29.3% (12/41)	14.6% (6/41)	5.6 – 1.6

6.2.1.4. Time period

The overall caries results and the breakdown by time period are displayed in Table 6.7. The results by time period are displayed in Figure 6.8 and demonstrate a peak in the prevalence of caries in the Roman period, occurring in 25.2% (124/493) of teeth compared to only 8.4% (40/476) in the Hellenistic

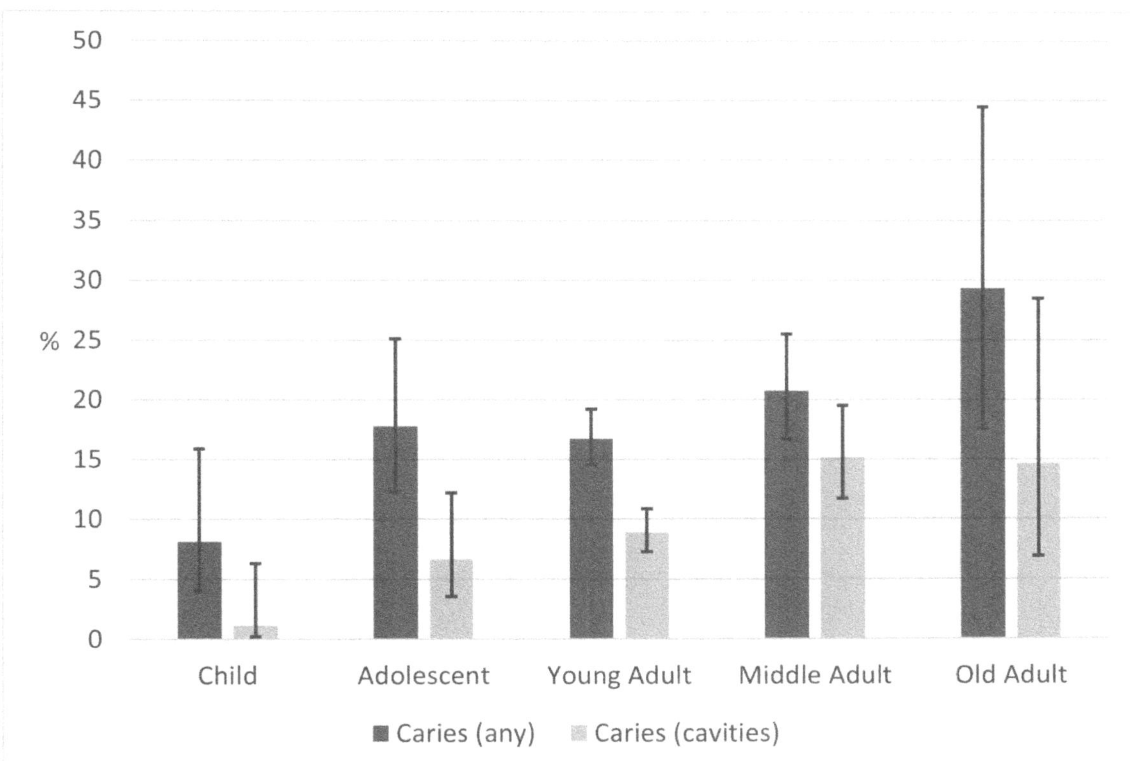

Figure 6.6. Prevalence of caries and cavities for the age groups with 95% confidence interval error bars.

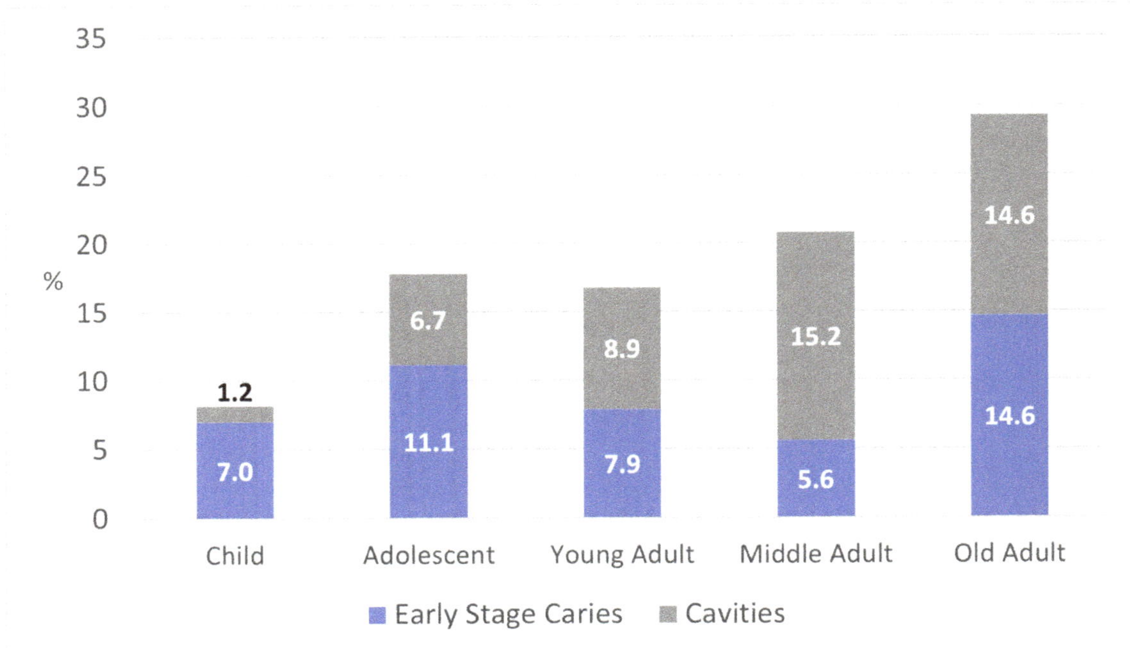

Figure 6.7. Prevalence of early stage caries and cavities (stacked to show total caries prevalence) for the age groups.

Table 6.7. Caries counts and scores by tooth for each time period.

	Caries (any)	Caries (cavity)	Caries Score (total)	Caries mean score (by all teeth)	Caries mean score (by carious teeth)	Total Teeth
Hellenistic	40	30	277	0.6	6.9	476
Roman	124	63	731	1.5	5.9	493
Late Antique	110	58	623	1.0	5.7	603
Total (all periods)	274	151	1631	1.0	6.0	1572

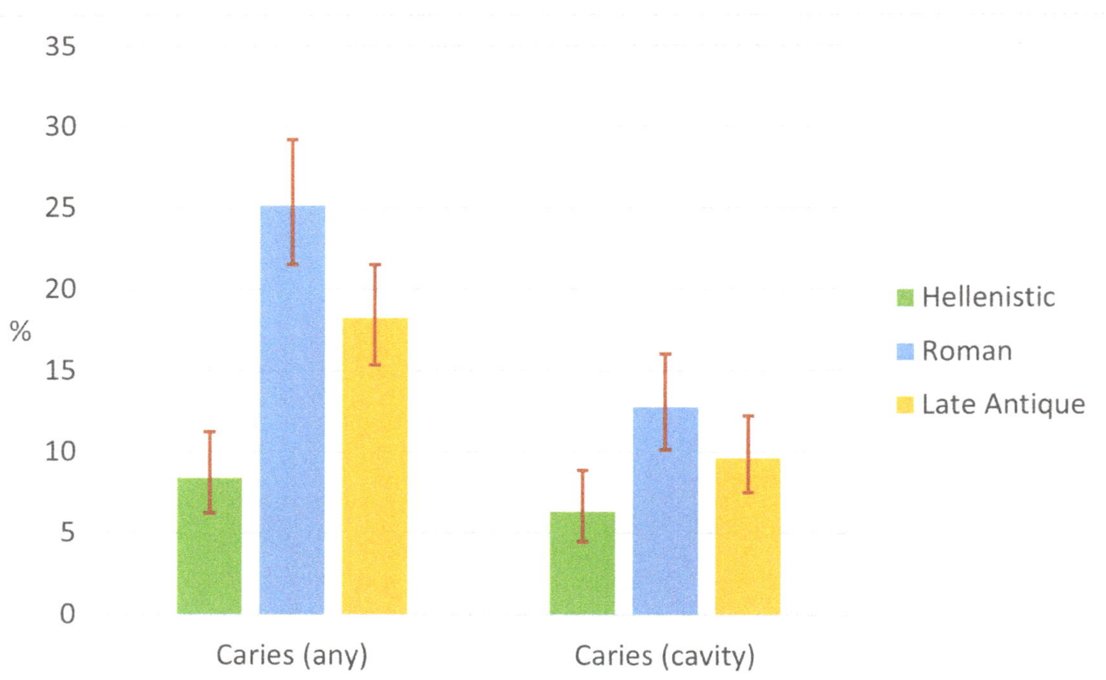

Figure 6.8. Prevalence of caries and cavities by tooth for each time period with 95% confidence interval error bars.

period and 18.2% (110/603) in the Late Antique period. The difference between caries prevalence for the three time periods was statistically highly significant ($X^2 = 47.7$, $p = 0.00$), as can also be seen from the confidence intervals in Figure 6.8 which do not cross over for caries. Although there is less difference for cavities prevalence, the same pattern can be observed, with 6.3% (30/476) for the Hellenistic period, 12.8% (63/493) for the Roman period and 9.6% (58/603) for the Late Antique period.

The severity of carious lesions, at a first glance, appears to be greatest in the Hellenistic period, with the smallest difference between the occurrence of any-caries versus cavitous-caries meaning relatively fewer occurrences of caries in the initial stages and more severe lesions (i.e. larger and penetrating deeper into the tooth through the enamel and into the dentine and pulp chamber, or in the case of the root, through the cementum and into the root canal). This is also demonstrated in the average caries score per carious tooth of 6.9 for the Hellenistic period, 5.9 for the Roman period and 5.7 for the Late Antique period. However, it should also be considered that due to the fact the surface condition of the Hellenistic teeth was often observed to be more degraded, that this result could be due to a difficulty in observing the early manifestations of caries in some teeth. While surface degradation of teeth was particularly common in the Hellenistic assemblage, if the destruction of enamel was deemed to have reached an unscorable extent, these teeth were not recorded, and this preservation phenomenon was not exclusive to Hellenistic graves and was noted from several other graves. Nevertheless, there is a suspicious lack of early stages for Hellenistic teeth which is likely due to preservation issues (e.g. Figure 6.9). Additionally, if the average caries score is divided by the total number of teeth (carious and non-carious) the Hellenistic period has the lowest score (0.6), the Roman period has the highest score (1.5) and the Late Antique score was intermediate (1.0). This indicates the cumulative effect of the existence of caries and the severity of the lesions, and suggests that caries was worst in the Roman period.

In order to control for the differences in age categories represented, the results by age group for each time period are presented in Table 6.8, with the caries (any) prevalences displayed in Figure 6.10 and the cavities results in Figure 6.11. These results support the collective results in indicating that caries was lowest in the Hellenistic period and highest in the Roman period and shows that the overall time period results have not been skewed by the demographics of the groups. It also enables a comparison of a single age group across the time periods. The largest sample size was for the Young Adults and it is clear from the caries results that this group follows the pattern of a peak in caries in the Roman period, though the cavities Young Adult results

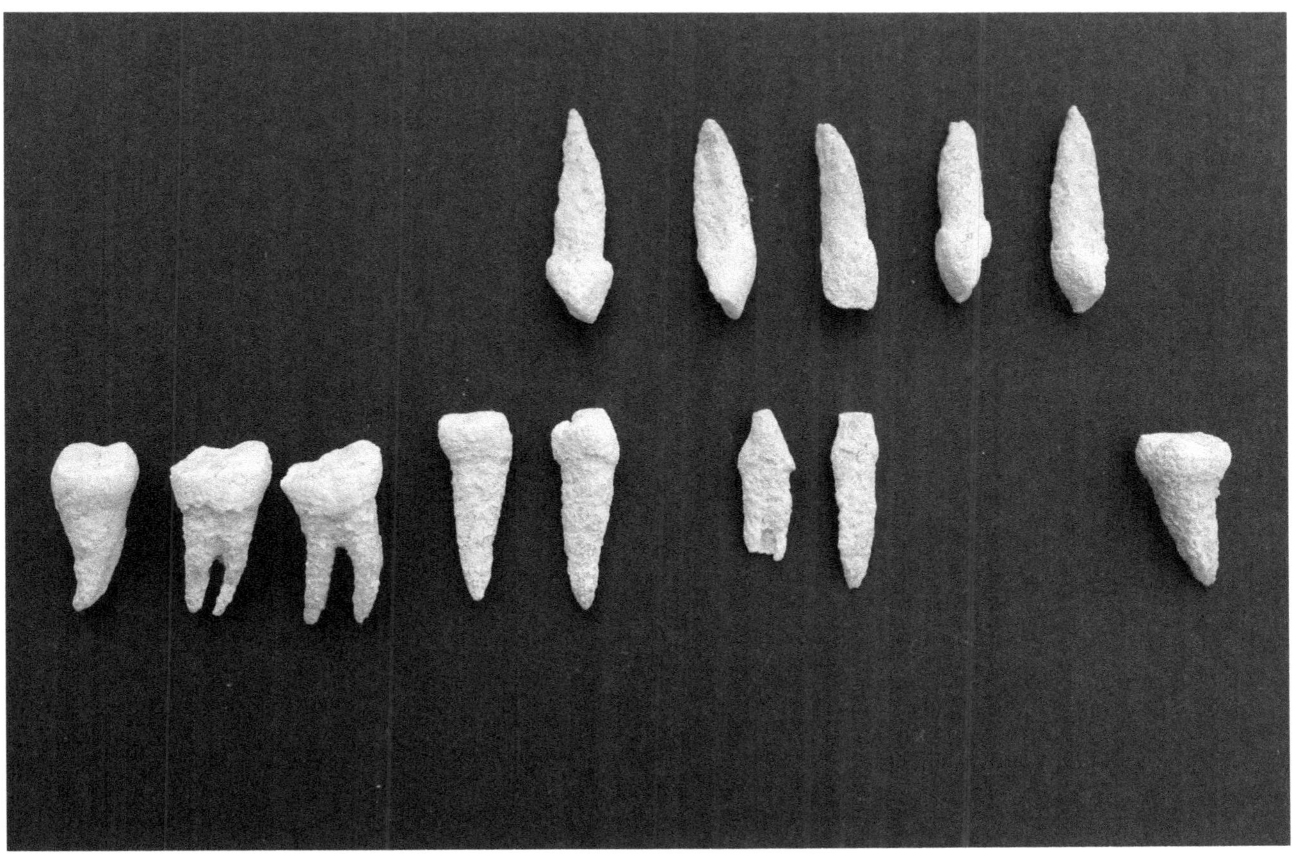

Figure 6.9. Poor enamel surface preservation of Hellenistic teeth. Unit 12, Individual 1. KMF/78 Tomb 39.

Table 6.8. Caries and cavities counts and prevalences (%) and total tooth counts for each age group by time period.

		Hellenistic	Roman	Late Antique
Child	Caries (any)	0	0	7
	%		0.0	9.6
	Caries (cavity)	0	0	1
	%		0.0	1.4
	Total teeth	0	15	73
Adolescent	Caries (any)	1	20	3
	%	3.3	28.6	8.8
	Caries (cavity)	1	7	1
	%	3.3	10.0	2.9
	Total teeth	30	70	34
Young Adult	Caries (any)	20	69	80
	%	6.3	24.4	20.3
	Caries (cavity)	15	32	43
	%	4.7	11.3	10.9
	Total teeth	318	283	394
Middle Adult	Caries (any)	21	33	13
	%	17.5	29.5	14.3
	Caries (cavity)	16	23	10
	%	13.3	20.5	11.0
	Total teeth	120	112	91
Old Adult	Caries (any)	0	5	7
	%	0.0	35.7	70.0
	Caries (cavity)	0	3	3
	%	0.0	21.4	30.0
	Total teeth	17	14	10

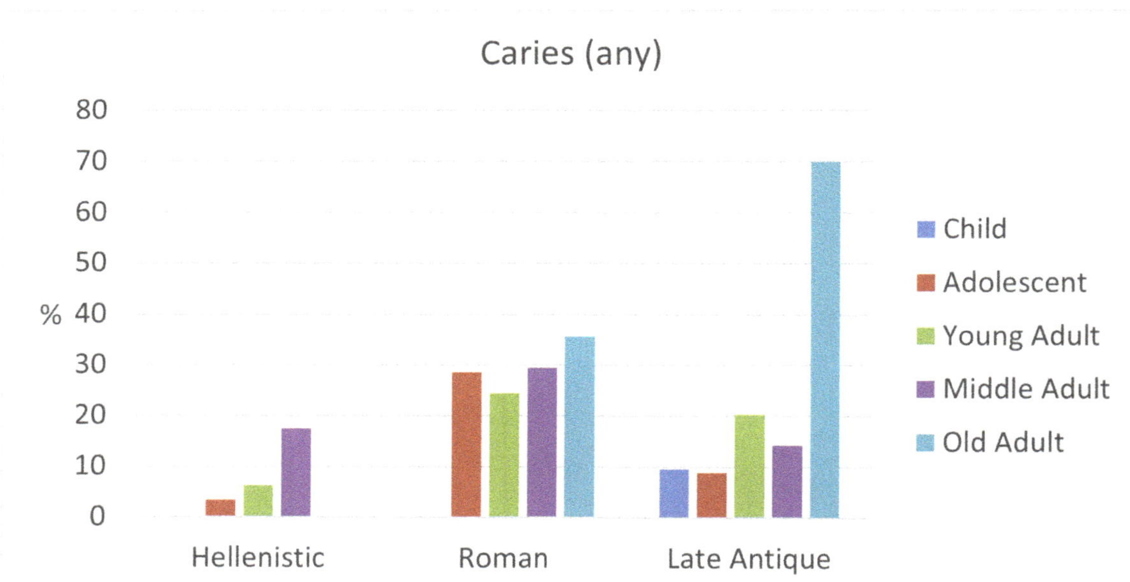

Figure 6.10. Caries (any, Hillson score 1–8) prevalence for each age group by time period.

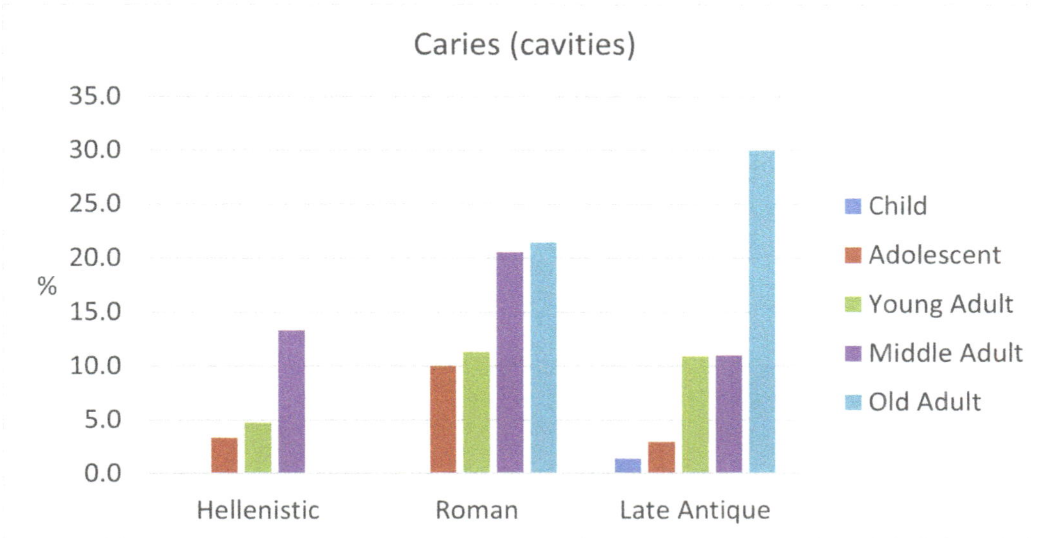

Figure 6.11. Caries (cavities, Hillson score 3–8) prevalence for each age group by time period.

show the Roman and Late Antique groups to be almost identical.

Though a focus on change over time is at the centre of this project, an understanding of what other variables are at work, affecting the health and diet of the population, can help to give insight into the nature of these changes, which is why an intrapopulation investigation is also carried out to investigate differences by sex, age group, tomb type, cemetery and location, to, in turn, give insight into how the evolving urban environment affected different aspects of society.

6.2.1.5. Sex

As shown by Figure 6.12 males have higher frequencies of caries than females, with 18.1% (80/441) of male teeth having caries, compared to 12.5% (78/626) of female teeth. This was a statistically significant difference according to a chi-square test ($X^2 = 6.6$, $p = 0.01$), though there is a slight overlap of the confidence intervals. This pattern prevails with the early manifestations of caries excluded, with 9.8% (43/441) of male teeth displaying cavities compared to 7.2% (45/626) of female teeth.

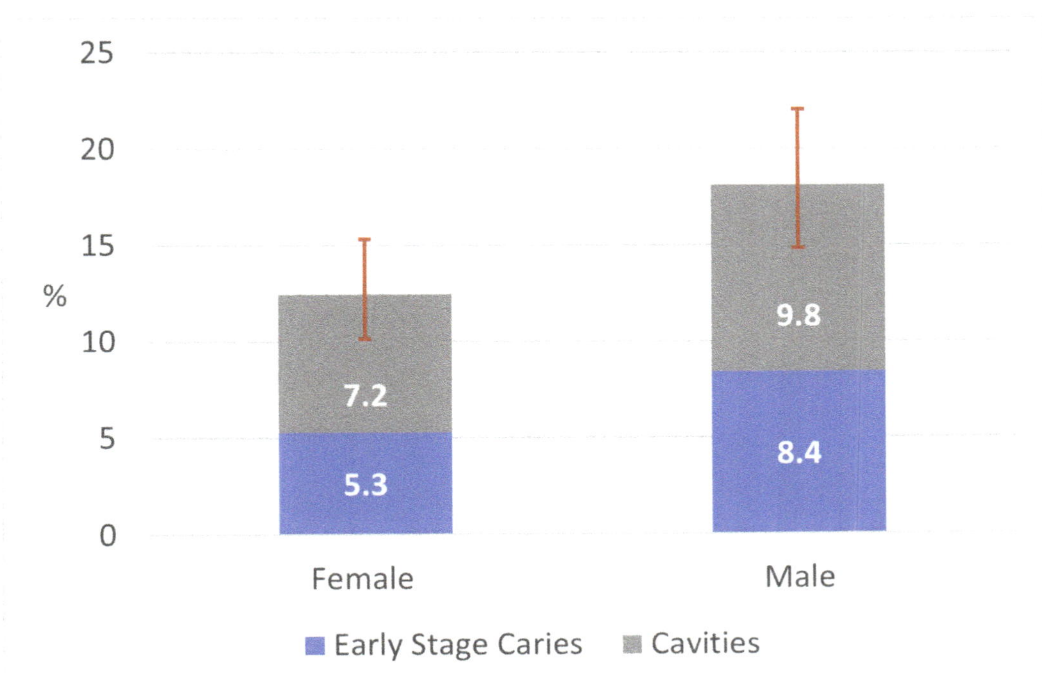

Figure 6.12. Prevalence of early stage caries and cavities (stacked to show total caries prevalence with 95% confidence interval error bars) by tooth for the sexes.

Table 6.9. Prevalence of caries, cavities and carious scores for the sexes.

	Teeth with caries	Teeth with cavities	Average Score (per carious tooth – for all teeth)
Female	12.5% (78/626)	7.2% (45/626)	6.4 – 0.8
Indeterminate	25.0% (7/28)	17.9% (5/28)	3.9 – 1.0
Male	18.1% (80/441)	9.8% (43/441)	6.9 – 1.3

When observing the difference in caries prevalence between the sexes within each time period, there is a mixed picture (Table 6.10). If the cavity level of caries is observed, the pattern of males having a higher occurrence of cavities prevails, though only marginally so for the Late Antique teeth and the confidence intervals for males and females within each time period have substantial overlap, suggesting no significant difference (Figure 6.13). However, with large numbers of Roman Female and Late Antique Male teeth having early-stage caries (Score 1 or 2) the results for the complete range of caries are very mixed with males having higher caries prevalence in the Hellenistic and Late Antique periods but the females having the greater caries prevalence in the Roman period and the highest overall occurrence of caries with 23.7% (Figure 6.14). The only significant difference between the sexes was for caries (any) in the Late Antique period, as can be seen from the non-overlapping confidence intervals in Figure 6.14.

Table 6.10. Prevalence of caries, cavities and carious scores for the sexes by time period.

	Teeth with Caries	Teeth with cavities	Average Caries Score (by carious tooth – for all teeth)
Hellenistic Female	6.0% (16/268)	4.5% (12/268)	6.8 – 0.4
Hellenistic Male	9.5% (10/105)	6.7% (7/105)	3.8 – 0.4
Roman Female	23.7% (46/194)	10.3% (20/194)	3.8 – 0.9
Roman Male	21.2% (25/118)	16.1% (19/118)	13.6 – 2.9
Late Antique Female	9.9% (16/162)	8.0% (13/162)	13.3 – 1.3
Late Antique Male	21.5% (45/209)	8.6% (18/209)	4.0 – 0.9

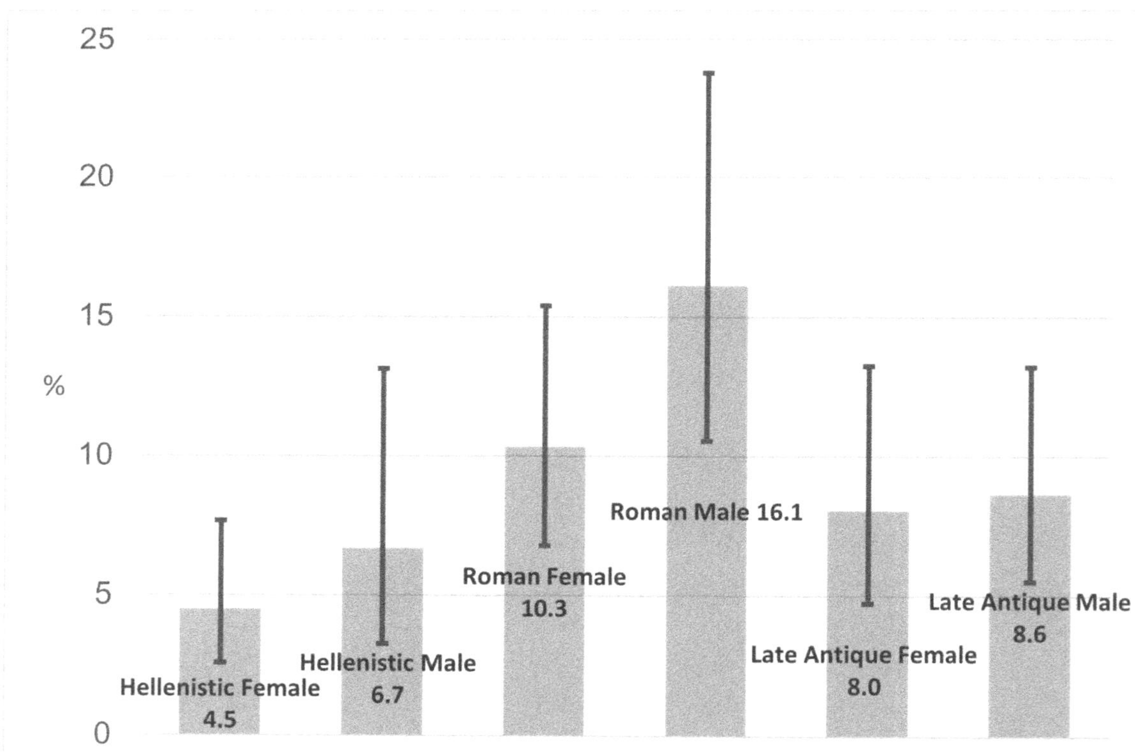

Figure 6.13. Prevalence of cavities for the sexes by time period with 95% confidence interval error bars.

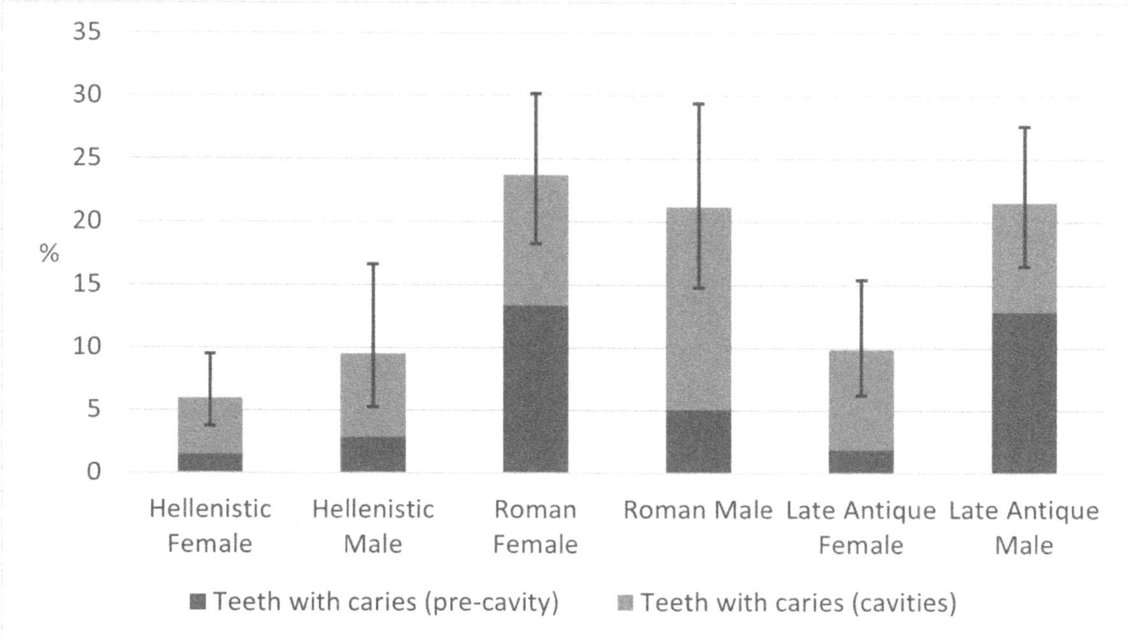

Figure 6.14. Prevalence of early stage caries and cavities (stacked to show total caries prevalence with 95% confidence interval error bars) for the sexes by time period.

The large numbers of Roman Female and Late Antique Male teeth with early-stage caries, is conversely reflected in the highest average caries scores being for the Roman Male and Late Antique Female groups (Table 6.10). Though cavities can be said to be the more reliable measure (compared to including the early caries stages), as poor surface condition can lead to missing the early manifestations, there is no reason why the teeth from the same contexts (e.g. Roman male and female) should have different surface preservation. This does not adequately explain the dramatic difference in early-stage caries between females and males in either the Roman or Late Antique periods. Nor can age differences be held accountable for this difference as there was not a dramatic difference in the age profiles of males and females in these time periods.

6.2.1.6. Tomb type

Though it is not really possible to compare the social significance of different types of tomb architecture across different times periods, Figure 6.15 and Table 6.11 present an overview of the caries prevalence for the tomb types for all the time periods combined. The tomb types are listed in order of supposed social status, based on perceived elaborateness and complexity of construction, as well as size and visibility.

There is a general pattern of higher caries prevalence in the more complex tombs, with the pit and cist caries confidence intervals not overlapping with the Built,

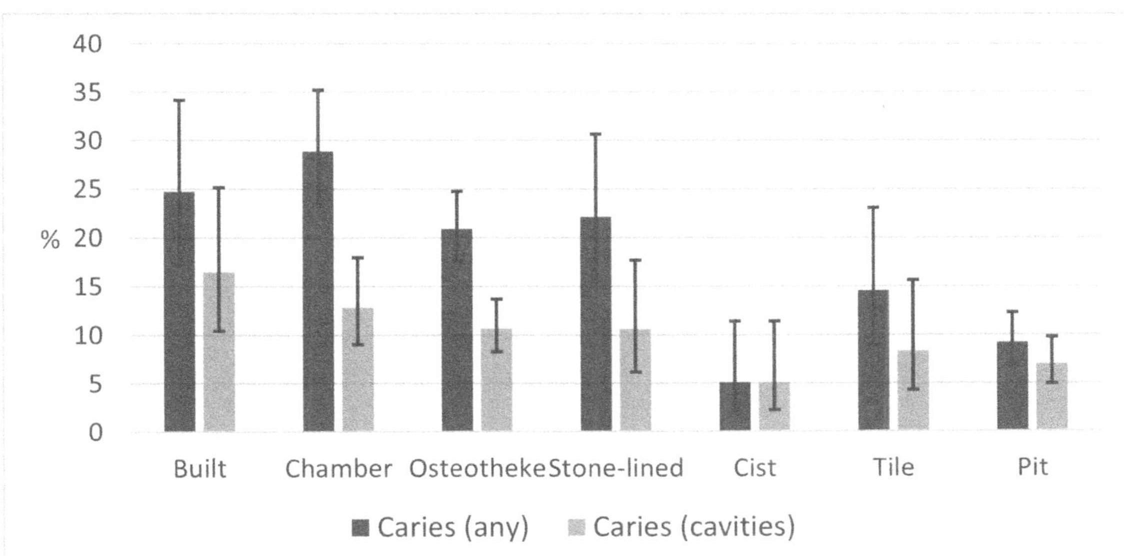

Figure 6.15. Prevalence of caries and cavities for the tomb types in all time periods with 95% confidence interval error bars.

Chamber, Osteotheke or Stone-lined ones. There are slight discrepancies between the caries (any stage) and cavities (caries score 3+) trends. The cavities prevalence has a subtle but consistent trend of having fewer cases of cavities as the tomb forms become simpler, from 16.5% of teeth from built tombs to 7% of teeth from pit graves. The 'any-stage' caries results are more variable with the chamber tomb teeth (28.9%) having a higher prevalence than those in the built tombs (24.7%), and the stone-lined tombs (22.1%) having a slightly higher prevalence than the osteothekai (20.9%). It should, however, be stressed that the ordering on these tombs is highly subjective and the mixing of tombs from different time periods may also confuse the attempt to order tombs by social status. These first four tomb categories (Built, Chamber, Osteotheke, Stone-lined) are all quite elaborate tomb forms. This Cist group is somewhat anomalous as it is a small sample size which included the Krevatina Roman cist grave which unusually contained no carious teeth. However, the survival and/or retrieval of teeth from this tomb was not good as only 18 teeth (all mandibular) of a possible 128 (from 4 adult individuals, each with 32 teeth) survived.

Table 6.11. Prevalence of caries, cavities and carious scores for the tomb types.

	Teeth with Caries	Teeth with Cavities	Average Caries Score (by carious tooth – for all teeth)
Built	24.7% (24/97)	16.5% (16/97)	11.1 – 2.7
Chamber	28.9% (63/218)	12.8% (28/218)	4.7 – 1.4
Osteotheke	20.9% (104/497)	10.7% (53/497)	4.9 – 1.0
Stone-lined	22.1% (25/113)	10.6% (12/113)	3.8 – 0.8
Cist	5.1% (5/98)	5.1% (5/98)	23.0 – 1.2
Tile	14.6% (14/96)	8.3% (8/96)	5.9 – 0.9
Pit	9.2% (41/445)	7.0% (31/445)	7.6 – 0.7

The tomb type results have also been presented by age group in Table 6.12, with the caries (any) results displayed in Figure 6.16, and the cavities in Figure 6.17. The sample sizes become too small for some of the groups (Built, Stone-lined, Cist, Tile) but it is important to keep in mind the impact that different demographic compositions may

Table 6.12. Caries and cavities counts and prevalences (%) and total tooth counts for each age group by tomb type.

		Built	Chamber	Osteotheke	Stone-lined	Cist	Tile	Pit
Child	Caries (any)	0	0	7	0	0	0	0
	%	0.0		9.6	0.0		0.0	
	Caries (cavity)	0	0	1	0	0	0	0
	%	0.0		1.4	0.0		0.0	
	Total teeth	8	0	73	1	0	6	0
Adolescent	Caries (any)	0	7	3	13	0	0	1
	%		25.9	15.8	54.2	0.0	0.0	3.3
	Caries (cavity)	0	2	1	5	0	0	1
	%		7.4	5.3	20.8	0.0	0.0	3.3
	Total teeth	0	27	19	24	14	20	30
Young Adult	Caries (any)	15	49	77	4	2	2	20
	%	25.9	29.5	22.2	6.9	5.6	5.6	6.8
	Caries (cavity)	9	20	41	3	1	1	15
	%	15.5	12.0	11.8	5.2	2.8	2.8	5.1
	Total teeth	58	166	347	58	36	36	294
Middle Adult	Caries (any)	4	8	9	9	4	13	20
	%	21.1	27.6	19.6	27.3	8.0	37.1	18.0
	Caries (cavity)	4	7	6	5	4	8	15
	%	21.1	24.1	13.0	15.2	8.0	22.9	13.5
	Total teeth	19	29	46	33	50	35	111
Old Adult	Caries (any)	5	0	7	0	0	0	0
	%	41.7	0.0	70.0				0.0
	Caries (cavity)	3	0	3	0	0	0	0
	%	25.0	0.0	30.0				0.0
	Total teeth	12	2	10	0	0	0	17

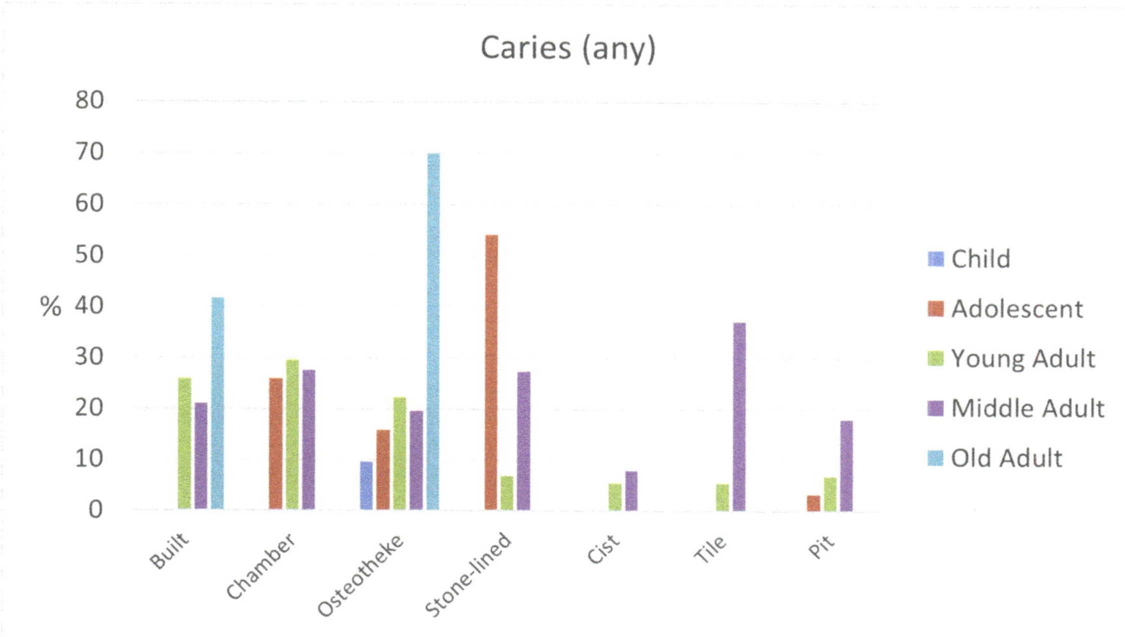

Figure 6.16. Caries (any) prevalence for each age group by tomb type.

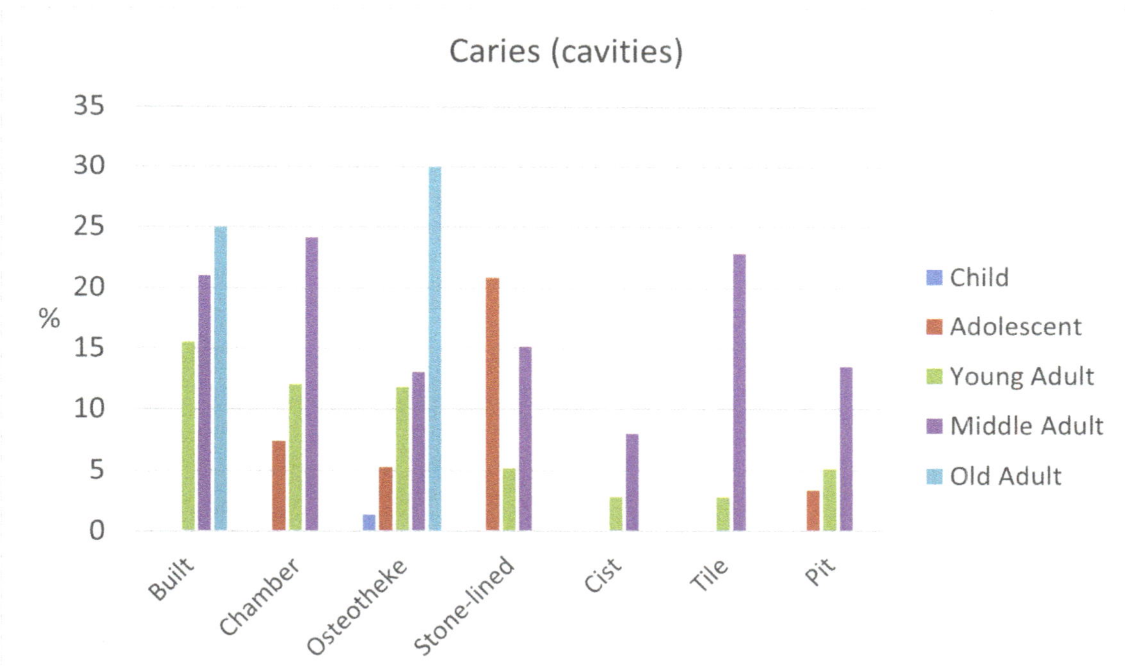

Figure 6.17. Caries (cavities) prevalence for each age group by tomb type.

have on the comparison of the tomb type groups. The built tomb group also has a relatively high proportion of Old Adult teeth which may accentuate the overall caries prevalence. Referring back to Table 6.4 for the proportions of tooth types, it is possible that the built tomb caries result has also been raised by the high proportion of molars (61.9%) making up the sample, with very few incisors or canines. The Tile grave is the only group to have more teeth in the Middle Adult than in the Young Adult category and considering the small sample size of this group, this has a significant effect in raising the overall caries prevalence for this group.

There are often a number of different and overlapping variables affecting the results. Investigating each in turn and also investigating a combination of variables, in so far as the sample size will allow (i.e. by sex or by tomb type within a single time period), can help to identify which are the significant variables impacting the results. This is possible for looking at caries prevalence within the Roman period for the different tomb types (Table 6.13 and Figure 6.18). However, as observed for the results from other analyses, there was not enough diversity in tomb type or cemetery location to do much of this sort of investigation for either the Hellenistic or Late Antique periods. As this is the time period when there was the greatest diversity in tomb form (in terms of the present assemblage), it would be expected that there might be significant differences in caries rates between the different tomb types.

The highest caries rates were in the rock-cut chamber tombs with 28.9% of teeth showing signs of the disease. The chamber tomb teeth were followed by those from the stone-lined tombs (26.7%), the built tombs (24.7%), and then the tile graves (19.7%). By far the lowest caries prevalence was amongst the cist tomb teeth with 4.8%. The only statistically significant differences between any pairs of tomb types were for Cist and Chamber groups ($X^2 = 5.4$, $p = 0.02$), as demonstrated by the confidence intervals not overlapping (Figure 6.18). However, this result should be considered with caution, considering it is by far the smallest sample size and the fact that only one tomb is represented (the Krevatina cist mentioned earlier, in Section 6.2.1.6).

Table 6.13. Prevalence of caries, cavities and carious scores for the Roman tomb types.

Tomb type	Teeth with caries	Teeth with cavities	Average Caries Score (by carious tooth – for all teeth)
Built	24.7% (24/97)	16.5% (16/97)	11.1 – 2.7
Chamber	28.9% (63/218)	12.8% (28/218)	4.7 – 1.4
Stone-lined	26.7% (24/90)	12.2% (11/90)	3.8 – 1.0
Cist	4.8% (1/21)	4.8% (1/21)	5.0 – 0.2
Tile	19.7% (12/61)	11.5% (7/61)	6.1 – 1.2

When the cavities rates are observed, other than the Cist tomb result, a slight trend emerges of increased caries prevalence with increased perceived-complexity of tomb type, with the highest cavities prevalence coming from the Built tomb teeth with 16.5% but these were not statistically significant differences. The average caries scores follow this same trend of higher scores (more severe lesions) for the more elaborate, complex tomb types for the Built, Chamber and Stone-lined categories. This is particularly pronounced for the Built tomb teeth, which had an average score of 11.1 by carious tooth and 2.7 for all teeth. The Tile grave average caries scores are an exception to the trend with noticeably elevated scores, particularly by carious tooth with an average score of 6.1. The reservations about the tooth type and age group compositions of these groups made earlier in this section (6.2.1.6) for all tomb types also applies here.

The wide confidence intervals in Figure 6.18 demonstrate the uncertainty in the reliability of these results due to the small sample sizes but that generally there was no significant difference in caries between these Roman tomb types.

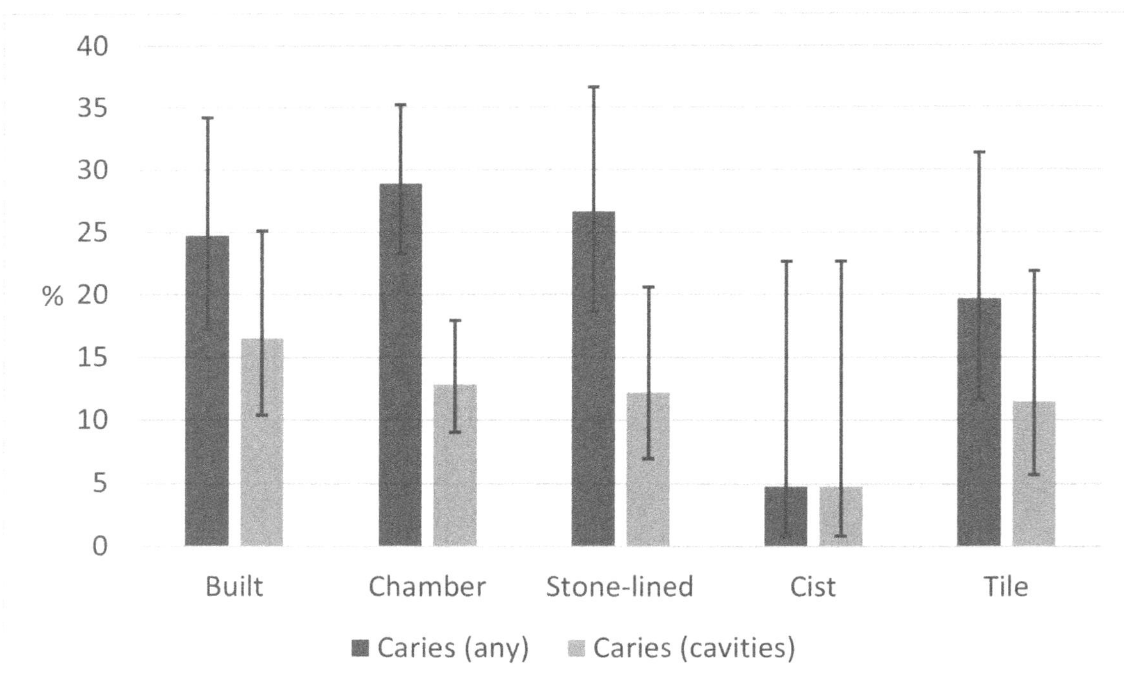

Figure 6.18. Prevalence of caries and cavities for the Roman tomb types with 95% confidence interval error bars.

6.2.1.7. Cemetery

The North Cemetery is the only cemetery that has skeletal remains from all three time periods. Each time period in the cemetery has been represented as a different cemetery for the following analysis, represented in Figure 6.19 and Table 6.14. The Krevatina, Spilia and Topana cemeteries are represented in the skeletal and dental record by a single tomb each. One of the most striking features of the graph (Figure 6.19) is the difference between the caries (any) and cavities at Monastiriako Kephali, demonstrating a very large number of teeth (23.4%) had early-stage (score 1 or 2) caries. The Monastiriako Kephali caries result was significantly higher than caries in any of the North Cemetery groups, as is demonstrated by the non-overlapping confidence intervals. The Sanatorium teeth also had over half of the carious teeth in the early stages of the manifestation of the disease (13.2% of all teeth). The Hellenistic North Cemetery and Spilia rock-cut chamber tomb had the fewest cases of early-stage caries. The Topana built tomb had the highest cavities prevalence (20.8%). The Topana group had a very small sample size and, referring back to Table 6.4, it also had a very high proportion of molars (62.5%) and very few incisors or canines, which may be the cause of this elevated result. Caries in general, and particularly cavities, were lowest in the North Cemetery in all three time periods.

Table 6.14. Prevalence of caries, cavities and carious scores for the cemeteries.

	Teeth with Caries	Teeth with Cavities	Average Caries Score (by carious tooth – for all teeth)
Monastiriako Kephali	35.2% (45/128)	11.7% (15/128)	3.5 – 1.2
Krevatina	0% (0/18)	0% (0/18)	0
North Cemetery (Hellenistic)	8.7% (42/484)	6.8% (33/484)	7.5 – 0.7
North Cemetery (Roman)	18.3% (17/93)	10.8% (10/93)	5.4 – 1.0
North Cemetery (Late Antique)	18.2% (107/588)	9.7% (57/588)	5.8 – 1.0
Sanatorium Basilica	25.7% (39/152)	12.5% (19/152)	4.6 – 1.2
Spilia	17.3% (9/52)	13.5% (7/52)	8.1 – 1.4
Topana	29.2% (14/48)	20.8% (10/48)	16.4 – 4.8

These results have also been presented by age group in Table 6.15, with the caries (any) results displayed in Figure 6.20, and the cavities in Figure 6.21. The sample sizes for several groups (Krevatina, Roman North Cemetery, Spilia and Topana) become far too small for any reliable analysis. The Roman North Cemetery is the only group with more Middle Adults than Young Adults and although the overall caries score is quite low, this may elevate the result in comparison with the other cemeteries. The Sanatorium group also has a high proportion of Middle and Old Adults represented in comparison with Young Adults, relative to the distributions of these age groups in the other cemeteries. The very high numbers of early stage caries compared to cavities in the Monastiriako Kephali group can in part be attributed to the high numbers of Young Adults compared to very few Middle Adults and no Old Adults. This suggests that this group does have a representatively high overall caries rate despite being largely younger individuals, potentially representing a higher sugar content in the diet than the other cemetery groups.

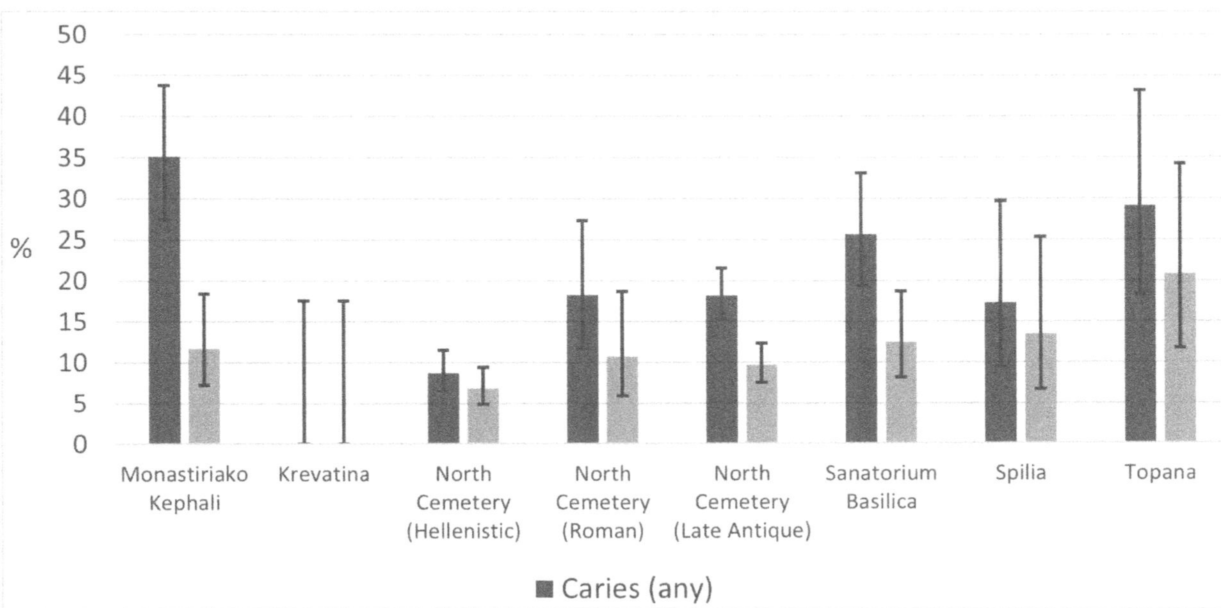

Figure 6.19. Prevalence of caries and cavities for each cemetery with 95% confidence interval error bars.

Table 6.15. Caries and cavities counts and prevalences (%) and total tooth counts for each age group by cemetery.

		Mon. Kephali	Krev.	NCH	NCR	NCLA	Sana.	Spilia	Topana
Child	Caries (any)	0	0	0	0	7	0	0	0
	%				0.0	9.6	0.0		
	Caries (cavity)	0	0	0	0	1	0	0	0
	%				0.0	1.4	0.0		
	Total teeth	0	0	0	12	73	3	0	0
Adoles.	Caries (any)	1	0	1	0	3	19	0	0
	%	20.0		3.3	0.0	8.8	42.2		
	Caries (cavity)	1	0	1	0	1	6	0	0
	%	20.0		3.3	0.0	2.9	13.3		
	Total teeth	5	0	30	20	34	45	0	0
Young Adult	Caries (any)	42	2	20	4	79	4	6	12
	%	38.5	15.4	6.3	14.8	20.3	6.6	15.8	30.8
	Caries (cavity)	13	1	15	2	43	3	5	8
	%	11.9	7.7	4.7	7.4	11.0	4.9	13.2	20.5
	Total teeth	109	13	318	27	390	61	38	39
Middle Adult	Caries (any)	3	0	21	14	13	11	3	2
	%	23.1	0.0	17.5	40.0	14.3	33.3	23.1	20.0
	Caries (cavity)	2	0	16	9	10	7	3	2
	%	15.4	0.0	13.3	25.7	11.0	21.2	23.1	20.0
	Total teeth	13	8	120	35	91	33	13	10
Old Adult	Caries (any)	0	0	0	0	7	5	0	0
	%			0.0	0.0	70.0	38.5		
	Caries (cavity)	0	0	0	0	3	3	0	0
	%			0.0	0.0	30.0	23.1		
	Total teeth	0	0	17	1	10	13	0	0

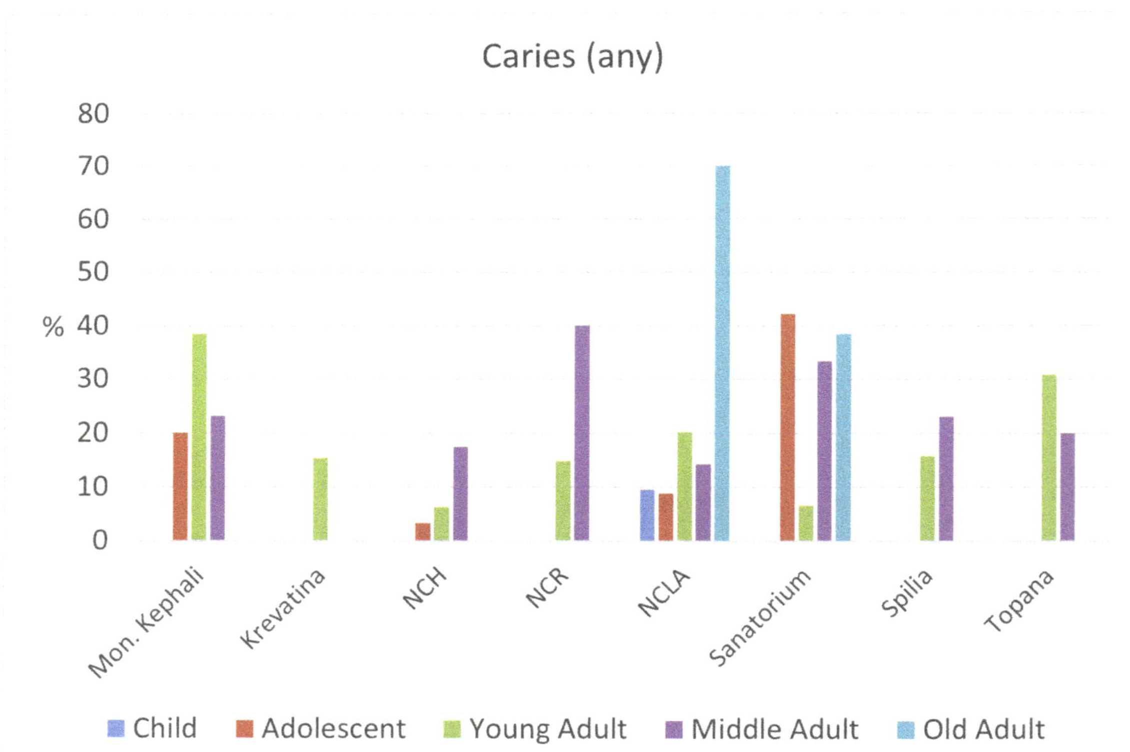

Figure 6.20. Caries (any) prevalence for each age group by cemetery.

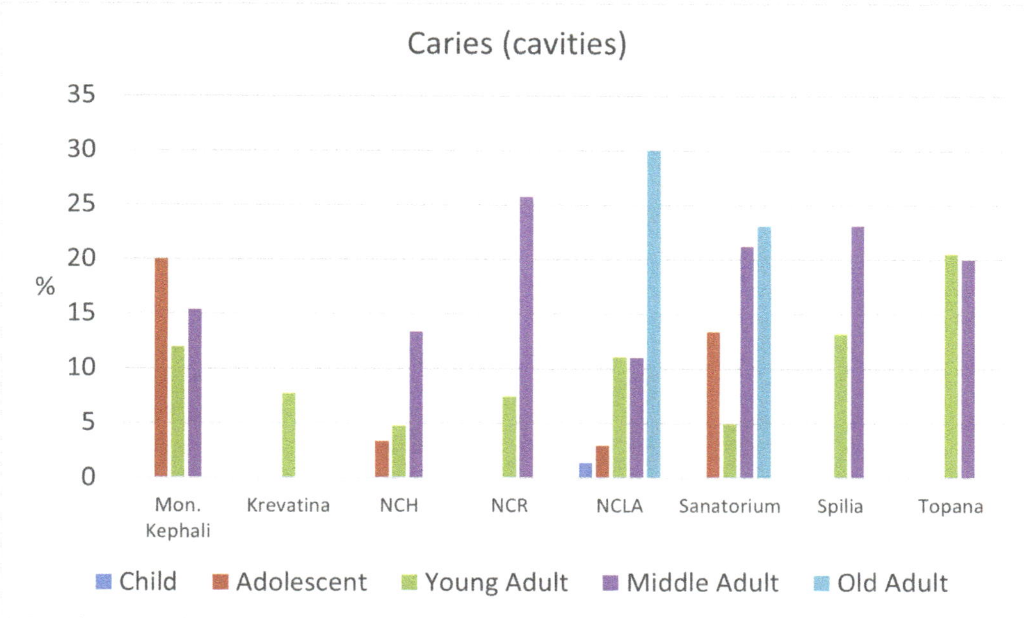

Figure 6.21. Caries (cavities) prevalence for each age group by cemetery.

6.2.1.8. Location

The cemetery results for caries and cavities prevalence can also be grouped into broader categories of location within the valley, by North and South. The North had lower caries and cavities rates than the south (Table 6.16 and Figure 6.22). The difference in caries or no caries for North and South was statistically highly significant ($X^2 = 15.12, p = 0.00$), whereas the cavities results were not significantly different ($X^2 = 0.55, p = 0.46$) as can be seen from the confidence intervals in Figure 6.22. However, when these results, for the North and South regions of the valley,

Table 6.16. Prevalence of caries, cavities and carious scores for the region of the valley (north and south).

	Teeth with Caries	Teeth with Cavities	Average Caries Score (by carious tooth – for all teeth)
North	16.0% (219/1365)	9.5% (129/1365)	6.6 – 1.1
South	27.3% (54/198)	11.1% (22/198)	4.3 – 1.2

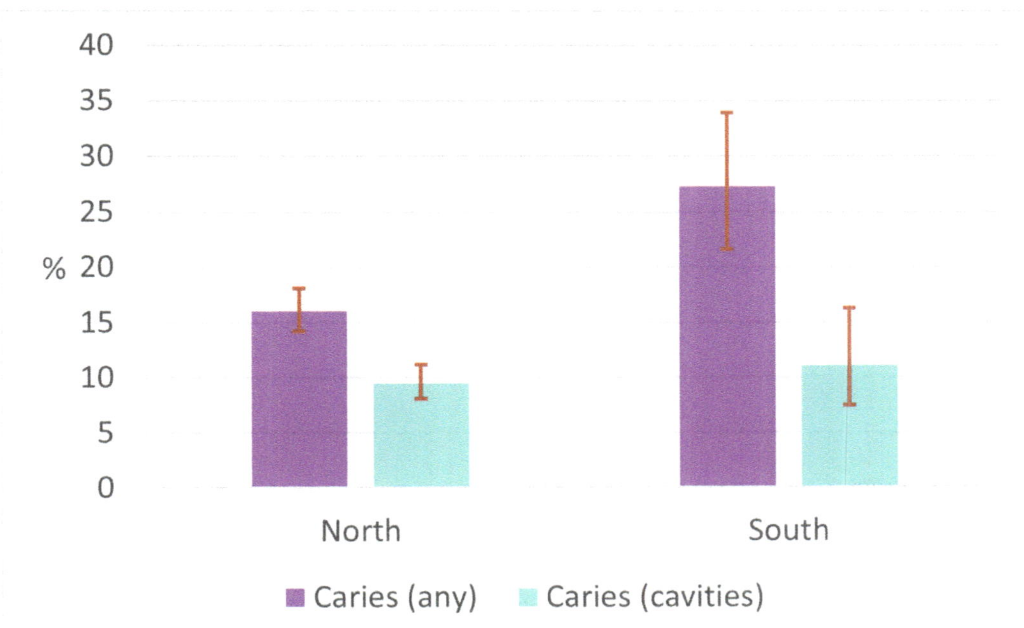

Figure 6.22. Prevalence of caries and cavities from tombs of all time periods by north-south location of the Knossos valley with 95% confidence interval error bars.

are looked at only within the Roman period (Table 6.17 and Figure 6.23), the difference is much less substantial, and is, in fact, reversed for cavities prevalence with a higher cavities rate in the North (13.3%) compared to the South (11.1%). These differences between caries and cavities rates for the Roman North and Roman South are not statistically significant (caries: $X^2 = 0.72$, $p = 0.40$, cavities: $X^2 = 0.53$, $p = 0.47$). This demonstrates that the lower caries rates in both the Hellenistic and Late Antique periods (all tombs of these periods are in the North) bring the North values down rather than this being a regionally defined pattern.

6.2.2. Calculus

Calculus was the most commonly occurring dental condition amongst the Knossos assemblage when assessed by tooth. Unfortunately, scoring by individual was not possible. Some level of calculus was found on 36.9% (576/1559) of all recorded teeth, the majority of which were only slight deposits (21.4% of all teeth) with only 3.3% (52/1559) of teeth having heavy deposits (Table 6.20). The calculus results were considered by the same variables as the caries results.

6.2.2.1. Tooth type

Calculus would be expected to be most common of the lingual surfaces of incisors and the buccal surfaces of the molars, next to the salivary glands (Hillson 1996, 255). However, while almost half of all incisors had some form of calculus deposit, the molars had the lowest prevalence of calculus for any of the tooth types (Table 6.18). The canines were close behind the incisors in terms of calculus prevalence, and the premolars were similar to the molars, with only a slightly higher prevalence. As calculus is not well understood, it is not clear why these results differ from the expected distribution of calculus within the dentition. Whether this is due to conditions in the mouth or preservation conditions (the latter being less likely), there is a clear pattern of higher calculus rates in the incisors and canines and lower calculus rates in the premolars and molars within the assemblage.

6.2.2.2. Age group

Permanent teeth for all age groups were scored for calculus (Table 6.19 and Figure 6.24). Unsurprisingly, there were relatively few cases of calculus on the children's permanent teeth and no cases of moderate or heavy calculus as these teeth would not have been erupted for long enough at the time of death for any substantial plaque deposits to have mineralised and developed. The same goes for the adolescent teeth, which have slightly more cases of calculus and a very small number of moderate and heavy deposits but numbers were still quite low compared to the adult categories.

Table 6.17. Prevalence of caries, cavities and carious scores for the region of the valley (north and south) for the Roman tombs.

	Teeth with Caries	Teeth with Cavities	Average Caries Score (by carious tooth – for all teeth)
Roman North	23.9% (70/293)	13.3% (39/293)	7.2 – 1.7
Roman South	27.3% (54/198)	11.1% (22/198)	4.3 – 1.2

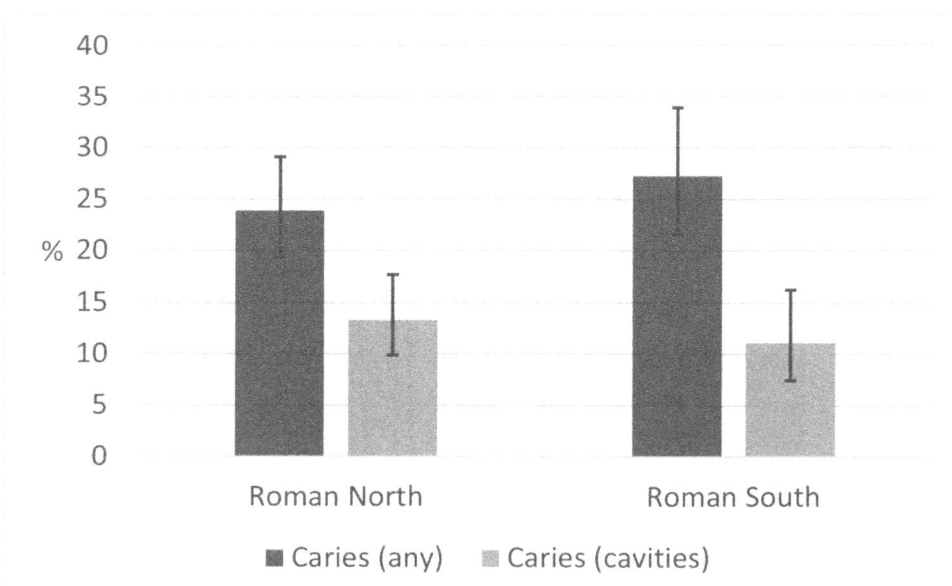

Figure 6.23. Prevalence of caries and cavities from Roman tombs by north-south location of the Knossos valley with 95% confidence interval error bars.

Table 6.18. Calculus scores (1,2,3), counts (*n*) and prevalences (%) for each tooth type.

	No. of teeth (*n*)	1 Slight	2 Moderate	3 Heavy	Calculus (1+2+3)
Incisor	325	25.8% (84)	16.0% (52)	6.2% (20)	48.0% (156)
Canine	167	25.7% (43)	14.4% (24)	6.0% (10)	46.1% (77)
Premolar	375	20.5% (77)	9.6% (36)	3.5% (13)	33.6% (126)
Molar	692	18.8% (130)	11.3% (78)	1.3% (9)	31.4% (217)

Table 6.19. Calculus scores, counts and prevalences for the age groups.

	0 (no calculus)	1 (slight)	2 (moderate)	3 (heavy)	No. of teeth	No. with calculus	% with calculus
Child	68	8	0	0	76	8	10.5%
Adolescent	115	14	2	2	133	18	13.5%
Young Adult	592	243	125	32	992	400	40.3%
Middle Adult	180	55	64	16	315	135	42.9%
Old Adult	27	13	0	0	40	13	32.5%

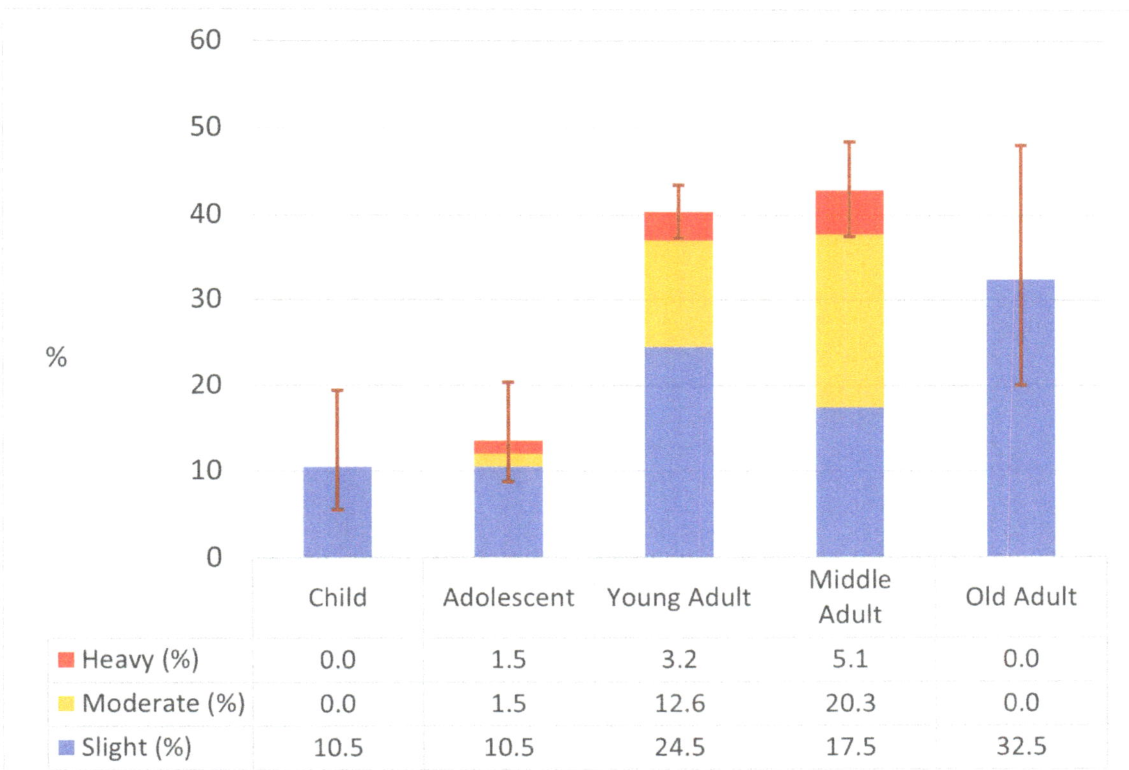

Figure 6.24. Prevalence of slight, moderate and heavy calculus deposits (stacked to show overall calculus prevalence with 95% confidence interval error bars) by tooth for the age groups.

Table 6.20. Calculus scores, counts and prevalences for each time period.

	0 (no calculus)	1 (slight)	2 (mod.)	3 (heavy)	No. of teeth	No. with calculus (1+2+3)	% with calculus (1+2+3)
Hellenistic	390	64	25	5	484	94	19.4%
Roman	324	70	75	18	487	163	33.5%
Late Antique	269	200	90	29	588	319	54.3%
Totals	**983**	**334**	**190**	**52**	**1559**	**576**	**36.9%**

The results do not show as clear an age-progressive pattern as might be expected. In part this is an issue with ageing individuals from dental attrition and the majority falling into the Young Adult age category, therefore not getting great enough resolution across a large proportion of adult life. There was, however, an increase in the occurrence of calculus from the Young Adult category to the Middle Adult category, but there is substantial overlap of the confidence intervals, demonstrating this was not a significant difference ($X^2 = 0.64$, $p = 0.43$).

There was a decline in the occurrence of calculus for the Old Adult category compared to the two younger adult age categories, with no cases of moderate or heavy calculus, though – again – this was not a statistically significant difference ($X^2 = 1.78$, $p = 0.41$). It is likely that due to the high levels of wear that calculus was worn or chipped off Old Adult teeth. Additionally, it is important to note that the Old Adult category has a very small sample size, represented by only 40 teeth, compared to the Young Adult category, for example, which had 992 teeth. In the age group specific analysis of the other variables, the Middle and Old Adult groups are combined to increase the sample size in an attempt to clarify patterns in calculus manifestation (Figures 6.28, 6.34 and 6.38).

6.2.2.3. Time period

The prevalence of calculus appears to have increased over time, from 19.4% (94/484) in the Hellenistic period, to approximately a third of teeth, 33.5% (163/487), in the Roman period and affecting over half of teeth recorded for the Late Antique period at 54.3% (319/588) (Figure 6.25). Heavy calculus deposits were not very common for any time period (Figure 6.26) but were most common in the Late Antique period, occurring in almost 5% of teeth. For both the Hellenistic and Late Antique periods slight deposits were most common and heavy deposits least common but in the Roman period, this data would suggest a relatively greater likelihood to have a moderate calculus deposit on a tooth with 15.4% of teeth having moderate calculus deposits compared to 14.4% with slight deposits. This suggests that the Hellenistic diet was least likely to trigger calculus formation, while the Late Antique diet was the most conducive to its formation. Though the occurrence of calculus in the Roman period was intermediate to the preceding and succeeding time periods, it seems that the Roman diet was more likely to produce a slightly heavier ('moderate') deposit. The differences between grades 0-3 of calculus formation ($X^2 = 163.21$, $p = 0.00$) and for calculus or no calculus ($X^2 = 141.92$, $p = 0.00$) were both highly statistically significant.

The calculus results for the time periods were also analysed by age group, as presented in Table 6.21 and Figure 6.27. Figure 6.28 compares the adult age groups, combining the Middle and Old Adults to improve the sample size. There is a clear trend of increased calculus, both with increased age within each time period and across the time periods.

6.2.2.4. Sex

The occurrence of calculus was more common in males than in females, with just over half of male teeth affected, 51.8% (219/423), compared to just over a third of female teeth, 34.7% (218/628) (Figure 6.29). This was a highly significant difference as can be seen from the confidence interval bars in Figure 6.29 and supported by a chi-square test ($X^2 = 30.3$, $p = 0.00$). However, while amongst male teeth slight deposits were by far the most common type of calculus, decreasing numbers of moderate deposits and very few heavy deposits, this trend was less obvious for female calculus deposits, with heavy deposits more common in female teeth than male teeth (Heavy deposits: Female 4.8%, Male 2.6%) (Figure 6.30).

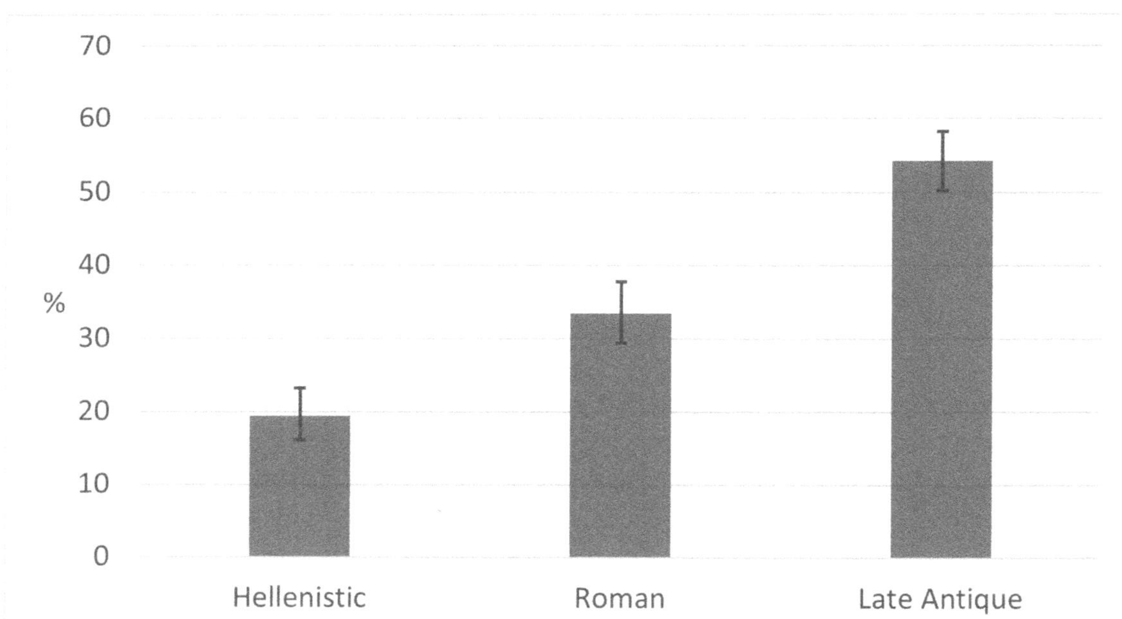

Figure 6.25. Prevalence of calculus by tooth for each time period with 95% confidence interval error bars.

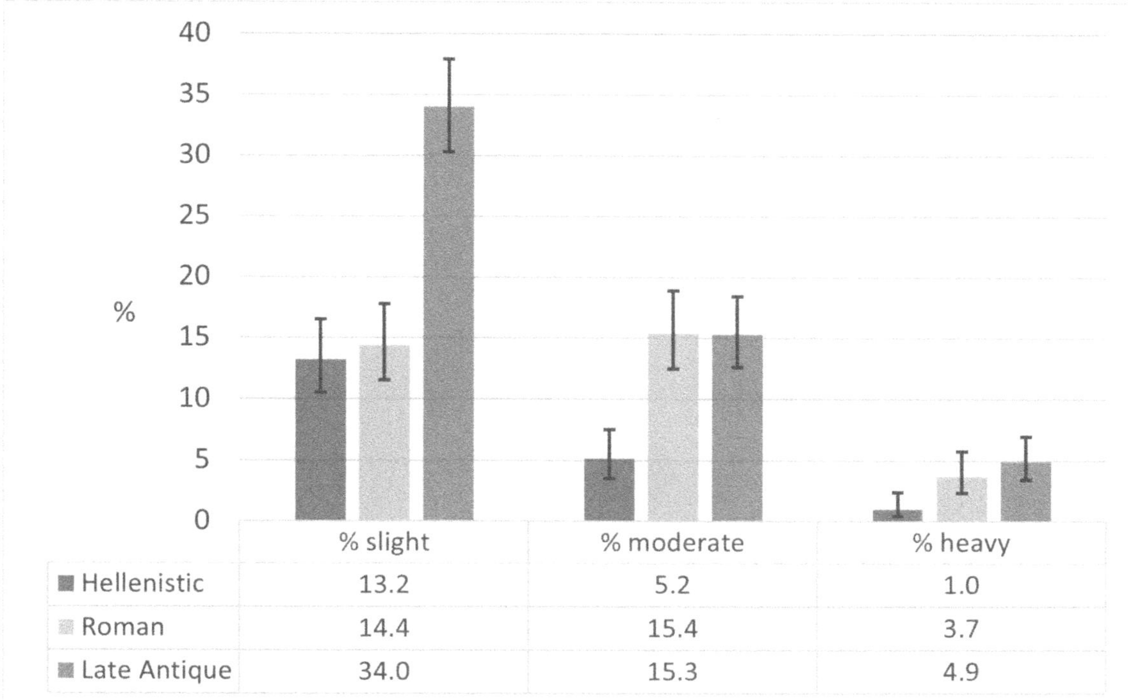

Figure 6.26. Prevalence of slight, moderate and heavy calculus deposits by tooth for each time period with 95% confidence interval error bars.

Table 6.21. Numbers of teeth with calculus, total numbers of teeth and percentage of teeth with calculus for each age group by time period.

		Hellenistic	Roman	Late Antique
Child	Calculus	0	0	8
	Teeth	0	13	63
	%		0.0	12.7
Adolescent	Calculus	0	7	11
	Teeth	30	70	33
	%	0.0	10.0	33.3
Young Adult	Calculus	64	101	235
	Teeth	319	279	394
	%	20.1	36.2	59.6
Middle Adult	Calculus	25	53	57
	Teeth	118	108	89
	%	21.2	49.1	64.0
Old Adult	Calculus	5	0	8
	Teeth	17	14	9
	%	29.4	0.0	88.9

Calculus prevalence was looked at for the sexes within each time period (Table 6.23 and Figure 6.31) and in each case the males had higher overall levels of calculus than the females. The trend of increased calculus prevalence over time is also evident when looked at for each sex. The female results go from 19.1% in the Hellenistic period, to 33.7% in the Roman period, to 62.9% in the Late Antique period. The male results were higher in each case but followed the same trend from 29.1% in the Hellenistic period, to 43% in the Roman period, to 67.6% in the Late Antique period.

The difference between females and males in the Hellenistic and Roman periods was approximately 10%, though the overlapping confidence intervals suggest these were not

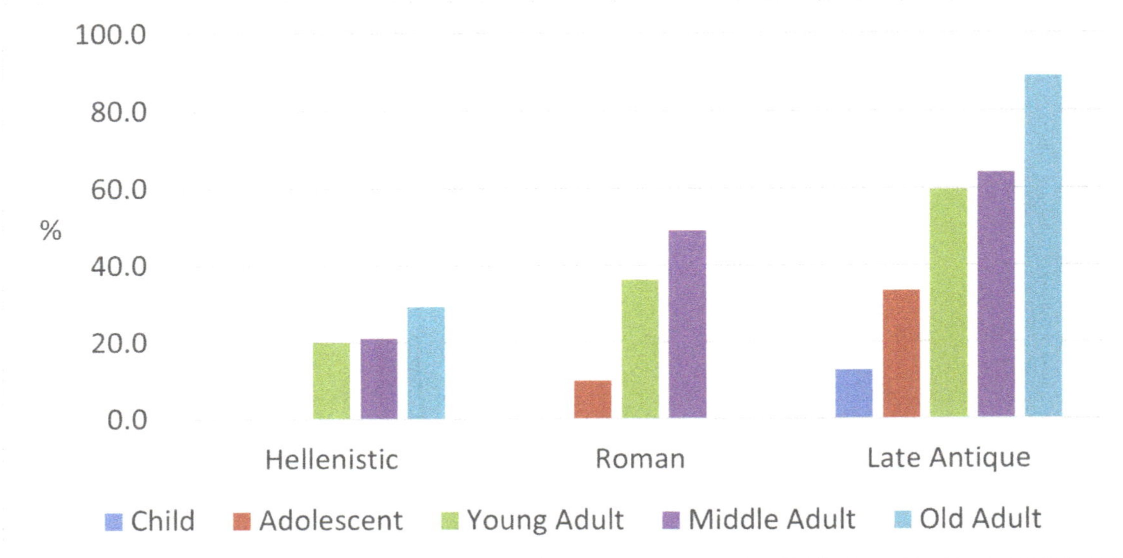

Figure 6.27. Calculus prevalence for each age group by time period.

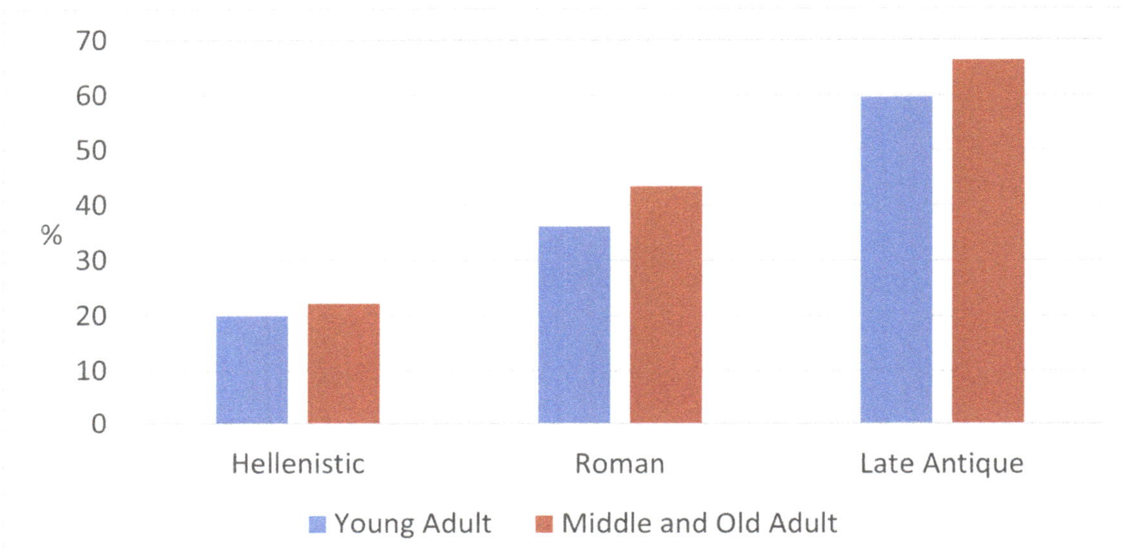

Figure 6.28. A comparison of calculus prevalence in Youngs Adults and Middle and Old Adults combined by time period.

Table 6.22. Calculus scores, counts and prevalences for the sexes.

	0 (no calculus)	1 (slight)	2 (moderate)	3 (heavy)	No. of teeth	No. with calculus	% with calculus
Female	410	100	88	30	628	218	34.7%
Male	204	136	72	11	423	219	51.8%

significant differences. The difference in the occurrence of calculus between Late Antique females (62.9%) and males (67.6%) was less than 5% and was again not statistically significant. The Late Antique males (47.5%) had far more cases of slight calculus than females (27.7%), while females had larger proportions of moderate (Females: 25.8%, Males: 17.2%) and heavy (Females: 9.4%, Males: 2.9%) calculus. The Hellenistic and Roman cases of slight, moderate and heavy calculus were much more proportionate between the sexes. Although there were no Hellenistic male teeth with heavy calculus deposits, there were also very few cases amongst the female teeth. Similar to the Late Antique case, the Roman females had more heavy deposits than the males, but numbers were low for both sexes as there were generally very few heavy calculus deposits. There were significant differences between the females across the three time periods.

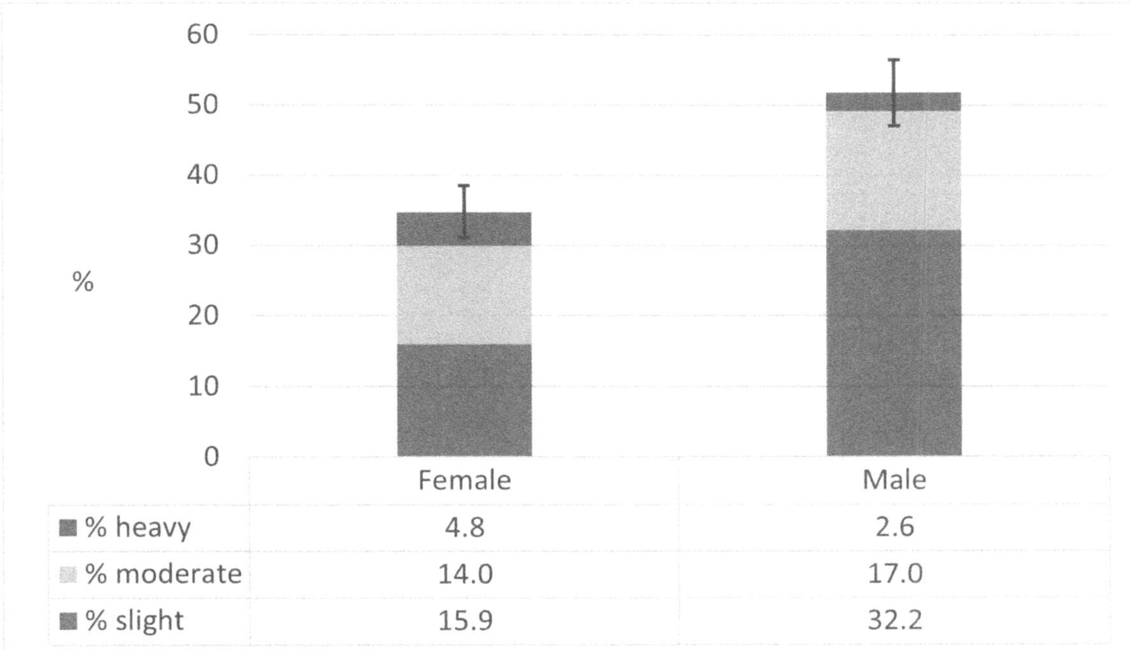

Figure 6.29. Prevalence of slight, moderate and heavy calculus deposits (stacked to show overall calculus prevalence) by tooth for the sexes.

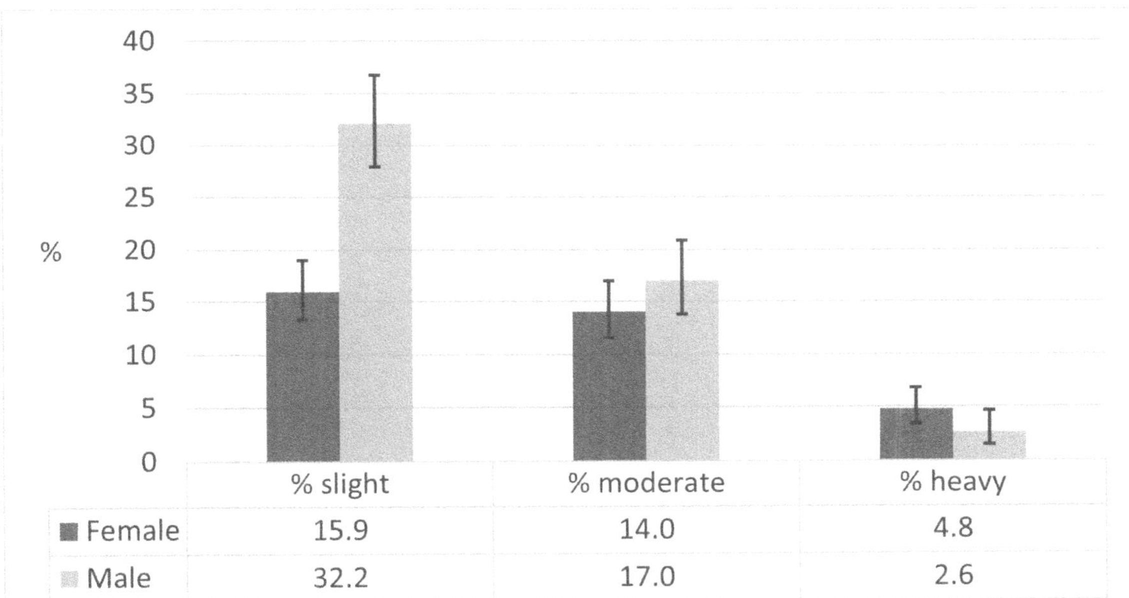

Figure 6.30. Prevalence of slight, moderate and heavy calculus deposits by tooth for the sexes with 95% confidence interval error bars.

Table 6.23. Calculus scores, counts and prevalences for the sexes in each time period.

	0 (no calculus)	1 (slight)	2 (mod.)	3 (heavy)	No. of teeth	No. with calculus	% with calculus
Hellenistic Female	220	33	14	5	272	52	19.1%
Hellenistic Male	73	20	10	0	103	30	29.1%
Roman Female	128	23	34	8	193	65	33.7%
Roman Male	65	19	27	3	114	49	43.0%
Late Antique Female	59	44	41	15	159	100	62.9%
Late Antique Male	66	97	35	6	204	138	67.6%

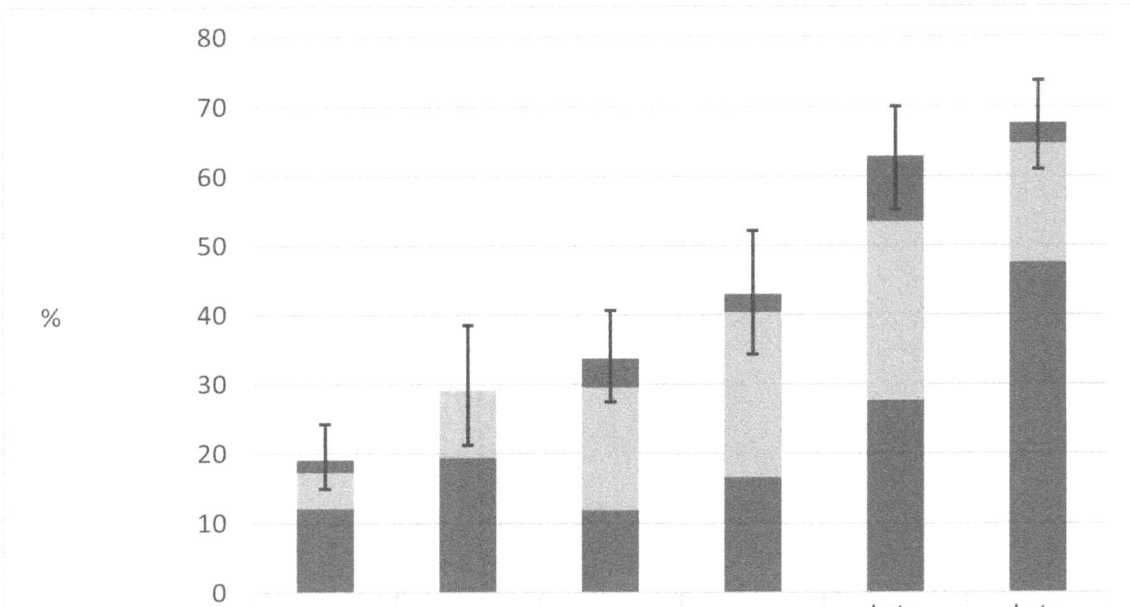

	Hellenistic Female	Hellenistic Male	Roman Female	Roman Male	Late Antique Female	Late Antique Male
Heavy (%)	1.8	0.0	4.1	2.6	9.4	2.9
Moderate (%)	5.1	9.7	17.6	23.7	25.8	17.2
Slight (%)	12.1	19.4	11.9	16.7	27.7	47.5

Figure 6.31. Prevalence of slight, moderate and heavy calculus deposits (stacked to show overall calculus prevalence with 95% confidence interval error bars) by tooth for the sexes in each time period.

For the males, there was a significant difference between the Roman and Late Antique calculus prevalences but the confidence intervals have significant overlap in a comparison of the Hellenistic and Roman periods (Figure 6.31).

6.2.2.5. Tomb type

As has been discussed previously, it is impossible to directly compare the social significance of tomb types from different time periods. Nevertheless, to give an overview of the results for all the different tomb types across the time periods they are presented below in Table 6.24 and Figure 6.32 and have been ordered roughly from the most complex and elaborate tombs to the simplest grave forms.

There is no apparent trend by proposed tomb complexity, with the lowest calculus prevalence coming from the chamber tombs (19.3%) and the highest from the cist graves (71.1%). With a range of 51.8% it is not surprising that the difference between the results was statistically highly significant, either for presence or absence of calculus ($X^2 = 194.46$, $p = 0.00$, see confidence intervals in Figure 6.32) or for calculus scores 0-3 ($X^2 = 289.08$, $p = 0.00$). The chamber tombs had the lowest calculus prevalence (19.3%), followed closely by the pit graves (19.9%), with the majority of occurrences in both cases being slight calculus deposits.

The cist grave results not only had the highest overall calculus prevalence but also the highest prevalence of

Table 6.24. Calculus scores, counts and prevalences for each tomb type.

	0 (no calculus)	1 (slight)	2 (mod.)	3 (heavy)	No. of teeth	No. with calculus	% with calculus
Built	62	12	14	6	94	32	34.0%
Chamber	180	27	12	4	223	43	19.3%
Osteotheke	241	172	54	18	485	244	50.3%
Stone-lined	49	32	33	2	116	67	57.8%
Cist	28	20	38	11	97	69	71.1%
Tile	60	12	13	5	90	30	33.3%
Pit	362	59	26	5	452	90	19.9%

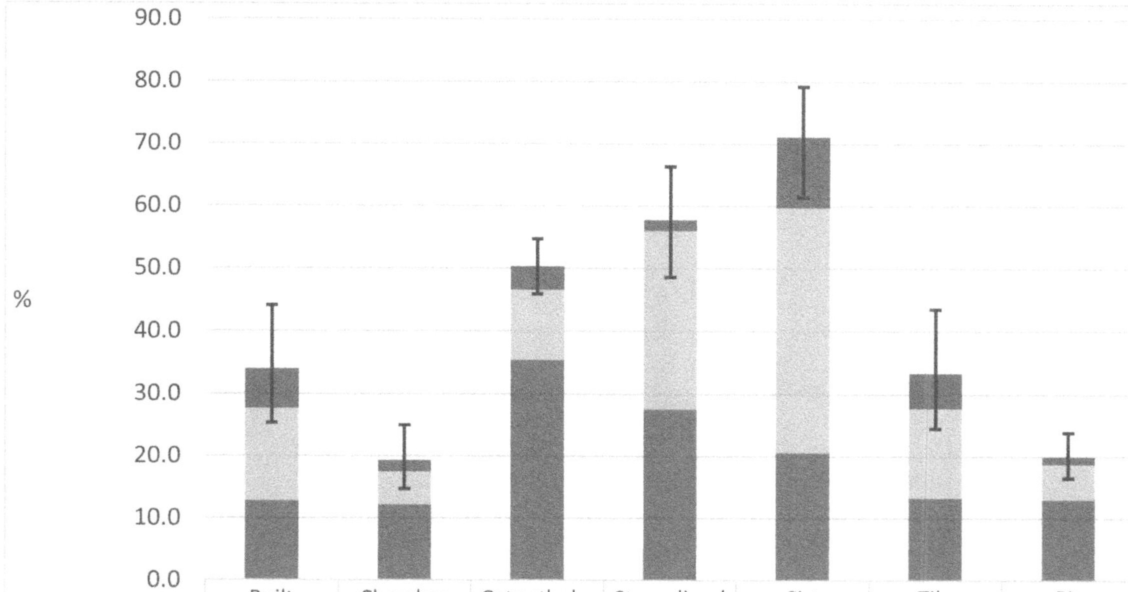

	Built	Chamber	Osteotheke	Stone-lined	Cist	Tile	Pit
Heavy (%)	6.4	1.8	3.7	1.7	11.3	5.6	1.1
Moderate (%)	14.9	5.4	11.1	28.4	39.2	14.4	5.8
Slight (%)	12.8	12.1	35.5	27.6	20.6	13.3	13.1

Figure 6.32. Prevalence of slight, moderate and heavy calculus deposits (stacked to show overall calculus prevalence with 95% confidence interval error bars) by tooth for the tomb types.

moderate (39.2%) and heavy (11.3%) deposits. There was, however, a larger percentage of cases of slight deposits in both the osteothekai (35.5%) and stone-lined tombs (27.6%), compared to the cist graves (20.6%). The fact that the highest three results for overall calculus prevalence come from the three types of stone-lined tombs (the so-called osteothekai, stone-lined tombs and cist graves), may go towards making a case for the notion that there is no social difference between these tomb types and that they are only divided due to inconsistencies in different excavators' recordings. However, the caries results show a far lower prevalence for the cist graves than for the osteothekai and stone-lined tombs, though this inconsistency could be due to the small sample size.

The results are also presented for the age groups in Table 6.25 and Figure 6.33, with a comparison of the Young Adults to a combination of Middle and Old Adults

Table 6.25. Numbers of teeth with calculus, total numbers of teeth and percentage of teeth with calculus for each age group by tomb type.

		Built	Chamber	Osteotheke	Stone-lined	Cist	Tile	Pit
Child	Calculus	0	0	8	0	0	0	0
	Teeth	8	0	63	1	0	4	0
	%	0.0		12.7	0.0		0.0	
Adolescent	Calculus	0	0	7	4	4	3	0
	Teeth	0	27	19	24	13	20	30
	%		0.0	36.8	16.7	30.8	15.0	0.0
Young Adult	Calculus	24	35	202	39	26	15	59
	Teeth	56	164	348	59	36	36	293
	%	42.9	21.3	58.0	66.1	72.2	41.7	20.1
Middle Adult	Calculus	7	8	19	25	39	12	25
	Teeth	17	29	46	33	48	31	111
	%	41.2	27.6	41.3	75.8	81.3	38.7	22.5
Old Adult	Calculus	0	0	8	0	0	0	5
	Teeth	12	2	9	0	0	0	17
	%	0.0	0.0	88.9				29.4

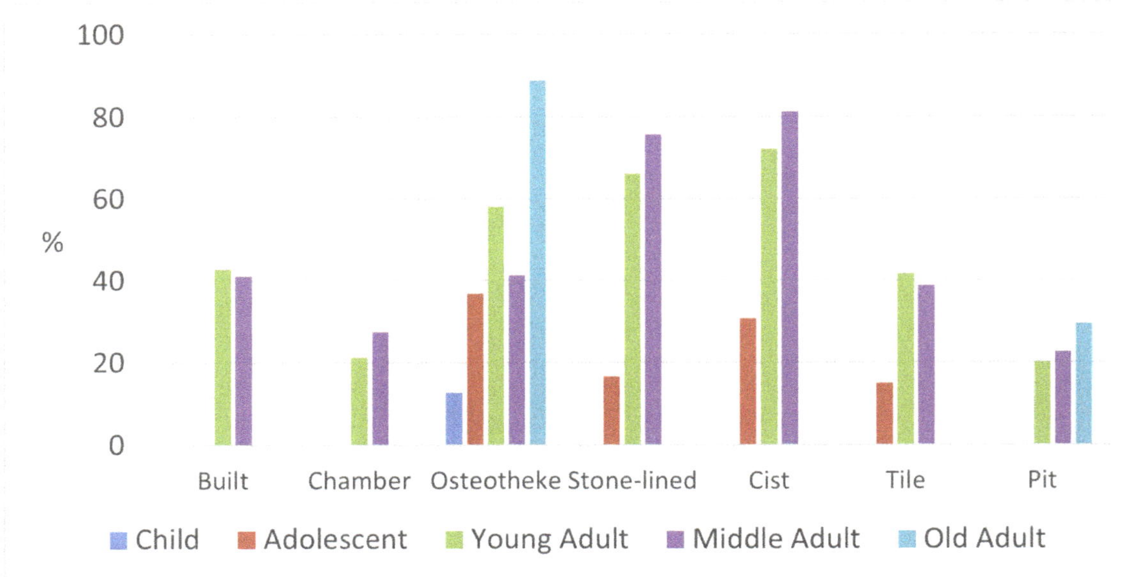

Figure 6.33. Calculus prevalence for each age group by tomb type.

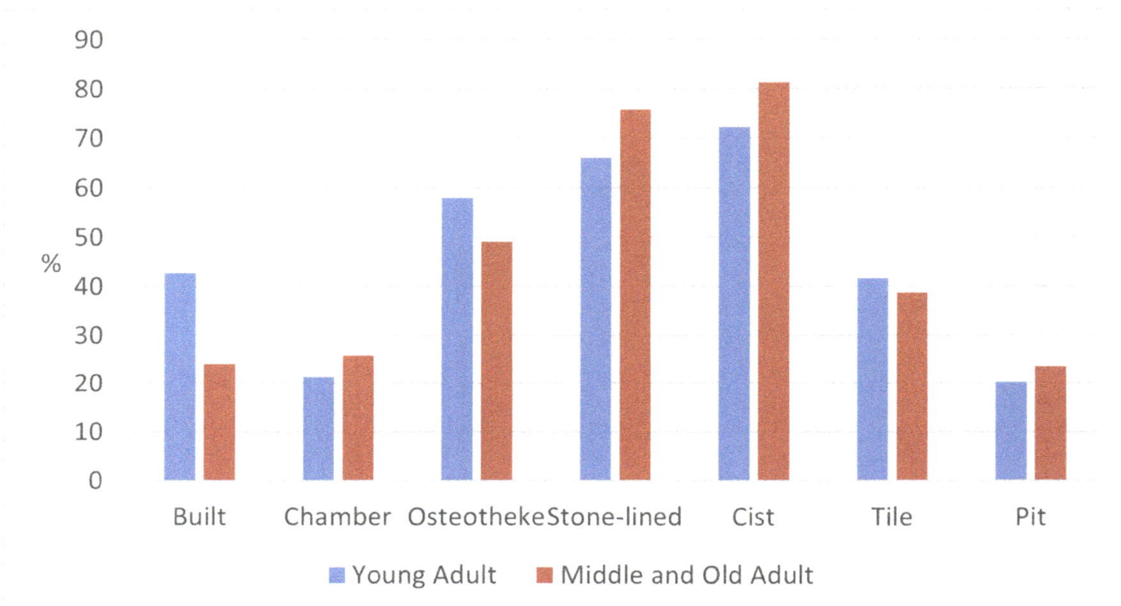

Figure 6.34. A comparison of calculus prevalence in Youngs Adults and Middle and Old Adults combined by tomb type.

in Figure 6.34. Many of these samples become too small for a meaningful analysis but some similar patterns to the caries analysis were noted such as a relatively high number of Old Adult teeth in the Built tomb group and a larger number of teeth in the Middle Adult group than that of the Young Adults for the Cist grave group and almost as many Middle as Young Adult teeth for the Tile grave group.

Roman tomb types were also compared to take a more detailed look within a single time period, which was not possible for the Hellenistic or Late Antique periods (Table 6.26 and Figure 6.35). A similar general pattern can be observed, with the cist grave (66.7% – there was only one cist grave studied for the Roman period: Unit 105) and stone-lined tombs (53.3%) having the highest levels of calculus and the chamber tombs (19.3%) having the lowest calculus prevalence. There is no trend by perceived tomb complexity or elaboration. The difference between the calculus prevalence for the different tomb types in the Roman period was, however, statistically highly significant, either on a presence-absence basis ($X^2 = 49.1$, $p = 0.00$) or for calculus scores 0-3 ($X^2 = 67.91$, $p = 0.00$). The cist graves and stone-lined tombs have the highest levels of both slight and moderate calculus deposits but the built tombs and tile graves have higher levels of heavy deposits. However, sample sizes become so small for the heavy deposits that these results cannot be taken as necessarily representative.

Table 6.26. Calculus scores, counts and prevalences for each Roman tomb type.

	0 (no calculus)	1 (slight)	2 (mod.)	3 (heavy)	No. of teeth	No. with calculus	% with calculus
Built	62	12	14	5	93	31	33.3%
Chamber	180	26	13	4	223	43	19.3%
Stone-lined	42	19	27	2	90	48	53.3%
Cist	7	5	9	0	21	14	66.7%
Tile	33	7	13	5	58	25	43.1%

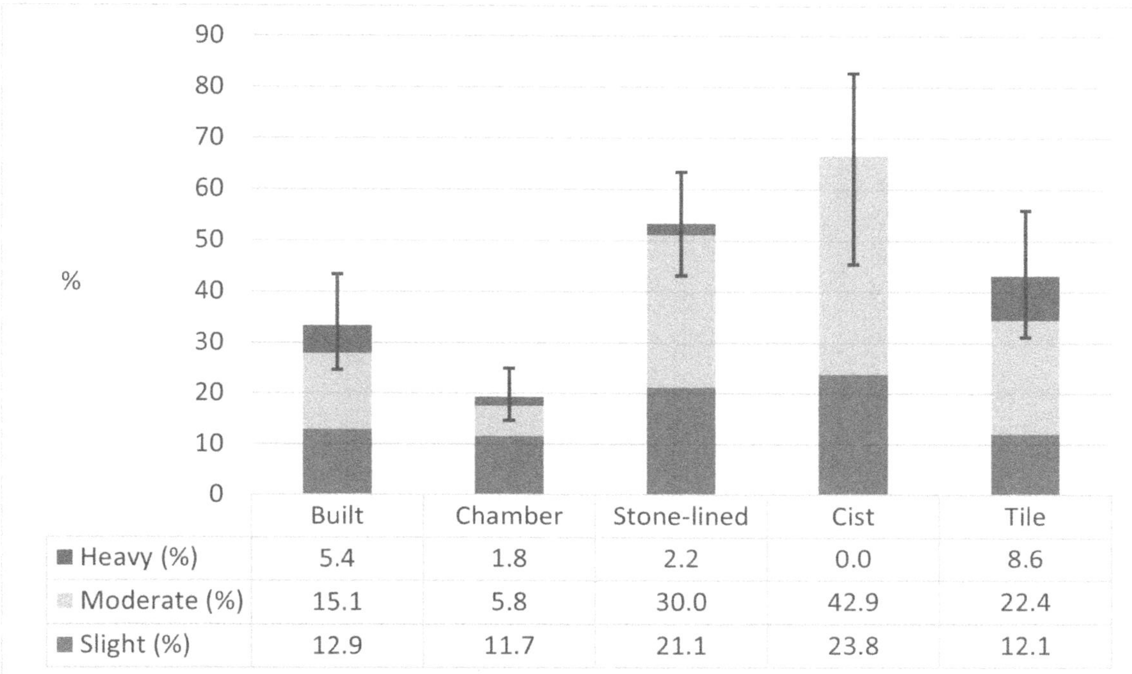

Figure 6.35. Prevalence of slight, moderate and heavy calculus deposits (stacked to show overall calculus prevalence with 95% confidence interval error bars) by tooth for each Roman tomb type.

6.2.2.6. Cemetery (Location)

The cemetery location is something that is important to consider in terms of the social significance of what it may have meant to be buried in a particular cemetery but it can also be a factor to consider preservation issues too. Preservation conditions within cemeteries can also be very localised and tomb form can play an important role. However, it is prudent to bear this notion in mind due to the fact that the North Cemetery Hellenistic assemblage and Spilia material had some of the worst surface conditions for the teeth and the bones were both more fragmented and often had poorer surface conditions. These are the two assemblages with the lowest calculus prevalence, and while it may not be the primary factor for the low calculus rates it is likely to be a contributing factor.

The calculus results for each cemetery are presented in Table 6.27 and Figure 6.36. The Krevatina cist grave (Unit 105) produced the overall highest levels of calculus (66.7%) for any cemetery but was a small sample size and was represented by only one tomb. After this the next highest cemetery group was the Late Antique North Cemetery but this and the Hellenistic North cemetery need to be considered separately from the discussion of the remaining Roman cemetery groups. Excluding the Krevatina grave, the Roman cemeteries with the highest calculus deposits are those from the north of the valley, Topana (47.6%), the North Cemetery (37%) and the Sanatorium cemetery (35.3%). The southern cemeteries, both comprised of rock-cut chamber tombs, had lower levels of calculus (Monastiriako Kephali 28.9%, Spilia 13%). The Topana cemetery (represented by a single Roman barrel-vaulted masonry built tomb: Unit 104) also had the highest levels of heavy deposits (9.5%), though the sample size was small. The Roman North Cemetery group also had a sizeable proportion of heavy calculus deposits (6.5%), and all three of these northern cemeteries had a higher proportion of moderate calculus (Sanatorium 20.3%, North Cemetery 19.6%, Topana 19%) than the southern cemeteries (Monastiriako Kephali 9.4%, Spilia 3.7%). Several significant differences can be identified from the confidence intervals bars in Figure 6.36 which do not overlap. However, within

Table 6.27. Calculus scores, counts and prevalences for each cemetery.

	0 (no calculus)	1 (slight)	2 (mod.)	3 (heavy)	No. of teeth	No. with calculus	% with calculus
Monastiriako Kephali	91	22	12	3	128	37	28.9%
Krevatina	7	5	9	0	21	14	66.7%
North Cemetery Hellenistic	390	64	25	5	484	94	19.4%
North Cemetery Roman	58	10	18	6	92	34	37.0%
North Cemetery Late Antique	269	200	86	29	584	315	53.9%
Sanatorium	99	21	31	2	153	54	35.3%
Spilia	47	4	2	1	54	7	13.0%
Topana	22	8	8	4	42	20	47.6%

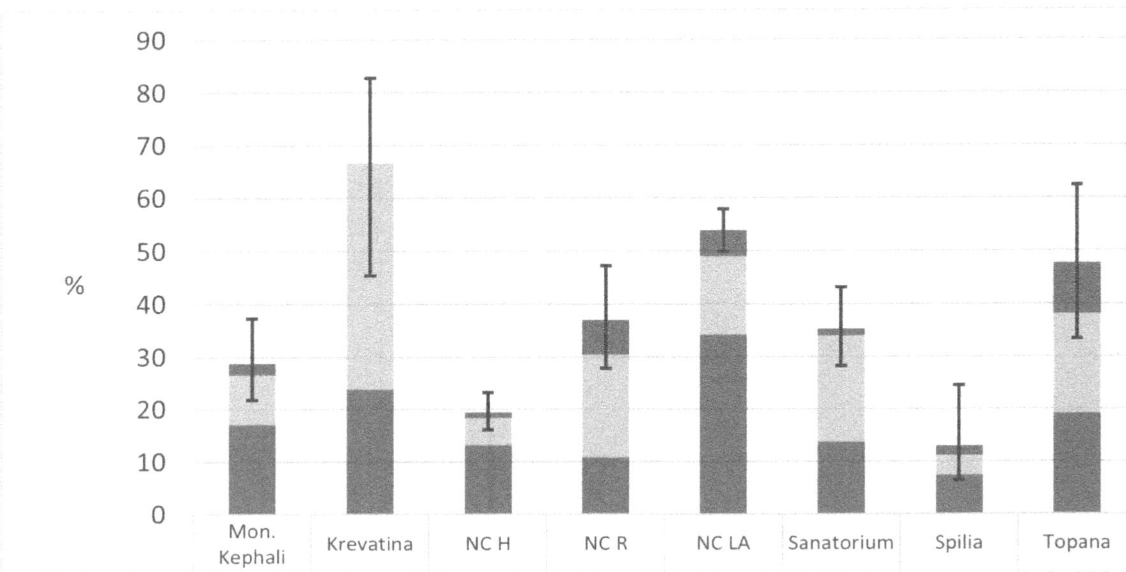

	Mon. Kephali	Krevatina	NC H	NC R	NC LA	Sanatorium	Spilia	Topana
Heavy (%)	2.3	0.0	1.0	6.5	5.0	1.3	1.9	9.5
Moderate (%)	9.4	42.9	5.2	19.6	14.7	20.3	3.7	19.0
Slight (%)	17.2	23.8	13.2	10.9	34.2	13.7	7.4	19.0

Figure 6.36. Prevalence of slight, moderate and heavy calculus deposits (stacked to show overall calculus prevalence with 95% confidence interval error bars) by tooth for each cemetery.

the Roman period these significant differences involve either Krevatina at the upper end of the scale, or Spilia at the lower end of the scale of calculus prevalence and these sample sizes are very small and based on a small number of individuals from a single tomb in each case. Within the North Cemetery, there are significant differences between each time period with calculus increasing over time

The difference in presence of calculus for the northern cemeteries combined and the southern cemeteries combined was also statistically significant (X^2 = 4.36, p = 0.03). The combined numbers of teeth with and without calculus for the cemeteries from the north and south of the valley are displayed in Table 6.28. The difference in calculus prevalence amongst the Roman cemeteries was also statistically highly significant for both the presence or absence of calculus (X^2 = 26.1, p = 0.00) and for scores 0-3 (X^2 = 45.69, p = 0.00).

These results are also presented for the individual age groups (Table 6.29, Figures 6.37–38), although for some of the smaller samples (especially Krevatina, Roman North

Table 6.28. Numbers of teeth with and without calculus for Roman tombs from cemeteries in the north and south of the valley.

	Calculus (present)	No calculus (absent)
Northern cemeteries	179	108
Southern cemeteries	145	58

Table 6.29. Numbers of teeth with calculus, total numbers of teeth and percentage of teeth with calculus for each age group by cemetery.

		Mon. Kephali	Krev.	NCH	NCR	NCLA	Sana.	Spilia	Topana
Child	Calculus	0	0	0	0	8	0	0	0
	Teeth	0	0	0	12	63	1	0	0
	%				0.0	12.7	0.0		
Adolescent	Calculus	0	0	0	3	11	4	0	0
	Teeth	5	0	30	20	33	45	0	0
	%	0.0		0.0	15.0	33.3	8.9		
Young Adult	Calculus	29	11	64	15	231	27	5	18
	Teeth	108	13	319	27	390	61	37	37
	%	26.9	84.6	20.1	55.6	59.2	44.3	13.5	48.6
Middle Adult	Calculus	7	3	25	16	57	23	1	3
	Teeth	13	8	118	32	89	33	13	9
	%	53.8	37.5	21.2	50.0	64.0	69.7	7.7	33.3
Old Adult	Calculus	0	0	5	0	8	0	0	0
	Teeth	0	0	17	1	9	13	0	0
	%			29.4	0.0	88.9	0.0		

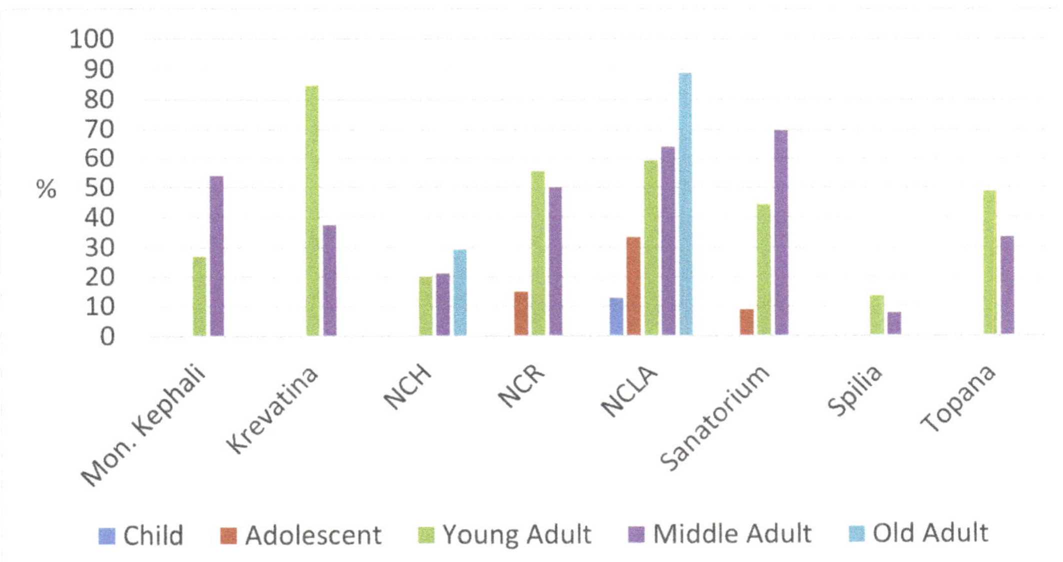

Figure 6.37. Calculus prevalence for each age group by cemetery.

Cemetery, Spilia and Topana), breaking the sample down further produces meaningless results. Some similar age group biases to those noted in the caries analysis (Section 6.2.1.7). The Sanatorium cemetery has a relatively high proportion of Middle and Old Adults compared to the other cemeteries, while the Monastiriako Kephali cemetery has very few Middle Adult teeth and none in the Old Adult category.

6.2.3. Antemortem tooth loss

Antemortem tooth loss rates look remarkedly low compared to other assemblages where the teeth can all or largely be scored in their sockets. The fragmentary nature of the material, with many loose teeth and fragmented or missing maxillae and mandibles, underscores the antemortem tooth loss rates for the population. Though this makes it difficult to compare to more complete dentitions from comparative studied assemblages, intrapopulation comparisons are still viable.

6.2.3.1. Time period

The prevalence of antemortem tooth loss (AMTL) for the different time periods supports the caries data in

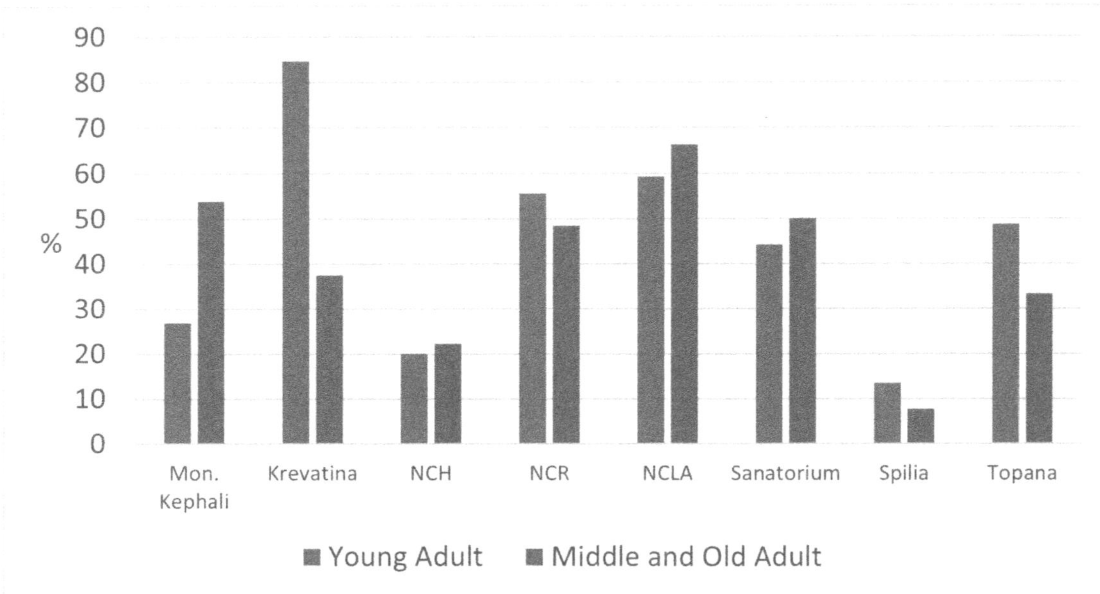

Figure 6.38. A comparison of calculus prevalence in Youngs Adults and Middle and Old Adults combined by cemetery.

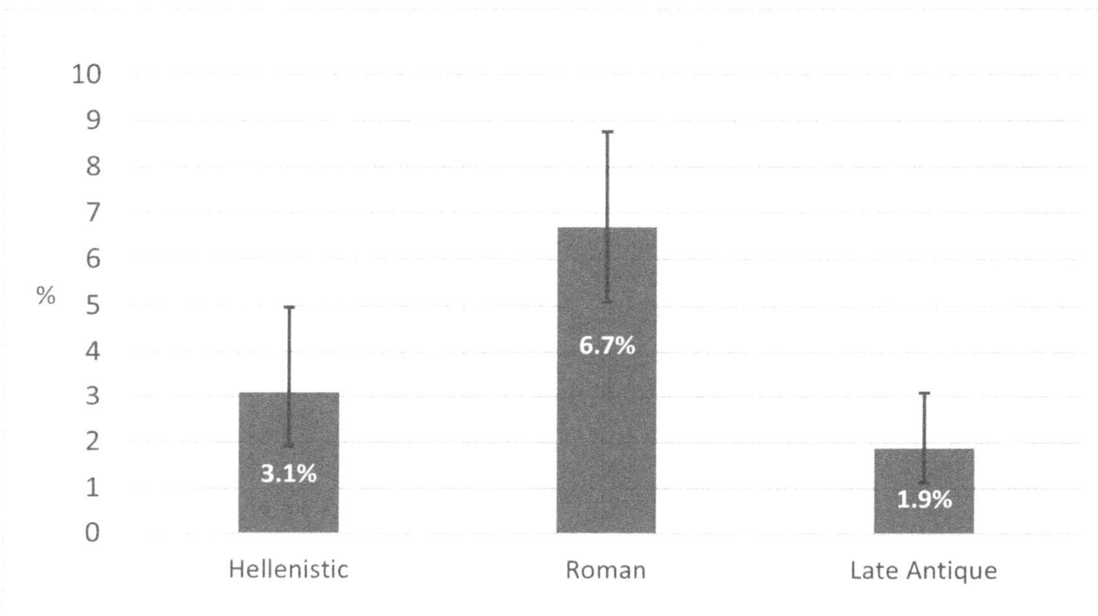

Figure 6.39. Prevalence of antemortem tooth loss (AMTL) by time period with 95% confidence interval error bars.

indicating that the Roman period had the worst dental conditions. For the Roman period 6.7% (48/717) of recordable spaces (teeth and sockets) displayed evidence of AMTL, but only 3.1% (16/517) for the Hellenistic period and 1.9% (15/798) for the Late Antique period. These results are displayed in Table 6.30 and Figure 6.39. The difference between the time periods was statistically highly significant ($X^2 = 24.6$, $p = 0.00$), as displayed by the non-overlapping confidence intervals in Figure 6.39.

Table 6.30. Counts and prevalence of antemortem tooth loss (AMTL) for each time period.

	AMTL	Present	Total teeth/ sockets	% AMTL
Hellenistic	16	501	517	3.1%
Roman	48	669	717	6.7%
Late Antique	15	783	798	1.9%

6.2.3.2. Sex

Antemortem tooth loss was more common in males, with 5.4% (31/573) recordable teeth or sockets showing remodelling, than in females, with antemortem tooth loss in 3.2% (25/791) of teeth or sockets. These results are displayed in Table 6.31 and Figure 6.40. The difference between the sexes was not significant as the confidence interval error bars for the sexes overlap.

Table 6.31. Counts and prevalence of antemortem tooth loss (AMTL) for the sexes.

	AMTL	Present	Total teeth/ sockets	% AMTL
Female	25	766	791	3.2%
Male	31	542	573	5.4%

6.2.3.3. Age group

The prevalence of antemortem tooth loss with increased age should be highly positively correlated. This is the case between the Young and Middle adult age categories with a dramatic increase from a very small number of cases, 1.2% (14/1180), in the Young Adults' dentitions, to 13.6% (65/478) for the Middle Adults (Table 6.32 and Figure 6.41). This difference was statistically highly significant (X^2 = 117.08, p = 0.00), as can be seen from the wide gap between the confidence intervals.

The Old Adult group, however, has a surprisingly low prevalence of antemortem tooth loss, occurring in only 2.2% (1/45) of recordable (and ageable) teeth and sockets. The wide confidence interval demonstrates the unreliability

Table 6.32. Counts and prevalence of antemortem tooth loss (AMTL) for each age group.

	AMTL	Present	Total teeth/ sockets	% AMTL
Young Adult	14	1180	1194	1.2%
Middle Adult	65	413	478	13.6%
Old Adult	1	45	46	2.2%

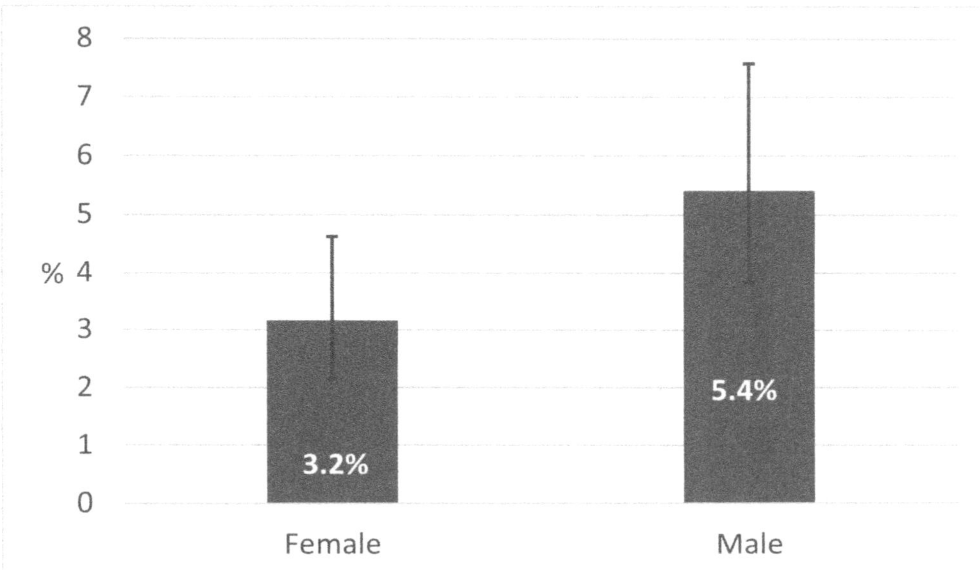

Figure 6.40. Prevalence of antemortem tooth loss (AMTL) by sex with 95% confidence interval error bars.

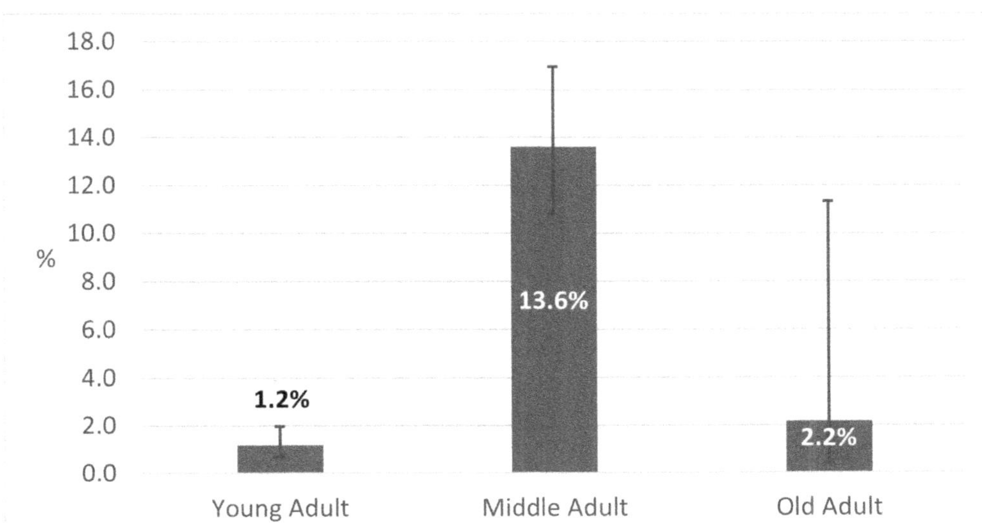

Figure 6.41. Prevalence of antemortem tooth loss (AMTL) by age group with 95% confidence interval error bars.

of the result and this can be explained in part by two methodological considerations. Firstly, this is an extremely small sample size and therefore it is impossible to say that the result is truly representative of this age group in the population. Secondly, in cases of gross antemortem tooth loss, where no teeth or other ageing characteristics exist, the dentition cannot be assigned to a specific adult age category, although it is highly likely that it should belong in the Old Adult category. One particularly blatant case of this is the mandible, Element 1935 from Unit 4 (Figure 6.42), which had complete remodelling of every socket other than the lower right third molar (LRM3), which appears to have been lost post-mortem leaving nothing by which to age the individual other than to say it was an adult. If this mandible alone was included in the antemortem tooth loss count for the Old Adult group, the prevalence would be 25.8% (16/62) as illustrated in Figure 6.43. This demonstrates the volatility of results with such small sample sizes.

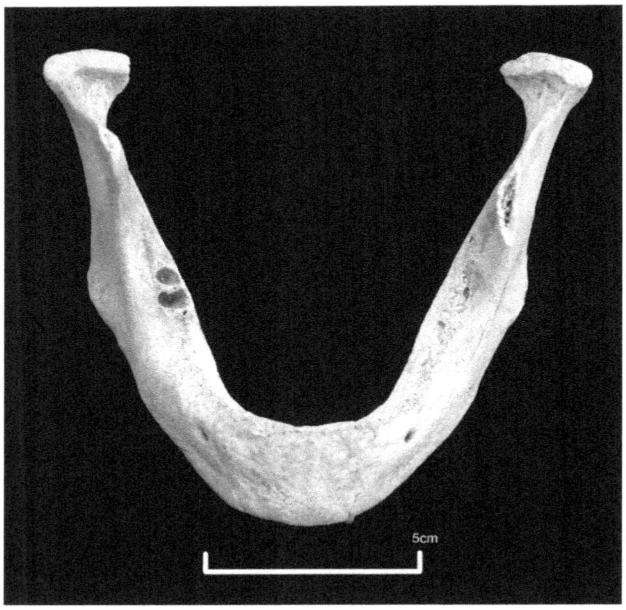

Figure 6.42. Unit 4, Element 1935. Mandible of a presumed-old adult with almost complete remodeling of the alveolar margin after antemortem tooth loss.

6.2.3.4. Tomb type

The antemortem tooth loss results for the different tomb types, for all the time periods are displayed in Table 6.33 and Figure 6.44. The cist grave antemortem tooth loss

Table 6.33. Counts and prevalence of antemortem tooth loss (AMTL) for each tomb type. AMTL= remodelling or remodelled sockets; Present=teeth or sockets with no remodelling (lost postmortem); total teeth and sockets= AMTL + Present; % AMTL= AMTL/Total teeth and sockets x 100.

	AMTL	Present	Total teeth and sockets	% AMTL
Built	8	162	170	4.7%
Chamber	6	281	287	2.1%
Osteotheke	13	652	665	2.0%
Stone-lined	7	146	153	4.6%
Cist	20	132	152	13.2%
Tile	12	116	128	9.4%
Pit	14	462	476	2.9%

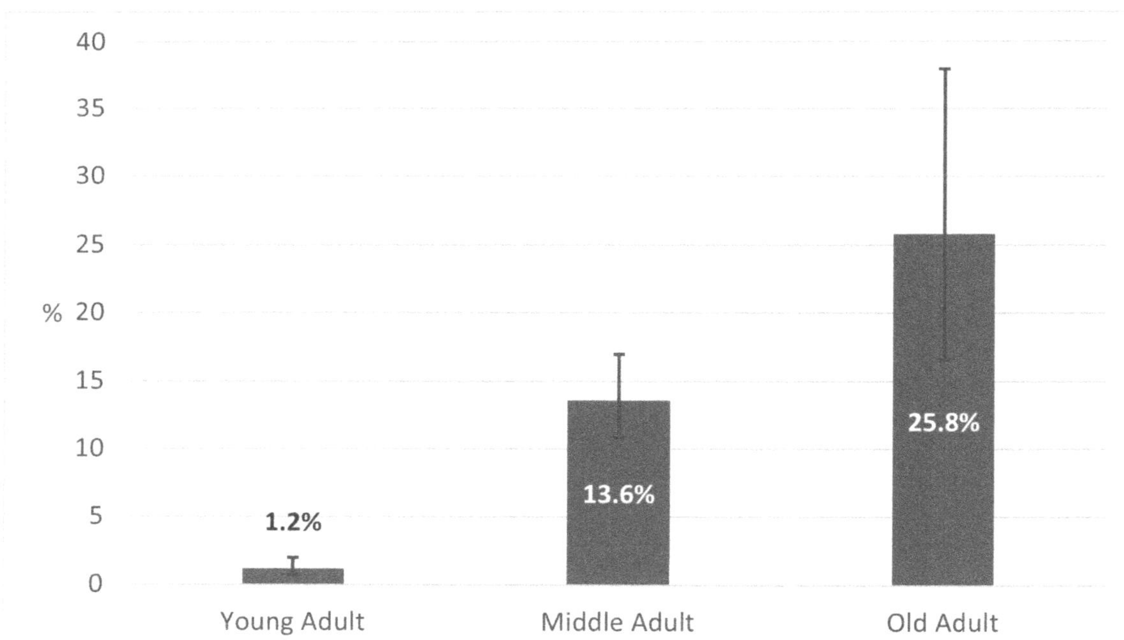

Figure 6.43. Alternative prevalence of antemortem tooth loss by age group (including Unit 4, Element 1935 as Old Adult) with 95% confidence interval error bars.

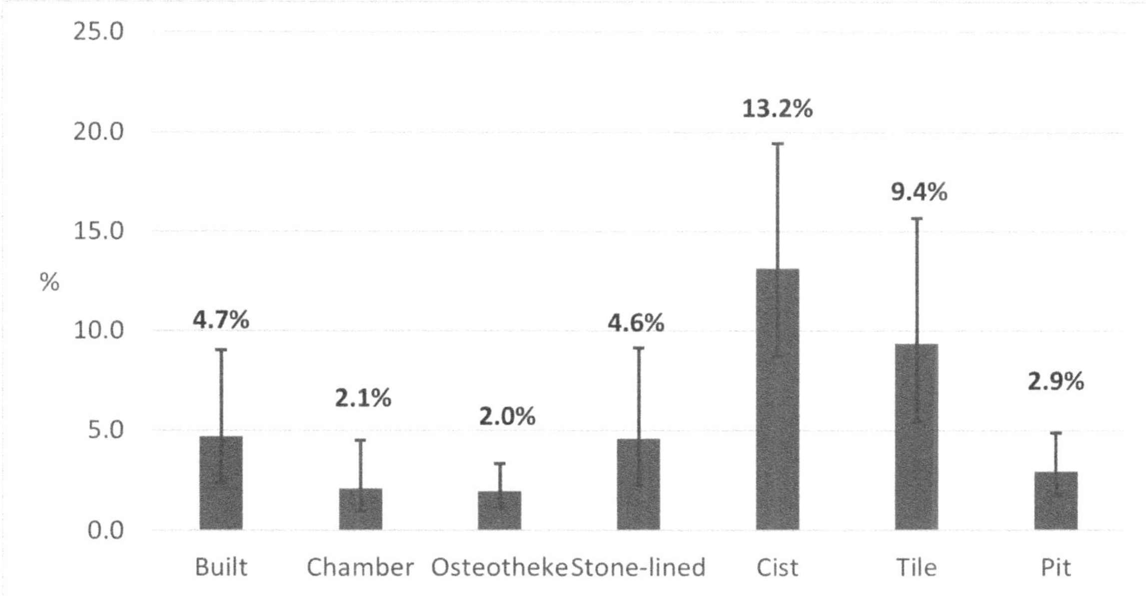

Figure 6.44. Prevalence of antemortem tooth loss (AMTL) by tomb type with 95% confidence interval error bars.

prevalence is significantly elevated due to the Roman Krevatina cist grave which had one individual (Unit 105, Individual 3, Middle Adult, indeterminate sex), out of the four in the grave, with the majority of teeth lost antemortem (17/20).

The tile grave assemblage had relatively high antemortem tooth loss prevalence, with 9.4% (12/128) compared to the remaining tomb types. The built and stone-lined tomb results were next highest, at 4.7% (8/170) and 4.6% (7/153) respectively. Antemortem tooth loss occurred in 2.9% (14/476) of recordable sockets for the pit graves. The lowest rates of antemortem tooth loss were from the rock-cut chamber tombs with 2.1% (6/287) and the stone osteothekai with 2% (13/652). There were no significant differences between the groups, as determined by the confidence intervals in Figure 6.44, other than those involving the Cist and Tile groups which are the least reliable samples, evidenced by having the widest confidence intervals. No pattern can be discerned in association with the perceived social status of the tomb type.

Narrowing the focus to look at only the Roman tomb types, presented in Table 6.34 and Figure 6.45, the pattern that emerges is similar to what was observed for the overall tomb type results. The Krevatina cist grave (Unit 105), discussed above, is the only Roman cist grave and therefore this result is even more exaggerated without the increased sample size created by the Late Antique cist grave (Unit 91). The tombs are then ordered from highest to lowest antemortem tooth loss rates, as Tile 11.4%, Stone-lined 6%, Built 4.7% and Chamber 2.1%, displaying no association with the perceived social status of the tomb by its elaboration or complexity.

Table 6.34. Counts and prevalence of antemortem tooth loss (AMTL) for each Roman tomb type.

	AMTL	Present	Total teeth/ sockets	% AMTL
Built	8	162	170	4.7%
Chamber	6	281	287	2.1%
Stone-lined	7	110	117	6.0%
Cist	18	37	55	32.7%
Tile	10	78	88	11.4%

6.2.3.5. Cemetery (Location)

The antemortem tooth loss results are presented for the different cemeteries in Table 6.35 and Figure 6.46. These are all Roman period cemeteries other than the North Cemetery, which has been divided up into its Hellenistic, Roman and Late Antique phases. The Krevatina cemetery is represented by the single cist grave and this elevated value has been discussed above in the results section for the tomb types. The Spilia group, represented by one rock-cut chamber tomb (Unit 109), had no cases of antemortem tooth loss as almost all of the teeth from this tomb were recorded loose with only a few small fragments of maxillae and mandibles surviving.

In a similar pattern to the calculus results, the northern cemeteries (the North Cemetery, Topana and Sanatorium) had higher antemortem tooth loss rates (8%, 6.7% and 3.7% respectively) than the southern Monastiriako Kephali cemetery (3.3%). However, the difference between the Sanatorium and Monastiriako Kephali results is negligible. Other than the Krevatina

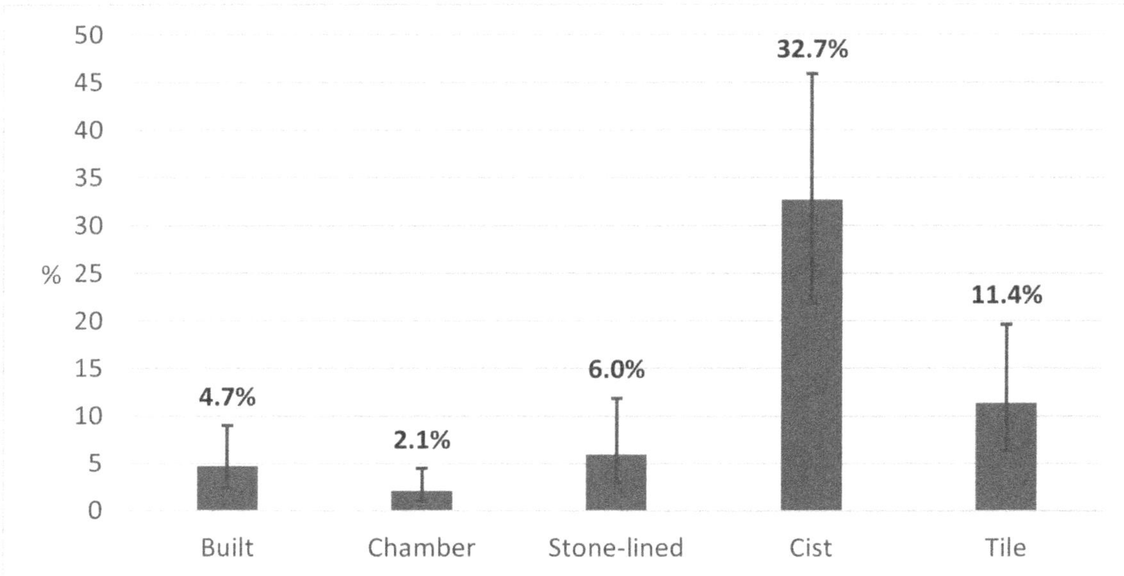

Figure 6.45. Prevalence of antemortem tooth loss (AMTL) by Roman tomb type with 95% confidence interval error bars.

Table 6.35. Counts and prevalence of antemortem tooth loss (AMTL) for each cemetery.

	AMTL	Present	Total teeth/ sockets	% AMTL
Monastiriako Kephali	5	147	152	3.3%
Krevatina	18	37	55	32.7%
Hellenistic North Cemetery	16	500	516	3.2%
Roman North Cemetery	11	127	138	8.0%
Late Antique North Cemetery	15	779	794	1.9%
Sanatorium	8	207	215	3.7%
Spilia	0	52	52	0.0%
Topana	7	98	105	6.7%

tomb, the only significant difference identified from the confidence intervals (Figure 6.46) was between the Roman and Late Antique North Cemetery groups. A comparison of northern (North, Sanatorium and Topana) and southern (Monastiriako Kephali) cemeteries was also not statistically significant (X^2 = 4.74, p = 0.32).

Excluding the Spilia result, the Hellenistic and Late Antique North cemetery groups have a lower prevalence of antemortem tooth loss than any of the Roman cemeteries. This was reflected in the overall assessment of antemortem tooth loss by time period.

6.3. Discussion

6.3.1. Time period

Dental health was at its worst in the Roman period with the prevalence of both caries and antemortem tooth loss at their highest. Calculus rates were higher in the Late Antique period (in just over half the teeth recorded) than in the Roman period, which had calculus on approximately one-third of teeth. This suggests that the Roman diet was more cariogenic than in the preceding or succeeding periods, which is likely to represent a high carbohydrate diet of starchy foods such as wheat. Wheat is likely to have been the staple food across all these time periods and the difference in the Roman period may have been a greater addition of sugars to the diet, in the form of fruit, wine, and honey, or could be due to improved preparation techniques and technologies producing a more refined and sticky carbohydrate diet. The distribution of caries by zones of the teeth (Section 6.2.1.2) suggests a higher level of sugar in the diet than in many archaeological agricultural societies, as caries often occurred in teeth prior to the exposure of dentine from wear or of the root from continual eruption.

The Hellenistic period had remarkably low levels of caries and calculus compared to the later time periods. While the problem surrounding the preservation condition of most of the Hellenistic graves was discussed in the results section (6.2.1.4) as a possible confounding factor in the recording of carious lesions and calculus deposits, this is unlikely to account for this level of difference between these different groups of teeth. Not only was the Hellenistic material assessed and deemed suitable for study but there were some Roman contexts studied that were in a similar state of preservation. Hellenistic Knossos was a large, complex urban centre that at least to some extent, had a centralised, administrated food production and distribution system

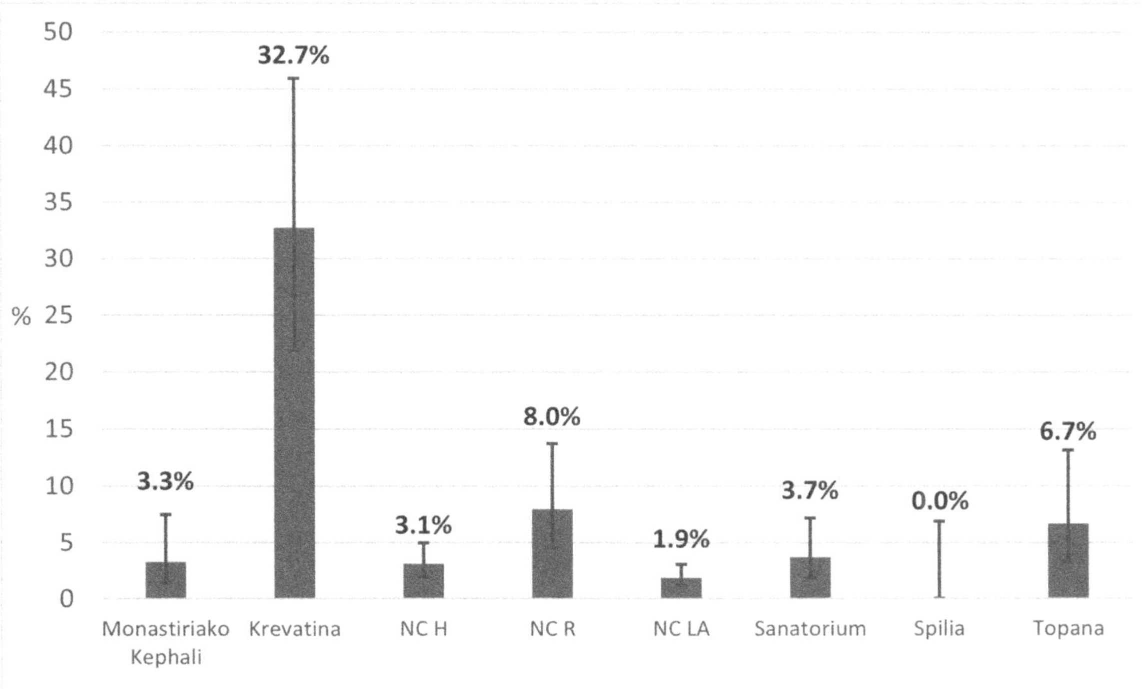

Figure 6.46. Prevalence of antemortem tooth loss (AMTL) by cemetery with 95% confidence interval error bars.

in the form of the *syssitia*. This did not continue into the Roman period therefore it is possible that food types, preparation techniques and technologies could have been somewhat different. It is possible that with the change in ownership of the 'Capuan lands' (the agricultural land to the south of Knossos) and the establishment of a colonist community, that there was a change in types of foods being produced and being desired by the resident population, such as fruit and honey, which could account for the increase in caries in the Roman period, though there is evidence for fruit consumption and honey production from earlier periods too. The change in the economy of Crete at this transition meant that a great deal more food would have been accessed through trade (Chaniotis 1999, 211). The difference in caries prevalence may also be due to groups of differing social status being represented in the Hellenistic and Roman graves represented by the assemblage. The Hellenistic assemblage was heavily dominated by females and the tomb forms were simpler than in the later periods representing a potentially lower social class (if other more elaborate tomb types existed in the Hellenistic period, as they did at Chania). Females (generally and for the Hellenistic period specifically) and pit grave individuals had lower caries rates than males or those buried in the later, more elaborate tomb forms.

The Late Antique period sees a fall in caries rates compared to the Roman period though the prevalence is still higher than it was in the Hellenistic period. Calculus prevalence, though predominantly light deposits, sees a dramatic increase in the Late Antique period, occurring in over half the teeth. The isotopic analysis indicated a higher animal protein component in Late Antique diets, which could partially explain this change in dental disease from the Roman period. The urban occupation in this period was steadily contracting in extent and the settlement would have had a significantly smaller population than in the Hellenistic and Roman periods. A centralised food production system and mass crop production (e.g. vines) for overseas trade may no longer have existed to the same extent. The amphora dumps at Knossos in the north (imports) and the south (local) appear to essentially be Early Roman (Trainor 2019) and the large-scale production and exportation of wine seems to have come to an end by c. AD 300 (Marangou 1999, 278), though amphora production did continue at Knossos (as well as at Gortyn and Eleutherna) into the Late Antique period (Frend and Johnston 1962, 229; Hayes 2001, 434; Gallimore 2015, 209). A return to a family or household level of food production and small-scale, local trade may have enabled a more diverse diet to be accessible and affordable. Cariogenic cereals will have remained the staple food in this time period but the higher caries rates in the Late Antique period compared to either the Hellenistic period or comparative Late Antique Cretan assemblages (Bourbou 2010, 47) may be explained by higher levels of sugars in the diet. If the Roman colonists, other sorts of migrants or merchants introduced higher levels of fruit or honey into the diets, these foods may have remained part of the diet into the Late Antique period. Evidence for Roman ceramic beehives is abundant on Crete, particularly in the west and centre of the island, though it was unclear whether this was on a scale for mass export or if the honey and wax was produced on a subsistence level (Francis 2016, 84). There is sparse evidence for Hellenistic beekeeping at Knossos but such evidence tends to be late Hellenistic and is generally uncommon throughout Crete until the Roman period though it is possible non-ceramic hives were used

(Homann-Wedeking 1950; Eiring 2001; Francis 2016). A small number of examples from Gortyn, Eleutherna and Sphakia demonstrate change in ceramic beehive shape in the Late Antique period and attest to continued honey production on Crete in this time period, though ceramic beehives are not known beyond the Early Byzantine period (Francis 2016, 89).

The study of a Late Roman (4th century AD) farmhouse at Pigi Athinas in Central Macedonia produced similarly high levels of calculus by tooth (49.8%) compared to the Knossos results but also had a remarkably high caries prevalence (21.9%) which led to the conclusion that not only were there evidently high levels of sugars and starches in the diet but that the contribution of environmental and geological factors to the occurrence of calculus needs to be investigated further (Tritsaroli 2014). The calculus results from Late Antique/Early Byzantine populations on Crete ranged from 4.5% at Eleutherna to 32.6% at Kefali, while the caries results (presumably comparable to the Knossos cavities results) ranged from 2.1% at Gortyn to 8.3% at Kefali (Bourbou 2010). The dramatically higher antemortem tooth loss results, ranging from 12.7% of teeth/sockets at Middle Byzantine Kastella to 42.9% at Kefali, demonstrate better preservation of the jaws compared to the Knossos assemblage. Few comparable studies have produced such high calculus results as have been observed at Knossos, but the Pigi Athinas and Kefali results show that such levels are not unprecedented in agricultural populations. It is unclear what the cause of such a range of calculus levels could be but it may be attributed to non-dietary factors such as use of the teeth as tools or the habitual chewing of substances.

6.3.2. Sex

There was a significant difference detected between females and males for caries, calculus and antemortem tooth loss, with males having a higher prevalence of all three conditions. No significant difference was detected for male and female diets from the stable isotope analysis, but this demonstrates the value of using multiple methods for the determination of aspects of ancient diets. The pattern of males having worse dental health generally prevails within each time period, though a more nuanced interpretation of both the caries and calculus data is required. Male cavities rates are higher than the female equivalent in each time period, though only marginally so for the Late Antique period. However, there are remarkably high rates of early-stage caries (score 1 or 2) for both Roman females and Late Antique males, resulting in the Roman females having an overall higher caries prevalence than the males and causing the Late Antique males to have a more elevated prevalence over the females. Calculus rates are consistently higher in males than females across the time periods but in every time period women have a higher prevalence of heavy calculus deposits. Antemortem tooth loss numbers were too small to give reliable results for the sexes within each time period, but the overall results showed that males had higher rates of antemortem tooth loss supporting the caries and calculus data.

Comparisons of caries in females and males across a broad range of archaeological populations temporally and geographically have demonstrated the opposite trend, with females having higher rates of caries, though this is most pronounced in hunter-gatherer populations (Larsen 2015, 73). This generally took the form of males having a greater amount of animal-sourced protein in their diets, which does not seem to be the case for either of the sexes at Knossos from the isotope results. The dental results, however, indicate some differences in diet between males and females and the caries data, in particular, the severity levels of lesions suggest that the nature of this difference varied within each time period. These differences could have taken the form of either differences in food preparation, with differential access to more or less refined foods, or in access to specific foodstuffs, such as the more cariogenic sugary foods, or could reflect different eating habits, in terms of frequency of meals, as more frequent consumption of carbohydrates is linked to higher caries rates (Arcella *et al.* 2002; Punitha *et al.* 2015)

The pattern of females having higher caries rates compared to males, due to labour division in hunter-gatherer societies, and this prevails in some Mediterranean agricultural populations (Masotti *et al.* 2013; Michael and Manolis 2014). The study of Archaic (7th century) to Roman (2nd century) Almyros on Corfu, found that 13.6% of females and 4.3% of males had carious teeth, though these results are from only 32 individuals across 9 centuries (Michael and Manolis 2014). However, many similar studies have found no significant difference between the sexes in terms of dental diseases (Belcastro *et al.* 2007; Bonsall and Pickard 2015). Results from late 10th-early 11th century Korytiani, West Greece, however, demonstrated a similar pattern to Knossos with males having higher levels of both caries and calculus, though in each case the overall prevalence was lower (caries: males 4.5%, females 3.6%; calculus: males 9.9%, females 5.0%) (Papageorgopoulou and Xirotiris 2009). A number of studies of Byzantine assemblages scoring caries by individual also demonstrated that males had a higher frequency of caries than females (Bourbou and Tsilipakou 2009; Bourbou 2010; Gnes *et al.* 2018). These examples demonstrate the difficulty of comparing results, scored by tooth, by individual or unspecified, from different studies.

These examples of studies showing different patterns of caries for males and females, suggests either regional or local differences in the social organisation of dining, whether due to cultural preferences or economic prosperity and availability of resources. Regional differences in dining practices are known from the Greek world with the *syssitia* (mandatory communal meals for citizens) being uncommon but not unique to Knossos, being reported also at Sparta, Miletus, Thebes and Carthage (Beer 2010, 107). However, the *syssitia*, which would have entailed males and females eating separately, did not endure into the Roman period, though Roman sumptuary laws were introduced to limit lavish expenditure. Such laws are attested in written sources to have been unpopular and may have been adhered to more rigorously in some cities than in others (Beer 2010). At Classical Athens, women ate separately from men and were not present at the symposium (Dalby 1996, 5). Although it seems to have been more common for women to have been present at the Roman dinner (with texts generally referring to banquets for the elite and therefore may not have applied habitually or throughout society), there were often different arrangements and roles for men and women and women do not appear to have been as numerous as men (Wilkins and Hill 2006, 74–75).

6.3.3. Age group

It is important to keep in mind that caries is a strongly age progressive disease and therefore, it could be the case that higher rates of caries or more severe lesions are due to individuals living longer. However, with a third of all adults (by MNI) unaged, and almost half of adults from both built and stone-lined tombs unable to be assigned to a specific adult age category, it is difficult to assess whether the proportions of individuals assigned to each age category are representative of the entire assemblage (not to mention the entire population). From the proportions of adults that can be assigned to the three adult age categories, Young, Middle and Old, there is no clear pattern of adults in the more elaborate tombs – or the tombs with higher rates of or more severe caries – living longer.

The general pattern for caries, calculus and antemortem tooth loss is that they are increasingly common with age from childhood to middle adulthood. The deviation of the Old Adult results from the expected value can be explained by the high levels of wear and antemortem tooth loss amongst older individuals, as well as the extremely small sample size of this category.

6.3.4. Tomb type

Nearly all Hellenistic individuals came from pit graves (with a small number of tile graves also represented in the assemblage) and conversely, all pit graves studied were Hellenistic in date. Similarly, the majority of Late Antique individuals came from the stone-lined osteothekai (and the osteothekai were exclusively Late Antique), with a small number from stone-lined or cist graves. Although it is stated in the results section that the social significance of tomb types from different time periods cannot be compared, the caries results demonstrate a trend of decreased caries prevalence with decreased tomb complexity (i.e. assumed lower social status). This is not supported by the calculus results which show no trends in association with tomb complexity. The highest calculus results came from the osteothekai, stone-lined tombs and cist graves, which may indicate their similarity in terms of social status, but is most indicative of the dietary change in the later Roman and Late Antique periods, as none of these burials was any earlier than the second-half of the 3rd century AD. Additionally, the antemortem tooth loss results show no trends or patterns in relation to tomb type which may demonstrate the conflicting caries and calculus results, with tooth loss being caused by both caries and periodontal disease.

It can sometimes be difficult to tell which variable is significant in observing differences, in this case, in dental disease. For example, the Hellenistic assemblage comes exclusively from the North Cemetery and consists largely of narrow pit graves cut into the soft kouskouras rock and a smaller number of tile graves. Therefore, whatever the phenomenon observed for the Hellenistic period, it is necessary to consider that it may be a cemetery specific or grave type specific phenomenon rather than being affected by the larger scale urban processes, such as population size and density, subsistence strategies, off-island connectivity, or political administration, changing between these time periods. For this reason, if variables can also be observed within a single time period without sample sizes becoming too small in the different groups, it can be more demonstrative of which variable is most responsible for any observation of change or difference. This is possible for looking at dental diseases within the Roman period for the different tomb types.

It might be expected, if the supposition about the tomb types in relation to social status is correct, that caries rates might be higher in the simpler tomb forms, as the lower echelons of society would more likely have eaten an unvaried and predominantly carbohydrate diet of cereal based foods. Meanwhile a more elite diet being consumed by those buried in the monumental built tombs and rock-cut chamber tombs might be more varied, including a greater variety of plant foods, such as legumes and vegetables, as well as animal proteins. However, this is not the pattern that emerges from the teeth studied here. The results show a general pattern of higher caries in the more complex tombs, both for a comparison of tomb types within the Roman period and including the earlier and later tombs. When the caries zone patterning is also considered, with caries appearing on the zones of the tooth that may suggest an accelerated caries rate compared to a standard high-starch diet of an agricultural population, eating cereal staples, it appears likely that there was a significant sugar component in the diet. The elite members of society, assumed to be represented by the more complex tomb forms, particularly the monumental built tombs and rock-cut chamber tombs of the Roman period, were more likely to have had access to such luxury foodstuffs.

This is perhaps the opposite of what might be hypothesised under the assumption that the lower levels of society would have had a simpler and more exclusively carbohydrate diet, as has been found to be the case in many societies (Phillip L. Walker and Hewlett 1990; Shimada *et al.* 2004; Winkler *et al.* 2017). In these cases, the more elite members of society are interpreted as having had better living conditions and access to resources, with a greater animal-protein component in the diet. However, the converse has also often been observed, with the same pattern that has been noted at Knossos (Leigh 1935; Suzuki *et al.* 1967; Sakashita *et al.* 1997; Larsen 2015, 77–78). This has been found to be the case when the high-status individuals had more access to sugars or consumed softer, more refined, sticky foods than the lower-status individuals, which results in increased incidences of caries (Larsen 2015, 77). In reality, the staple in all diets at Knossos is likely to have been wheat, but it may be the case that those being buried in the more elaborate tomb forms had access to additional cariogenic foods such as honey, figs and other fruits.

The caries rate for cist graves is remarkably low; however, it is important to note that this result is based on 18 mandibular teeth from four individuals in a single grave and therefore may not be representative. This tomb (Krevatina cist: Unit 105) seems to be somewhat unusual in a variety of respects not least of which includes the fact that its inhabitants appear to have had very few carious teeth, despite two of the individuals being in the Middle Adult age category. This was a Late Roman tomb in an area which had in the Early Roman period been part of the settlement and therefore represents a new cemetery (other Late Roman cist and tile graves have been reported in this area) at this time, and therefore may represent a non-traditional burying group.

6.3.5. Cemetery (Location)

There was no consistent pattern that prevailed for the occurrence of the different dental conditions across the different cemeteries. For the Roman period, there seemed to be a slight north/south divide for calculus and antemortem tooth loss, with both conditions being higher in the cemeteries in the north of the valley (North Cemetery, Topana and Sanatorium), compared to those in the south (Monastiriako Kephali, Spilia and Krevatina). While the difference in the presence of calculus for the northern and southern cemeteries was statistically significant, the results for antemortem tooth loss were not as distinctly different. Additionally, the caries results did not reflect a similar pattern, with the Monastiriako Kephali (south) and Topana (north) cemeteries having the highest results and the North Cemetery (in each time period) having the lowest caries rates. Of these conditions, caries is the most intimately connected with diet therefore it is unlikely that individuals being buried to the north and south of the settlement had significantly different diets.

Tomb type is a clearer indicator of social status than cemetery location. Even in the comparative example of Imperial period cemeteries near Rome, at Lucus Feroniae and Isola Sacra, the former being composed largely of slaves, war veterans and manual labourers and the latter a more "middle class" urban population, these cemeteries can be as easily defined by tomb type as by location, the former consisting of pit graves and the latter of monumental tombs (Manzi *et al.* 1999). In this case the social status of the interred individuals is more clearly defined than at Knossos. The two cemeteries can also be differentiated by their dental health with Lucus Feroniae having a higher caries prevalence (6.1%) and fewer teeth with calculus (26.9%) compared with Isola Sacra, which produced a caries prevalence of 4.0%, with calculus occurring in 33.9% of teeth. The difference in caries between these two 1st–3rd century AD cemeteries was, however, much less significant than when compared to the nearby 7th century AD Lombard cemetery at La Selvicciola (caries: 12.6%), though calculus (27.1%) remained similar as it is less heavily dictated by dietary factors. The caries data suggest that status differences within the Imperial Roman population were less significant than large scale socio-economic changes over time in influencing dietary differences. Although a relationship between diet and social status at Knossos is indicated tentatively by the correlation between caries and complexity of tomb type, this pattern does not prevail in the other dental conditions nor in the cemetery/location results. Therefore, similar to the situation observed in the cemeteries surrounding Rome from Imperial to Early Medieval times, socio-economic changes over time appear to be more significant than status differences within the Roman period (at least going by the status indicators that are available).

6.4. Conclusions

It can be observed in the dental data that there are changes in diet from Hellenistic to Roman times and again between the Roman and Late Antique periods. There is no close dating for some of the tombs in this study, and none can be dated to the second half of the 1st century BC or the first half of the 1st century AD, around the time after the Roman conquest of Crete and the subsequent establishment of a colony at Knossos. This makes it difficult to discern exactly when the changes in diet occurred, whether in the Late Hellenistic period, around the time of the Roman conquest, or if they were associated with the establishment of a colony at the site. The change between the Hellenistic and Roman periods in the dental results was manifested by an increase in caries, calculus and antemortem tooth loss, demonstrating a general decline in dental health in the later period. This is due to increased consumption of cariogenic carbohydrates. As wheat, olive oil and wine would have been the staple foods in both time periods and the isotope data does not suggest a significant difference in meat consumption between these time periods, this is likely to have taken the form of either a change in food preparation techniques or increased sugary foods in the diet. The former would be represented by the greater refinement of cereals for bread or porridge resulting in a finer, stickier grain. There is evidence at Knossos – and elsewhere on Crete – for a change in cookware ceramics, with a change in the preferential shape from the casseroles of local or regional fabrics in the Hellenistic period, to cook pots being preferred in the Roman period, as well as a greater variety of shapes and a greater number of imports during the 2nd and 3rd centuries (Hayes 1971; 1983; Sackett 1992; Gallimore 2015). However, it cannot be determined whether the contents of such pots would have changed significantly. The latter change, supported by the caries-zone analysis of the teeth, would have taken the form of an increased component of foods such as sweetened wine, honey, figs, dates and other fruit in the diet. This could be due to either increased connectivity making certain foods more readily available or the cultural influence of incomers (merchants/migrants/colonists) to Roman Knossos.

The isotope results indicated a slight increase in animal sources of protein in the later Roman and Late Antique periods and the associated dental data, with decreased caries and tooth loss and increased calculus, support this suggestion. This may be due to a reduction in pressure on resources and a greater number of people living above basic subsistence levels, though the movement of the Knossian people to Heraklion may have meant the pressure on resources in the wider area did not change. It could also be due to increased prosperity, which would have suffered considerable set-backs for some time following the Roman conquest. There appeared to have been broad prosperity during the 2nd and 3rd centuries AD, as suggested by the public building works and mosaics in public and private settings, and also attested in the 4th–6th centuries from the basilica churches and mosaics. Meat production requires more land and involves the wasteful conversion of plant calories into animals (Jongman 2007b). Therefore, whether due to decreased pressure on resources or increased prosperity, an increase in the meat component in the diet seems likely. Such changes demonstrate that the changing urban environment and the social changes that concurrently occurred were substantial enough to have a significant impact on the lives, lifestyles, physical wellbeing, and health of the inhabitants of Knossos.

Within each time period, there was a degree of variation by demographic and social characteristics. A difference in diet between the sexes was more apparent from the dental results than it was from the isotope data. For each dental condition, males had the higher prevalence demonstrating poorer dental hygiene and access to more cariogenic foods and potentially different dietary habits, in terms of eating more frequently than females. Most Classical Greek and Roman written sources suggest a division of labour, with women doing the majority of food preparation and frequently eating separately but many sources also mention a division in male and female dining at banquets (Dalby 1996, 6; Wilkins and Hill 2006, 76). The different diets of females and males, indicated by the dental disease results, suggest that meals adhered to social rules even after the dissolution of the *syssitia*. Dental conditions generally followed the expected trend of being age progressive with the exception of the Old Adult category which was generally explicable by the effects of high wear, tooth loss, calculus chipping and the sample size being small and potentially unrepresentative. The social differences can only really be assessed for the Roman period where there was a greater diversity of tomb types and cemetery locations to use as potential social status criteria. While the caries data show a trend of decreasing caries alongside decreasing tomb complexity, the antemortem tooth loss and calculus results do not match this trend. It would be expected that individuals of higher social status (buried in the more complex tombs) would have a lower prevalence of caries due to a more diverse diet, compared to a more exclusively cereal-based diet. However, the opposite may indicate that the uppermost social classes had greater access to sweeteners, such as honey and fruit, or alternatively, that the lower social classes are entirely absent from the Roman sample, given that no pit graves and only a few tile graves were included in the sample.

Without a larger and more intact dental assemblage it is hard to be certain that patterns and trends observed are representative. Ideally, complete dentitions with a typical ratio of lip and cheek teeth would be used rather than loose teeth, making the results more easily comparable across different populations. However, this would dramatically decrease sample sizes. The results, particularly for caries and calculus had quite large sample sizes for many of the variables, and therefore even if the results are not easily compared with other studies, the comparisons over time and by demographic and social characteristics are valid within the Knossos assemblage. More systematic studies of dental disease alongside stable isotope analyses for Greek and Roman populations will help to create a picture of variations in diet between and within populations.

7

Activity: Joint Disease and Entheseal Changes

7.1. Introduction to activity-related pathology

Throughout much of the history of osteoarchaeology, as a discipline, scholars have attempted to reconstruct activity or occupation from the human skeleton. Methods have included the observation of joint diseases, entheseal changes (often called musculoskeletal stress markers in the past), non-metric traits such as squatting facets (features on the distal tibia and upper surface of the talus from habitual kneeling or squatting) and external auditory exostoses (a bone spur or partial or complete bony overgrowth of the ear canal thought to be caused by habitual swimming in cold water), and cross-sectional geometry of long bones. This endeavour has been fraught with hazards as scholars have often been over-ambitious in the depth and specificity of this reconstruction (Jurmain 1977; 1980; Merbs 1983; Walker and Hollimon 1989; Larsen *et al.* 1995; Hershkovitz *et al.* 1996; Capasso *et al.* 1999). It is not possible to make blanket statements about specific 'occupations' of individuals, inferred from bone lesions. Similar bone lesions can have a variety of different aetiologies, and the same activity can manifest itself differently in different individuals. However, what can be attempted, on a palaeoepidemiological level, is a general assessment of activity levels in the population, to differentiate between a heavy manual labouring lifestyle and an inactive one. This can be insightful for identifying changes over time in society in terms of labour division: gender-based and within different subsets of society being buried in particular tomb types or cemeteries. This chapter presents the results of the analysis of joint diseases (focusing on osteoarthritis and intervertebral disc disease) and entheseal changes, in making an attempt to identify broad changes in activity and lifestyle over time and between different subsets of the population.

The two types of articular joints found in the human body are called amphiarthrodial or syndesmoses and diarthrodial or synovial. Syndesmosis joints are somewhat mobile but serve primarily to stabilize specific regions of the skeleton; these include the pubic symphysis, distal tibiofibular joint and intervertebral bodies. Synovial joints are found at the ends of bones that articulate with each other within a fibrous capsule and the articular surfaces are covered with a highly lubricated hyaline cartilage and synovial membrane which allow full mobility; these include the major joints of the limbs (Larsen 2015). The deterioration of articular joints, which involves the bone and surrounding tissues, can be caused by a variety of conditions and circumstances. Osteoarthritis (only at synovial joints) is the most commonly occurring joint disease, though it often occurs in association with other diseases. While in some cases this can be coincidental, there are some conditions that appear to be directly related, including Paget's disease and osteoporosis (Waldron 2009, 39). The clinical and epidemiological literature employ a confusing array of terms, definitions and mixed consensus of aetiology. It can be agreed upon that it is a multifactorial degenerative disorder involving focal, progressive loss of articular cartilage, often accompanied by marginal osteophyte lipping and articular surface deterioration from bone-on-bone contact (Felson 2003). Although the cause of the manifestation of osteoarthritis is not known with certainty, contributing factors include age, genetics, sex, race, body weight, trauma, and, most importantly, movement (Waldron 2009, 28). There is considerable disagreement on the relative importance of these different factors but a mechanical loading environment due to activity features prominently.

Intervertebral disc disease (IVDD) is the other main form of joint disease focused on in this chapter, although Schmorl's nodes, diffuse idiopathic skeletal hyperostosis (DISH), and ankylosing spondylitis also feature. The vertebrae are articulated by fibrous discs and the degeneration of the disc is particularly associated with ageing and tends to occur equally in both sexes (Waldron 2009, 43). The narrowing of the disc space between the vertebral bodies is accompanied by marginal osteophytes (bone growth around the edges of the vertebral bodies) and pitting on the superior and inferior surfaces of the vertebral bodies, most often in the lower cervical and lumbar spine (Waldron 2009, 43). Schmorl's nodes (recognised as an indentation in the vertebral surface lined with cortical bone) occur when the vertebral endplate (upper and lower surface of the vertebral bodies) is damaged allowing the vertebral disc to herniate into the damaged hollow. There are many possible causes but it has been observed that they are particularly common in individuals imposing high impact on the lower thoracic and lumbar regions of the spine, such as elite athletes (Waldron 2009, 45). Ankylosing spondylitis is the most common of a group of erosive arthropathies known as the seronegative spondyloarthritides. The main feature of erosive arthropathies (joint diseases) is the loss of bone, as opposed to the proliferation of new bone which is the main feature of osteoarthritis and intervertebral disc disease (proliferative arthropathies). Ankylosing spondylitis affects the pelvis, sacrum, vertebrae, and ribs, as well as causing erosions and bony ankylosis (stiffening, fusion and immobility) at entheses. The disease often begins with sacroiliitis and the sacroiliac joints can become symmetrically fused and the vertebrae become fused creating an effect known as 'bamboo spine'. The erosive lesions of the vertebral bodies may not be visible due to the ankylosing of the spine (Waldron 2009, 57–59). Though its occurrence is not activity related, it is mentioned to differentiate these spinal lesions from those caused by intervertebral disc disease and DISH.

Waldron, Rogers and colleagues distinguish some individuals as 'bone formers' (Waldron and Rogers 1990; Rogers *et al.* 1997; Waldron 2009, 72). These are individuals who are more predisposed to produce heterotopic ossification (growth of bone in the non-skeletal tissues) and to ossify costal cartilages, the thyroid cartilage and other soft tissues. They are more likely to produce prominent osteophytic and enthesophytic bone growth. DISH appears to represent an extreme expression of bone forming, with the production of new bone onto the anterior longitudinal ligament of the spine and ossification of extra-spinal entheses and ligaments and other soft tissues (Waldron 2009, 73). This causes bone formation that looks like melted candle wax down only the right-hand side of the vertebrae, due to the descending aorta on the left (Ciocci 1987; Waldron 2009, 73). DISH has been associated with obesity in modern cases and with a rich, monastic diet in the medieval period. Though the aetiology is not fully understood, there is a clear association between DISH and the state of nutrition enjoyed by those with a rich (plentiful, high calorie and diverse) diet, but it should not be assumed that every individual with DISH is necessarily a monk or high-status individual (Waldron 2009, 75).

Entheses, or muscle attachment sites, are visible throughout the skeleton in the form of tuberosities and rugosities on the bones at the point where the tendon or ligament of the muscle is attached. Entheseal changes, referred to in the past as 'musculo-skeletal stress markers' (MSMs), are alterations at the enthesis and can involve both the formation and destruction of bone. These entheseal changes can take the form of various types of bone protrusions or enthesophytes (isolated bone spur, longitudinal or shapeless protrusions, marginal ridges), fine or macro porosity, surface discontinuity or furrowing, or complete loss of original morphology (Villotte *et al.* 2016).

As a bone forming condition, entheseal changes vary in their manifestation between different individuals, with 'bone-formers' being genetically more inclined to form bone at such sites than others (Waldron 2009, 72). Therefore, there may not always be a direct correspondence between rigorous activity or heavy loading at an enthesis and the production of new bone. Entheseal changes often occur in conjunction with other bone forming diseases including DISH and seronegative spondyloarthropathies (including ankylosing spondylitis). The production of new bone at an enthesis can be a direct structural response of the bone to the forces acting on it, according to the principles of biomechanics, which can include strenuous or repetitive daily activity, traumatic incidents, or particular body conformations or postural requirements. It can be difficult or impossible to identify whether the activity is habitual or exceptional, and duration, frequency and intensity of activity, degree of mechanical overloading, and age of onset are all contributing factors to the manifestation of lesions (Luttmann *et al.* 2003; Jurmain *et al.* 2012, 532). Age-at-death and body mass are also contributing factors in the occurrence of entheseal changes and this sort of multifactorial aetiology is to be expected with activity-related changes. Two major age-related phases have been identified that affect entheseal changes. One is around 30-35 years of age, related to decreased resistance of the tendon leading to poorer tendinous vascularisation and hydration (Rodineau 1991; Bard 2003). The other occurs over 50 years of age as entheses undergo tissue disruption (at least for the fibrocartilaginous entheses) and major bony changes (Villotte 2008; Cardoso and Henderson 2009; Villotte *et al.* 2010; Jurmain *et al.* 2012, 538). The young age-at-death of many of the adults in the assemblage means an assessment of the entheseal changes is more likely to be activity-related.

It was claimed in the past that osteoarthritis was the most useful of all diseases for reconstructing the life style of early populations (Wells 1982, 152), but in more recent literature the focus has been on the multifactorial nature of the condition. At Roman Isthmia the difference between the shoulder and vertebral osteoarthritis in the rural and urban assemblages (higher in rural), was interpreted as being due to their greater exposure to agricultural labour work (Rife 2012). Patterns of osteoarthritis have sometimes been proposed for individuals of known occupation, such as manual labourers, farmers, ballet dancers, and in unusual circumstances a correlation between patterns of joint disease and a highly specific activity have been identified, such as for the hand joints of weavers and cotton mill workers or the case of a cello player (Hadler *et al.* 1978; Ciranni and Fornaciari 2003; Larsen 2015). However, it is one thing to know an individual's occupation and work backwards from that and it is unsurprising that individuals doing repetitive or heavy loading activities will manifest certain patterns of joint disease. It is another matter to purport to be able to identify a specific occupation from a pattern of joint disease due to the multitude of factors that can cause the same lesions and the multifactorial influences (genetic, environmental, and behavioural) all contributing to the manifestation of the disease. Additionally there is "no convincing evidence of a consistent relationship between a particular occupation and a particular form of osteoarthritis" and Waldron reaffirms this earlier statement by stating emphatically that "occupation cannot be deduced from lesions in the skeleton" (Waldron 1994, 94; 2007, 11). Some specific articular modifications are linked more to specific physical activities, while others are more age-related phenomena (Stirland 2000; Waldron 2012). Age is, of course, an important factor and in urbanised industrial populations osteoarthritis or IVDD are rarely seen in individuals below forty years of age, but archaeological assemblages tend to have relatively high occurrences even amongst older juveniles and young adults (Larsen and Hutchinson 1999; Arden and Nevitt 2006; Waldron 2009,

31). Regardless of cause, owing to disability from loss of movement, osteoarthritis would have had substantial economic, social, and behavioural costs, as well as the negative impact on individual lifestyles (Corti and Rigon 2003; Sharma *et al.* 2006).

This chapter does not assign occupations or identify specific activities but aims to identify general activity levels in seeking differences over time and between subsets of the population. Sexual dimorphism is often identified in osteoarthritis but with a wide range of variation. Some studies show females to have higher prevalences of the disease (Rife 2012), some find no significant differences between the sexes (Rojas-Sepúlveda *et al.* 2008), but most frequently males show a consistently greater prevalence of osteoarthritis than females, regardless of subsistence strategy or socio-economic complexity (Waldron 1992; Sofaer Derevenski 2000; Klaus *et al.* 2009; Novak and Šlaus 2011). Differences can often be identified in many aspects of health between individuals of different social status due to the inequality in health and quality of life in hierarchical societies. Higher status individuals are often exposed to less demanding activities, while the lower echelons of society may be engaged in more heavy manual labour (Larsen 2015). Temporal trends have been identified due to changes in workload and activity, often in relation to subsistence, from foraging to farming, and changes in weaponry and fishing equipment.

7.2. Methodology

A variety of joint diseases were recorded, with a particular focus on osteoarthritis and intervertebral disc disease, which are relatively commonly occurring conditions and were systematically recorded. Cases of less common joint conditions, such as erosive ankylosing spondylitis, DISH and Schmorl's nodes, were also noted when they occurred. Entheseal changes were the other main movement-related pathological lesions recorded, which are also commonly occurring and manifest themselves on a continuous scale from normal to prominent bony changes.

Diagnoses of joint diseases were based on 'operational definitions'. These are criteria that must be fulfilled in order for a disease to be recognised. Some lesions can be pathognomonic of a condition (i.e. they match this disease and no other) but normally this is not the case and for a disease to be said to be present a particular number of major or minor criteria are fulfilled (Waldron 2009, 6).

7.2.1. Osteoarthritis

Using Waldron's (2009) operational definition for osteoarthritis, the presence or absence of osteoarthritis was determined by recordable joint. The presence of osteoarthritis was confirmed if eburnation (a pathognomonic feature of osteoarthritis, observed as a hardened, shiny patch on the joint surface caused by bone-on-bone friction when the cartilaginous part of the joint has worn away), or any two of the following lesions could be observed: marginal osteophytes (new bone growth around the edges of the joint surface), new bone or pitting on the joint surface, alteration in the joint contour (Waldron 2009, 34). Examples of these criteria are presented in Figures 7.1–2.

Joints without osteoarthritis were also recorded to give an overall count of all scoreable adult joint surfaces, in order to calculate the prevalence of the condition. Calculating prevalences of disease is an important feature

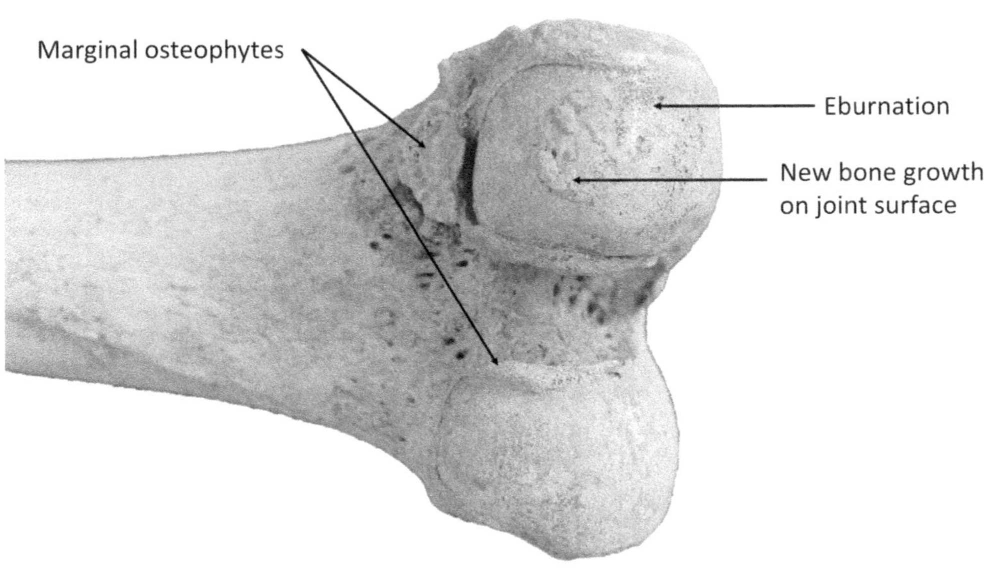

Figure 7.1. Distal femur (Unit 4, Individual 705) demonstrating some of the key criteria for osteoarthritis.

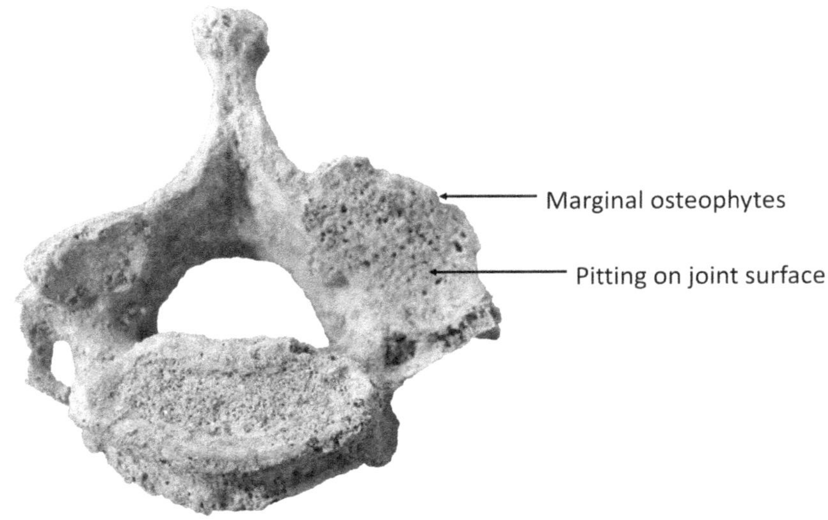

Figure 7.2. Cervical vertebra (Unit 4, Individual 1577) demonstrating some of the key criteria for osteoarthritis on the inferior articular facet joint.

of the palaeoepidemiological approach, for comparing the different groups within the population by time period, sex, tomb type, and cemetery. The significance of the differences between the different groups is determined using 95% confidence intervals and chi-square tests.

7.2.2. Intervertebral disc disease (IVDD)

The operational definition for the presence of IVDD involves pitting on the inferior or superior surface of vertebral bodies and marginal osteophytes (Waldron 2009, 43). Figure 7.3 shows some examples of these features. Like for osteoarthritis, all scoreable vertebral bodies with and without IVDD were recorded. Having counts of both the total numbers of recordable adult vertebrae and vertebrae with IVDD meant that the prevalence of the disease could be obtained. Calculating the prevalence of the disease enables a comparison of the different groups within the population.

7.2.3. Other arthropathies

Schmorl's nodes are recognised as an indentation in the superior or inferior surface of the vertebral bodies, lined with cortical bone (Waldron 2009, 45). These were recorded as prevalences out of the total numbers of adult vertebral bodies counted.

Ankylosing spondylitis is defined as the bilateral fusion of vertebrae at both the vertebral bodies and arches with no

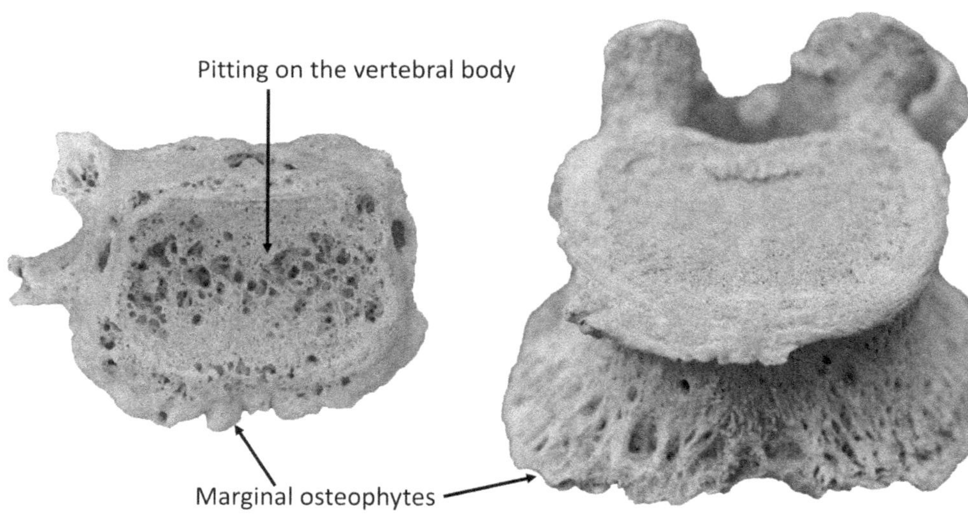

Figure 7.3. Cervical vertebra (Unit 91, Individual 240) and thoracic vertebra (Unit 4, Individual 1666) demonstrating some of the key criteria for IVDD.

Table 7.1. Enthesis sites recorded and the bone on which they can be found.

Enthesis (muscle attachment site)	Bone
Costal impression/tuberosity	Clavicle
Deltoid tuberosity	Humerus
Bicipital tuberosity	Radius
Pronator ridge	Ulna
Ischial tuberosity	Ischium
Gluteal line	Femur
Patellar ligament	Patella
Tibial tuberosity	Tibia
Calcaneal tuberosity	Calcaneus

skip lesions, symmetrical fusion of both sacroiliac joints, and if visible, erosions may occur in the vertebral bodies and peripheral joints (Waldron 2009, 59). In practice, due to the commingled nature of the assemblage it was generally recognised by fully fused vertebrae. DISH is defined as the ossification and fusion of contiguous vertebrae confined to the right side of the vertebral bodies in the thoracic region and ossification into extra spinal entheses and ligaments (Waldron 2009, 77). As there were very few cases of either ankylosing spondylitis or DISH observed in the assemblage, these were reported as incidences rather than prevalences.

7.2.4. Entheseal changes

Entheseal changes are defined as either new bone formation or bone destruction at an enthesis (Jurmain *et al.* 2012, 535). These were recorded as 'absent', 'minor' or 'prominent' at a variety of sites throughout the skeleton. The sites were selected for their tendency to survive relatively intact, ease of recording, and likelihood to produce results related to common activity. Sites were recorded bilaterally at the skeletal sites listed in Table 7.1. Total numbers of these entheses were recorded in order to calculate prevalences of entheseal changes for the different groups within the population by time period, sex, tomb type and cemetery.

7.3. Results

The results section is organised by joint disease (osteoarthritis, intervertebral disc disease, and then other arthropathies), followed by entheseal changes. 'Other arthropathies' includes Schmorl's nodes, ankylosing spondylitis and diffuse idiopathic skeletal hyperostosis (DISH). For the statistical testing of differences between a joint or enthesis having or not having a pathological condition the chi-square test was generally employed, except in cases where the sample size was extremely small and the Fisher's exact test was employed instead or as well as the chi-square test. The inclusion of 95% confidence intervals in the bar charts is also a simple and effective method of determining whether the differences between the prevalences of the diseases were significantly different between the groups being compared.

7.3.1. Osteoarthritis

Osteoarthritis was recorded on 9.5% (831/8703) of all recorded joint surfaces.

7.3.1.1. Time period

Osteoarthritis was recorded on 19.2% (74/385) of joints recorded for Hellenistic individuals, 7.7% (303/3933) of Roman period joint surfaces, and 10.4% (454/4385) of joints from the Late Antique period (Figure 7.4). The differences between the time periods were highly statistically significant (Hellenistic v. Roman: X^2=58.37, p=0.000; Roman v. Late Antique: X^2=17.59, p=0.000), as demonstrated by the non-overlapping confidence intervals in Figure 7.4.

Figure 7.5 presents the prevalence of osteoarthritis by joint or anatomical region of collective joints for each time period.[21] The jaw (temporomandibular joint) has very low levels of osteoarthritis in every time period from 0% (0/36) in the Hellenistic period, to 3% (2/66) in the Roman period, and 3.8% (4/105) in the Late Antique period.

The articular facet joints of the cervical vertebrae (48%) and lumbar vertebrae (38%) for the Hellenistic period show the highest prevalence of osteoarthritis of any joint surfaces and are dramatically higher results than for the same joints in the later time periods, which were 13% for both cervical and lumbar vertebrae from the Roman period and 11% for both cervical and lumbar vertebrae from the Late Antique period. However, the Hellenistic sample sizes were extremely low for both cervical (n=27) and lumbar (n=8) vertebrae compared to over 100 of each type (142 cervical, 108 lumbar) from the Roman period and over 200 of each type (236 cervical, 210 lumbar) for the Late Antique period. The prevalence of osteoarthritis in the thoracic vertebrae was much more similar across all three time periods at 13% in both the Hellenistic (n=16) and Late Antique (n=399) periods and 14% in the Roman period (n=189). However, the sample size for the Hellenistic period is, again, very poor. The prevalence of osteoarthritis is marginally higher for each type of vertebrae in the Roman period compared to the Late Antique. This difference was not statistically significant (X^2=0.34, p=0.56). The only statistically significant differences for comparing all three time periods were between the cervical vertebrae (X^2=27.98, p=0.000), and for all the vertebrae combined (X^2=22.46, p=0.000). The statistically significant differences between the Hellenistic

[21] Appendix D displays tables of raw numbers of joint surfaces recorded and those with osteoarthritis, as well as the percentages and cumulative totals for joint areas. Appendix D can be accessed at https://doi.org/10.30861/9781407360355-AppendixD

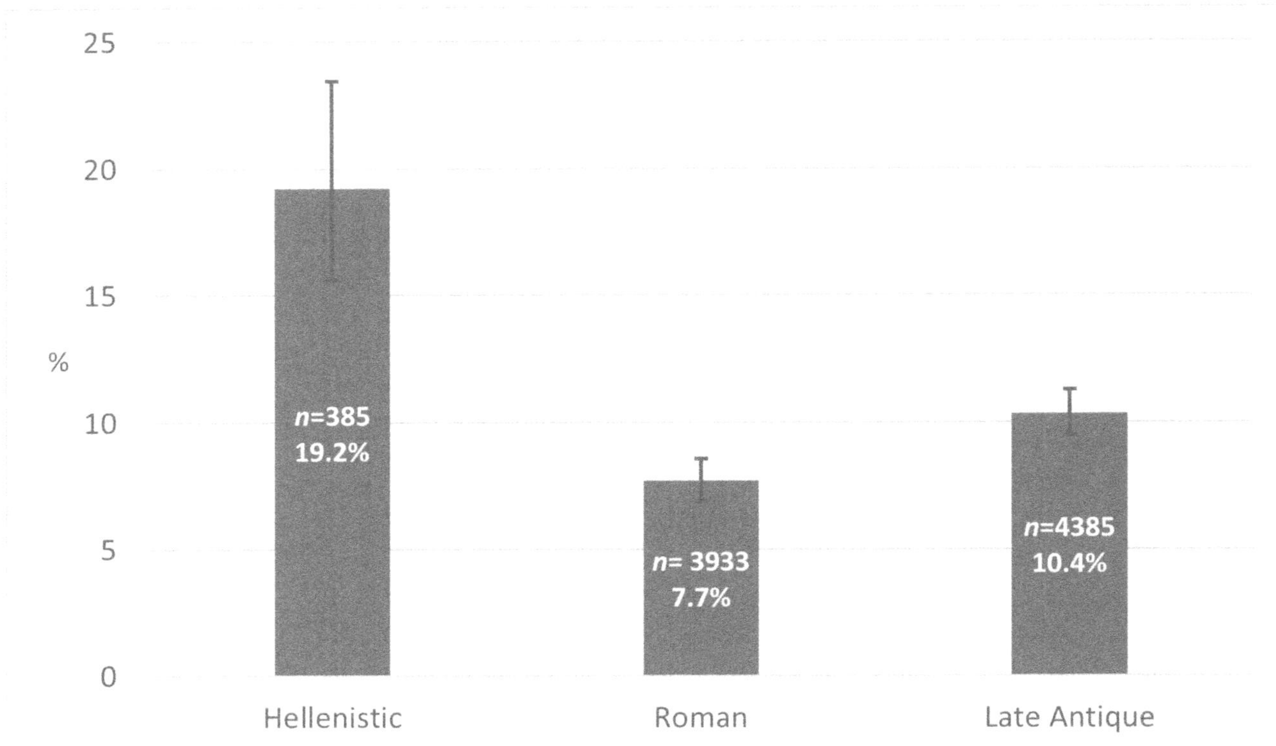

Figure 7.4. Percentage of osteoarthritis present for all joint surfaces combined in each time period with sample sizes (*n*) and 95% confidence interval error bars.

and Roman periods were for the cervical vertebrae (X^2=19.06, p=0.000) and for all the vertebrae combined (X^2=17.0, p=0.000), and between the Hellenistic and Late Antique periods were for the cervical vertebrae (X^2=26.45, p=0.000), lumbar vertebrae (X^2=4.83, p=0.03), and for all the vertebrae combined (X^2=22.36, p=0.000).

Contrary to the results for the vertebrae, the prevalence of osteoarthritis in the shoulder (proximal humerus, glenoid facet of scapula, acromial facet of scapula and distal clavicle) and sternal (manubrium, proximal clavicle) joints was lower in the Hellenistic period than the later periods. However, there were only 11 joints in the shoulder region and 4 in the sternal region recorded (see Appendix D: Table 5 for raw numbers by joint surface). For all the shoulder and sternal joints, there was a slightly higher prevalence of osteoarthritis in the Late Antique period compared to the Roman period, though this was not statistically significantly different, and looking solely at the shoulder region the prevalence of osteoarthritis was higher in the Roman period, while the sternal region showed higher levels of osteoarthritis in the Late Antique period. No differences were statistically significant, either for all three time periods or any two time periods, for the shoulder joints, sternal joints or all of them combined.

The incidence of osteoarthritis in the joints of the upper limb, at the elbow (distal humerus, proximal radius, proximal ulna), wrist (distal radius, distal ulna), and in the hands (proximal and distal metacarpals and phalanges) are all highest in the Hellenistic period and lowest in the Roman period. As with the previously mentioned cases, the sample sizes are by far the smallest in the Hellenistic period for these joints compared to the later time periods (elbow n=16, wrist n=3, metacarpals n=81, phalanges n=66). However, the Hellenistic results are consistently higher and there is a slightly more reliable sample size for the joints of the hands. The difference in the prevalence of osteoarthritis in each set of upper limb joints between the Hellenistic and Roman assemblages is statistically significant (elbow: X^2=5.06, p=0.02, wrist: X^2=5.77, p=0.02, metacarpals: X^2=48.45, p=0.000, phalanges: X^2=16.51, p=0.000), though the confidence intervals for the elbow and wrist are particularly wide for the Hellenistic sample and overlap with the Roman confidence intervals, suggesting these samples were too small to be confident in a significant difference. The difference between elbow or wrist osteoarthritis is not statistically significant for the Roman and Late Antique periods, nor for the Hellenistic period compared to the Late Antique period. The difference between the prevalence of osteoarthritis in the metacarpals and phalanges is statistically significant between the Roman and Late Antique periods (metacarpals: X^2=5.80, p=0.02, phalanges: X^2=5.67, p=0.02), as well as for a comparison of the Hellenistic and Late Antique periods (metacarpals: X^2=21.12, p=0.000, phalanges: X^2=6.52, p=0.01).

Osteoarthritis was recorded in the lower limb for the hips (acetabulum of pelvis, proximal femur), knees (distal femur, proximal tibia, patella), ankles (distal tibia, distal fibula, talus), and feet (proximal and distal metatarsals and phalanges). The joints of the lower limb show the same pattern as for the upper limb, with the highest prevalence of osteoarthritis occurring in the Hellenistic period, except for the ankle (0/28) and metatarsals (0/13) where no examples were recorded, and for each lower limb joint the Roman prevalence of osteoarthritis was the lower than for the Late Antique period (Figure 7.5). The lack of recorded examples of osteoarthritis in Hellenistic ankles or metatarsals may again be due to the small sample sizes, particularly in light of these joints having the lowest prevalence of osteoarthritis in the Roman and Late Antique periods too. For the Roman period osteoarthritis was recorded in 1.3% (3/229) of ankle joint surfaces and 2.6% (14/533) of metatarsals, while for the Late Antique period the prevalence was 3.3% (8/241) for ankles and 3.8% (19/504) for metatarsals. The difference between osteoarthritis prevalence of the lower limb joints was not statistically significant between any of the time periods, other than the significant difference in the osteoarthritis prevalence of the knee between the Hellenistic and Roman periods (X^2=9.27, p=0.002). There were no other statistically significant differences in the occurrence of osteoarthritis in any of the lower limb joints as demonstrated by the overlapping confidence intervals (Figure 7.5).

7.3.1.2. Sex

For the assessment of the difference in osteoarthritis between the sexes, the sample size is severely reduced due to the large numbers of unsexed elements. Osteoarthritis was recorded in 7.6% (31/408) of female joint surfaces and 15.6% (129/827) of male joint surfaces (Figure 7.6). The difference between the osteoarthritis prevalence in females and males was statistically highly significant (X^2=15.51, p=0.000).

Appendix D gives a full listing of numbers of each joint type, both those with osteoarthritis and the total numbers of joint surfaces recorded. Figure 7.7 demonstrates that there was no female osteoarthritis recorded for the cervical vertebrae (0/21), shoulders (0/12), hands (0/65), ankles (0/21) or metatarsals (0/18). This could in part reflect the smaller sample size, but the pattern of osteoarthritis throughout the body indicates differences in activity between males and females. Females had a higher prevalence of osteoarthritis in the jaw (4.8%, 4/83), elbows (16%, 4/25), wrists (20%, 1/5), and hips (16%, 13/79),

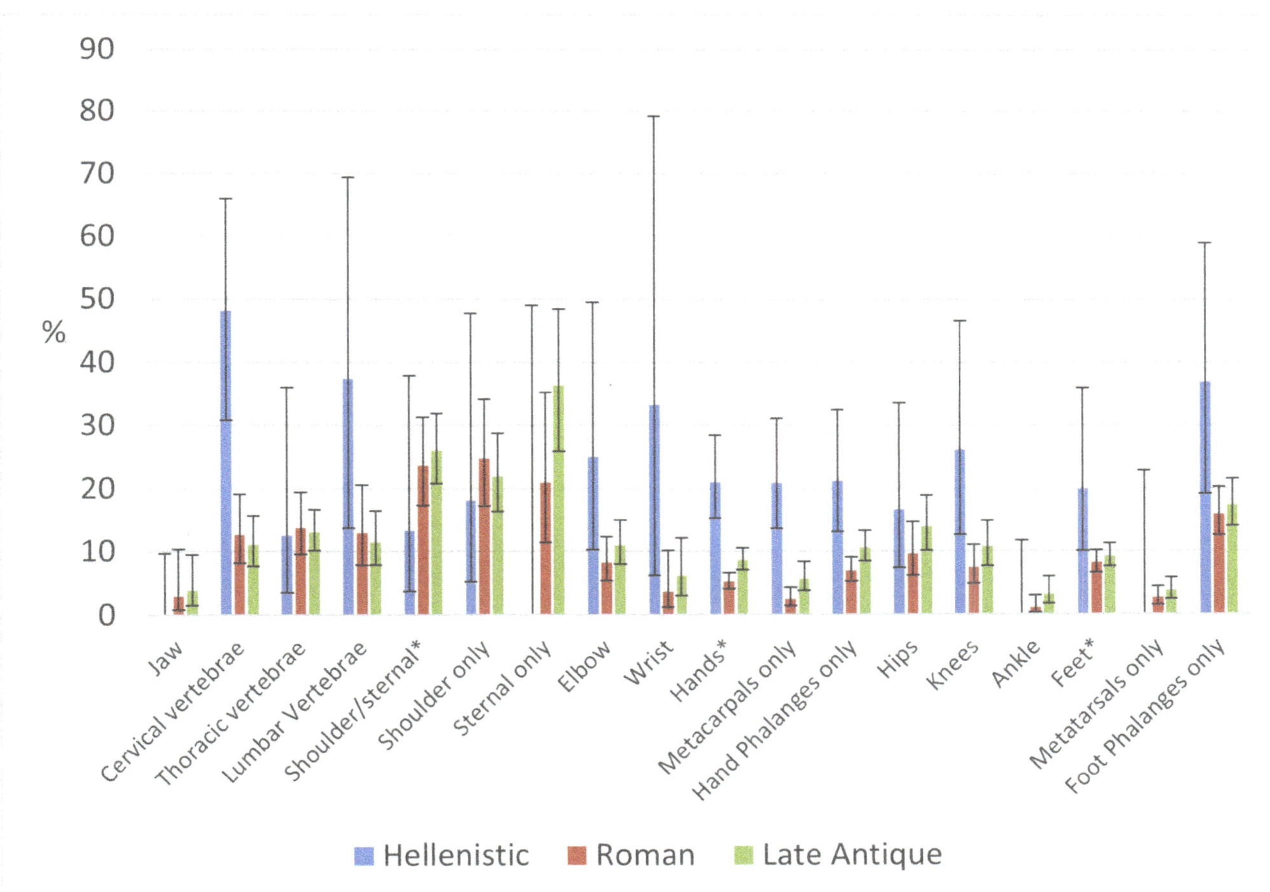

Figure 7.5. Percentage of osteoarthritis present by joint/area of collective joints for each time period with 95% confidence interval error bars. * denotes joint areas which are broken down further into the following two categories in each case, e.g. 'Feet' is a combined result for both the metatarsals and foot phalanges. Sample sizes (*n*) are presented in Table 7.2.

Table 7.2. Counts and prevalence (%) of osteoarthritis present and numbers of joints recorded (*n*) by joint/area of collective joints for each time period.

	Hellenistic			Roman			Late Antique		
	OA	Joints (*n*)	% OA	OA	Joints (*n*)	% OA	OA	Joints (*n*)	% OA
Jaw	0	36	0.0	2	66	3.0	4	105	3.8
Cervical vertebrae	13	27	48.1	18	142	12.7	26	236	11.0
Thoracic vertebrae	2	16	12.5	26	189	13.8	52	399	13.0
Lumbar Vertebrae	3	8	37.5	14	108	13.0	24	210	11.4
Shoulder/sternal*	2	15	13.3	33	140	23.6	61	235	26.0
Shoulder only	2	11	18.2	24	97	24.7	37	169	21.9
Sternal only	0	4	0.0	9	43	20.9	24	66	36.4
Elbow	4	16	25.0	20	244	8.2	33	301	11.0
Wrist	1	3	33.3	3	83	3.6	7	114	6.1
Hands*	31	147	21.1	63	1215	5.2	88	1020	8.6
Metacarpals only	17	81	21.0	12	481	2.5	23	407	5.7
Hand Phalanges only	14	66	21.2	51	734	6.9	65	613	10.6
Hips	5	30	16.7	18	188	9.6	33	237	13.9
Knees	6	23	26.1	21	284	7.4	30	280	10.7
Ankle	0	29	0.0	3	291	1.0	9	282	3.2
Feet*	7	35	20.0	77	939	8.2	87	947	9.2
Metatarsals only	0	13	0.0	14	533	2.6	19	504	3.8
Foot Phalanges only	7	19	36.8	55	345	15.9	67	385	17.4

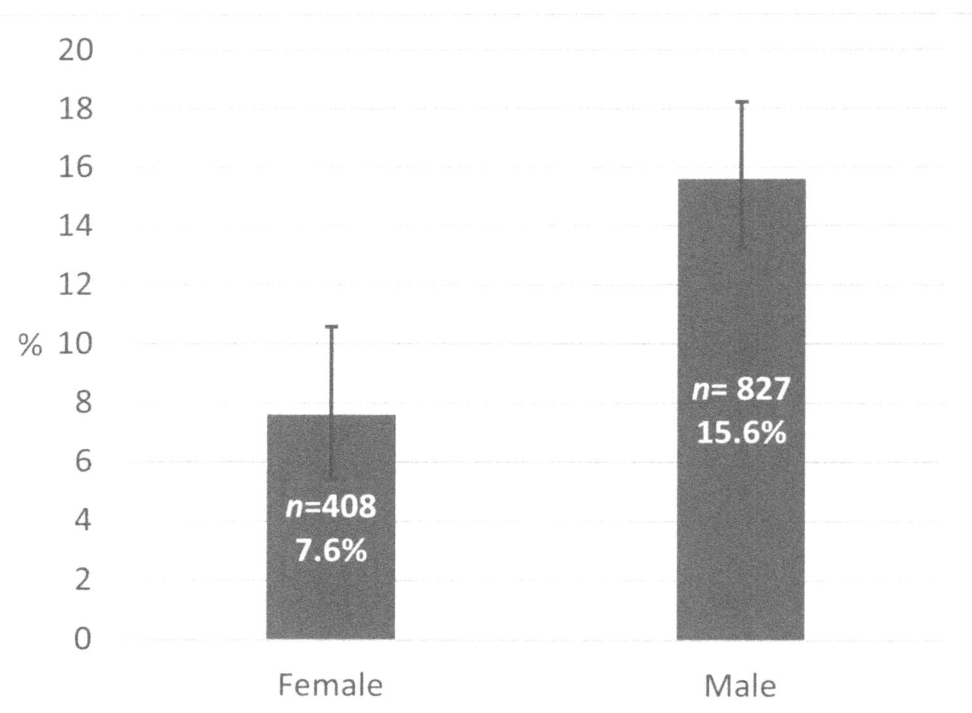

Figure 7.6. Percentage of osteoarthritis present for all joint surfaces combined for both sexes, with sample sizes (*n*) and 95% confidence interval error bars.

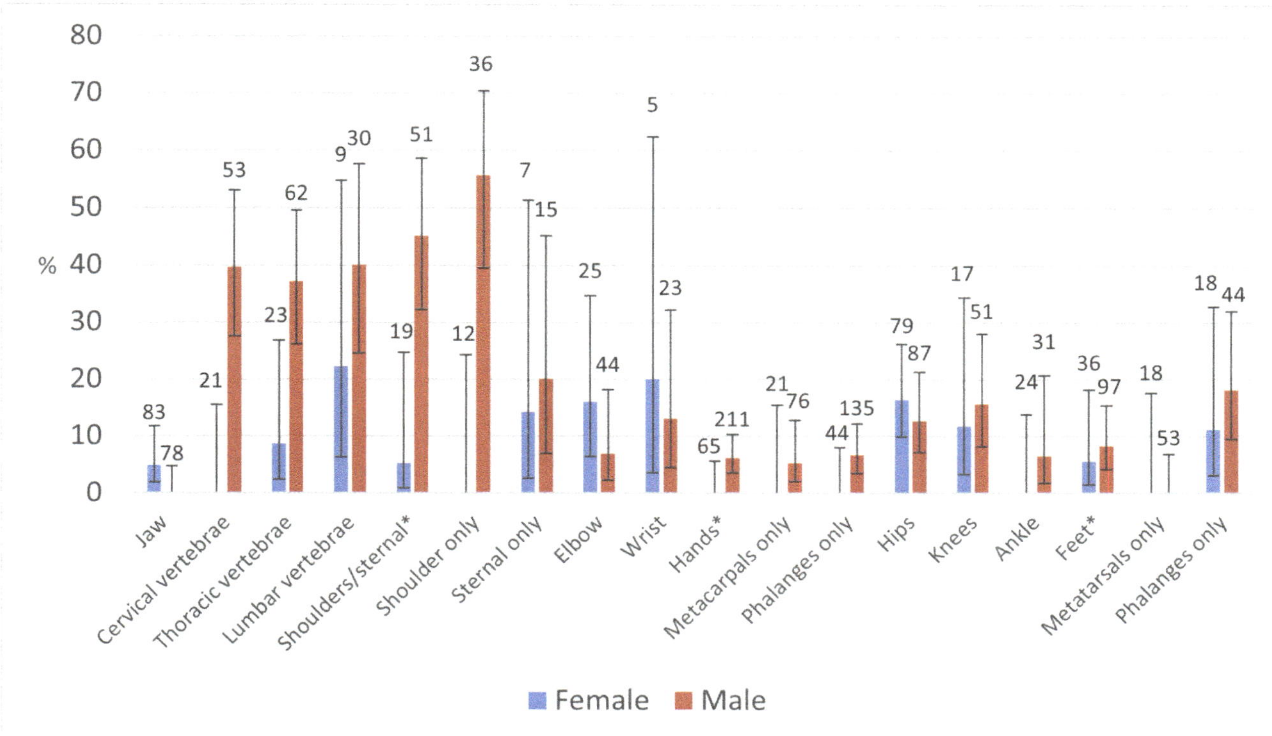

Figure 7.7. Percentage of osteoarthritis present by joint/area of collective joints for males and females with 95% confidence interval error bars and sample sizes (*n*). * denotes joint areas which are broken down further into the following two categories in each case, e.g. 'Hands' is a combined result for both the metacarpals and hand phalanges.

compared to the male jaw (0%, 0/78), elbows (7%, 3/44), wrists (13%, 3/23), and hips (13%, 11/89). These were not, however, statistically significant differences (elbow: X^2=1.47, p=0.22, Fisher's p=0.25, wrist: X^2=0.16, p=0.69, Fisher's p=1, hips: X^2=0.49, p=0.486), as indicated by the substantial overlap of confidence intervals (Figure 7.7).

Males have remarkably higher osteoarthritis levels than females for the cervical vertebrae (40%, 21/53), thoracic vertebrae (37%, 23/62), lumbar vertebrae (40%, 12/30) and shoulders (56%, 20/36). These were statistically highly significant differences in each case, other than for the lumbar vertebrae (X^2=0.95, p=0.33, Fisher's p=0.44): for the cervical vertebrae (X^2=11.62, p=0.001), thoracic vertebrae (X^2=6.52, p=0.01), and shoulders (X^2=11.43, p=0.001). The only other area that produced a statistically significant difference in osteoarthritis for males and females was the hands (X^2=3.95, p=0.047), for which there were no cases amongst the females (0/65), but it occurred in 6% (13/211) of male joints. For the remaining joints, of the sternal area, knees, ankles and feet, the prevalence of osteoarthritis for females and males was not significantly different.

The sample sizes become very small for looking at the sexes by time period. Certain elements are overrepresented in an assessment of joint disease between the sexes in a largely commingled assemblage. Only elements that are in close association with sexable traits of the skull and pelvis appear in the sexed sample, other than for isolated individuals where other elements can be associated with the sexable elements. This occurs for the previous overall assessment of females and males, but the problem is accentuated for the sexes within each time period due to the reduction of the sample size. The Late Antique sample, in particular, which was almost entirely commingled remains, is represented largely by the joints of the skull and pelvis. This is particularly the case for the Late Antique female result which is almost exclusively representative of osteoarthritis of the pelvis. Quite high levels of hip osteoarthritis in females could explain why the overall female prevalence of osteoarthritis (11.5%) appears to be higher than that of the males (7.8%). This is contrary to the Hellenistic and Roman periods, which have a significantly higher prevalence of osteoarthritis amongst the males and are better represented by a range of joints.

Figure 7.8 displays the results for the occurrence of osteoarthritis in females and males within each time period. The difference between the prevalence of osteoarthritis in Hellenistic females (7.2%, 8/111 joint surfaces) and Hellenistic males (24.3%, 28/115) was statistically significant (X^2=12.39, p=0.000). In the Roman period, the males (15%, 70/443) also had a statistically significantly higher prevalence of osteoarthritis (X^2=15.72, p=0.000) than the females (5.0%, 11/218). The Late Antique female (11.5%, 9/78) and male (7.8%, 21/269) difference in results for osteoarthritis was not statistically significant (X^2=1.07, p=0.30) and it is likely that the female result is biased, as previously mentioned.

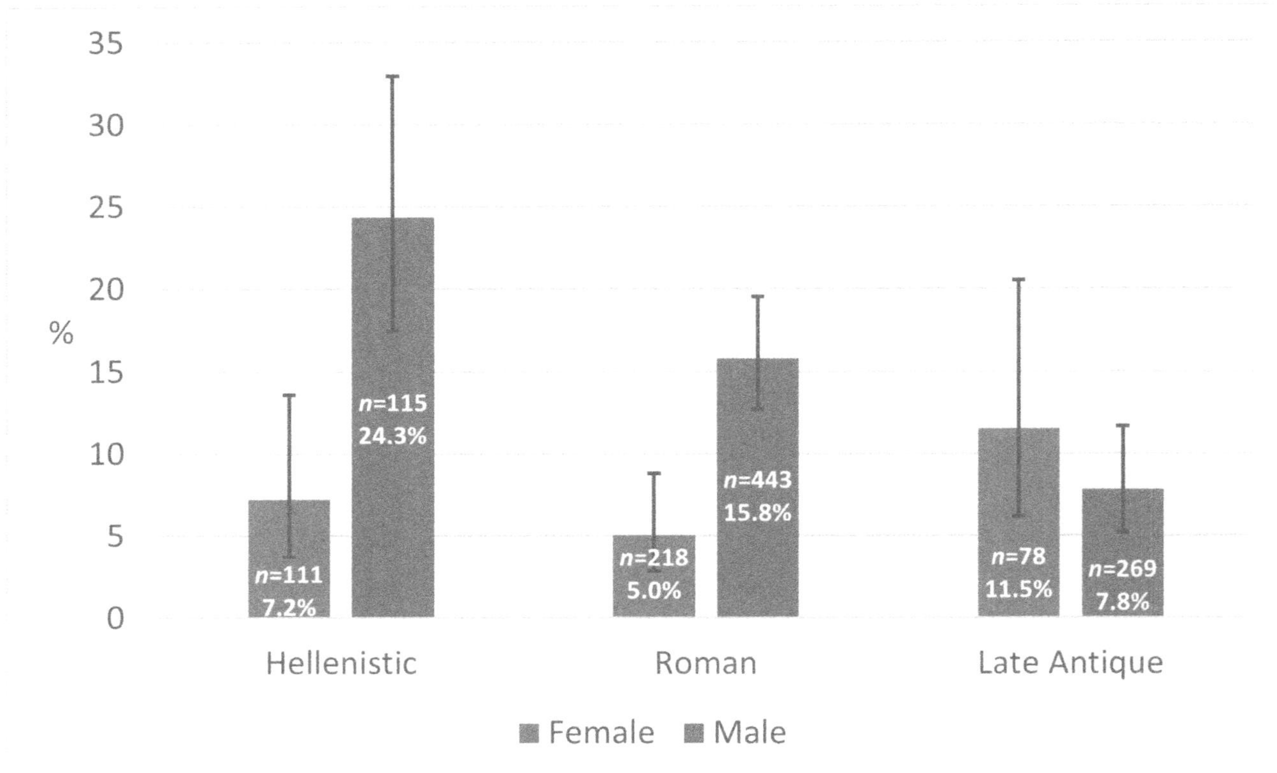

Figure 7.8. Prevalence of osteoarthritis for females and males within each time period, with sample sizes (*n*) and 95% confidence interval error bars.

The male results demonstrate a decline in osteoarthritis over time. The difference in the prevalence of osteoarthritis for the three time periods was statistically significant (X^2=36.02, p=0.000) yet demonstrates a different pattern for the time periods combined (Section 7.3.1.1, Figure 7.4). The prevalence of female osteoarthritis also declines from the Hellenistic to Roman period, which was a statistically significant difference (X^2=31.42, p=0.000). However, there was an increase in osteoarthritis recorded for the Late Antique sample. Although this result is unreliable and likely biased, the difference between this result and the female results for the Hellenistic and Roman osteoarthritis is statistically significant (X^2=31.68, p=0.000).

7.3.1.3. Tomb type

The osteoarthritis results for each tomb type are summarised in Table 7.3 and displayed in Figure 7.9. The lowest prevalence of osteoarthritis was found in the built tombs (3.8%), while the highest prevalence came from the cist graves (15.6%), closely followed by the pit graves (15.1%). The most reliable sample sizes come from the built tombs, chamber tombs and osteothekai, while the tile grave sample size was the smallest. There is no clear pattern of the distribution of osteoarthritis across the tomb types, which have been ordered in terms of perceived complexity but also tend to be indicative of a time period. The more complex tomb forms, the built and chamber tombs of the Early Roman period, the stone-lined tombs of the Late Roman-Late Antique periods and the osteothekai of the Late Antique period, generally have a lower prevalence of osteoarthritis compared to the simpler tomb forms, the cist, tile and pit graves (tile and pit graves largely representing the Hellenistic-Early Roman, the only cist graves being the Late Roman Krevatina grave (Unit 105) and the Late Antique KMF Tomb 309 (Unit 91)). The osteothekai having quite a high prevalence of osteoarthritis and the tile grave prevalence being low are the main anomalies to this vague pattern. The difference between the combined results for the complex tomb types compared to the simpler tomb types was statistically highly significant (X^2=32.38, p=0.000). The difference between all of the tomb types (each as an individual variable) was also highly significant (X^2=118.74, p=0.000). A comparison of the Hellenistic and Early Roman simple tombs (pit vs. tile) proved to have a statistically significant difference in osteoarthritis prevalence (X^2=7.09, p=0.008), as did the comparisons of the other Early Roman tombs (built vs. chamber: X^2=26.62, p=0.000, and built vs. chamber vs. tile: X^2=105, p=0.000). The difference in osteoarthritis prevalence between the Late Roman and Late Antique tomb types also proved to be statistically significant (osteotheke vs. stone-lined vs. cist: X^2=26.61, p=0.000).

A feature of the graphs for the prevalence of osteoarthritis for each joint (Figure 7.10) is that the tomb types with small sample sizes produce quite erratic results, with high and low extreme prevalences. This is particularly notable

Table 7.3. Numbers of joint surfaces with evidence of osteoarthritis, the total numbers of recorded joint surfaces, and the percentage of joint surfaces with osteoarthritis for each tomb type (for all time periods combined).

	Osteoarthritis (OA)	Total joint surfaces (*n*)	% OA
Built	54	1428	3.8
Chamber	144	1750	8.2
Osteotheke	417	3718	11.2
Stone-lined	33	564	5.9
Cist	82	526	15.6
Tile	17	220	7.7
Pit	63	418	15.1

for both the tile and cist grave results. The high number of joints with 0% osteoarthritis within the tile grave sample is likely due to many of the joints having very small sample sizes (see Appendix D for the raw data). The cist results are also a little erratic, though generally high in keeping with the overall highest prevalence of osteoarthritis. Some of the cist results were remarkably high (thoracic and lumbar vertebrae, hips, foot phalanges) while other joints had a remarkably low prevalence of osteoarthritis compared to the other tomb types (cervical vertebrae, hands, knees, ankles, metatarsals). Both the tile and cist graves are represented by a relatively small number of individuals, so particularly high or low results may be heavily influenced by a small number of individuals who were either highly osteoarthritic throughout their joints or entirely free from the condition. However, with a vastly different prevalence of osteoarthritis within closely connected joints, particularly the spine and feet, this suggests that the cist tomb results may also be affected by too small a sample size for the results to be fully reliable.

In keeping with the overall pattern, the joints from the built tomb group tend to have very low frequencies of osteoarthritis, often the lowest in comparison with the other tomb forms. The contemporary chamber tombs have fairly low-to-middling results in comparison to the other tomb form but almost invariably demonstrate a higher prevalence of osteoarthritis than the built tombs, with the exception of the elbow. For the majority of joints the difference in the prevalence of osteoarthritis for the built and chamber tombs was not statistically significant, but for a number of joints or groups of joints there was a statistically significant difference: cervical vertebrae (X^2=5.36, p=0.02, Fisher's p=0.02), hand phalanges (X^2=5.39, p=0.02), ankles (X^2=8.29, p=0.004), metatarsals (X^2=4.78, p=0.03).

The stone-lined tomb results often rival those of the built tombs for having the lowest occurrence of osteoarthritis, though, like the tile grave results, they show a degree of instability, with very high results for the shoulder and knees but most other results being towards the lower end

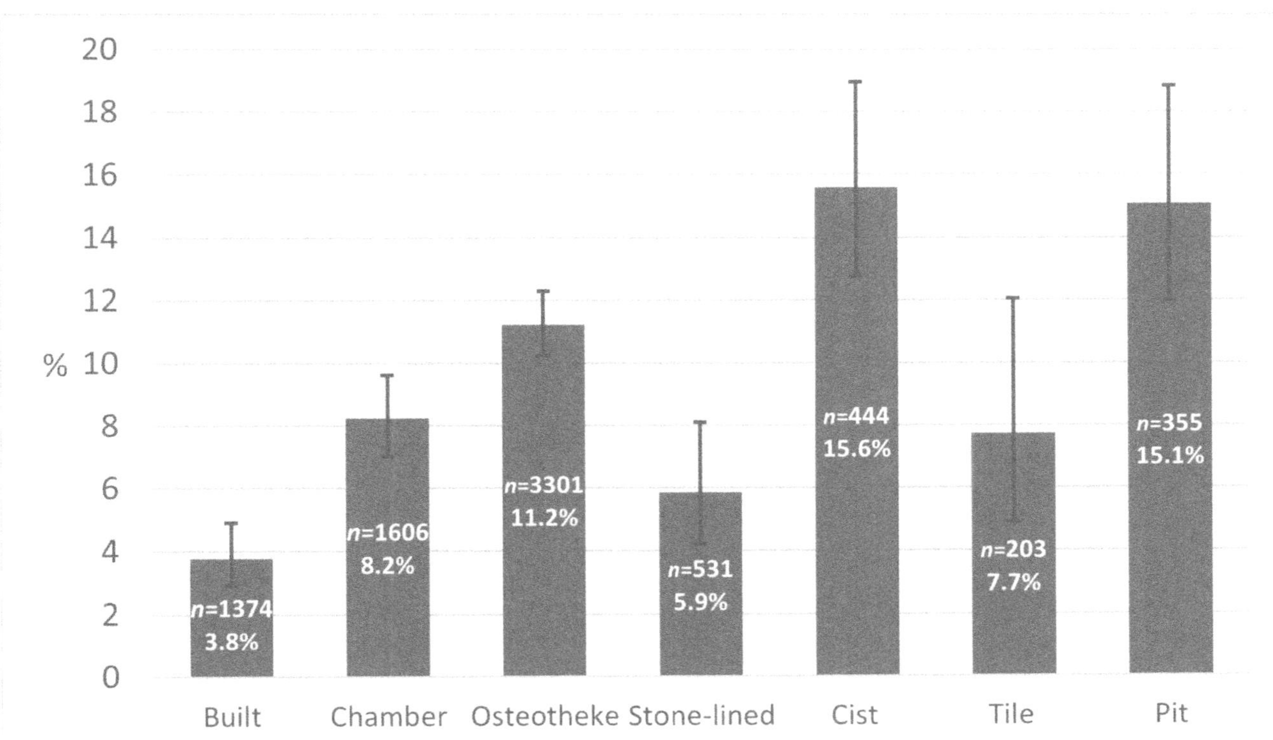

Figure 7.9. Prevalence of osteoarthritis for each tomb type, for all time periods combined, with sample sizes (*n*) and 95% confidence interval error bars.

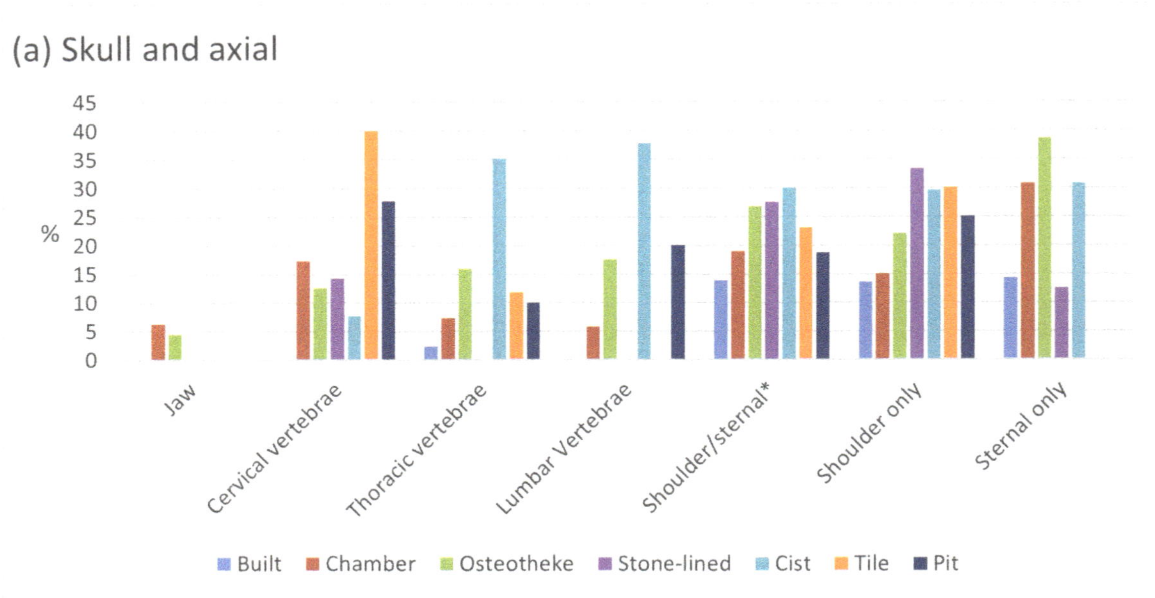

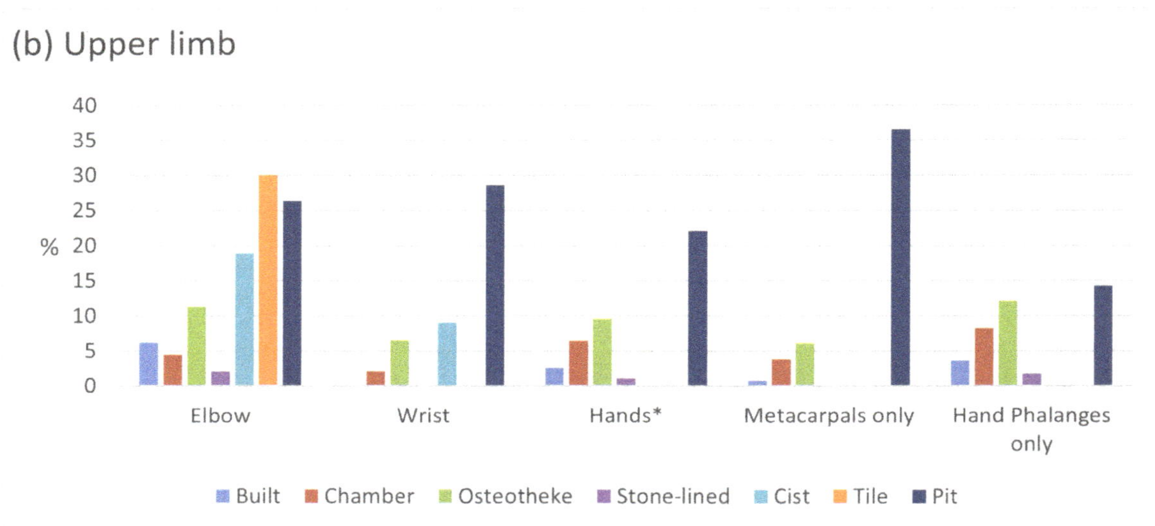

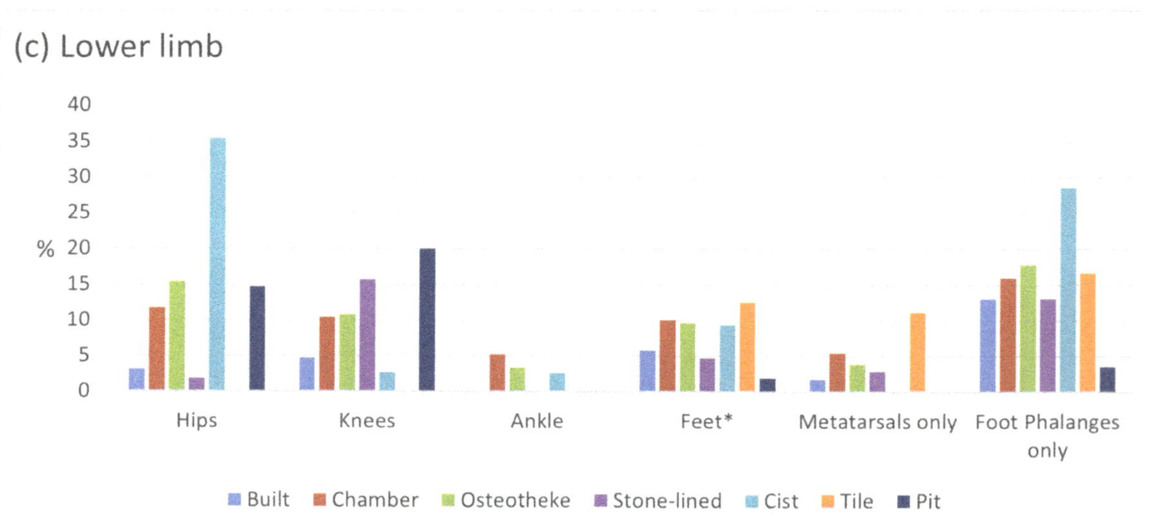

Figure 7.10. Prevalence of osteoarthritis for each joint/joint region by tomb type for (a) the skull and axial skeleton, (b) the upper limb, and (c) the lower limb. * denotes joint areas which are broken down further (into the following two categories in each case).

of the spectrum of osteoarthritis prevalence across the tomb types. The osteoarthritis results for the pit graves are generally high but also demonstrate a degree of instability due to the small sample sizes for many joint categories. The wrist, metacarpals, hand phalanges and knees produced higher levels of osteoarthritis for the pit grave group than for any other tomb type but other joints (sternal region, ankle, metatarsals) produced no evidence for osteoarthritis.

The osteotheke results tend to be middling to high, matching the overall summary result for all the joints combined, in which it had the third highest prevalence of the tomb types. In a comparison with the stone-lined tombs (despite the problems mentioned above regarding sample size), which are closest to the osteothekai temporally and in terms of construction, several joints proved to have a statistically significant difference in osteoarthritis prevalence: the thoracic vertebrae (X^2=3.92, p=0.048), lumbar vertebrae (X^2=4.97, p=0.03), elbows (X^2=3.98, p=0.046), hand phalanges (X^2=5.71, p=0.02), and hips (X^2=6.95, p=0.01). In each of these cases, and in fact for all joints other than the knees (an insignificant difference), the osteothekai had a higher prevalence of osteoarthritis.

7.3.1.4. Cemetery (location)

Due to the larger sample size for joint surfaces than for elements in the other analyses (dental disease etc.), a more detailed breakdown of the cemeteries by time period could be carried out. Table 7.4 demonstrates the differences in sample size between the different cemeteries and the overall prevalence of osteoarthritis in each. The Spilia cemetery (a single Roman rock-cut chamber tomb) does not feature at all, as no joint surfaces survived for recording, with this tomb being largely represented by teeth.

The results for osteoarthritis prevalence are also displayed in Figure 7.11 and demonstrate that the Hellenistic North Cemetery and Late Roman Krevatina tomb had the highest prevalence of osteoarthritis (both 18.6%), while the Roman built tomb at Topana (2.6%) had the lowest levels of osteoarthritis. The Roman Sanatorium cemetery (n=84, represented by only one tomb: KSM/61 GEOM T.1, Unit 93), and the Late Antique Monastiriako Kephali 'cemetery' (n=103, represented by only the KOP/79 single burial, Unit 108) had particularly low sample sizes. The Roman Topana tomb (n=230, MK/61 T.1, Unit 104), Late Roman Krevatina tomb (n=290, Unit 105), Hellenistic North Cemetery (n=322, represented by 55 tombs) and Roman North Cemetery (n=430, represented by 10 tombs, though predominantly by the built tombs, T.33 [Unit 68] and T.58 [Unit 71]) also had fairly low sample sizes. The most reliable sample sizes came from the Late Antique North Cemetery (n=4182), the Roman Monastiriako Kephali cemetery of rock-cut tombs (n=1658), and the Late Roman Sanatorium Basilica cemetery (n=1256).

Table 7.4. Numbers of joint surfaces with evidence of osteoarthritis, the total numbers of recorded joint surfaces, and the percentage of joint surfaces with osteoarthritis for each cemetery in each time period.

	Osteoarthritis (OA)	Total joint surfaces (n)	%
Hellenistic North Cemetery	60	322	18.6
Roman North Cemetery	27	430	6.3
Roman Monastiriako Kephali	140	1658	8.4
Roman Topana	6	230	2.6
Roman Sanatorium	6	84	7.1
Late Roman Krevatina	54	290	18.6
Late Roman Sanatorium	64	1256	5.1
Late Antique North Cemetery	449	4182	10.7
Late Antique Monastiriako Kephali	4	103	3.9

As the KOP/79 tomb (Late Antique Monastiriako Kephali) represents only one individual, there is little value in comparing it to the likely-contemporary Late Antique North cemetery. The KOP/79 individual had osteoarthritis in 3.9% of his joints (although he was in the Young Adult category), while the prevalence of osteoarthritis in the Late Antique North Cemetery was 10.7% of joint surfaces. This was the highest result after the 18.6% prevalence for both the Hellenistic North Cemetery and the Late Roman Krevatina grave, and with the largest sample size, is the most reliable result.

Besides the Late Antique Monastiriako Kephali result (3.9%), the lowest results for osteoarthritis prevalence came from the Roman Topana tomb (2.6%), the Late Roman Sanatorium cemetery (5.1%) and the Roman North Cemetery (6.3%). These are a mixture of Early-Middle Roman (Topana and North Cemetery) and Late Roman (Sanatorium) but are all found to the north of the settlement and represent cemeteries largely of substantial built or stone-lined tombs.

The remaining, middling results for osteoarthritis by joint, from the two cemeteries not yet mentioned, were 7.1% in the Roman Sanatorium KSM/61 rock-cut chamber tomb, and 8.4% in the Roman Monastiriako Kephali rock-cut chamber tomb cemetery. There was, however, a statistically significant difference (X^2=9.71, p=0.008)

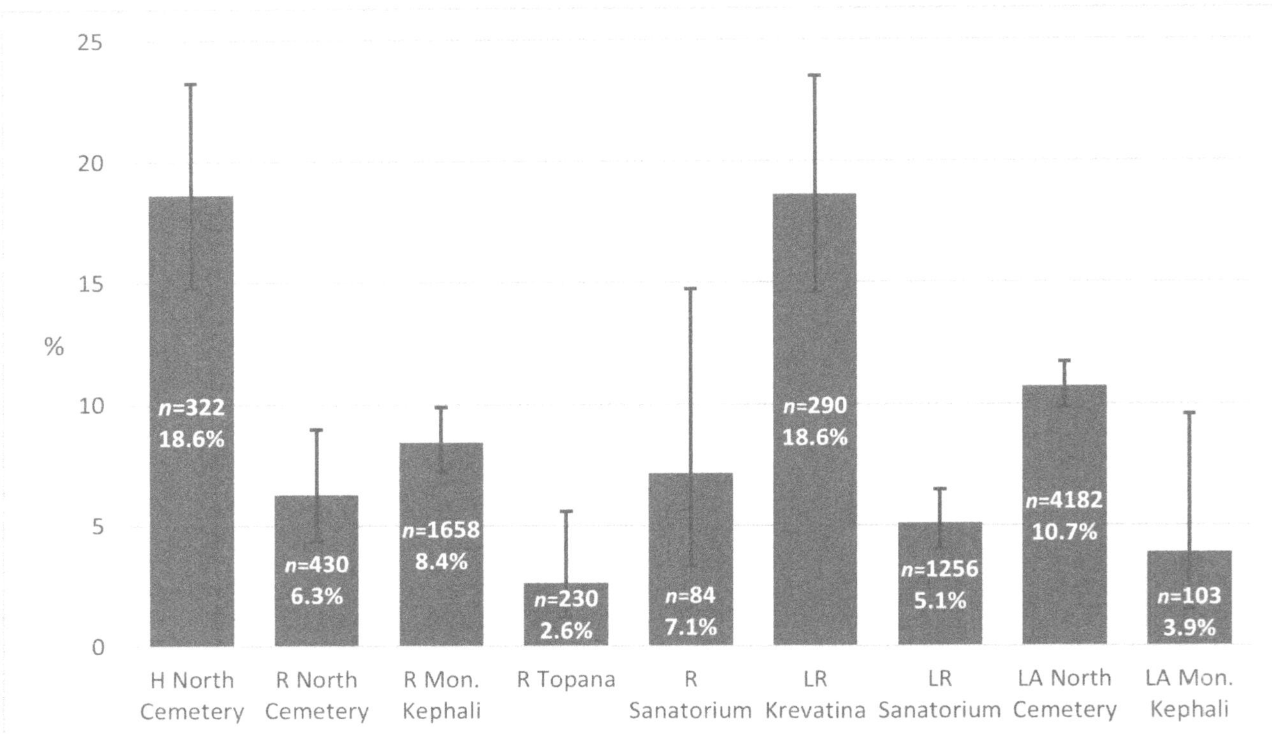

Figure 7.11. Prevalence of osteoarthritis for each cemetery in each time period with sample sizes (*n*) and 95% confidence interval error bars.

between these likely-contemporary chamber tombs, though the KSM/61 tomb is located to the north of the settlement while the Monastiriako Kephali tombs are to the south of the settlement.

A comparison of osteoarthritis prevalence of the Hellenistic and Roman periods in the North Cemetery proved to be statistically significantly different (X^2=27.47, p=0.000). Within the Roman period (1st-2nd centuries), the prevalence of osteoarthritis between the cemeteries (three to the north and one to the south) was significantly different (X^2=11.06, p=0.01). For a comparison of each pair of cemeteries the results were significantly different, other than a comparison of the Topana and Sanatorium cemeteries, both to the north of the settlement (X^2=3.44, p=0.06) which, perhaps due to the smaller sample sizes, could not be deemed significantly different, and for the North Cemetery and Monastiriako Kephali cemetery (X^2=2.17, p=0.14). The Late Roman (3rd-4th centuries) cemeteries at Krevatina and the Sanatorium had significantly different osteoarthritis results (X^2=61.13, p=0.000), with the southern Krevatina result higher than the northern Sanatorium result. The Late Antique North Cemetery and Monastiriako Kephali KOP/79 tomb produced a statistically significant difference in osteoarthritis (X^2=4.99, p=0.03), though not highly significant, with the North Cemetery having the higher prevalence of the condition. A comparison of the Late Roman Sanatorium cemetery and Late Antique North Cemetery produced a more highly significant difference (X^2=35.98, p=0.000). Both were to the north of the settlement, but the later cemetery produced the higher prevalence of osteoarthritis.

Figure 7.12 displays the results by joint or group of joints for each cemetery. The lowest three sample sizes were excluded due to the samples becoming so small for each joint as to be meaningless, though the raw numbers for the Roman Topana, Roman Sanatorium and Late Antique Monastiriako Kephali cemeteries can be found alongside the others in Appendix D. The Late Roman Krevatina cemetery was the next lowest sample size and its results for osteoarthritis by joint do appear quite erratic (with many of the highest results for some joints and many having a 0% prevalence), though these results come from only four individuals. The same is true of the Hellenistic North Cemetery results by joint (the next smallest sample size), though a large number of individuals are represented by this small sample (i.e. often an individual will be represented by only a single joint surface). These two cemeteries had the highest overall prevalence of osteoarthritis.

In the overall results the southerly Roman Monastiriako Kephali cemetery (8.4%) had a higher prevalence of osteoarthritis than the Roman North Cemetery (6.3%), though this was not a statistically significant difference. For the thoracic vertebrae, shoulder, and elbow joints, however, the North cemetery had the higher prevalence, and the results for the sternal and feet joints are very close to being the same. This supports the lack of significant difference between the osteoarthritis prevalence. However, for an overall discussion of the combined results for

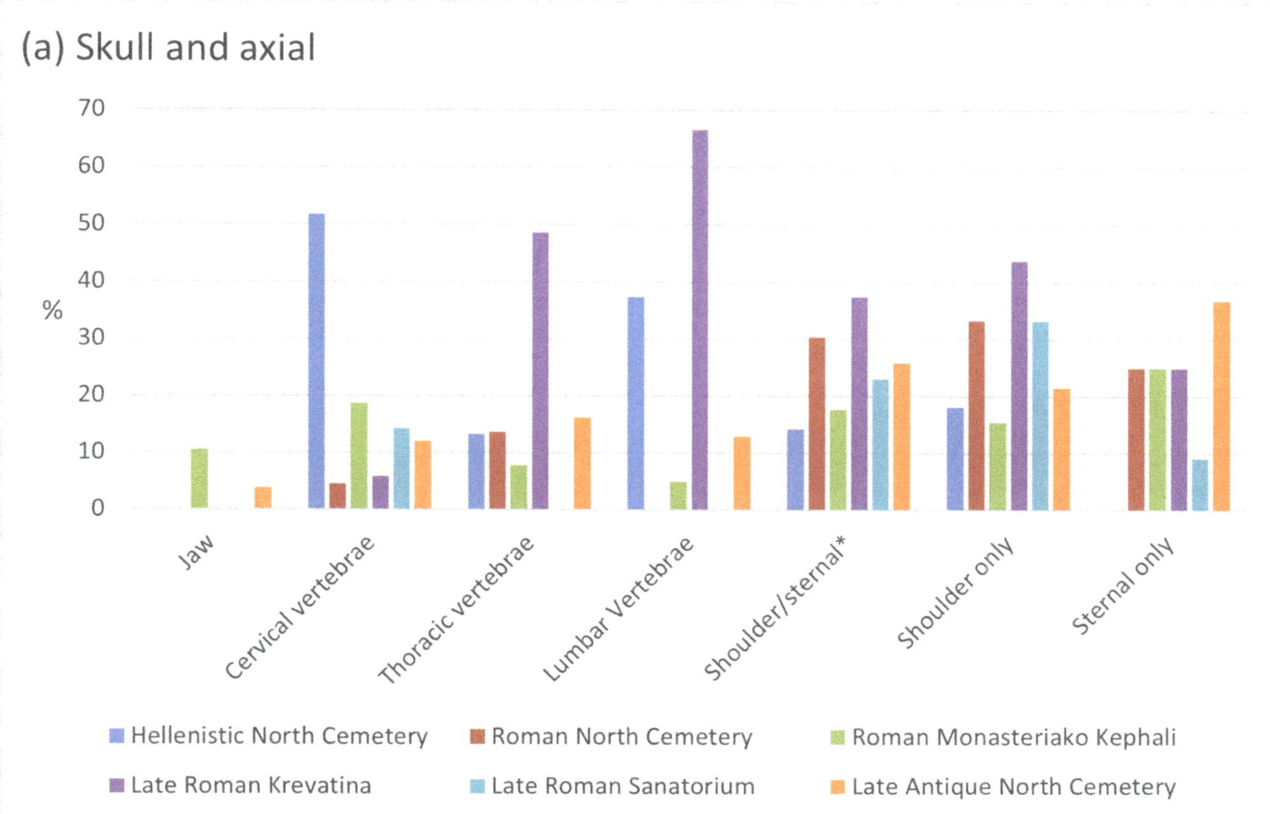

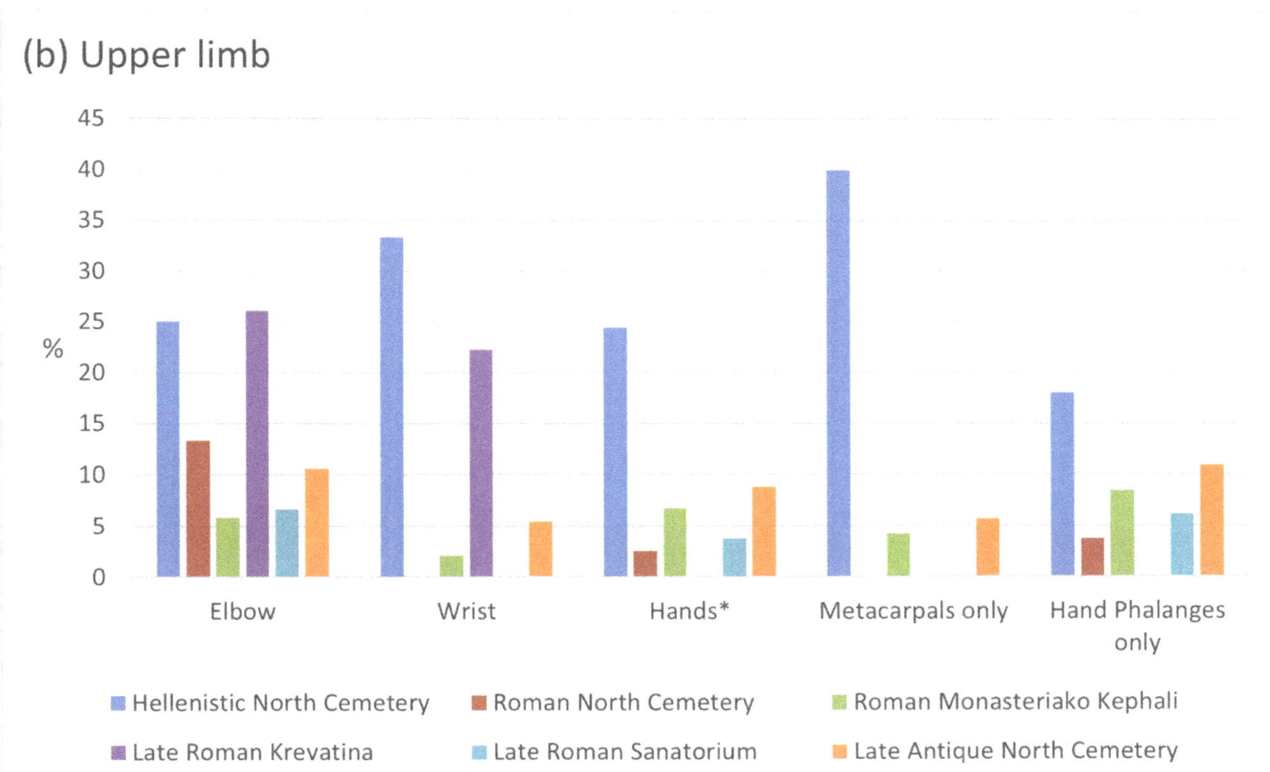

Figure 7.12. Prevalence of osteoarthritis for each joint/joint region by cemetery for (a) the skull and axial skeleton, (b) the upper limb, and (c) the lower limb. * denotes joint areas which are broken down further (into the following two categories in each case).

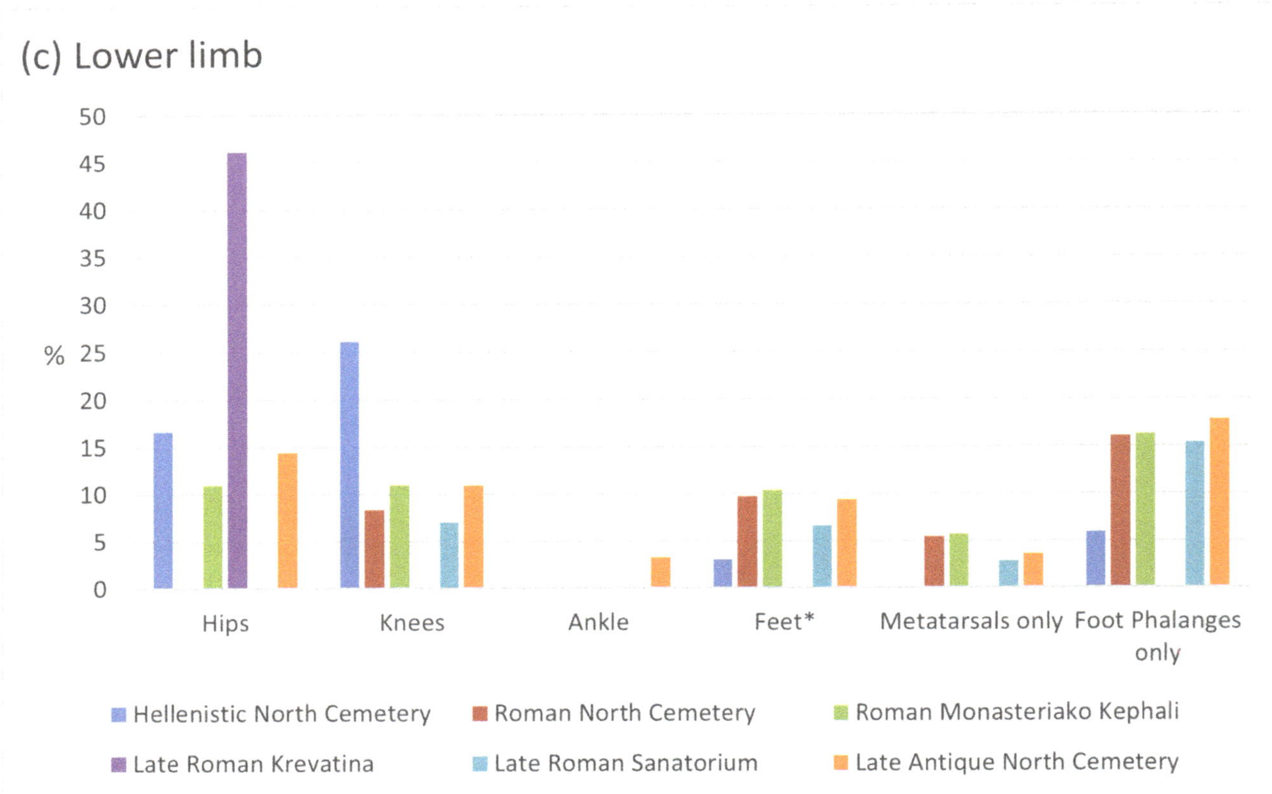

Figure 7.12. (*Continued*)

cemeteries from the north and south of the settlement, see the discussion below in association with Figure 7.13.

A comparison of the overall osteoarthritis results for the Late Roman Sanatorium (5.1%) and Late Antique North Cemetery (10.7%) produced a significantly higher result for the North Cemetery. The cervical vertebrae and shoulder joints were the only incidences for which the Sanatorium cemetery had a higher prevalence of osteoarthritis.

Figure 7.13 shows the combined results from the cemeteries to the north and south of the settlement for different date ranges within the Roman and Late Antique periods (no comparison was possible for the Hellenistic period). For the 1st–2nd centuries, the North result was represented by the Roman North Cemetery, Roman Topana and Roman Sanatorium cemeteries, and the South result by only the Roman Monastiriako Kephali cemetery. The 1st–4th centuries were represented by the above, with the addition of the Late Roman Sanatorium cemetery results for the North and the Late Roman Krevatina results for the South. For the 3rd-7th centuries, the North was represented by the Late Roman Sanatorium cemetery and Late Antique North Cemetery, while the South was represented by a much smaller sample, combining the Late Roman Krevatina and Late Antique Monastiriako Kephali graves. There appears to both be a clear pattern of increased osteoarthritis over time and a higher prevalence amongst the southerly burials compared to those of the north. The differences in osteoarthritis prevalence between the three date ranges for both the north (X^2=50.86, p=0.000) and south (X^2=56.75, p=0.000) were statistically significant, as were the differences within each date range between the north and south burials (1st–2nd C. X^2=7.63, p=0.006; 1st–4th C. X^2=32.8, p=0.000; 3rd–7th C. X^2=11.76, p=0.001).

7.3.2. Intervertebral disc disease

Intervertebral disc disease (IVDD) was recorded in 50.3% of scorable vertebrae. A total of 1364 vertebral bodies (excluding the C1, including the sacrum) were recorded for IVDD.

7.3.2.1. Time period

Figure 7.14 shows the prevalence of IVDD by time period. Similar to osteoarthritis, from the Hellenistic period (50%, 30/60) to the Roman period (44.7%, 238/532) the prevalence of IVDD decreases, and then increases in the Late Antique period (54.1%, 418/772). However, the difference is smaller than for osteoarthritis, and in the case of IVDD, the Late Antique has a higher prevalence than the Hellenistic (which was the other way around for osteoarthritis). The Hellenistic period is, however, represented by a very small sample size for the number of individuals that it represents (adult MNI=70, each with 24 vertebrae would give a potential sample size of 1680 vertebrae). Figure 7.15, which shows the prevalence of IVDD by vertebral region, demonstrates that the Hellenistic results are higher than the Late Antique for

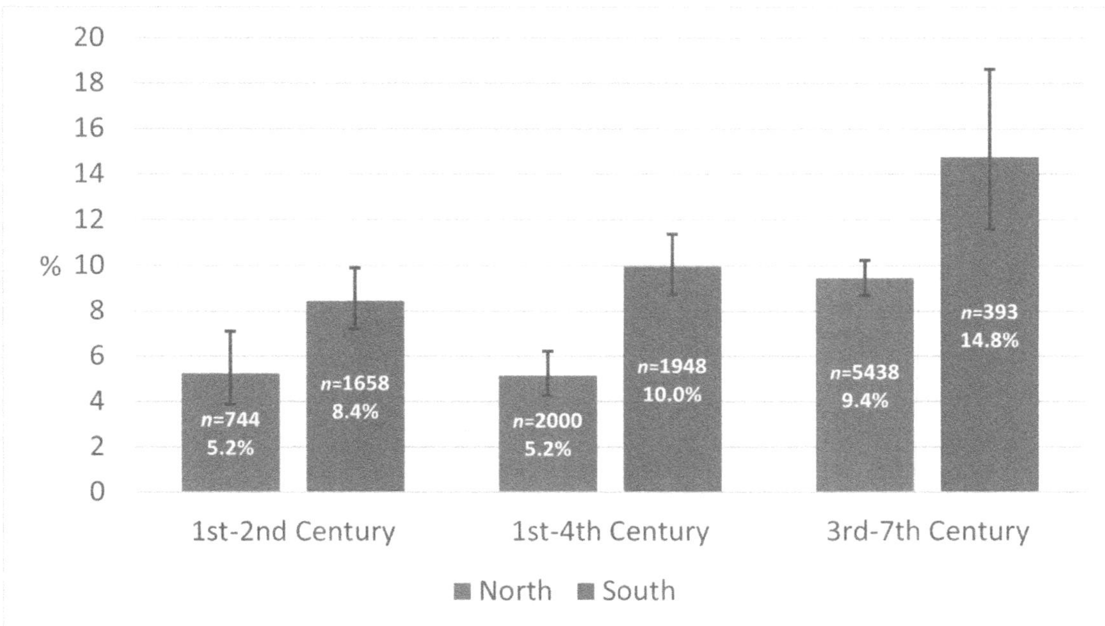

Figure 7.13. Prevalence of osteoarthritis for the cemeteries to the north and south of the settlement for Roman and Late Antique date ranges, with sample sizes (*n*) and 95% confidence interval error bars.

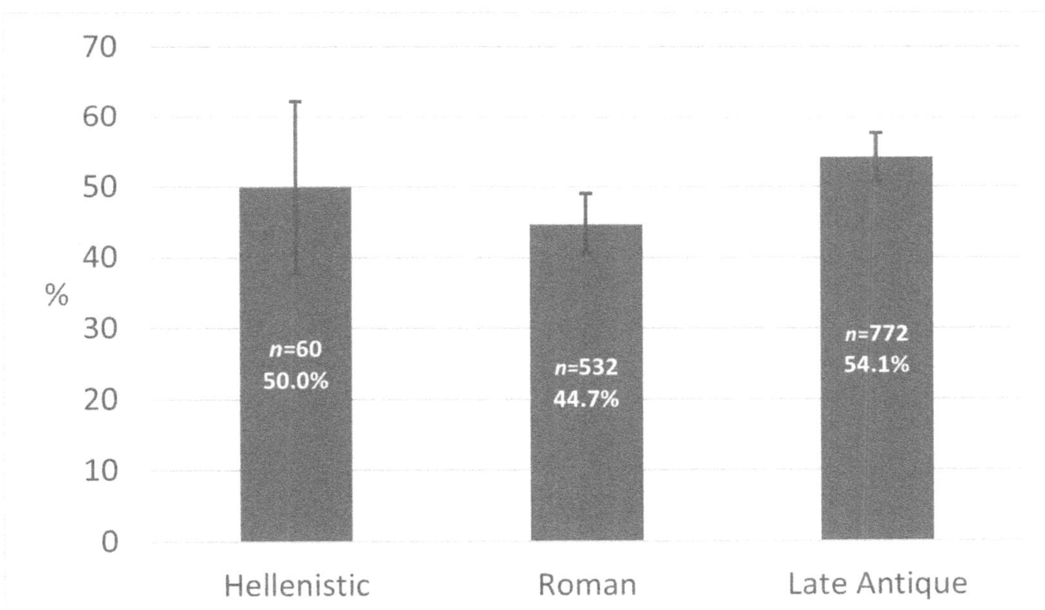

Figure 7.14. Prevalence of intervertebral disc disease (IVDD) for each time period with sample sizes (*n*) and 95% confidence interval error bars.

both the thoracic and lumbar vertebrae. The confidence interval error bars (Figure 7.14) suggest no significant difference between the Hellenistic period and either of the later periods, though the difference between the Roman and Late Antique periods is a significant difference, as the 95% confidence intervals do not overlap. For each vertebral region, the Roman result was the lowest, supporting the overall lowest prevalence for this time period.

7.3.2.2. Sex

Figure 7.16 shows the prevalence of IVDD for females (31.0%, 18/58) and males (69.0%, 98/142), and demonstrates a significantly higher result for the males. These are small sample sizes as only 200 vertebrae could be assigned a sex out of the total 1364 recorded. Though the sample sizes for each vertebral region are even smaller,

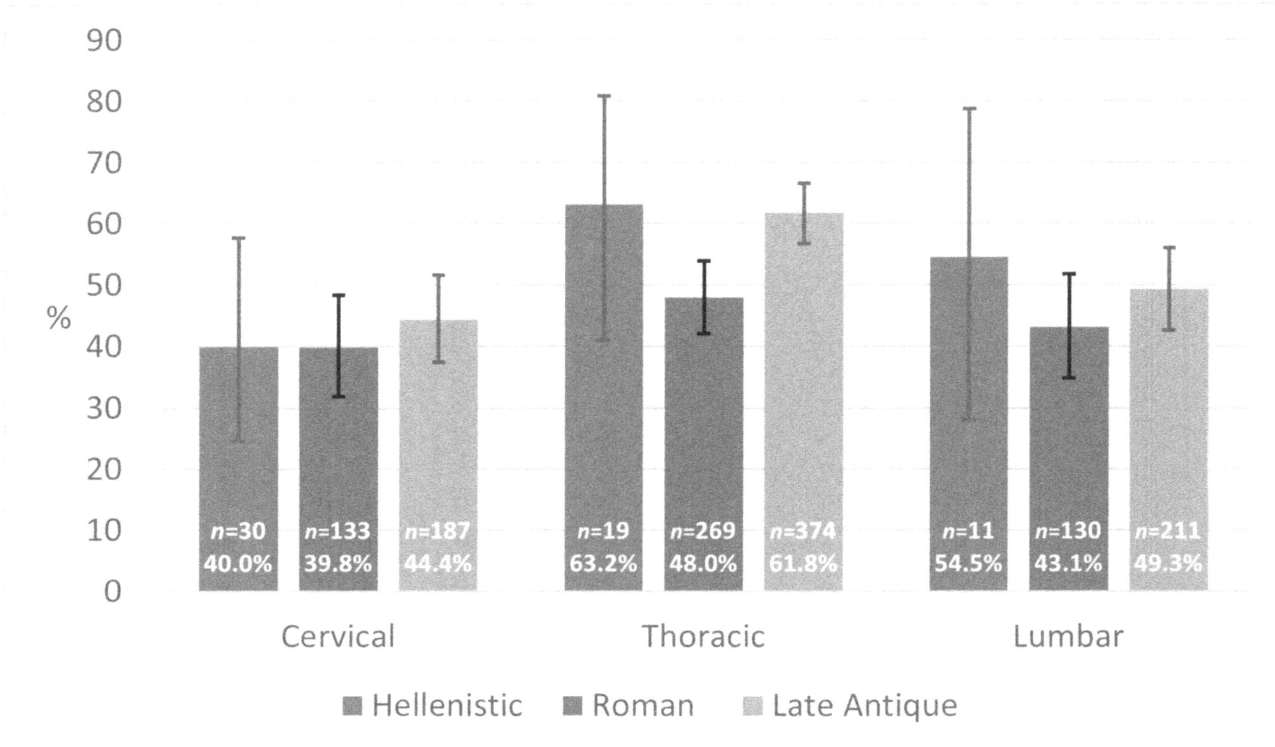

Figure 7.15. Prevalence of intervertebral disc disease (IVDD) for the cervical, thoracic and lumbar regions of the spine in each time period with sample sizes (*n*) and 95% confidence interval error bars.

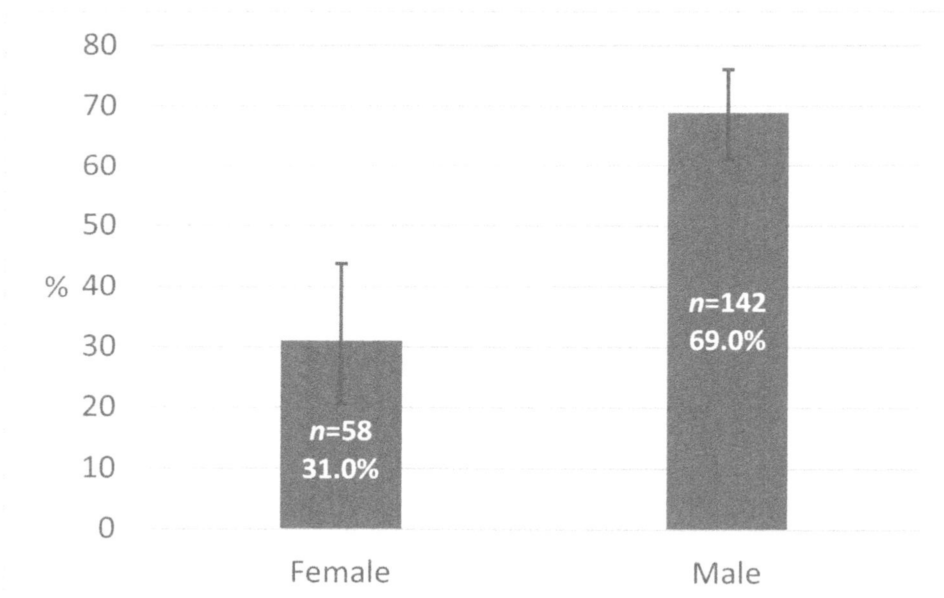

Figure 7.16. Prevalence of intervertebral disc disease (IVDD) for females and males with sample sizes (*n*) and 95% confidence interval error bars.

the pattern of males having higher IVDD than females is supported by the results displayed in Figure 7.17. Males also had higher osteoarthritis of the vertebral articular facets for all vertebral regions compared to females (Section 7.3.1.2). The sample size was too small to look at the difference in IVDD between the sexes within each time period.

7.3.2.3. Tomb type

The prevalence of IVDD for each tomb type for all time periods is displayed in Table 7.5 and Figure 7.18. The highest prevalence of IVDD came from the tile graves (64.9%) and the lowest from the built tombs (35.7%). There is some indication of lower disc disease in the more

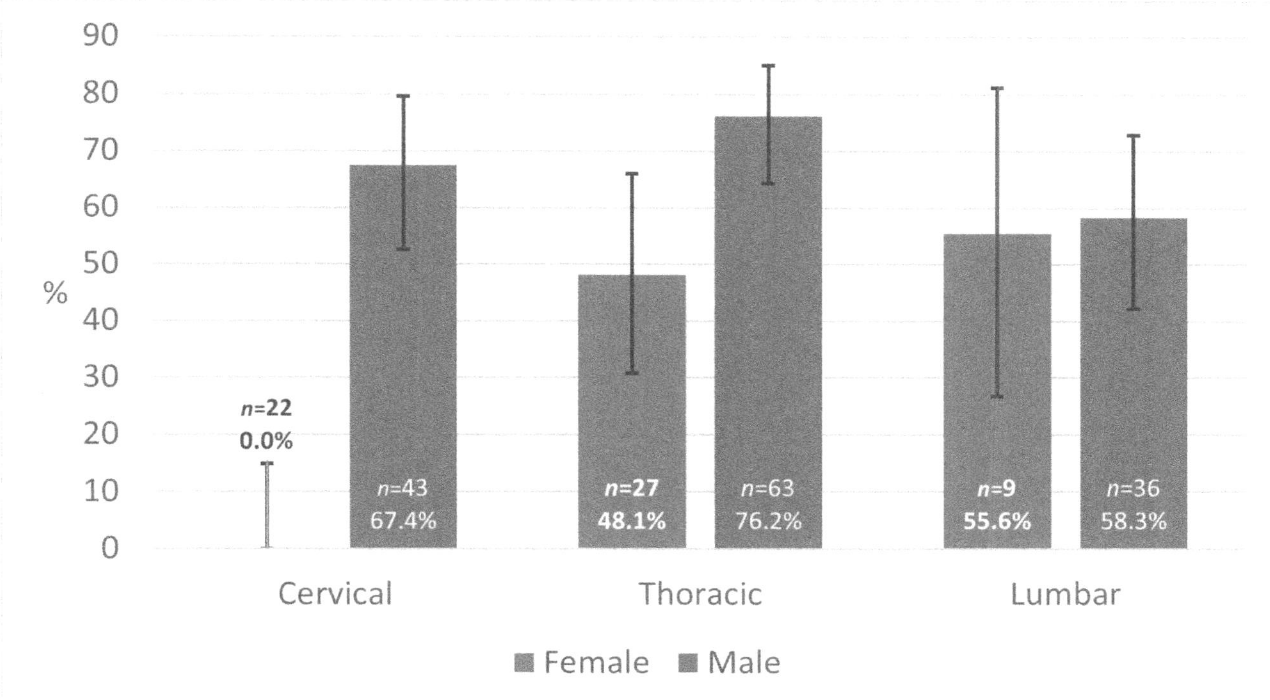

Figure 7.17. Prevalence of intervertebral disc disease (IVDD) for each region of the spine, for the sexes with sample sizes (*n*) and 95% confidence interval error bars.

Table 7.5. Numbers of vertebral bodies displaying intervertebral disc disease (IVDD), total numbers of vertebral bodies recorded, and the percentage of vertebral bodies with IVDD.

	IVDD	Total vertebrae (*n*)	%
Built	35	98	35.7
Chamber	134	301	44.5
Osteotheke	325	619	52.5
Stone-lined	52	104	50.0
Cist	81	140	57.9
Tile	24	37	64.9
Pit	30	59	50.8

complex tombs (Built, Chamber, Stone-lined) and a higher incidence of IVDD for the cist and tile grave groups, but the pit graves (50.8%), as the simplest tomb type, are the main exception to the pattern with a fairly low prevalence of IVDD. The built tombs have the lowest IVDD result, though the confidence intervals suggest that there was no significant difference between this result and those of the chamber, stone-lined and pit groups. The p values from the chi-square statistical tests are summarised in Table 7.6 and demonstrate the statistically significant differences, though the 95% confidence interval error bars in Figure 7.18 are less optimistic in assigning these differences as being meaningful as the majority of tomb type prevalences have overlapping confidence intervals.

An assessment of IVDD for each region of the spine (cervical, thoracic and lumbar) shows a similar pattern of increasing disc disease with decreasing tomb complexity (Figure 7.19). The tombs with the smaller sample sizes have more dramatically different results for different parts of the spine due to the small sample size. Slightly different patterns do emerge amongst the tomb types, though these could also be sample size bias.[22] In most cases the thoracic vertebrae have the highest prevalence of IVDD but for the built tomb sample the lumbar vertebrae (39.4%) have the highest rates of IVDD. For the stone-lined tombs the cervical vertebrae (62.5%) have the highest occurrence of IVDD, though the result is only just ahead of that of the thoracic vertebrae, and for the osteothekai the thoracic and lumbar regions of the spine have almost identical rates of IVDD with the thoracic vertebrae only marginally higher.

7.3.2.4. Cemetery (location)

Table 7.7 and Figure 7.20 present the numbers and percentages of vertebrae with IVDD for each cemetery location within each time period. The Roman Sanatorium and Late Antique Monastiriako Kephali samples had extremely small sample sizes and the Monastiriako Kephali sample was represented by only one individual. The results for these samples are unrepresentative of the

[22] As with all the results for this chapter, the full tables of raw numbers and percentages can be found in Appendix D.

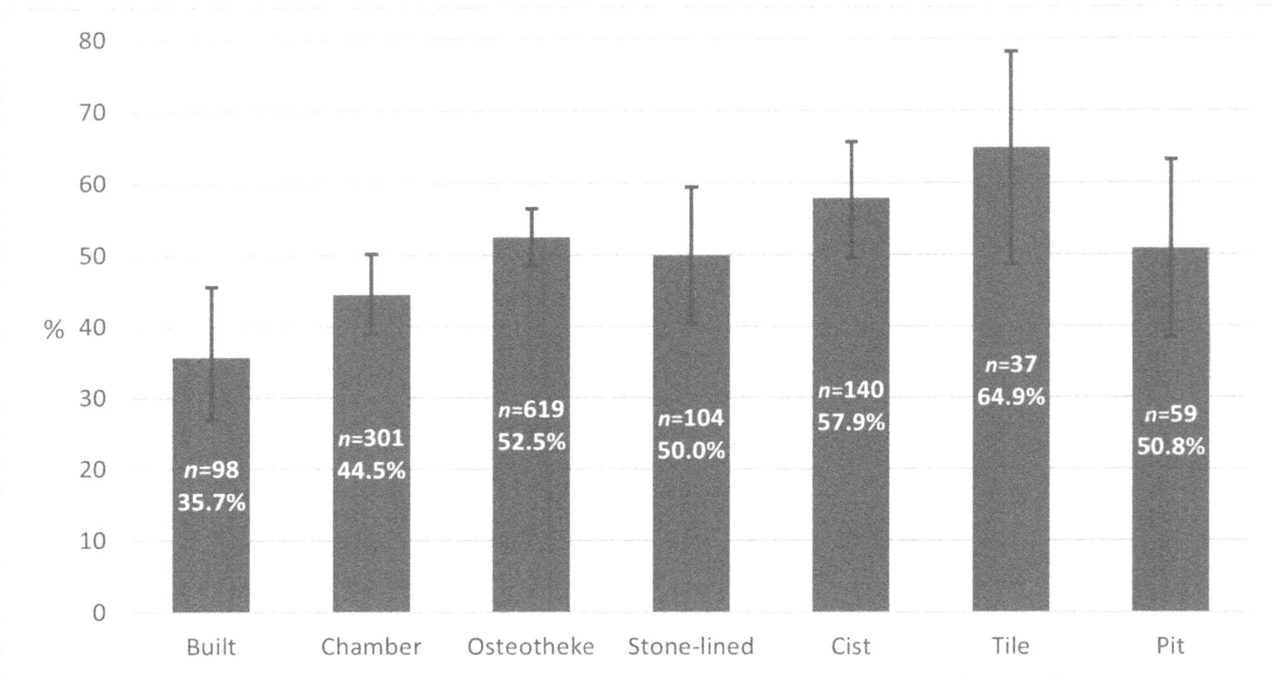

Figure 7.18. Prevalence of intervertebral disc disease by tomb type with sample sizes (*n*) and 95% confidence interval error bars.

cemetery groups and exaggerated to the high and low extremes. Excluding these samples from the discussion (and from Figure 7.21), the highest prevalence of IVDD was in the Hellenistic North Cemetery (61.2%) and the lowest was the Late Roman Sanatorium cemetery (33.8%). There was not a statistically significant difference between the Hellenistic and Roman North Cemetery samples (X^2=0.86, p=0.35), nor between any of the Roman (North Cemetery, Monastiriako Kephali, and Topana) cemeteries (X^2=0.17, p=0.92). The combined results for the cemeteries in the north (North Cemetery, Sanatorium, and Topana) and those in the south (Monastiriako Kephali) for the Roman period showed no statistically significant difference (X^2=0.82, p=0.37). The differences between the Late Roman and Late Antique (Krevatina, Sanatorium, and North Cemetery) samples were, however, statistically significant (X^2=5.7, p=0.02). The combined results for the cemeteries in the north (Sanatorium and North Cemetery) and those in the south (Krevatina and Monastiriako Kephali) for the Late Roman and Late Antique periods showed no statistically significant difference (X^2=1.72, p=0.19).

Figure 7.21 demonstrates the prevalence of IVDD for each region of the spine, for each cemetery, in each time period. This graph is included for the purposes of consistency, but the sample sizes have become small enough in many instances to be deemed unreliable. For the Hellenistic North Cemetery, Roman North Cemetery, and Late Roman Krevatina samples, IVDD increases with each region from the top to the bottom of the spine, while the Late Roman Sanatorium displays the opposite pattern of decreasing

Table 7.6. P values from chi-square tests for statistically significant differences (shaded) in intervertebral disc disease (IVDD) between pairs of tomb types.

	Built	Chamber	Osteotheke	Stone-lined	Cist	Tile	Pit
Built		0.13	0.002	0.006	0.002	0.001	0.002
Chamber	0.13		0.02	0.08	0.04	0.03	0.049
Osteotheke	0.002	0.02		0.06	0.41	0.29	0.42
Stone-lined	0.006	0.08	0.06		0.22	0.24	0.34
Cist	0.002	0.04	0.41	0.22		0.44	0.39
Tile	0.001	0.03	0.29	0.24	0.44		0.18
Pit	0.002	0.049	0.42	0.34	0.39	0.18	

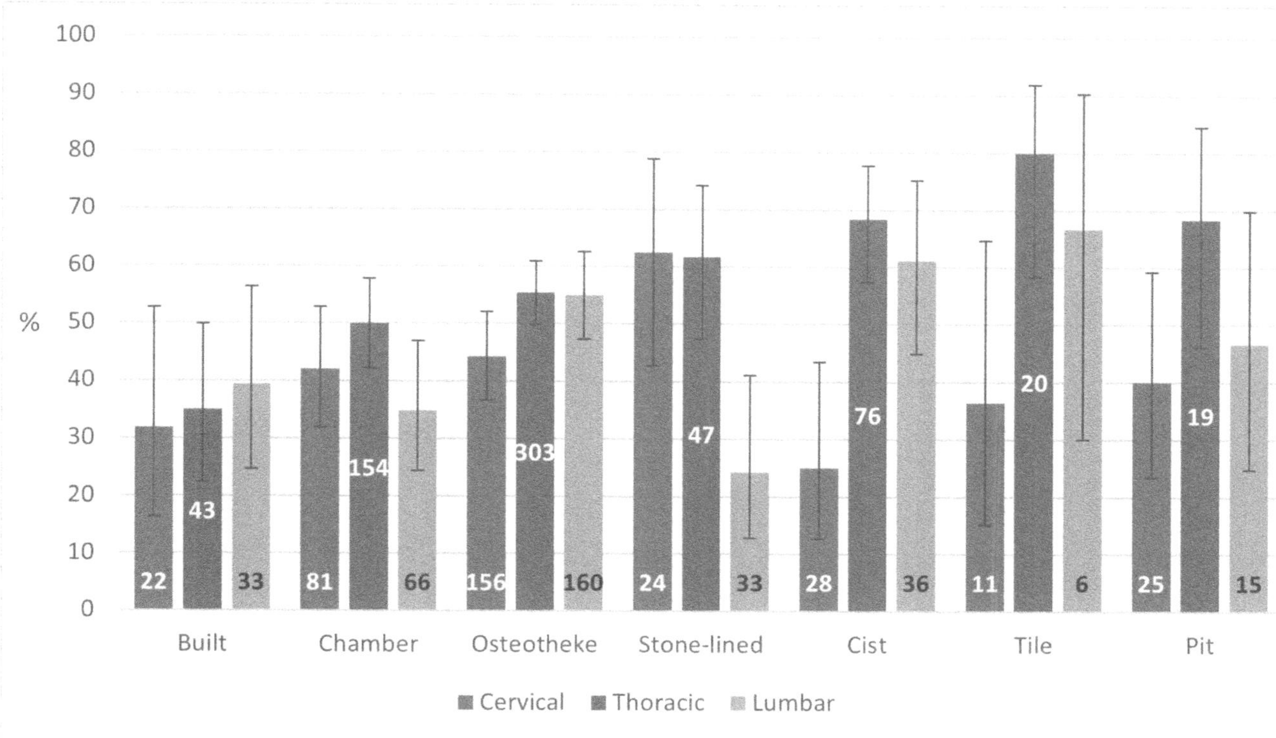

Figure 7.19. Prevalence of intervertebral disc disease (IVDD) for each region of the spine, for the tomb types with sample sizes (*n*) and 95% confidence interval error bars.

Table 7.7. Numbers of vertebrae with intervertebral disc disease, total numbers of vertebrae, and the percentage of vertebrae with intervertebral disc disease.

	IVDD	Total vertebrae (*n*)	%
Hellenistic North Cemetery	30	49	61.2
Roman North Cemetery	26	50	52.0
Roman Monastiriako Kephali	134	274	48.9
Roman Topana	19	39	48.7
Roman Sanatorium	0	14	0.0
Late Roman Krevatina	38	70	54.3
Late Roman Sanatorium	22	65	33.8
Late Antique North Cemetery	405	740	54.7
Late Antique Monastiriako Kephali	14	16	87.5

IVDD going down the spine. The Roman Monastiriako Kephali and Late Antique North Cemetery samples show a peak of IVDD in the thoracic spine, while the Roman Topana sample shows a lower prevalence of IVDD in the thoracic spine compared to either the cervical or lumbar regions.

7.3.3. Other arthropathies

7.3.3.1. Schmorl's nodes

A total of 52 incidences of Schmorl's nodes were recorded, though in a number of cases multiple incidences came from a single spine, with neighbouring vertebrae sometimes affected. The numbers are perhaps too few for the prevalences to be meaningful in most incidences but the counts, sample sizes of numbers of scoreable vertebrae, and the percentage of vertebral bodies with Schmorl's nodes are presented in the following tables, with the prevalences displayed in the following bar charts. Table 7.8 and Figure 7.22 show the results for each time period, Table 7.9 and Figure 7.23 display the Schmorl's nodes prevalence for females and males, Table 7.10 and Figure 7.24 present the results for each tomb type, and Table 7.11 and Figure 7.25 have the results for each cemetery or location within each time period. The results for the sexes are the least meaningful due to the extremely reduced sample size of sexed vertebrae.

The Hellenistic period had no cases of Schmorl's nodes recorded, but it also had by far the smallest sample size of vertebral bodies (Table 7.8). There was a Schmorl's nodes prevalence of 2.6% (14/532) for the Roman period, and of 4.9% (38/772) for the Late Antique period. This was a

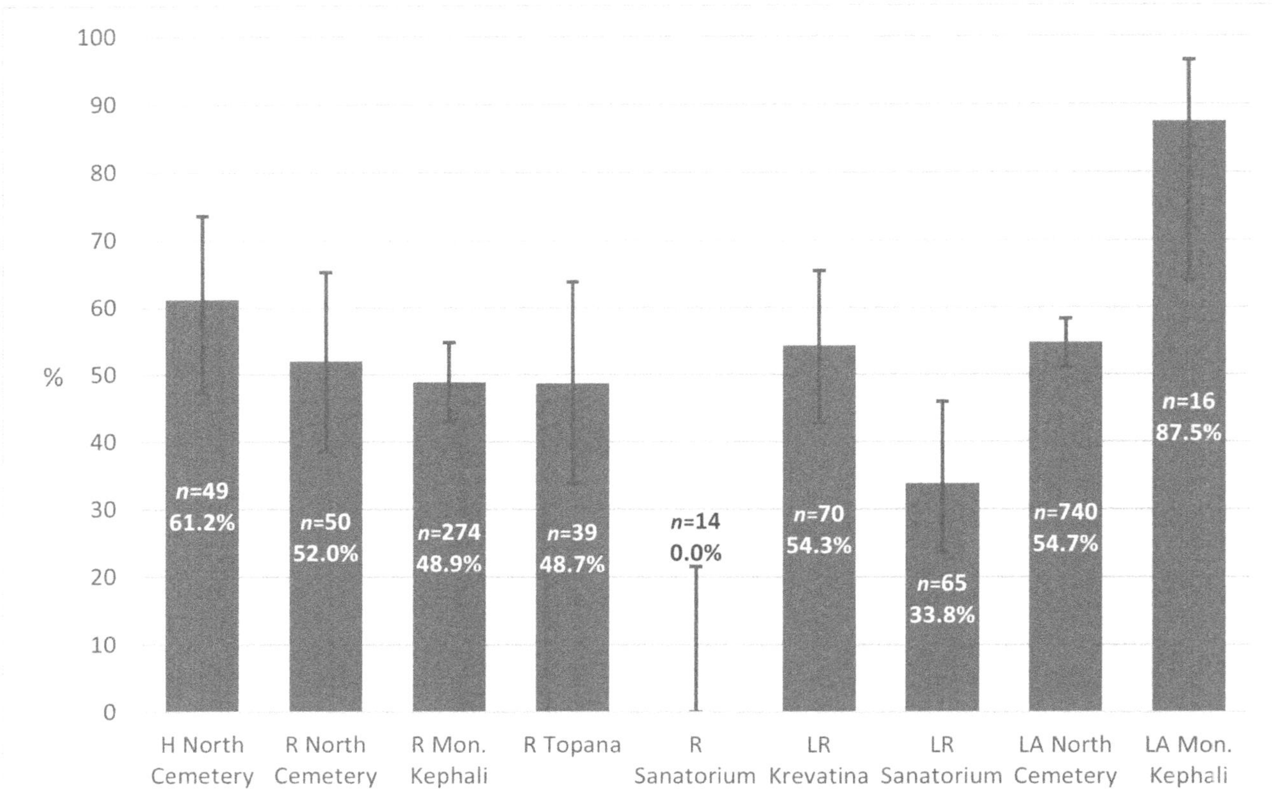

Figure 7.20. Prevalence of intervertebral disc disease (IVDD) for each cemetery or burial location in each time period with sample sizes (*n*) and 95% confidence interval error bars.

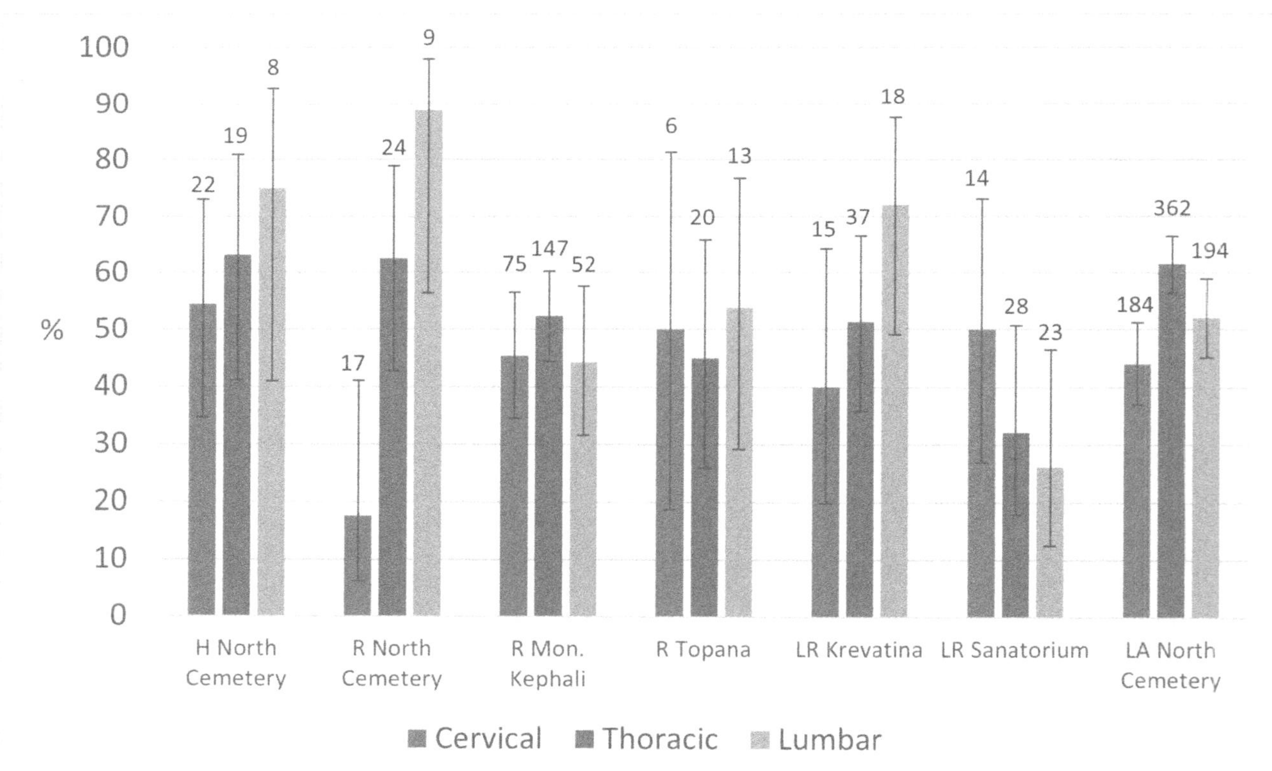

Figure 7.21. Prevalence of intervertebral disc disease (IVDD) for each region of the spine, in each cemetery with sample sizes (*n*) and 95% confidence interval error bars.

Table 7.8. Prevalence of Schmorl's nodes for each time period.

	Schmorl's nodes	Vertebral bodies	%
Hellenistic	0	60	0.0
Roman	14	532	2.6
Late Antique	38	772	4.9

Table 7.9. Prevalence of Schmorl's nodes for females and males.

	Schmorl's nodes	Vertebral bodies	%
Female	0	58	0
Male	4	142	2.8

statistically significant difference between the Roman and Late Antique results (X^2=4.32, *p*=0.04).

With slightly anomalous results at either end of the spectrum of tomb types from the built and pit tombs, the results otherwise showed a general trend of increased Schmorl's nodes with decreased tomb complexity. However, sample sizes are in many cases small and may not be fully representative, for example in the incidence of the highest result from the tile grave group (*n*=37) and the lowest result of no cases being recorded in the pit graves (*n*=59). There were, however, statistically significant differences between the tile and pit graves and between these groups compared with some other tomb types: Built v. Tile (X^2=11.53, *p*=0.04), Built v. Pit (X^2=14.49, *p*=0.02), Chamber v. Tile (X^2=11.54, *p*=0.02), Chamber v. Pit (X^2=14.54, *p*=0.01), Osteotheke v. Pit (X^2=9.61, *p*=0.048),

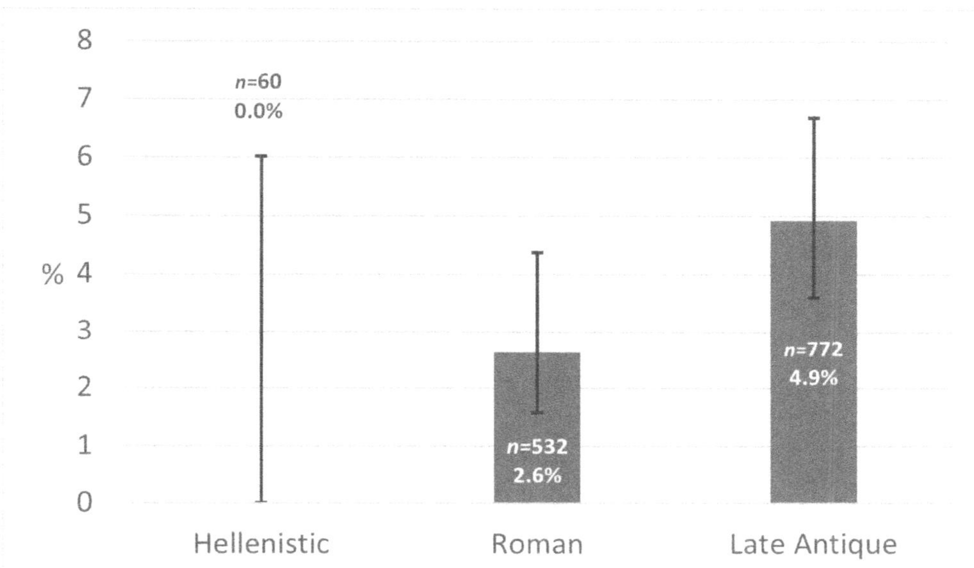

Figure 7.22. Prevalence of Schmorl's nodes for each time period with sample sizes (*n*) and 95% confidence interval error bars.

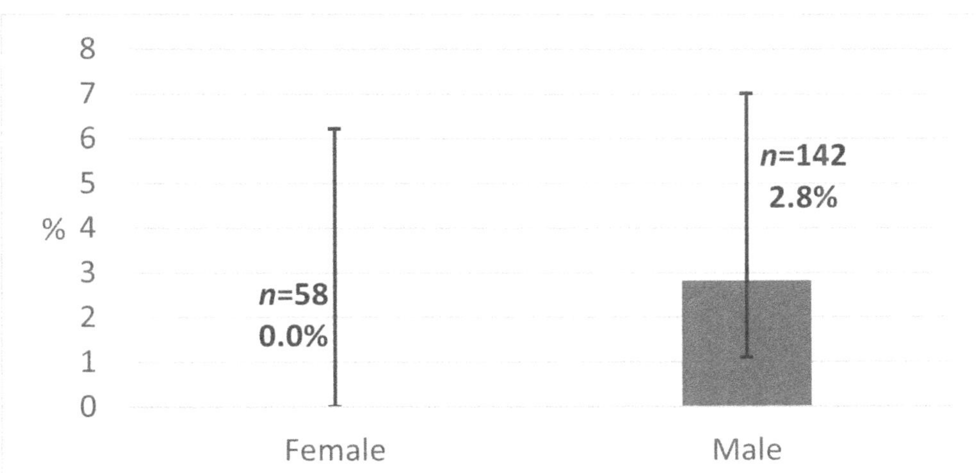

Figure 7.23. Prevalence of Schmorl's nodes for females and males with sample sizes (*n*) and 95% confidence interval error bars.

Table 7.10. Prevalence of Schmorl's nodes for each tomb type.

	Schmorl's nodes	Vertebral bodies	%
Built	4	98	4.1
Chamber	6	301	2.0
Osteotheke	23	619	3.7
Stone-lined	5	104	4.8
Cist	10	140	7.1
Tile	4	37	10.8
Pit	0	59	0.0

and Tile v. Pit (X^2=6.66, p=0.01). The differences in Schmorl's nodes prevalence between any other pair of tomb types was not statistically significant.

Though several of the cemetery groups had small sample sizes, there are interesting observations that can be made about this data. The Roman Monastiriako Kephali group only had 6 Schmorl's nodes in 274 vertebrae, a fairly reliable sample size. The scarcity of Schmorl's nodes in the assemblage from this burial group, suggests a lack of the types of activity that can cause this condition. Though details of the range of these activities are not known, Schmorl's nodes tend to be common in highly active individuals, such as athletes and farmworkers. This result

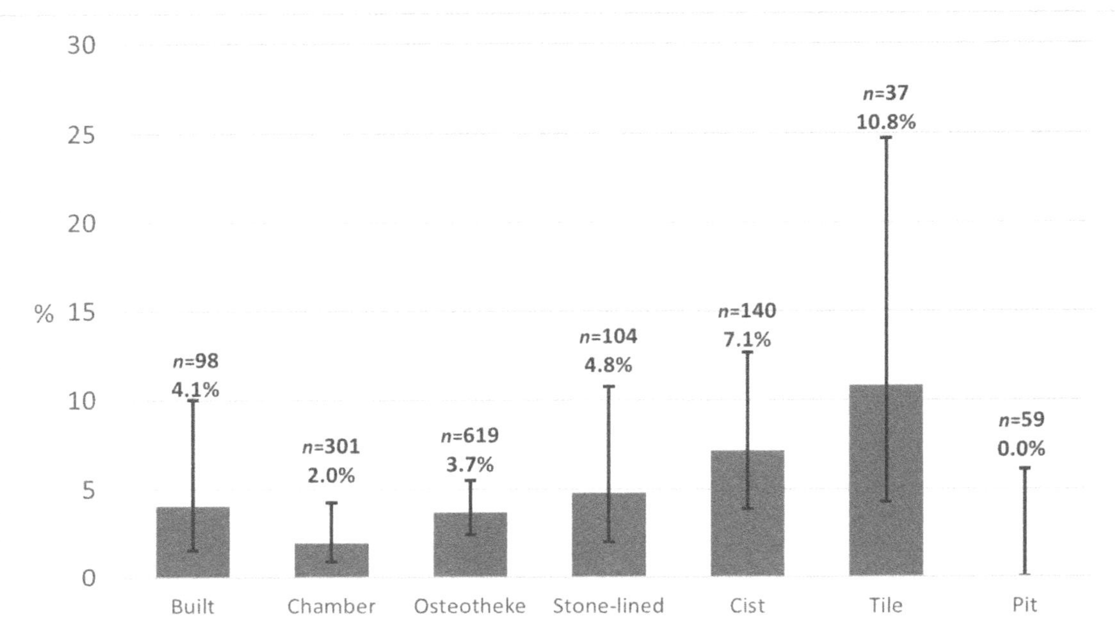

Figure 7.24. Prevalence of Schmorl's nodes for each tomb type with sample sizes (*n*) and 95% confidence interval error bars.

Table 7.11. Prevalence of Schmorl's nodes for each cemetery/location within each time period.

	Schmorl's nodes	Vertebral bodies	%
Hellenistic North Cemetery	0	49	0.0
Roman North Cemetery	4	50	8.0
Roman Monastiriako Kephali	6	274	2.2
Roman Topana	4	39	10.3
Roman Sanatorium	0	14	0.0
Late Roman Krevatina	0	70	0.0
Late Roman Sanatorium	0	65	0.0
Late Antique North Cemetery	38	740	5.1
Late Antique Monastiriako Kephali	0	16	0.0

was not significantly lower than for the other cemetery groups, as determined by the overlapping confidence intervals in Figure 7.25. The Late Antique North Cemetery (the largest sample size) had a higher prevalence of Schmorl's nodes, and although still a fairly low prevalence, this was notably higher than in the Roman Monastiriako Kephali group. Several other cemetery groups had a prevalence of zero, though sample sizes were quite low for these groups. The Krevatina cemetery had a decent sample size (n=70) considering it represents only four individuals, therefore, in this instance a zero result is meaningful. The Roman North Cemetery (8.0%) and Roman Topana (10.3%) groups had much higher prevalences but as these sample sizes were low, these results had wide confidence intervals, indicating that the difference was not significant.

7.3.3.2. Ankylosing spondylitis

Nine incidences of probable ankylosing spondylitis were recorded in the assemblage. None could be assigned to a

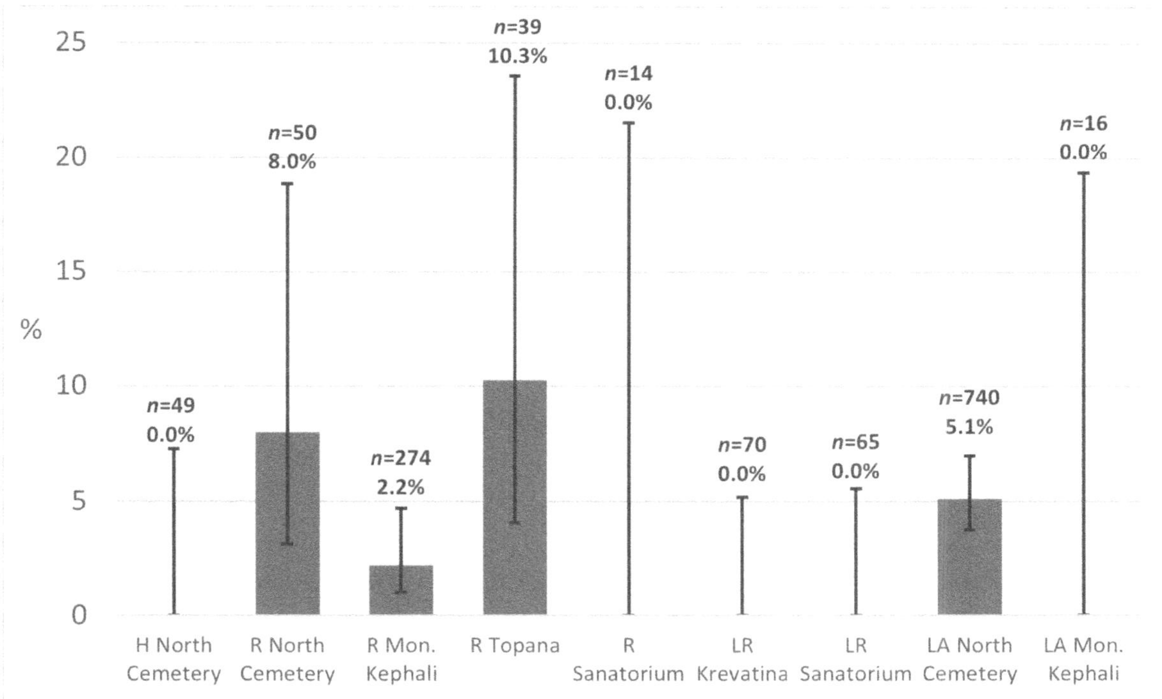

Figure 7.25. Prevalence of Schmorl's nodes for each cemetery/location within each time period with sample sizes (*n*) and 95% confidence interval error bars.

specific age (A= adult) or sex category (U= unknown). There were two cases in the lumbar vertebrae in the Roman Monastiriako Kephali rock-cut chamber tomb (Unit 5). The remaining examples all came from the North Cemetery osteothekai and the nearby Fortetsa Fork (Unit 4) osteotheke.

7.3.3.3. Diffuse idiopathic skeletal hyperostosis (DISH)

Three incidences of DISH were recorded across the entire assemblage and these are outlined with all their associated contextual information in Table 7.13. DISH was found in one of the four individuals, a young adult female, from

Table 7.12. Cases of ankylosing spondylitis.

Unit No.	Ind. no.	Unit Name	Vertebrae affected	Age	Sex	Time period	Tomb type	Cemetery
4	795	KFF74 T.1	2 thoracic vertebrae	A	U	LA	Osteotheke	LA North Cemetery
4	620	KFF74 T.1	2 lumbar vertebrae	A	U	LA	Osteotheke	LA North Cemetery
4	321	KFF74 T.1	2 thoracic vertebrae	A	U	LA	Osteotheke	LA North Cemetery
5	447	MK76 April	2 lumbar vertebral arches	A	U	R	Chamber	R Mon. Kephali
5	537	MK76 April	2 lumbar vertebral arches	A	U	R	Chamber	R Mon. Kephali
78	153	KMF78 T.151	L5 and sacrum	A	U	LA	Osteotheke	LA North Cemetery
78	86	KMF78 T.151	2 thoracic vertebrae	A	U	LA	Osteotheke	LA North Cemetery
84	485	KMF78 T.244	3 thoracic partial vertebral bodies	A	U	LA	Osteotheke	LA North Cemetery
85	340	KMF78 T.254	3 thoracic partial vertebral bodies	A	U	LA	Osteotheke	LA North Cemetery

Table 7.13. Cases of diffuse idiopathic skeletal hyperostosis (DISH).

Unit No.	Ind. no.	Unit Name	Vertebrae affected	Age	Sex	Time period	Tomb type	Cemetery
4	1925	KFF74 T.1	2 lumbar vertebrae	A		LA	Osteotheke	LA North Cemetery
88	46	KMF78 T.299	2 thoracic vertebrae	A		LA	Osteotheke	LA North Cemetery
105	4	1936/2 Krevatina	3 thoracic vertebrae	YA	F	R	Cist	LR Krevatina

the Late Roman Krevatina cist grave. The other two incidences of DISH observed in the assemblage were both from Late Antique osteothekai, both adults of unknown age or sex, one affected in the thoracic spine and the other in the lumbar vertebrae.

7.3.4. Entheseal changes

Of the selection of commonly affected enthesis sites selected for study, 1023 entheses were recorded. Of those, 297 (29%) displayed signs of either minor or prominent entheseal changes. The majority of cases recorded were minor manifestations.

7.3.4.1. Time period

The results for the prevalence of entheseal changes are displayed in Table 7.14 and Figure 7.26. Entheseal changes occurred in 41.9% (36/86) of entheses in the Hellenistic period. There was a substantial decline in their

Table 7.14. Numbers (*n*) of entheses recorded, and numbers and percentages with entheseal changes, within which, numbers and percentages of those that presented as minor or prominent entheseal changes, for each time period.

	Hellenistic	% Hellenistic	Roman	% Roman	Late Antique	% Late Antique
Minor	27	31.4	121	23.8	82	19.2
Prominent	9	10.5	31	6.1	27	6.3
Entheseal changes (any)	36	41.9	152	29.9	109	25.5
Entheses (*n*)	86		509		428	

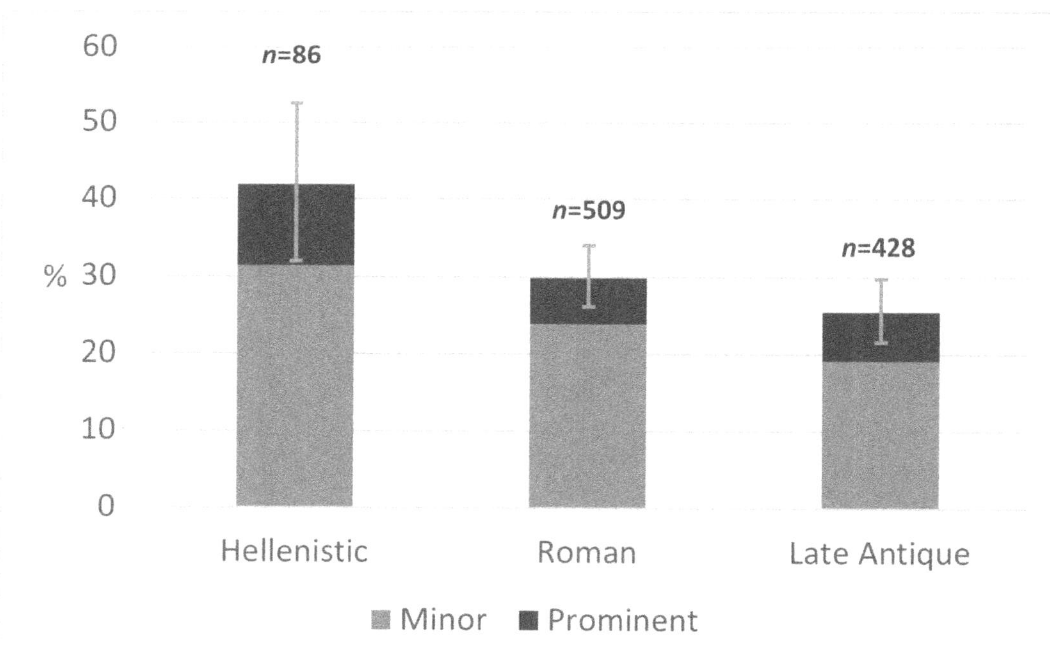

Figure 7.26. Prevalence of entheseal changes (minor and prominent) by time period with sample sizes (*n*) and 95% confidence interval error bars.

occurrence in the Roman period to 29.9% (152/509), and a further, smaller decline to 25.5% (109/428) in the Late Antique period. The difference between the Hellenistic and Roman periods was statistically significant (X^2=4.90, p=0.03), but the difference between the Roman and Late Antique periods was not statistically significant (X^2=2,24, p=0.13). The difference for comparing all three time periods together was statistically significant (X^2=9.68, p=0.008). The minor entheseal changes, which made up the majority of the observed lesions, followed the same pattern of decline over time, from 31.4% in the Hellenistic period, to 23.8% in the Roman period, to 19.2% in the Late Antique period. The less common prominent expressions of entheseal changes were most common in the Hellenistic period (10.5%) and were almost equal in their occurrence in the Roman (6.1%) and Late Antique (6.3%) periods.

7.3.4.2. Sex

Table 7.15 and Figure 7.27 display the entheseal change results for females and males. As with all analyses, the sample size is reduced for elements which can have their sex determined due to the large numbers of commingled remains. Males have a higher prevalence of entheseal changes (Males: 41%, Females: 30.1%) in general as well as a higher prevalence of both minor (Males: 34.4%, Females: 27.7%) and prominent (Males: 6.6%, Females: 2.4%) entheseal changes. The difference between the female and male entheseal change prevalences was not, however, statistically significant (X^2=2.51, p=0.11).

Table 7.15. Numbers (*n*) of entheses recorded, and numbers and percentages with entheseal changes, within which, numbers and percentages of those that presented as minor or prominent entheseal changes, for females and males.

	Female	Female %	Male	Male %
Minor	23	27.7	42	34.4
Prominent	2	2.4	8	6.6
Entheseal changes	25	30.1	50	41.0
Entheses (*n*)	83		122	

7.3.4.3. Tomb type

Table 7.16 and Figure 7.28 present the results for entheseal changes by tomb type. The highest prevalence is for the cist tombs with 43.3% (39/90) of entheses showing lesions, followed by the pit graves (41.3%, 31/75). There was no statistically significant difference in entheseal change prevalence between the cist and pit graves (X^2=0.07, p=0.80). The cist graves had few cases of prominent lesions (4.4%, 4/90), whereas the pit graves (13.3%, 10/75), followed by the chamber tombs (9.4%, 12/128), had the highest proportions of prominent entheseal changes. The built tombs had the lowest prevalence of entheseal changes overall (18.4%, 42/228), though almost a third of lesions were prominent. Stone-lined tombs (24.1%, 32/133) were the next lowest prevalence, followed closely by the

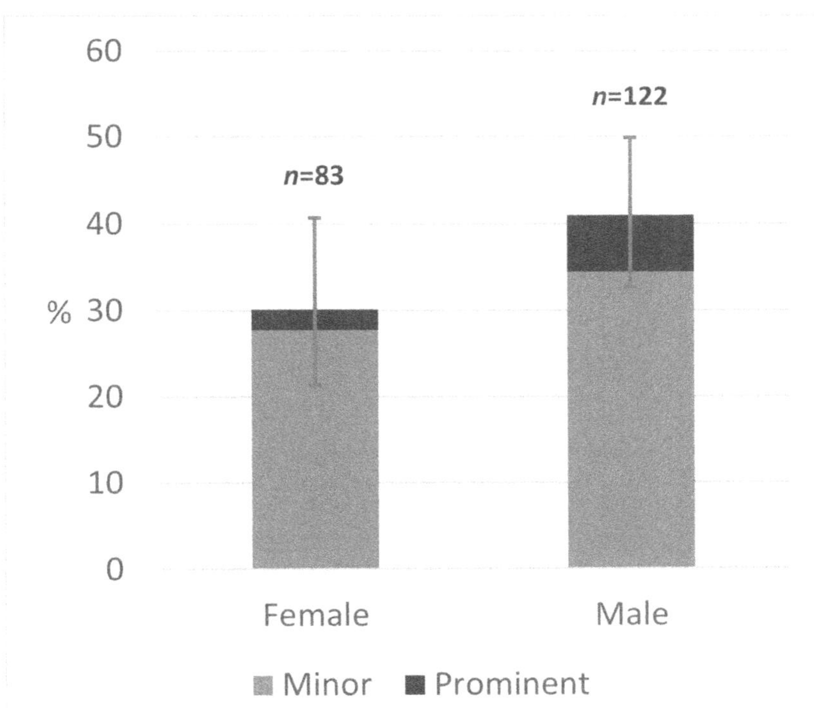

Figure 7.27. Prevalence of entheseal changes (minor and prominent) for females and males with sample sizes (*n*) and 95% confidence interval error bars.

Table 7.16. Numbers (*n*) of entheses recorded, and numbers and percentages with entheseal changes, within which, numbers and percentages of those that presented as minor or prominent entheseal changes, for the tomb types.

	Built		Chamber		Osteo.		S-L		Cist		Tile		Pit	
	No.	%	No.	%	No.	%	No.	%	No.	%	No.	%	No.	%
Minor	29	12.7	41	32.0	58	17.8	31	23.3	35	38.9	14	35.9	21	28.0
Prominent	13	5.7	12	9.4	26	8.0	1	0.8	4	4.4	1	2.6	10	13.3
Entheseal changes	42	18.4	53	41.4	84	25.8	32	24.1	39	43.3	15	38.5	31	41.3
Entheses (*n*)	228		128		325		133		90		39		75	

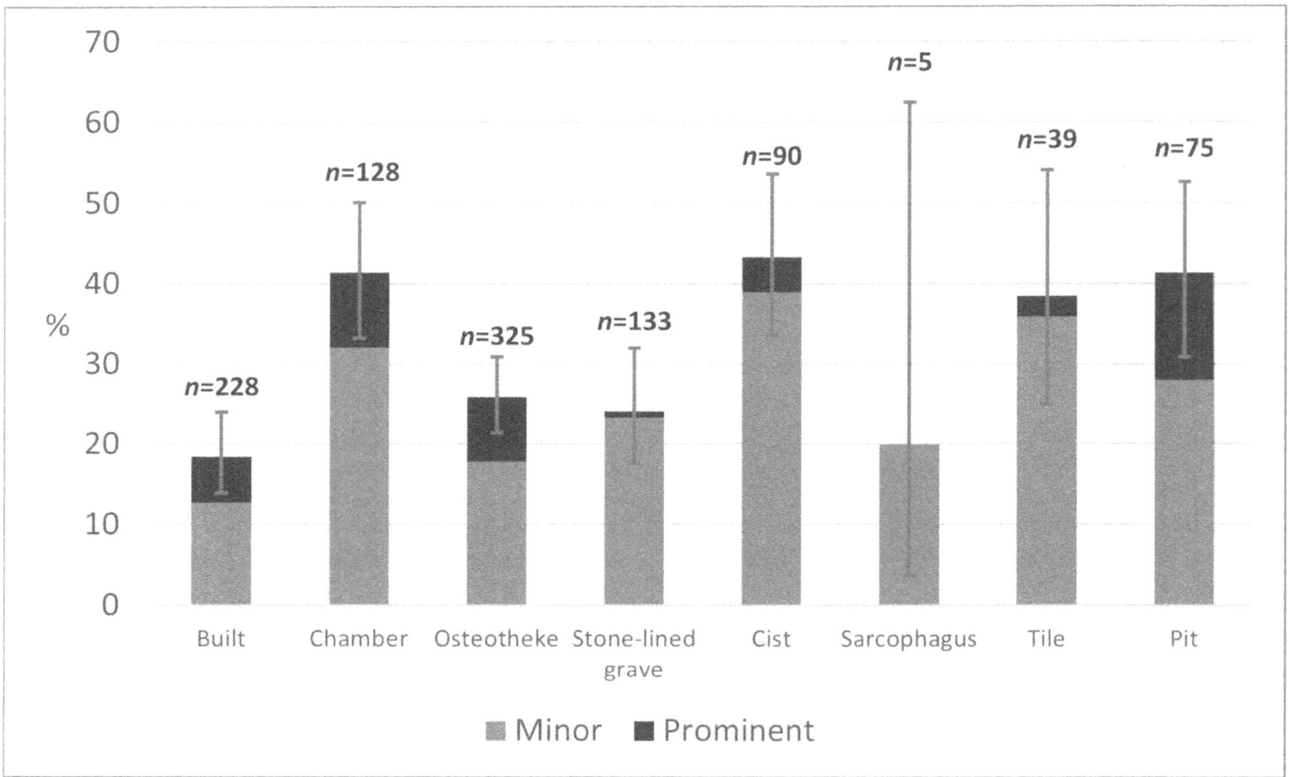

Figure 7.28. Prevalence of entheseal changes (minor and prominent) for the tomb types with sample sizes (*n*) and 95% confidence interval error bars.

osteothekai (25.8%, 84/325), with no significant difference between the two (X^2=0.16, p=0.69). The osteothekai, however, had a far higher proportion of prominent lesions with 8% (26/325) of entheses having prominent lesions, which was almost a third of all lesions (26/84), compared to only a single incidence (0.8%, 1/133 entheses, or 1/32 entheseal changes) in the stone-lined tombs. Tile graves (38.5%, 15/39) had a fairly high prevalence of entheseal changes, but a very small sample size. Chamber tombs (41.4%, 53/128) were the main exception to the pattern of the more complex tomb forms having lower prevalences of entheseal changes and the less complex tomb types having higher rates.

7.3.4.4. Cemetery (location)

Table 7.17 and Figure 7.29 display the results for the occurrence of entheseal changes between the different cemeteries or burial locations. The cemetery with the highest prevalence of entheseal changes was the Late Roman Krevatina cemetery (a single cist grave, Unit 105) with 66.7% (30/45) of entheses showing lesions. The lowest prevalence of entheseal changes came from the Topana cemetery (again a single tomb, Unit 104) with 11.1% (4/36) and half of all lesions (2/4) being prominent, but this sample size was very small.

The pattern for the North Cemetery over time reflects the overall pattern of a decline in entheseal change prevalence with each time period, from 41.9% (36/86) for the Hellenistic North Cemetery, to 29.9% (20/67) in the Roman North Cemetery, to 25.6% (106/414) in the Late Antique North Cemetery. The difference between the Hellenistic and Roman results was not statistically significant (X^2=2.34, p=0.13). This may in part be due to the fairly small sample sizes as a comparison of all three

Table 7.17. Numbers (*n*) of entheses recorded, and numbers and percentages with entheseal changes, within which, numbers and percentages of those that presented as minor or prominent entheseal changes, for the cemeteries/locations.

		Minor	Prominent	Entheseal changes	Entheses
Hellenistic North Cemetery	No.	27	9	36	86
	%	31.4	10.5	41.9	
Roman North Cemetery	No.	15	5	20	67
	%	22.4	7.5	29.9	
Roman Monastiriako Kephali	No.	30	12	42	104
	%	28.8	11.5	40.4	
Roman Topana	No.	2	2	4	36
	%	5.6	5.6	11.1	
Roman Sanatorium	No.	11	0	11	24
	%	45.8	0.0	45.8	
Late Roman Krevatina	No.	26	4	30	45
	%	57.8	8.9	66.7	
Late Roman Sanatorium	No.	37	8	45	233
	%	15.9	3.4	19.3	
Late Antique North Cemetery	No.	79	27	106	414
	%	19.1	6.5	25.6	
Late Antique Monastiriako Kephali	No.	3	0	3	14
	%	21.4	0.0	21.4	

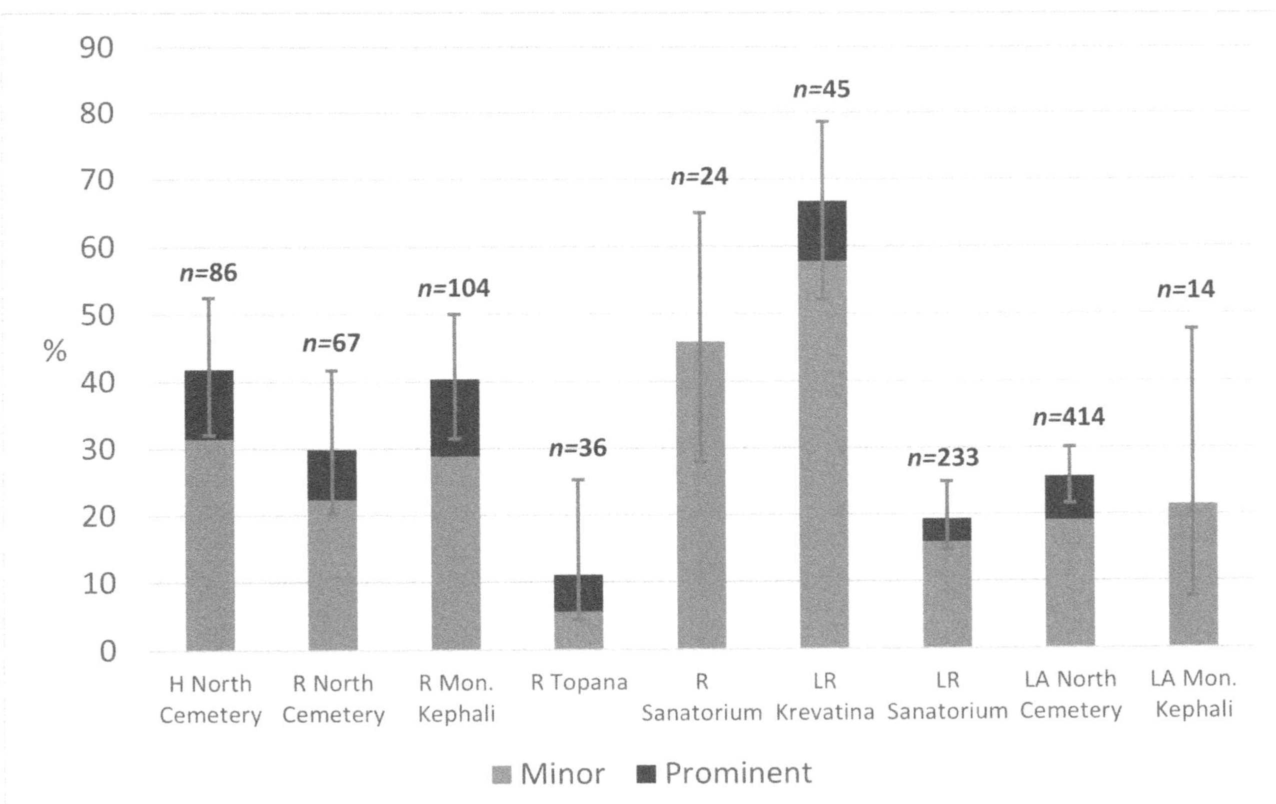

Figure 7.29. Prevalence of entheseal changes (minor and prominent) for the cemeteries/locations with sample sizes (*n*) and 95% confidence interval error bars.

time periods was statistically highly significant (X^2=66.13, p=0.000), as were the comparisons of the Late Antique results with each of those for the Hellenistic and Roman periods.

For the Roman period (1st–2nd centuries) the North Cemetery (29.9%, 20/67) has a lower prevalence of entheseal changes than the Monastiriako Kephali cemetery (40.4%, 42/104), though this was not a statistically significant difference (X^2=1.96, p=0.16). The Topana tomb (11.1%, 4/36) had the lowest and Sanatorium tomb (Unit 93, 45.8%, 11/24) the highest results for the Roman cemeteries. Although the Topana and Sanatorium samples were particularly low, the differences between them and each of the other Roman cemeteries were all statistically significant, with an overall chi-square result of X^2=12.38, p=0.006 for a comparison of all the Roman cemeteries. The combined results for the Roman northern cemeteries (North Cemetery, Topana and Sanatorium) had an entheseal changes prevalence of 27.6% and this was compared to the southern cemetery (Monastiriako Kephali) result of 40.4%, which was a statistically significant difference (X^2=4.23, p=0.04).

For the Late Roman period (3rd–4th centuries), the Krevatina cemetery (66.7%, 30/45) had a statistically significantly higher result (X^2=42.93, p=0.000) than the Sanatorium cemetery (19.3%, 45/233), despite the small sample size of the former. The difference between the Late Roman Sanatorium cemetery and the Late Antique North Cemetery (25.6%, 106/414) was not statistically significant (X^2=3.30, p=0.07), with both having quite low prevalences. The Late Antique Monastiriako Kephali result was also quite low (21.4%, 3/14), but only represented a single individual. The difference between the entheseal changes prevalence for the Late Roman-Late Antique (3rd–7th centuries) northern cemeteries combined (North Cemetery and Sanatorium: 23.3%) and the southern cemeteries combined (Krevatina and Monastiriako Kephali: 55.9%) was statistically significant (X^2=29.81, p=0.000).

7.4. Discussion

7.4.1. Time period

Osteoarthritis rates decreased from the Hellenistic to Roman periods, and then increased by a smaller, but nevertheless significant, margin in the Late Antique period. Amongst males there was a decline across the three time periods, with the lowest prevalence of osteoarthritis in the Late Antique period, though by contrast the Late Antique females had higher osteoarthritis levels than in any other period. Similar to the osteoarthritis levels, IVDD shows a pattern of decline in the Roman period, followed by increased incidences in the Late Antique. Schmorl's nodes were few but appeared to increase in occurrence across the time periods from Hellenistic to Late Antique. No incidence of Schmorl's nodes, DISH or ankylosing spondylitis was recorded for the Hellenistic period. However, the small numbers of vertebrae surviving from Hellenistic contexts may mean these results for vertebral pathology are not fully representative. There is, however, a clear pattern of lower levels of joint disease in the Roman assemblage. Entheseal change prevalence, however, decreased over time from the Hellenistic to Late Antique periods, though there was a significant decrease from the Hellenistic to Roman period, while the difference between the Roman and Late Antique periods was not significant. The social implications of these patterns of changes observed in the prevalence of joint disease and entheseal changes are discussed in the following paragraphs for each time period.

At no other site in Greece has there been a comparison of joint disease, entheseal changes or activity as inferred from the skeleton at a single site across these time periods. Bourbou (2005, 93) compared assemblages from Hellenistic Chania and Roman Sfakaki (near Rethymnon) and found that the Hellenistic sample had a higher prevalence of osteoarthritis than the Roman, similar to the pattern observed at Knossos between these time periods. However, the sample size was particularly small due to the poor preservation of many joint surfaces and the Hellenistic and Roman samples come from different sites, therefore there may have been various factors affecting joint disease differently in these different populations. Additionally, spondylosis (a broad term referring to degenerative conditions in the spine) and Schmorl's nodes were both found to have a slightly higher prevalence in the Roman Sfakaki sample. There are therefore no examples of studied assemblages from within a single site across these time periods for direct contrast and comparison.

The Hellenistic assemblage had high levels of osteoarthritis, IVDD and entheseal changes which dropped off significantly for osteoarthritis and entheseal changes, and to a smaller extent for IVDD, going into the Roman period. The question must be raised again about the subset of society that was being buried in the Hellenistic North Cemetery (female-dominant, simple graves with few grave goods) and how representative the assemblage is of the population at Knossos at that time. Does the simple burial type represent individuals of lower social status or was this the only burial type found at Hellenistic Knossos? The former suggestion – as well as the existence of more elaborate Hellenistic burials at Chania and Gortyn (Ioannidou-Karetsou 1974; Markoulaki and Niniou-Kindeli 1982; 2009; Tsigkou 2004; 2009; di Vita 2010) – would be supported by the higher levels of joint disease and entheseal changes, which would indicate a manual-labouring lifestyle. It is known that these North Cemetery pit and tile graves represented by the skeletal material are not the only burial type at Knossos, as some cists are also reported (Brock 1957; Hood and Smyth 1981), but it is not known whether there were any more elaborate tombs. Whether or not there was a range of social strata represented in the present assemblage, the Hellenistic results indicate that a sizeable proportion of the population were engaged in manual labour, such as agricultural labour, construction work, transportation of heavy goods, or military activities. Although it is mentioned that the cemetery was predominantly (two-thirds) female, the Hellenistic males had significantly higher levels of osteoarthritis than the females, therefore it is not the sex imbalance affecting the Hellenistic result in comparison to the later time periods.

The Roman assemblage generally has a lower prevalence of activity or movement-related pathological conditions which is likely to some extent to reflect the type of individual represented in the burial assemblage. The Roman assemblage is largely represented by individuals who were buried in ostentatious tombs and are likely to have been the elite members of society. A discussion of pathology by tomb type is found in Section 7.4.3. While it is unclear from the burial record what sort of subset or cross-section of society is represented by the Hellenistic assemblage, with the transition from a subsistence economy to a system more dependent on trade, it is possible that a smaller proportion of the population was engaged in manual labour, such as farm work, in the Roman period. It is also possible that these individuals had moved out of the urban areas to smaller settlements which was feasible due to peaceful relations on the island (Sanders 1982; Hayden *et al.* 1992). It is known that there would have been a large workforce required for the many building projects during the Roman period, which would have involved a great deal of physical labour, but it may be the case that such individuals are not represented in the skeletal assemblage. The apparent increase in average life expectancy (more individuals with a later age-at-death) in the Roman period should have had the opposite impact on the level of joint disease being recorded if age was the primary influencing factor, but with the opposite being the case (increased joint disease prevalence) this reinforces the significance of the difference between these time periods.

The Late Antique period had a higher prevalence of osteoarthritis, IVDD, and Schmorl's nodes than the Roman period. However, entheseal change rates were slightly reduced, though this was not a statistically significant difference and with any condition with a multifactorial aetiology it must be considered that other variables could be the more dominant factors in the manifestation of lesions. The difference in the manifestation of joint diseases and entheseal changes between the Roman and Late Antique periods appears to be less significant than the difference between the Hellenistic and Roman periods and this is likely to be due to the more gradual socio-economic changes during the Late Roman period. A break-down of the results into cemeteries with narrower time periods is discussed in Section 7.4.4. With fewer imports or exports known at or from Knossos in the Late Antique period this may have meant a return to subsistence living with more of the urban population engaged in manual labour. The increase in levels of joint disease and slight reduction in entheseal changes could be due to a certain level of increased activity across the entire assemblage without particularly heavy loading at the muscle attachment sites with the potential loss of the inactive elite class and hierarchical society of the Roman period.

Although based on a small number of examples from studies carried out by different investigators, a reduction in the levels of joint disease from sites in Greece from the Bronze Age to Archaic period was attributed to a change in the social environment and conditions of life, particularly working conditions due to the role played by physical labour in the occurrence of joint disease (Angel 1946, 91; Grmek 1989, 82). This sets a precedent for the changes in activity types or levels caused by major social or political changes across time to be observable from lesions in the skeleton. This is not only indicative of changes in labour, but osteoarthritis of the jaw (temporomandibular joint) shows changes in diet. Osteoarthritis was recorded in the temporomandibular joints of 25.5% (11/43) of the assemblage at Neolithic Çatalhöyük and 20% of individuals at Middle Bronze Age Lerna (Angel 1971a; 1971b), compared to 0%, 3% and 3.8% for Hellenistic, Roman and Late Antique Knossos respectively, demonstrating very low levels in each time period at Knossos. This illustrates a softer diet and more sophisticated food processing methods and technology in these historic periods at Knossos. Mention of joint diseases and entheseal changes in studies of Greek assemblages are nearly always reported by individual, therefore it is not possible to compare the different regions of the body but Angel states that the prevalence of osteoarthritis in the Bronze Age is substantially higher (as much as double for some joints) that of the Classical and Roman periods (Angel 1971b, 87, 89).

7.4.2. Sex

Males had higher rates of osteoarthritis, IVDD, Schmorl's nodes and entheseal changes than females. This tends to be the case for the majority of skeletal assemblages studied from prehistoric and historic times, regardless of the population's socio-political complexity or subsistence strategy (Larsen 2015). It is generally interpreted as being due to males commonly taking on more physical labour and heavy manual work than females, though there are exceptions, such as at Late Roman Isthmia (Rife 2012). Rife found that males tended to only show vertebral lesions in late adulthood, while females showed joint lesions, particularly in the spine and shoulders, throughout adulthood, which he claims indicates women were already involved in heavy lifting from a young age and were engaged in work at least as strenuous as men's (Rife 2012, 424, 428). This could indicate that females are naturally more predisposed to joint disease if both sexes are generally fairly inactive, which is supported by the fact that osteoarthritis is more common in females in modern populations (Srikanth *et al.* 2005; Cross *et al.* 2014; Kolhe *et al.* 2017).

Rife's results for the sexes are looked at by prevalence of joint disease by individual and therefore do not differentiate between an individual with early manifestations of joint disease in a single joint and individuals with advanced joint disease throughout the body. This is not an uncommon way of presenting the data from non-commingled assemblages and there is a discussion of the general prevalence of alterations/disease by joint but this does not bring in the demographic or other variables. The greater issue with these results as a comparative source is not differentiating between the types of joint diseases, which occurred in 78.6% (11/14) of females and 60% (6/10) of males. The osteoarthritis results from Early -Middle Byzantine Crete were also recorded by individual, with 3% (6/195) of females and 9% (18/195) of males exhibiting lesions in at least one joint (Bourbou 2010, 54). As would be expected for recording by individual rather than by joint, these results were slightly lower than the Knossos results (Females: 15.6%, Males: 7.6% of joint surfaces). This demonstrates the problems with comparing different sorts of assemblages as well as the problems caused by inconsistencies in recording methods.

Osteoarthritis of the elbows, wrists, and hips was higher in females than in males. Regarding the elbows and wrists, this could be due to the repetitive movements of activities more associated with the domestic domain such as food preparation and fabric manufacturing, supported by a similar pattern being observed elsewhere, particularly in the female elbow joint (Papageorgopoulou and Xirotiris 2009). Meanwhile the males having a higher prevalence of shoulder and spine osteoarthritis may be due to heavy lifting, which could be due to farming, construction work, or transportation of goods. Males also had significantly higher levels of hand osteoarthritis, which might be associated with more delicate or intricate repetitive movements, such as those ascribed to the possible female dominated activities above, as an explanation for the high levels of female wrist and elbow osteoarthritis. It is, however, possible that as well as heavy lifting, the male dominated activities could have involved intricate handiwork, such as wood-working, butchery, fishing, ceramic and other craft production. These are gross generalisations of gender-associated activities to give examples of the types of activities which could have led to one sex having significantly higher osteoarthritis than the other, and it should always be kept in mind that age, hormones (sex) and genes are key factors in an individual's propensity for osteoarthritis. As with the elbows and wrists, the difference in the osteoarthritis of the hips was not significantly different between the sexes, but the higher female prevalence could be explained by the child-bearing design of the female pelvis, both in terms of its direct function for this purpose and the fact that it is intended more for this purpose, while evolutionarily the male pelvis is designed for more efficient bipedal movement (i.e. walking and running).

7.4.3. Tomb type

The built tombs had the lowest rates of osteoarthritis, IVDD and entheseal changes. These are the most elaborate types of tombs known from these time periods at Knossos and they have been associated with the Roman colonists or Latin incomers due to the tomb form being new on Crete in the Early Roman period and a Latin inscription on one of these tombs at Knossos (Grammatikaki 2004). It may also be the case that some local elites adopted some new burial customs and use of Latin but whether migrant or local, it appears that the occupants of these built tombs from the Imperial Roman period generally had a more non-labouring life than other inhabitants of the city in the same time period or those in either the preceding or succeeding periods.

The cist, pit and tile graves tend to have the highest levels of joint disease and entheseal changes, though with the small sample size the tile grave results are a little erratic and unreliable. For osteoarthritis and IVDD the osteotheke results are also amongst the highest, alongside these simpler tomb forms, and the chamber tomb entheseal change results show comparably high levels to those of the simpler (pit, tile and cist) graves. The pit and tile graves of the Hellenistic and Early Roman periods are the simplest tomb types known from Knossos. It appears that the occupants of these graves tended to have quite high levels of joint disease and entheseal changes, which is likely to indicate that they had more physically taxing lifestyles than the majority of individuals being buried in more architecturally-complex tombs. The cist grave results are particularly elevated by the Krevatina grave, which is discussed further in Section 7.4.4.

The Late Antique osteotheke results are the third highest of any tomb type for both osteoarthritis and IVDD, and the Schmorl's node and entheseal change prevalences are relatively low. In each case, the osteothekai had the largest and most reliable sample size of any tomb type. As age is an important factor in the manifestation and expression of joint disease Figure 7.30 is included to demonstrate the percentage of Old and Middle adults coming from each tomb type. Too few individuals were recorded in the Old Adult category (n=18) to use this alone. The osteothekai have the largest number of the Middle and Old adults (n=30) from the assemblage, though this is a relatively small percentage of all adults. Although age affects both joint disease and entheseal changes, the numbers of older adults could go some way towards explaining the high levels of joint disease.

The chamber tombs had fairly low levels (below the means for the entire assemblage) of osteoarthritis, IVDD and Schmorl's nodes, but had a very high prevalence of entheseal changes (and of those, a substantial proportion of prominent changes). This would suggest that potentially the joint disease is less influenced by activity than entheseal changes or that other variables are more influential in the

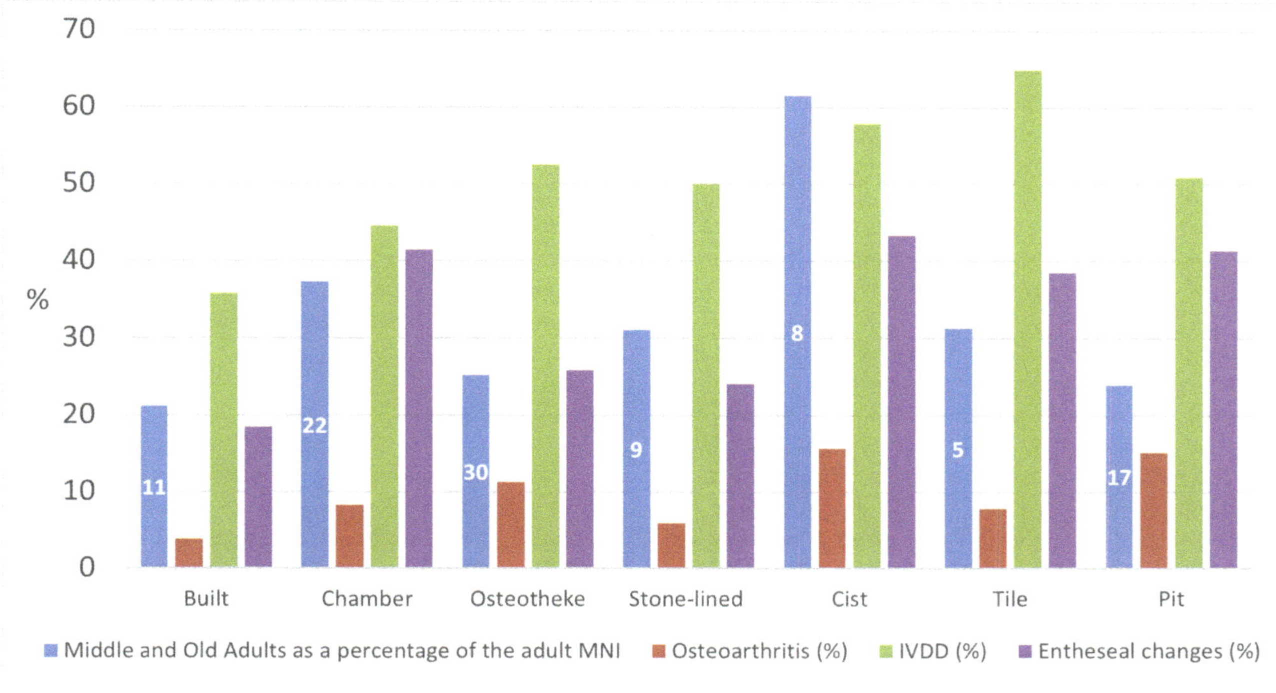

Figure 7.30. Old and Middle adults as a percentage of the MNI for each tomb type (labelled with the total number of Old and Middle Adults), in comparison with the levels of osteoarthritis (Figure 7.9), IVDD (Figure 7.18) and entheseal changes (Figure 7.28).

manifestation of either joint diseases or entheseal changes in this situation.

The low levels of osteoarthritis and entheseal changes in the stone-lined tombs, with middling results for the vertebral pathological conditions, indicates that these too, like the built tombs (though later in date), had occupants with a fairly inactive lifestyle. There were ornamental elements to some of these graves, including several *opus signinum* floors, the *opus Alexandrinium* covering of KSM Tomb 8 with a hole cut through a marble cover slab with a Late Minoan black steatite bowl inset for libations and marble veneering. The inclusion of glass vessels and silver and gold jewellery in a few tombs is also noteworthy in a time period known for a scarcity of grave goods. They were also large and built with substantial, dressed stone slabs and the association of many of these tombs (those from the Sanatorium cemetery) with the later basilica church is discussed further in Section 7.4.4. There were also built mausolea, a funerary enclosure, tile graves and pit graves in this cemetery. This diversity of tomb architecture could demonstrate that the common feature of the cemetery was religion rather than social status or wealth. Nevertheless, the level of tomb elaboration alongside the lack of joint disease and entheseal changes, suggests that the people being buried in these stone-lined tombs had experienced a relatively inactive life, without manual labour, and are likely to have been of quite a high level of social standing within the Knossos community.

It may seem obvious that different social groups of a population would have different activity patterns and therefore manifest different levels of joint disease, but not all populations are as diverse or hierarchical as they are likely to be in a large urban centre. At Isthmia, the uniformity in joint disease across the population was interpreted as depicting "a socially and economically homogenous community… in which the physical activities of agrarian survival were not differentiated by social class" (Rife 2012, 428). This is a very different picture to that which emerges from the Knossos results, which show significant differences in physical activity levels between different social groups, demonstrative of a large, hierarchical society and necessary for a functioning and successful economy at a major urban centre.

7.4.4. Cemetery (location)

There is only one cemetery for the Hellenistic period, but in a comparison with the Roman North Cemetery, the Hellenistic North Cemetery has higher incidences of osteoarthritis, IVDD and entheseal changes. This is consistent with the pattern noticed between the Hellenistic and Roman periods in general (Section 7.4.1).

For the earlier Roman period (1st–2nd centuries), the Topana cemetery (one built tomb) had the lowest prevalence of osteoarthritis, IVDD and entheseal changes (ignoring the Sanatorium 0% IVDD, based on the small sample size). The Roman Monastiriako Kephali rock-cut chamber tomb cemetery had the highest levels of osteoarthritis and entheseal changes, though the North Cemetery had slightly higher IVDD. Although the Monastiriako Kephali cemetery had the highest osteoarthritis prevalence, the only significant difference was with the Topana group. It was more a case of the Topana tomb having a remarkably low prevalence of osteoarthritis than any discernible patterns by wider cemetery group or region (north or south) of the city. Additionally, there were no significant differences between the IVDD results for these cemeteries.

The two Late Roman cemeteries (the Krevatina cist grave (Unit 105) and Sanatorium cemetery) produced very different (statistically significant) results, with very high levels of osteoarthritis, IVDD, and entheseal changes in the Krevatina grave, and low levels of each condition in the Sanatorium cemetery. No detail is known of the construction of the Krevatina cist grave, whether it was a substantially built or a simpler stone-lined construction, though its location was in a non-traditional burial area, that had been settlement until the earlier Roman period. Although the small sample size (MNI=4) may be the cause of the extent to which the results are elevated, they are consistently high across each of the conditions recorded in this chapter. This grave also produced one of the three examples of DISH (often associated with a high-status diet). This demonstrates how equating high levels of joint disease and entheseal changes with low social status, and the presence of DISH with high social status is a gross over-simplification. However, the Sanatorium cemetery produced very low levels of osteoarthritis, IVDD, and entheseal changes and there are indications of the individuals interred there having a certain prestige or high social status due to elements of tomb construction (Sections 3.4 and 7.4.3) and the fact that the later basilica appears to have been deliberately positioned to be associated with the earlier cemetery (Frend and Johnston 1962, 188).

For the Late Antique period, the majority of burials are from the North Cemetery, with only one other tomb from the Monastiriako Kephali area (KOP/79, Unit 108). With the majority of the Late Antique North Cemetery tombs being osteothekai, the discussion of this cemetery is fairly similar to that for the osteothekai in Section 7.4.3. The osteoarthritis and IVDD results are quite high, while the prevalence of entheseal changes is much lower relative to the other cemetery samples. The Late Antique Monastiriako Kephali (KOP/79) individual had significantly lower levels of osteoarthritis, higher levels of IVDD (because some degree of the disease was recorded in most of the individual's vertebrae) and slightly lower levels of entheseal changes. The KOP/79 tomb is a single, primary burial, and to the south-west of the settlement, while the North Cemetery burials are multiple, largely secondary interments (to the north of the settlement), and it therefore makes for an interesting comparison. It could be speculated that a single burial in a substantial stone-lined tomb could represent a higher status individual with a more inactive lifestyle, and that the large osteothekai of the North Cemetery represented a more standard burial type for the majority of the population, that would have included those with a more physically-demanding lifestyle. However, this interpretation is made to fit the results, which for the KOP/79 tomb cannot be taken to be representative of the burial type, tomb form or location. Additionally, it could be argued that the osteothekai are also substantial built or stone-lined tombs and the secondary burial requires an added process that demonstrates extra care and attention, or ceremony, by the living towards the dead, which can sometimes be an indication of status (see Section 3.4).

7.5. Conclusions

It seems likely that the changes in activity patterns observed across time from the prevalence of joint disease and entheseal changes in the skeletal assemblage are reflective of the societal groups represented in the skeletal material for each time period more than gross changes in the levels of manual labour being carried out across the population for each time period. However, it is also possible that the presence of these groups of differing activity levels in cemeteries close to the settlement represents changes in the composition and hierarchy of society. The idea of a more established urban elite in the Roman period may have meant that those involved in physical labour, particularly farm workers, may have moved away from the city or may simply have been buried further away from the city to make way for the conspicuous built tombs (mausolea) known largely from the north of the city and the rock-cut chamber tombs in the hillsides around the south of the valley. It seems likely that the Hellenistic assemblage represents a group of lower social status engaged in manual labour and buried in simple, unadorned graves. The difference in joint disease and entheseal changes between the Roman and Late Antique assemblages appears to represent a gradual transition from Imperial times into the later Roman period and through to the 7th century AD. The increase in joint disease alongside the reduction in population and a reduction in investment (of time, energy or wealth) in burials may represent a return to a more subsistence level of living.

It is important not to be overly simplistic in the interpretation of high rates of joint disease and entheseal changes as equating to low status individuals. There are high status pursuits that can involve heavy physical work, such as riding or hunting. Even sitting can cause large amounts of pressure on the lumbar spine (Nachemson 1966; van Deursen *et al.* 1999; Lengsfeld *et al.* 2000), though this explanation does not really extend to many other parts of the body, nor is there any distinctly different pattern observed for the lumbar joint diseases in the assemblage. Additionally, the multifactorial aetiology of osteoarthritis, IVDD and entheseal changes means that there are always other influences at work on the manifestation of lesions that must be factored into a consideration of the meaning of prevalence patterns.

The relationship between activity and joint disease is of course more complex than has generally been depicted in the comparison of the subgroups of the assemblage. In modern populations, age and obesity are two of the main causes of osteoarthritis, alongside activity. Osteoarthritis can occur in those who are inactive and obesity has been found to significantly affect the occurrence of osteoarthritis in the hands and knees (Grotle *et al.* 2008). Obesity is unlikely to have been a contributing factor on the prevalence of osteoarthritis in any premodern population. Referring to Chapter 4 on the demography of the assemblage, the majority of adults fall into the Young Adult age category and although the Hellenistic period had fewer adults in the Middle or Old Adult categories (see Section 4.3.2) than either the Roman or Late Antique periods, there were no significant differences in the adult age distribution of the assemblage across the time periods. Therefore, insofar as can be determined from the ageing data available for the assemblage, the different categories being compared had a similar age distribution.

Trauma is another analysis that is often included in this sort of study of activity and the link between social status and biological status (Robb *et al.* 2001; Bourbou 2005). This is due to the assumption that those involved in physical occupations are more likely to experience broken bones or other traumatic lesions from falls, or sharp or blunt force impacts (e.g. from farming equipment or weapons). There were so few incidences of trauma recorded in the Knossos assemblage that this analysis could not have added any meaningful results to the discussion of changes in activity and lifestyle across the time periods or between sub-groups of society at Knossos.

The majority of lesions on both joint surfaces and entheses in the assemblage were quite minor. Although most individuals did not live long enough for these joint and entheseal changes to be severely debilitating, the higher levels among certain groups of lower social standing or wealth are likely to have led to a harder life for these people, both due to the fact they were tasked with physical labouring and from the resultant effects of joint disease.

The analysis of joint diseases and entheseal changes as indicators of activity in the assemblage have enabled changes to be identified between the three time periods and within the Roman period for different groups of society. As with the previous analyses, there seems to have been a more dramatic transition from the Hellenistic to Roman period and a more gradual process of change into Late Antiquity. There were more significant differences between males and females than were observed in the dietary analyses, indicating a division of labour between the sexes. The lower prevalence of joint diseases and entheseal changes in the Roman period has been interpreted as an absence of the majority of manual labourers in the assemblage and the differences in these conditions between the different tomb types and cemetery locations supports the idea of a more hierarchical society in this time period with a more established urban elite. This is likely to have been implemented by the establishment of the colony and the presence of the colonists but there was probably also a local elite group, which would be supported by the diversity of tomb types in this time period, as well as the precedence of Greek over Latin in private inscriptions at the site (Baldwin Bowsky 2004b).

8

Development

8.1. Introduction

The investigation of childhood development within the assemblage is conducted using bone lengths and stature estimation. Adult long bone lengths are determined by growth processes during childhood development, including interruptions to growth caused by disease and malnutrition and 'catch-up' growth that occurs afterwards. Stature can be estimated from bone lengths to make different bones comparable, increasing the sample available across the different variables for the comparison of childhood growth. Other methods for the assessment of development could include the analysis of enamel hypoplasia, Harris lines of interrupted growth in long bones using radiographs, and skeletal indicators of diseases caused by malnutrition such as rickets or scurvy. The condition of the material did not lend itself to a systematic investigation of development at a palaeoepidemiological level using any of these methods.

Enamel hypoplasia would have been the most promising and informative alternative method but there are problems with recording lesions across the complete growth phase in damaged, worn and isolated teeth (Hillson 2014, 176). In teeth with wear, only an incomplete sequence can be recorded as the earliest developmental stages of the crown are lost to occlusal wear. Surface wear or polishing of the enamel means that even when observing the teeth microscopically lesions or delays in the laying down of enamel (larger gaps between perikymata) cannot be seen clearly the whole length of the tooth crown. There is also the question of where the threshold should be for the diagnosis of defects in terms of its size and visibility either by the eye or under the microscope. Hypoplastic defects are part of a continuum from microscopic to highly visible and certain parts of the crown are less likely to produce a prominent defect than others (Hillson 2014, 177). Particularly in areas of the tooth where the perikymata are more densely packed (towards the CEJ [cementoenamel junction]) growth disruptions cannot be identified using the standard approach of observing linear enamel hypoplasia with the naked eye (Hassett 2014, 463). This requires the use of scanning electron microscopy of high resolution epoxy resin casts (as enamel is translucent and diffracts the beam and therefore does not allow the perikymata to be clearly viewed). This is a highly time-consuming method which means a relatively small proportion of the assemblage can be analysed in comparison with simple surface observation techniques. Additionally, in commingled material where teeth are often loose and isolated, only the growth sequence of a single tooth can be traced rather than the growth of the whole dentition with matching lesions identifiable in neighbouring teeth.

Stature estimation techniques were developed in forensic anthropology for personal identification of human remains for individuals of known height. However, in archaeological contexts the purpose tends to be an assessment of development and nutrition. Growth is sensitive to environmental conditions and therefore final stature attained can act as an indicator of developmental conditions. Adequate nutrition is required to provide the energy for growth and in cases of insufficient nutritional intake, growth is retarded and stature measurements are smaller (Stinson 2012). Episodes of infectious disease can also impair growth either by impairing the absorption of nutrients, causing a reduction in food intake due to a change in energy needs, or via other mechanisms (Stephensen 1999; Mays 2016). The relationship between stature and nutrition is a net rather than gross measure. This means that not only does it reflect the balance in the growth account in light of the net nutritional conditions during that individual's growth years but can also reflect the conditions during their parents' and even grandparents' lives (Fogel *et al.* 1983, 450). The best evidence of this is the secular change during the 20th century with improvements in socioeconomic conditions resulting in gradually increasing heights (Bielicki 1986; Hoppa and Garlie 1998; Papadimitriou *et al.* 2002; Myburgh *et al.* 2017). However, stature is strongly controlled by genetic factors (McEvoy and Visscher 2009) and must therefore be investigated at a population level, rather than a comparison of individuals, controlling for the normal genetic variation in the range of statures. In controlling for the main variable in this way, the impact of nutrition and disease on the population, or any sub-group within it, can be assessed by comparing average values for groups in the population.

There are a number of ways to estimate living stature from human remains. If supine, articulated and undisturbed, the skeleton can be measured in the grave. This approach is flawed as it depends on precise positioning of the body and a complete lack of disturbance. The Fully method is often lauded as the most accurate method, as it involves measuring the height of the skull, vertebrae, femur, tibia, talus and calcaneus and entering these lengths into an equation which accounts for the thickness of the soft tissue between the bones (Fully 1956; Raxter *et al.* 2006). This method removes a great deal of the margin of error from the estimate but requires high level of preservation with all of the aforementioned bones in perfect condition. The most common method used in archaeological contexts therefore employs the separate measured lengths of single long bones and regression equations, which work on the assumption that there is a strong correlation between the length of each limb bone and an individual's stature. Similar equations have also been developed for segments of long bones but there is a much poorer correlation with stature than for complete long bones (Steele 1970; Simmons *et al.* 1990). In addition to long bones, metacarpals and metatarsals also have lengths which correlate with stature (Musgrave and Harneja 1978; Byers *et al.* 1989; Meadows and Jantz 1992; Ibrahim *et al.* 2017). This is a slightly weaker correlation than for long bones but as these smaller bones of the hands and feet have a much greater tendency to survive intact, the methods that have been developed to estimate stature from these bones have proved to be very useful with more fragmentary material.

Linear regression equations provide the best estimate for one measurement from another when the relationship between them is relatively simple. For stature estimation they work on the assumption that there is a strong correlation between the length of a bone and an individual's overall stature. These equations were originally developed using skeletal collections where individuals' actual living stature measurements were independently known. The most commonly used stature equations were calculated by Mildred Trotter and Goldine Gleser (Trotter and Gleser 1952; 1958; Trotter 1970; Trotter and Gleser 1977) working with the Terry Collection at Washington University (now housed at the Smithsonian Institute's National Museum of Natural History). This consisted of 1728 American 'Negro'[23] and American 'White' males and females, with ages-at-death ranging from 14 to 102 years (largely 20–80 years), and year of birth ranging from 1828 to 1943 (Hunt and Albanese 2005). The statures of the cadavers, which were largely unclaimed individuals from the local St Louis hospitals and morgues and donated to the medical school by the state, were measured after death and before embalming. In the case of the military personnel, stature was measured at the time of induction into military service. This collection was large enough to create sex- and race-specific equations that should give reliable stature estimates within each group and standard errors to indicate the level of accuracy.

The techniques are not without flaws, as the correlation between bone length and stature is not perfect and there are a number of variables affecting stature. The relationship between the measurement of a bone and the measurement of stature is not the same between individuals or even among different bones of the same body. An individual's stature, when estimated from the lengths of different bones within the body (demonstrated later in Section 8.4.3 by the KOP/79 individual), can vary by as much as 13cm (Ousley 1995, 769; Byers 2016, 242). Therefore, when using linear regression equations to calculate stature from a bone length, accuracy will vary between individuals and different bones within a single individual are likely to give different stature estimates (Ousley 2012). Two individuals with the same estimated stature (for example, the same length of femur) could in reality have had quite different measured statures from each other. However, the differences between the predicted stature (regression line) and actual stature follow the expectation of 'random errors' or normal variation and show which bones have a higher correlation with stature and using the same reference group for estimating stature removes any bias of the equation as it will be the same for all the estimates (Ousley 2012).

Stature estimation has been a standard feature of biological anthropology studies in Greece since the emergence of the discipline, but raw bone lengths tend not to be reported. The majority of these studies merely report stature means without considering the socioeconomic impact on stature or using the data for any further discussion. A selection of studies which present stature estimates for comparable assemblages of proximate geographic and temporal contexts are presented in Table 8.1. This demonstrates that the sample sizes tend to be small and the reporting of the number of individuals or bones that estimates are based on is often poor. It is also not always made clear which method has been used for stature estimation. A small number of studies have considered the socio-economic factors affecting final adult stature attained by individuals, including the Agelarakis and Agelarakis (1989) palaeopathological study of an assemblage from Middle and Late Byzantine Abdera in Northern Greece and Kron's studies of health, nutrition and living conditions in the Greco-Roman world in relation to wider considerations, such as agriculture and the economy (Kron 2005; 2012; 2018). Kron's comparison of Ancient Greek and Roman stature estimates with those reported for early modern and modern populations found that Greeks and Romans generally enjoyed better nutrition than all but the most developed modern societies (Kron 2005, 75). The present study aims to interpret the stature results from Knossos to reflect how the changing conditions in the city impacted on the living conditions, health and development of the population, thus reflecting on the nature and scale of the changes.

Though this is a study of developmental conditions, there are variables besides nutrition and disease affecting bone lengths and stature. As mentioned previously, these include genes, sex, race, geographic origins and environmental characteristics. Approximately 50 genes and regions of the genome are known to be involved in controlling stature and the pattern and pace of growth, with hundreds or possibly even thousands of further, smaller effects still unknown within the genome. Based on heritability, stature is thought to be c. 80% controlled by genes, with the remainder controlled by environmental conditions, including diet and disease exposure (McEvoy and Visscher 2009). The impact of disease on stature is also partially genetically controlled. Sex is a determining factor of stature and although there will always be an overlap in the stature of females and males in a population, the male average stature is always taller than that of the females. This variable

[23] These studies were conducted at a time when studies of 'race' were considered an important aspect of physical anthropology. The terminology is often outdated and is only used here to clarify, in reference to the source, which equations are being employed. Terms of 'race' are therefore quoted in inverted commas.

Table 8.1. Stature estimates for males and females from comparative sites and time periods. Where the study states which method was used for stature estimation, it has been noted. T&G 'w'= Trotter and Gleser American 'Whites', and it is assumed but not specified that Trotter 1970= Trotter and Gleser American 'Whites' formulae.

Site	Time period	Male mean (cm)	n	Female mean (cm)	n	Study	Method
Greece (various)	Early Iron	166.7	42	155.1	53	Bisel & Angel 1985	Trotter & Gleser 'w'
Greece (various)	Classical	170.5	52	156.2	30	Bisel & Angel 1985	Trotter & Gleser 'w'
Athens	Classical	165.6	3	155	1	Angel 1945	unknown
Greece (various)	Hellenistic	171.9	23	156.4	20	Bisel & Angel 1985	Trotter & Gleser 'w'
Sounion	Hellenistic	167.4	1			Angel 1945	unknown
Corinth	Hellenistic-Roman	165.8	4	148.3	5	Fox 2005	Eliakis *et al.* 1966
Paphos (Cyprus)	Hellenistic-Roman	171.1	9	155.9	7	Fox 2005	Eliakis *et al.* 1966
Greece (various)	Imperial Roman	169.2	18	158	19	Bisel & Angel 1985	Trotter & Gleser 'w'
Kerameikos, Athens	Roman	172.6	2	153.6	2	Lagia 2000	T&G 'w' as modified by Krogman and Iscan 1986
Athens	Roman	163.6	2	157.2	4	Angel 1945	unknown
Lerna Hollow, Corinth	Late Roman	170	3	160	1	Wesolowsky 1973	Trotter & Gleser 'w'
Gortyn, Crete	Early Byzantine	172.8	18	160.1	6	Mallegni 1988	Trotter & Gleser 'w'
Eleutherna, Crete	Early Byzantine	169	52	160	21	Bourbou 2004	Trotter 1970
Messene	Early Byzantine	170	23	150	12	Bourbou 2004	Trotter 1970
Kefali, Crete	Early Byzantine	165	8	148	2	Zygouri 2005	Trotter 1970
Aliki, Thasos	Early Byzantine	162		150		Buchet & Sodini 1984	Trotter 1970
Kastella, Crete	Middle Byzantine	161	2	154	2	Bourbou 2006; 2009	Trotter 1970
Stylos, Crete	Middle Byzantine	166	3			Bourbou 2003; 2009	Trotter 1970
Polystylon, Abdera	Middle-Late Byzantine	168		156		Agelarakis & Agelarakis 1989	Trotter & Gleser 'w'
Greece (various)	Byzantine Medieval	169.6	98	156.2	43	Bisel & Angel 1985	Trotter & Gleser 'w'

is controlled by investigating the sexes separately using sex-specific formulae. Stature formulae have traditionally been developed for specific racial groups. The relationship between bone lengths and stature varies by population, based on genetic and environmental differences between populations, therefore different regression equations are required. Differences have also been observed between geographically defined populations, even over relatively small distances, which may also be due to genetic differences or environmental issues, primarily disease incidence and nutrition (McEvoy and Visscher 2009, 300). For example, males born in Portugal in the 1970s were on average 11cm shorter than their Danish contemporaries, with the Portuguese females 6cm shorter than their Danish counterparts (Garcia and Quintana-Domeque 2007). It is difficult to distinguish whether genetic or environmental factors are more responsible for this sort of variation and the two are not mutually exclusive as genetic variants can determine the body's response to the environment, such as an episode of disease or how efficiently the body can process certain foods.

A population approach enables groups within the population to be compared using summary statistics (mean, standard error, degrees of freedom, standard deviation and 95% confidence intervals). As the population comes from a single site there is a degree of control over geographic and genetic variables. Just as stature has been used in modern populations as a measure of socio-economic living conditions and wellbeing, the aim of this analysis is to identify such differing conditions for people living at Knossos across the Hellenistic, Roman and Late Antique periods, with their differing social, economic and political contexts, and between different social groups within the population.

8.2. Methodology

8.2.1. Bone Lengths

Complete long bones (humerus, radius, ulna, femur, tibia and fibula), metacarpals and metatarsals were measured in order to assess developmental conditions. The long bones were measured as maximum lengths according to the descriptions given by Trotter and Gleser (1952, 472–73), including for the femur and tibia for which bicondylar and 'ordinary' lengths respectively are also described. The metacarpals and metatarsals were measured as interarticular lengths, from the apex of the capitulum to the midpoint of the articular surface, except for the fifth metatarsal which was measured to include the styloid process, according to the methods outlined in Section 8.2.2 for stature estimation (Musgrave and Harneja 1978; Byers *et al.* 1989). Measurements were taken using sliding calipers for the shorter bones (metacarpals and metatarsals) and a tape measure lain flat on the table was used for the longer bones of the limbs in the absence of an osteometric board available.

The assessment of bone lengths has to be conducted separately for each bone type and different bone types are not comparable, but this avoids the biases that occur in stature estimations. The results for bone lengths are presented as summary tables of descriptive statistics for each variable, including the mean, 95% confidence intervals, standard deviation, sample size (n), standard error of the mean (calculated from the standard deviation and sample size), and a Shapiro-Wilk normality test. These descriptive statistics were calculated for each variable using SPSS. Bone lengths are plotted for the categorical variables as stacked histograms, showing the number of bones (frequency) of each length and a normality curve. As well as the histogram normality curves, normality of the sample distribution is tested using the Shapiro-Wilk statistical test and the supporting check of Q-Q plots (included with the descriptive statistics in SPSS but not presented). This enables the assessment of whether it is reasonable to suggest that the sample is random and therefore representative of the population. The mean (dot) and 95% confidence intervals (whiskers) are presented as error bar plots for a clear comparison of the mean bone lengths for each categorical variable. If the confidence intervals of two mean values do not overlap a t-test for equal means is applied to confirm whether the difference was statistically significant. It was attempted to assess bone lengths separately for the sexes but due to the problems the bilateral metric sex estimation (Section 8.2.3) caused to the data distribution normality, they were also assessed with the sexes combined (see results in Section 8.3 for further descriptions of data problems).

8.2.2. Stature estimation

Due to the mixture of different types of bones measured and some bones being poorly represented, or not represented at all, for certain variables, stature estimates were employed as a secondary stage. This enables a greater sample size as all the measured bones are comparable on the same scale.

For the long bones the Trotter and Gleser (1952) regression equations for 'White' males and 'White' females were used as these have previously been deemed to be the best match for 'Caucasian' or European populations (Stewart 1979). Though it is not ideal to use standards based on a temporally and geographically distant population, appropriate reference collections or assemblages for developing such methods are extremely rare. The measurements were recorded in millimetres but were converted to centimetres for these equations. The equations employed are outlined in Table 8.2.

Table 8.2. Regression equations used for long bones for females and males, with measurements and standard errors (SE) in centimetres (Trotter and Gleser 1952; Trotter 1970).

Females	SE	Males	SE
3.36 Hum + 57.97	4.45	3.08 Hum + 70.45	4.05
4.74 Rad + 54.93	4.24	3.78 Rad + 79.01	4.32
4.27 Ulna + 57.76	4.30	3.70 Ulna + 74.05	4.32
2.47 Fem + 54.10	3.72	2.38 Fem + 61.41	3.27
2.90 Tib + 61.53	3.66	2.52 Tib + 78.62	3.37
2.93 Fib + 59.61	3.57	2.68 Fib + 71.78	3.29

Table 8.3. Regression equations used for each metacarpal (right and left) for females and males, with measurements and standard errors (SE) in centimetres (Musgrave and Harneja 1978).

Female	SE	Male	SE
2.25 LMet1 + 65.62	7.21	1.69 LMet1 + 94.76	5.49
2.61 LMet2 – 3.10	5.58	1.06 LMet2 + 100.06	5.79
2.25 LMet3 + 22.71	6.59	1.12 LMet3 + 98.21	5.82
2.26 LMet4 + 36.89	7.66	1.29 LMet4 + 96.86	5.79
2.27 LMet5 + 45.97	8.14	1.17 LMet5 + 109.35	6.30
1.16 RMet1 + 110.29	5.54	1.75 RMet1 + 92.04	5.80
1.35 RMet2 + 74.61	4.70	1.24 RMet2 + 88.13	5.84
1.29 RMet3 + 80.26	4.73	1.26 RMet3 + 88.80	6.01
1.35 RMet4 + 85.94	4.98	1.45 RMet4 + 87.19	5.95
1.52 RMet5 + 83.17	4.72	1.36 RMet5 + 99.38	6.20

The metacarpals were measured and regression formulae applied following the Musgrave and Harneja (1978) method. This method was developed from measuring the interarticular length of the metacarpals using sliding callipers from radiographs and the lengths adjusted to compensate for enlargement during the radiography process. The individuals were predominantly 'White' British citizens who were admitted to the Bristol Royal Infirmary with hand injuries. This study measured the bones interarticular length directly (i.e. not from radiographs) using sliding callipers. Different equations were developed and have been applied according to side and sex and are presented in Table 8.3. The original measurements, recorded in millimetres, were adjusted to centimetres for these equations.

Metatarsal lengths were also used for stature estimation following the method outlined by Byers *et al.* (1989). This method was developed using 66 skeletons from the Terry Collection at the Smithsonian Institute and 64 from the University of New Mexico's Maxwell Museum of Anthropology of known age, sex and race. Lengths were measured from the apex of the capitulum to the midpoint of the articular surface for the first to fourth metatarsals and both the functional and maximum (including tuberosity/styloid process) lengths for the fifth metatarsals. This study used the maximum length for the fifth metatarsal due to the greater ease of taking the measurement (rather than deciding on the midpoint of the articular surface) and as

Table 8.4. Regression equations used for each metatarsal for females and males, with measurements and standard errors (SE) in millimetres (Byers *et al.* 1989).

Female	SE	Male	SE
656 + 16.3 (Met1)	49.6	768 + 15.2 (Met1)	63.2
712 + 12.8 (Met2)	52.0	868 + 11.3 (Met2)	70.1
732 + 13.3 (Met3)	57.5	862 + 12.0 (Met3)	68.9
719 + 13.8 (Met4)	57.5	863 + 12.3 (Met4)	68.5
905 + 10.6 (Met5)	64.9	912 + 11.2 (Met5)	70.3

the standard errors for these equations were smaller. The equations for 'Euro-American' females and males were used as detailed in Table 8.4. Measurements and standard errors are in millimetres.

8.2.3. Sex estimation

As with all the other analyses the lack of age and sex information attributable to the majority of elements, due to their commingled state, poses a problem not only for the interpretation of bone lengths and stature but also for the process of estimating stature using sex-specific regression equations. There are methods for estimating sex from bone metrics and these have therefore been employed solely for this analysis. These methods are problematic as there is a great deal of overlap in stature and bone lengths of males and females. Using these measurements to estimate both sex and stature results in the average male stature being over-estimated (as any shorter male 'outliers' will be assumed to be female and the female regression formula applied) and the average female stature being under-estimated (due to the taller female 'outliers' being assumed to be male and the male regression formula being used). In situations where there was associated morphological sexing information associated with a measured bone, this overrode the metric sexing assessment. To determine the sex of the metacarpals and metatarsals the methods of Manolis *et al.* (2009) and Mountrakis *et al.* (2010) respectively were used. A clear cut-off point was employed half-way between the male and female mean values, without an indeterminate group or any cross-over. Though this is not a realistic separation of males and females, as there will always be an overlap in stature, it enabled the largest number of bones to be included for stature estimation. Without employing metric sex determination, only 21 bones, with sex determined morphologically from associated skull and pelvis traits, would have been available for analysis.

Sex was determined for the humeri and femora from measurements of the diameter of the head according to the method of Stewart (Stewart 1979), based on the Terry collection. The sex determination for the tibiae and fibulae was calculated in the same way as the metacarpals and metatarsals, by using a female-male cut-off point half way between the female and male maximum length means using the raw data from the Terry Collection Postcranial Osteometric Database (https://anthropology.si.edu/cm/terry.htm). These are not ideal standards to use, as the Terry Collection 'whites' group is made up of modern Americans and are therefore temporally and geographically distant but as they have been found to be a relatively good match for past European populations, this was deemed to be the best option to allow for sex-specific metric analysis to be conducted. As the measurements of the radius and ulna do not appear to be strongly sexually dimorphic (Bass 1995, 163, 172), the means of the Knossos radii and ulnae lengths were used as cut-off points to determine whether the male or female stature formulae should be applied.

8.2.4. Methodological problems

Besides the methodological problems discussed in the stature estimation literature generally (outlined by Ousley 2012) and referred to in the introduction (Section 8.1), there are some further issues within this line of analysis that should be mentioned. Different reference populations were used for the different methods used for the long bones, metacarpals and metatarsals which introduces a bias depending on which bone/method/reference collection is being used in each case. This is not a very significant problem considering the different scales of standard error for each bone type. However, it is preferable to use the raw bone lengths in an attempt to avoid the stature estimation problems.

Using metrics for sexing (as well as stature estimation) was necessary as very few measurable bones would have had a sex attributed to them due to the commingled nature of the assemblage. This creates a very divided and assymmetrical picture of females and males in the assemblage. It emphasises the extremes, elevating the male average and lowering the female average. Another issue that arises because of the commingled assemblage is that there are repeated estimations for single individuals from different bones. The extent of this repetition cannot be known.

8.3. Bone Length Results

The results for bone lengths are presented as a summary table of descriptive statistics, including the mean, 95% confidence intervals, standard deviation, sample size (n), standard error of the mean (calculated from the standard deviation and sample size), and a Shapiro-Wilk normality test, followed by stacked histograms with normality curves and error bar plots displaying mean bone lengths. The Hellenistic period is largely absent from the following results and discussion, as there were very few measurable Hellenistic bones. Where any do exist, they are included in the tables and graphs, but generally the sample size was too small even for descriptive statistics.

8.3.1. Time period

8.3.1.1. Humerus

The humerus bone length results are presented in Table 8.5 (descriptive and normality statistics), Figure 8.1 (stacked histograms) and Figure 8.2 (error bar plot). The

Table 8.5. Descriptive and normality statistics for humerus lengths for each sex/time period group.

Humerus Length (mm)				95% Confidence Interval			Shapiro-Wilk (normality)		
	n	Mean	Std. Error	Lower Bound	Upper Bound	Std. Dev.	Statistic	df	Sig. (*p*)
Female Roman	2	280	10.00	152.94	407.06	14.142			
Female Late Antique	10	294	5.434	281.71	306.29	17.185	0.910	10	0.280
Male Roman	9	328	3.711	319.66	336.78	11.133	0.957	9	0.771
Male Late Antique	2	338	17.00	121.99	554.01	24.042			

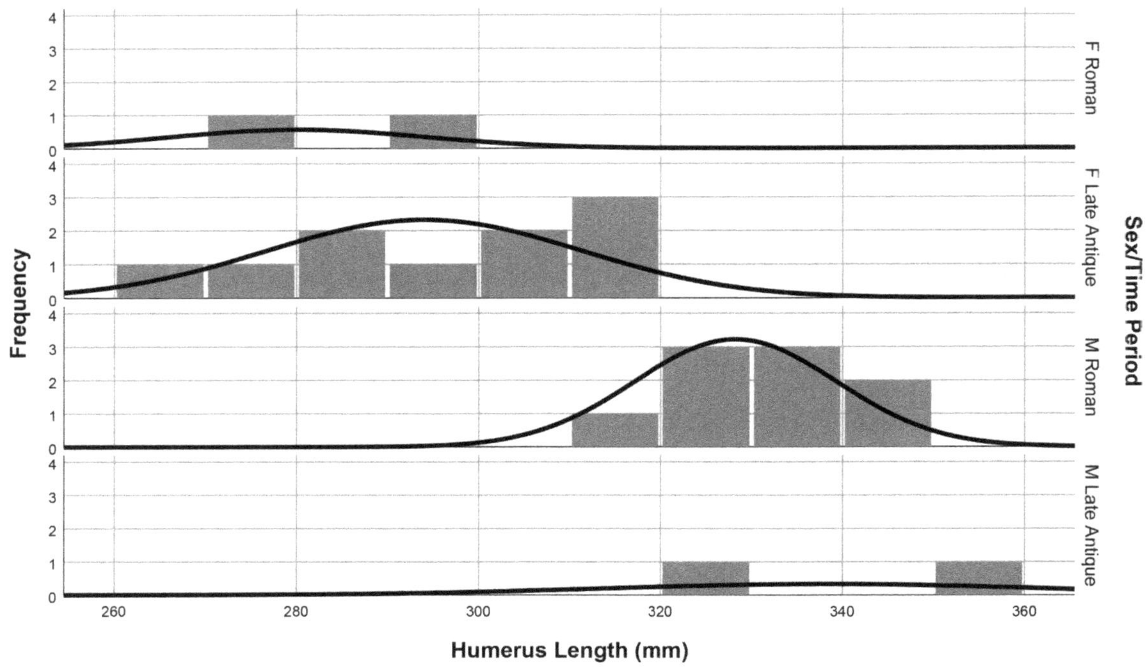

Figure 8.1. Stacked histograms showing the frequency of humerus lengths for each sex/time period group and including a normality curve to demonstrate expected values.

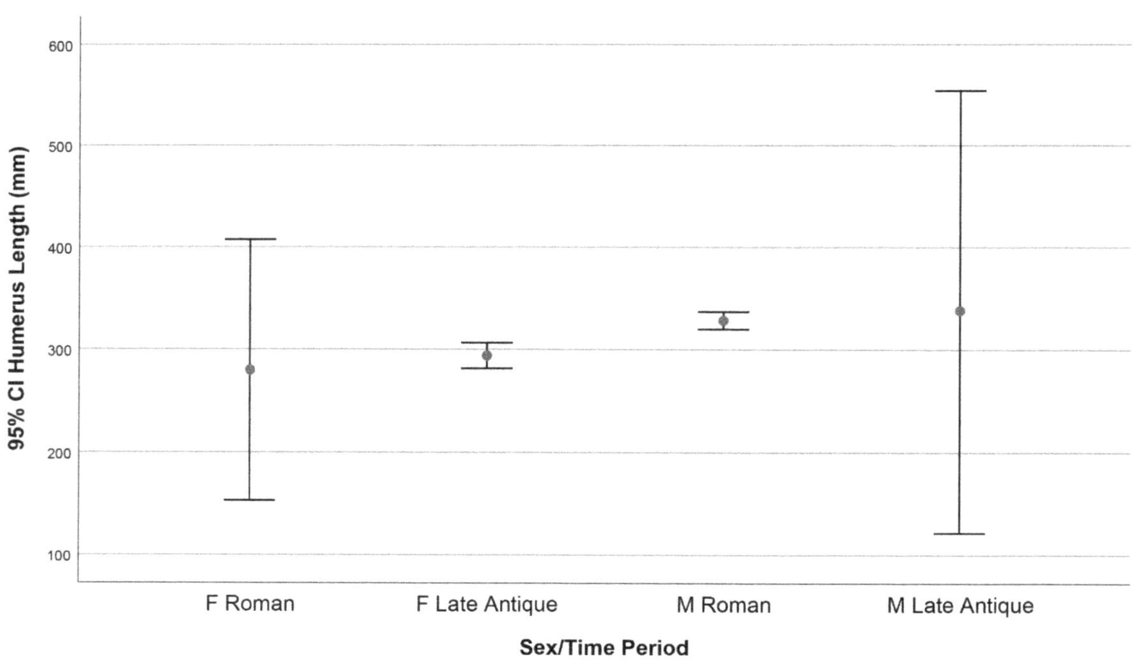

Figure 8.2. Error bar plots demonstrating mean humerus lengths for each sex/time period group, with 95% confidence intervals.

sample sizes, particularly for the Female Roman and Male Late Antique groups, are too small to allow for any comparison to be made or statistics to be assessed. The mean values for both females and males for a comparison of the Roman and Late Antique time periods are very similar with no significant difference. There is sexual dimorphism but this is unsurprising considering sex was generally determined metrically from the diameter of the humeral head.

8.3.1.2. Radius

Except for the Female Late Antique group, the other groups have a quite normal distribution of radius lengths (Shapiro-Wilk $p>0.05$) and could represent a random sample that is representative of the population, although the sample sizes are quite small (Table 8.6). The difference between the time periods for females and males showed the opposite patterns, with the Female Late Antique mean radius length being higher than the Roman mean, while the Male Roman mean radius length was higher than the Male Late Antique mean value (Figures 8.3–4). In both cases however, there was substantial overlap in the 95% confidence intervals, demonstrating no significant difference could be determined in radius lengths between the time periods from this sample.

8.3.1.3. Ulna

The Shapiro-Wilk scores (Table 8.7) suggest that the distribution of ulna lengths for each sex/time period group was strongly normal. However, the normality curves on the histograms (Figure 8.5) demonstrate that due to the very small sample sizes, the randomness and representativeness of these samples cannot be determined. Although the means for both sexes were higher in the Late Antique samples compared to the Roman ones, the 95% confidence interval whiskers in Figure 8.6 show a large degree of overlap suggesting no significant difference in ulna lengths between the time periods.

Table 8.6. Descriptive and normality statistics for radius lengths for each sex/time period group.

Radius Length (mm)				95% Confidence Interval			Shapiro-Wilk (normality)		
	n	Mean	Std. Error	Lower Bound	Upper Bound	Std. Deviation	Statistic	df	Sig. (*p*)
Female Roman	6	208.17	4.246	197.25	219.08	10.400	0.893	6	0.335
Female Late Antique	7	216.57	3.741	207.42	225.72	9.897	0.795	7	0.037
Male Roman	7	255.07	6.205	239.89	270.26	16.418	0.963	7	0.840
Male Late Antique	11	238.27	4.766	227.65	248.89	15.806	0.934	11	0.449

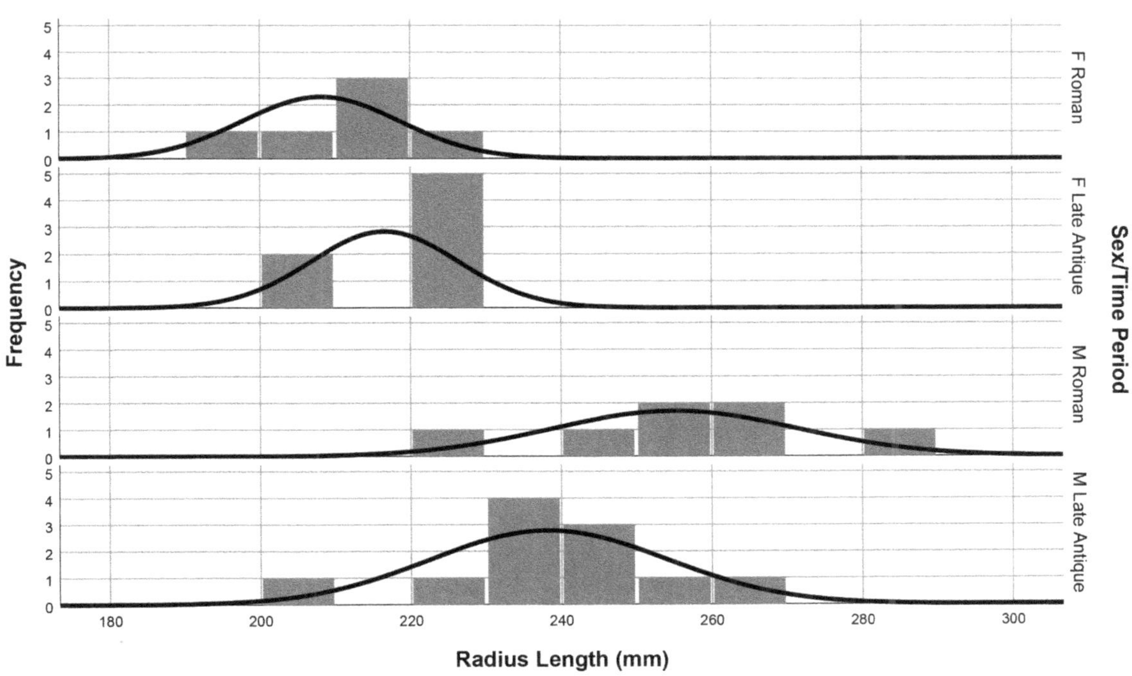

Figure 8.3. Stacked histograms showing the frequency of radius lengths for each sex/time period group and including a normality curve to demonstrate expected values.

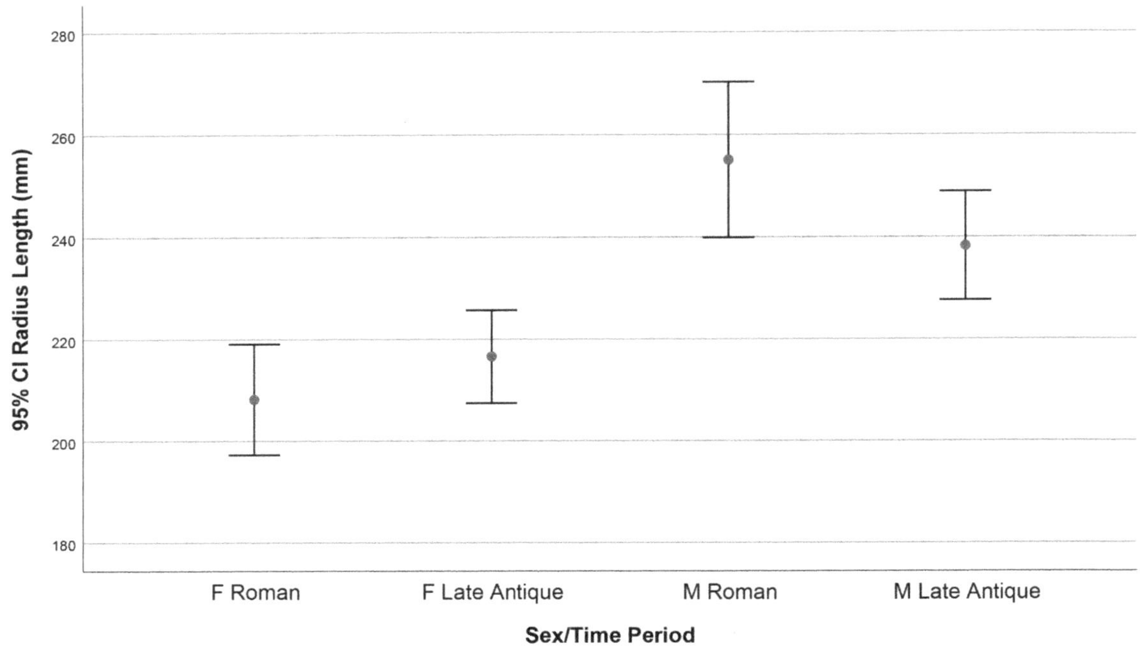

Figure 8.4. Error bar plots demonstrating mean radius lengths for each sex/time period group, with 95% confidence intervals.

Table 8.7. Descriptive and normality statistics for ulna lengths for each sex/time period group.

Ulna Length (mm)				95% Confidence Interval			Shapiro-Wilk (normality)		
	n	Mean	Std. Error	Lower Bound	Upper Bound	Std. Deviation	Statistic	df	Sig. (*p*)
Female Roman	3	222.67	4.096	205.04	240.29	7.095	0.974	3	0.688
Female Late Antique	5	233.20	6.711	214.57	251.83	15.007	0.906	5	0.446
Male Roman	3	266.67	4.485	247.37	285.96	7.767	0.932	3	0.497
Male Late Antique	3	273.00	11.358	224.13	321.87	19.672	0.983	3	0.747

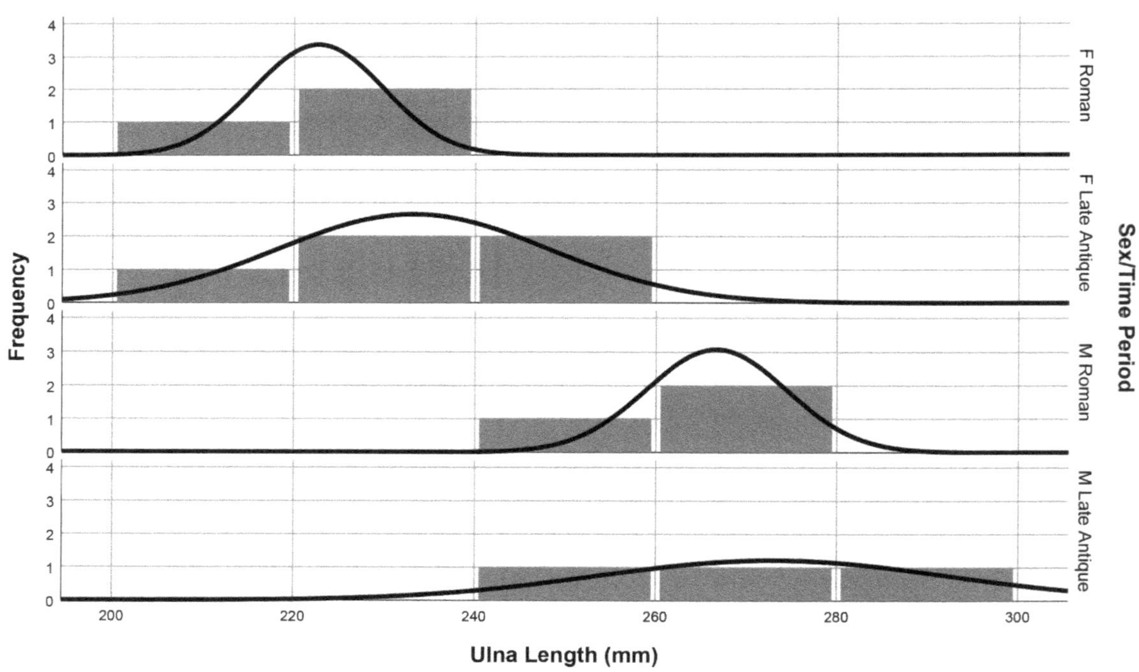

Figure 8.5. Stacked histograms showing the frequency of ulna lengths for each sex/time period group and including a normality curve to demonstrate expected values.

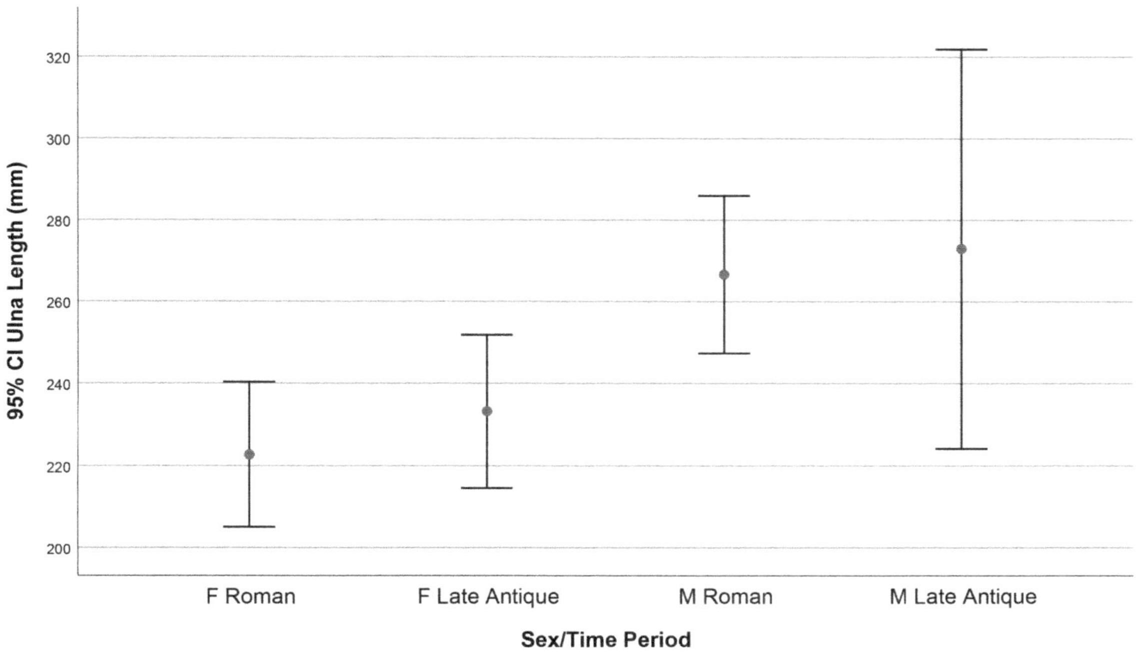

Figure 8.6. Error bar plots demonstrating mean ulna lengths for each sex/time period group, with 95% confidence intervals.

8.3.1.4. Femur

Each sex/time period group has a normal distribution of femur lengths, according to the Shapiro-Wilk test (Table 8.8), but as the sample sizes are small, the normality curves on the histograms show that the bars are not always a very close match to the curve (Figure 8.7). The Hellenistic period is represented in the female group. The female femur lengths show the highest mean value in the Roman period with both the Hellenistic and Late Antique mean femur lengths c.2cm shorter, however, the 95% confidence intervals still have a substantial amount of crossover (Figure 8.8). The comparison of the male groups shows the Late Antique mean to be only marginally lower than the Roman mean value and with very similar confidence interval bounds, there can be no significant difference determined.

8.3.1.5. Tibia

Other than the Female Hellenistic group with a sample size, the tibia has the best sample sizes of the limb bones across the Roman and Late Antique groups, and the Shapiro-Wilk test suggests that these have a normal distribution indicative of a random (representative) sample (Table 8.9). The normality curves on the histograms do, however, show quite a ragged distribution, except for the Male Late Antique lengths distribution which matches the curve most neatly (Figure 8.9). The non-neat and non-normal distributions of these groups was also visible on the Q-Q plots. For both females and males, the Late Antique mean values were lower than the Roman means although only marginally so for the males which demonstrate no significant difference (Figure 8.10). Conducting a t-test to compare the Female Roman and Female Late Antique means produced a mean difference of 18.6mm with 95% confidence intervals of −2.2mm to 39.6mm. As the confidence intervals cross zero, it is unlikely there is any difference in the female tibia lengths between these time periods.

8.3.1.6. Fibula

Unfortunately, the small sample sizes mean that no comparison of fibula lengths by the female or male time period categories are possible. The Hellenistic period had no

Table 8.8. Descriptive and normality statistics for femur lengths for each sex/time period group.

Femur Length (mm)				95% Confidence Interval			Shapiro-Wilk (normality)		
	n	Mean	Std. Error	Lower Bound	Upper Bound	Std. Deviation	Statistic	df	Sig. (*p*)
Female Hellenistic	3	388.33	6.009	362.48	414.19	10.408	0.923	3	0.463
Female Roman	6	409.50	12.943	376.23	442.77	31.703	0.962	6	0.836
Female LA	4	386.63	5.064	370.51	402.74	10.127	0.811	4	0.123
Male Roman	8	447.63	6.887	431.34	463.91	19.478	0.948	8	0.693
Male LA	8	444.13	6.090	429.72	458.53	17.225	0.844	8	0.083

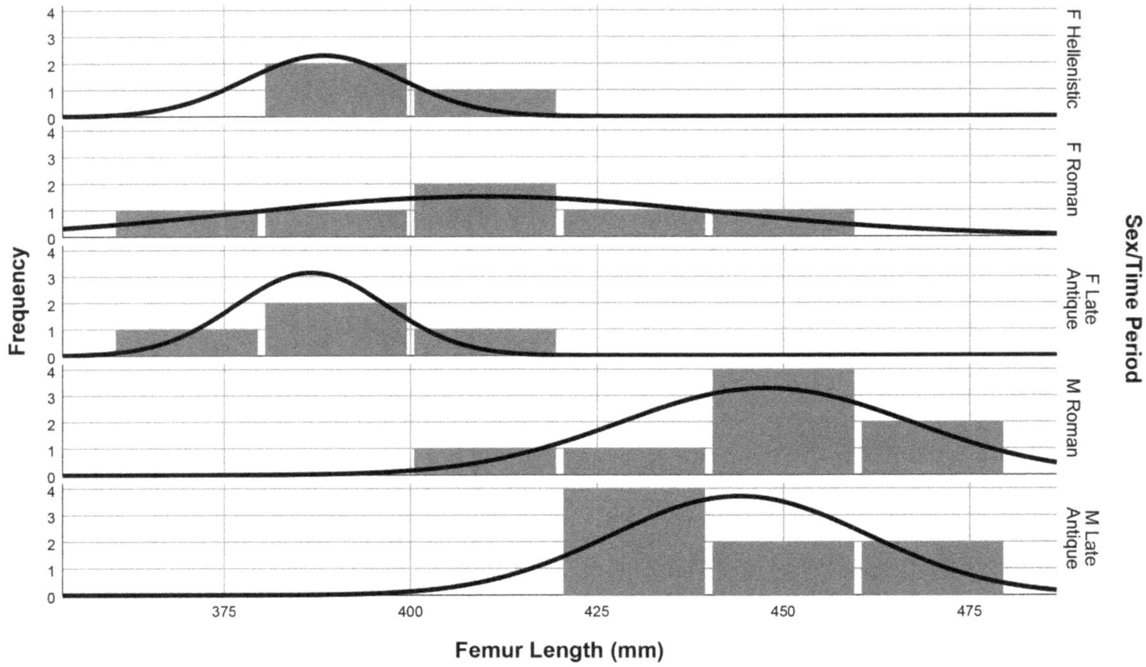

Figure 8.7. Stacked histograms showing the frequency of femur lengths for each sex/time period group and including a normality curve to demonstrate expected values.

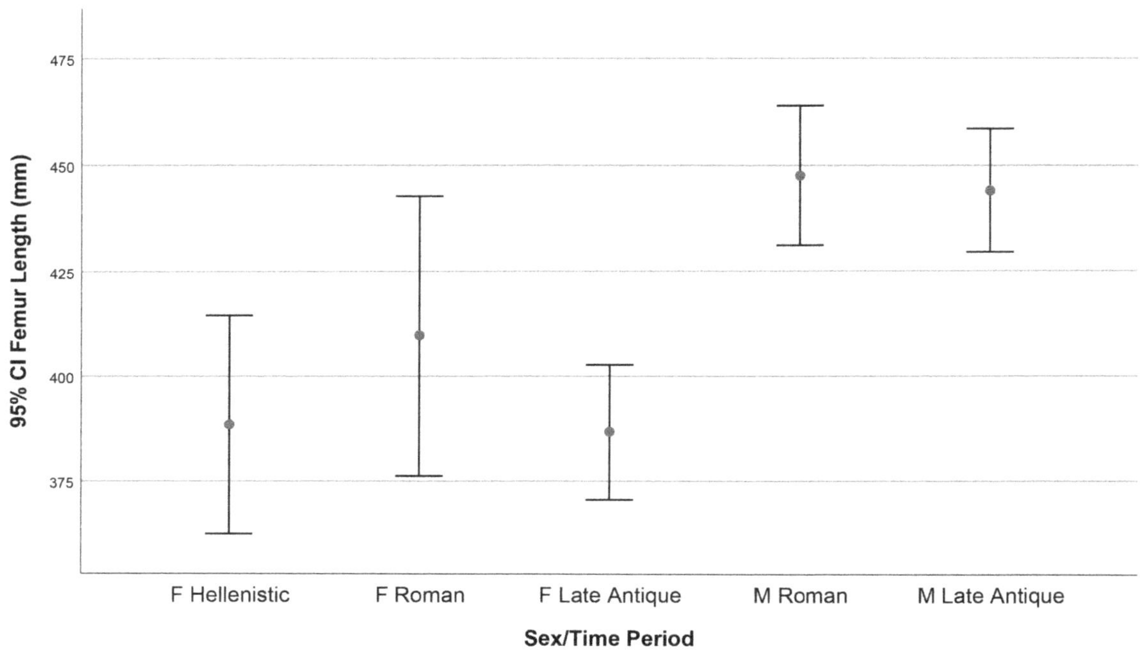

Figure 8.8. Error bar plots demonstrating mean femur lengths for each sex/time period group, with 95% confidence intervals.

Table 8.9. Descriptive and normality statistics for tibia lengths for each sex/time period group.

Tibia Length (mm)				95% Confidence Interval			Shapiro-Wilk (normality)		
	n	Mean	Std. Error	Lower Bound	Upper Bound	Std. Deviation	Statistic	df	Sig. (*p*)
Female Hellenistic	1								
Female Roman	8	352.13	4.984	340.34	363.91	14.096	0.884	8	0.205
Female Late Antique	8	333.50	8.339	313.78	353.22	23.586	0.870	8	0.152
Male Roman	8	382.88	6.261	368.07	397.68	17.707	0.876	8	0.173
Male Late Antique	11	379.09	6.168	365.35	392.83	20.457	0.942	11	0.549

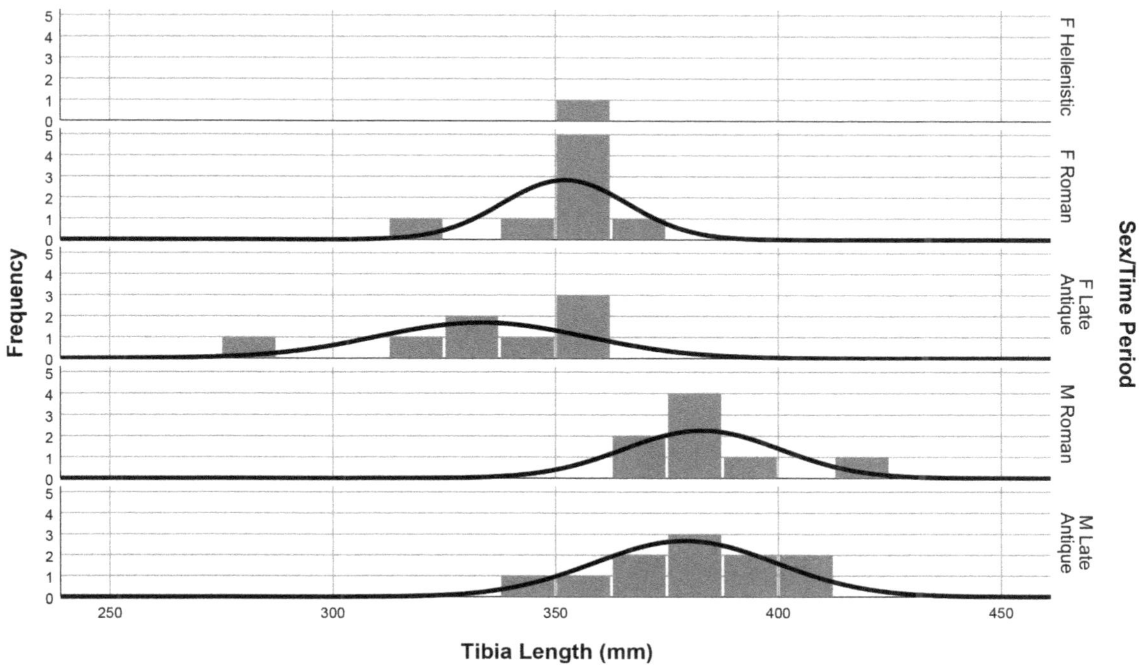

Figure 8.9. Stacked histograms showing the frequency of tibia lengths for each sex/time period group and including a normality curve to demonstrate expected values.

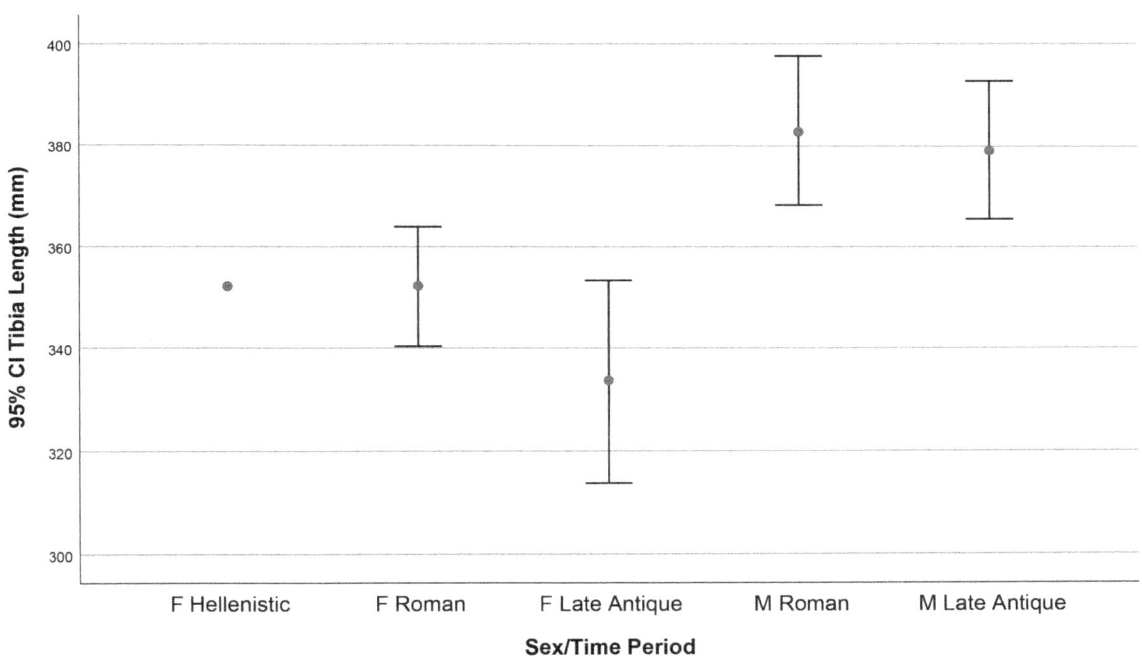

Figure 8.10. Error bar plots demonstrating mean tibia lengths for each sex/time period group, with 95% confidence intervals.

measurable fibulae and the Late Antique groups had only one for each the female and male categories. The available fibula length results are presented in Table 8.10, the histograms in Figure 8.11 and the error bar plot in Figure 8.12.

8.3.1.7. First metacarpal

The metacarpals and metatarsals offer improved sample sizes than the limb bones as they survive complete more readily. Unfortunately, the Hellenistic period remains underrepresented. The results for the first metacarpal by sex/time period group are presented in Table 8.11, as stacked histograms (Figure 8.13), and as error bar plots (Figure 8.14). It is clear from the Shapiro-Wilk tests and histograms that the metacarpal lengths for these groups are not normally distributed. Even the Male Roman group which has a Shapiro-Wilk $p>0.05$, does not match the normality curve very closely in the histogram. The error bar plots demonstrate very little difference between the means of either females or males in a comparison of the Roman

Table 8.10. Descriptive and normality statistics for fibula lengths for each sex/time period group.

Fibula Length (mm)				95% Confidence Interval			Shapiro-Wilk (normality)		
	n	Mean	Std. Error	Lower Bound	Upper Bound	Std. Deviation	Statistic	df	Sig. (*p*)
Female Roman	8	336.25	5.561	323.10	349.40	15.728	0.899	8	0.283
Female Late Antique	1								
Male Roman	4	369.00	5.017	353.03	384.97	10.033	0.706	4	0.014
Male Late Antique	1								

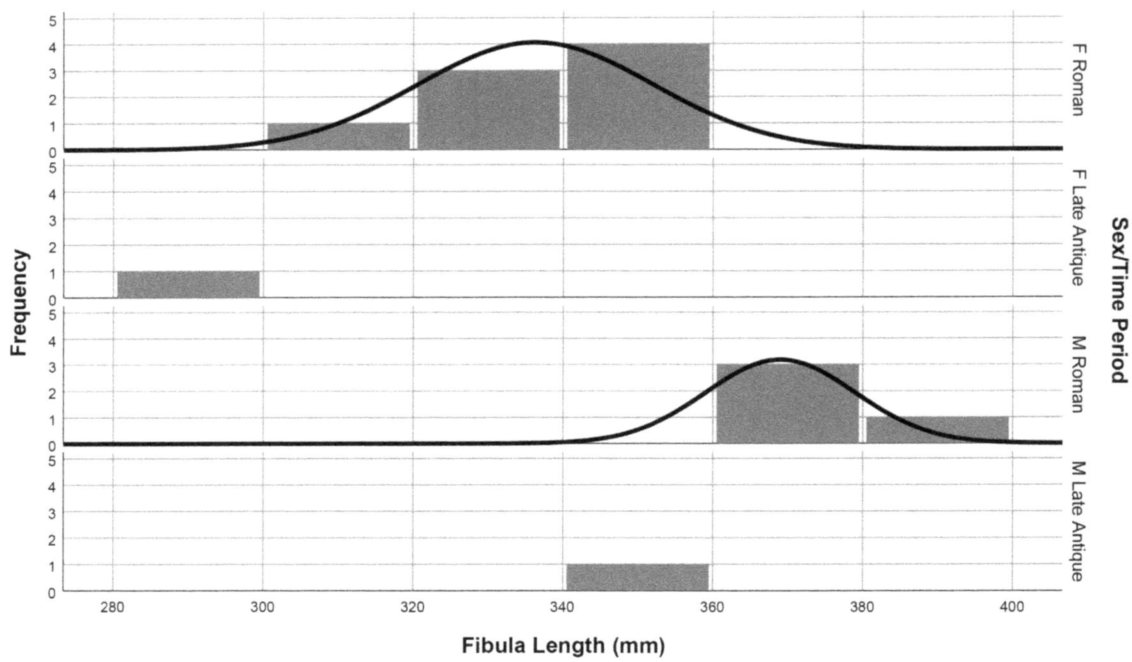

Figure 8.11. Stacked histograms showing the frequency of fibula lengths for each sex/time period group and including a normality curve to demonstrate expected values.

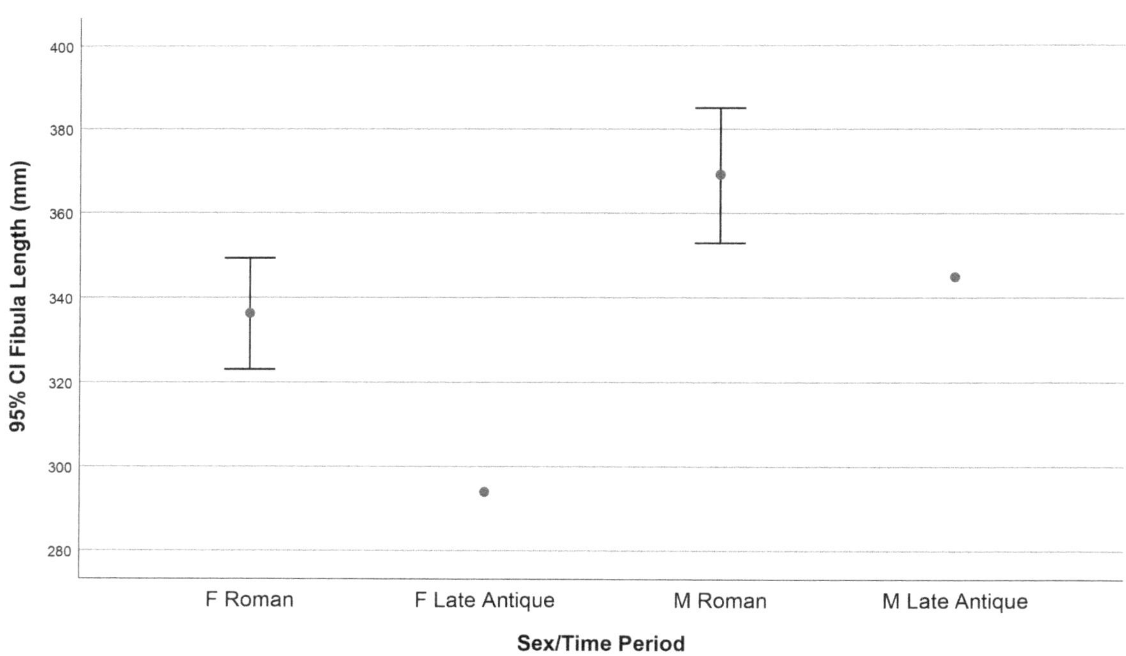

Figure 8.12. Error bar plots demonstrating mean fibula lengths for each sex/time period group, with 95% confidence intervals.

Table 8.11. Descriptive and normality statistics for first metacarpal lengths for each sex/time period group.

First Metacarpal Length (mm)				95% Confidence Interval			Shapiro-Wilk (normality)		
	n	Mean	Std. Error	Lower Bound	Upper Bound	Std. Deviation	Statistic	df	Sig. (*p*)
Female Hell.	1								
Female Rom.	20	41.00	0.334	40.30	41.70	1.496	0.837	20	0.003
Female LA	14	40.50	0.442	39.55	41.45	1.653	0.747	14	0.001
Male Hell.	1								
Male Roman	19	45.89	0.616	44.60	47.19	2.685	0.934	19	0.201
Male LA	34	46.13	0.439	45.23	47.02	2.560	0.912	34	0.010

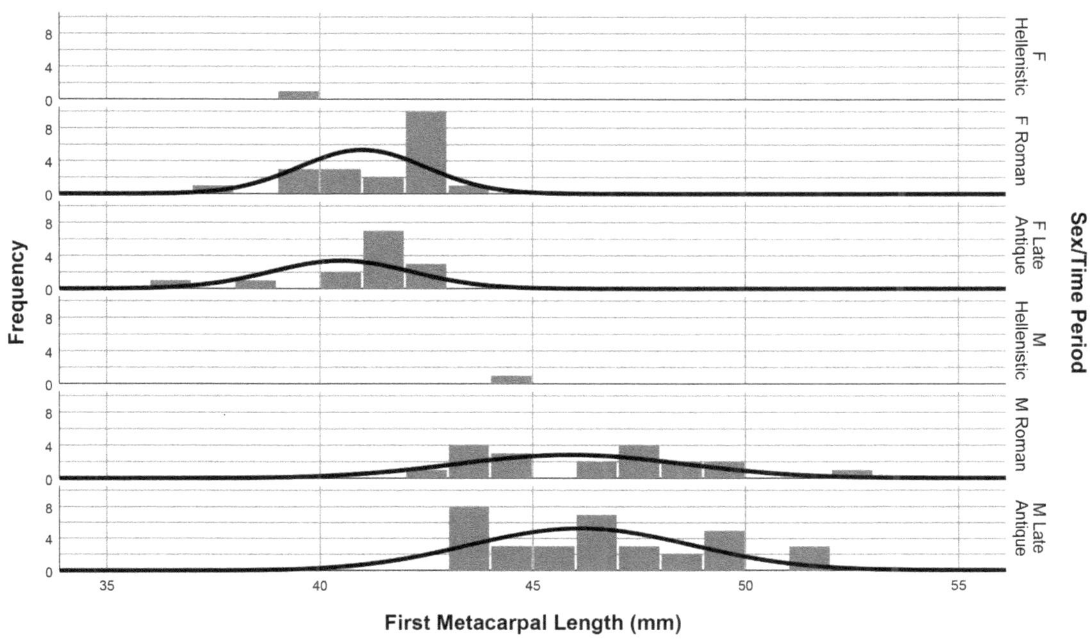

Figure 8.13. Stacked histograms showing the frequency of first metacarpal lengths for each sex/time period group and including a normality curve to demonstrate expected values.

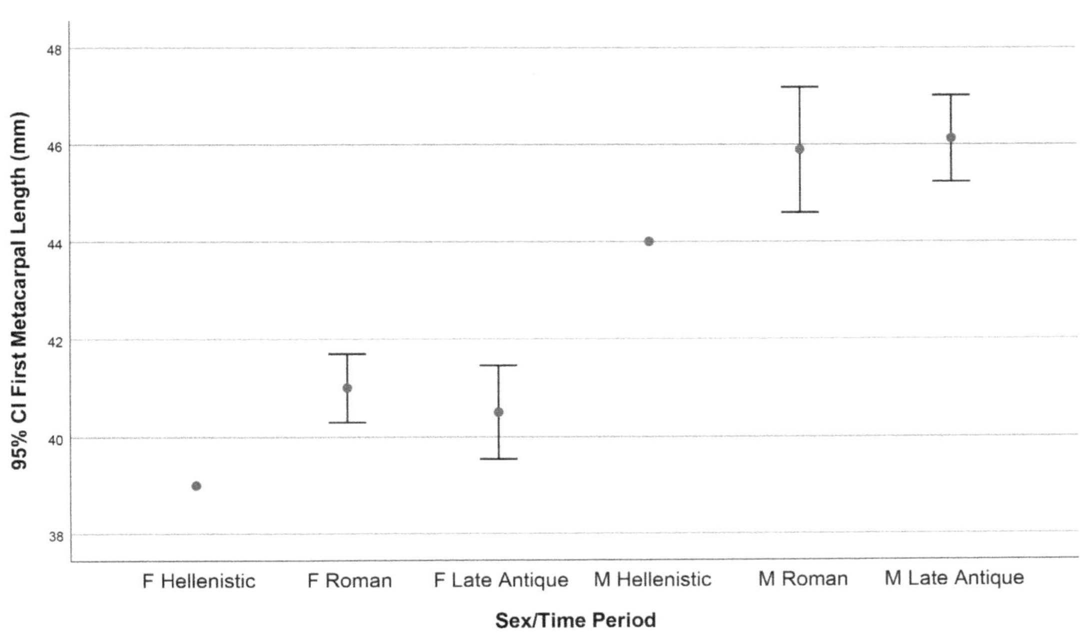

Figure 8.14. Error bar plots demonstrating mean first metacarpal lengths for each sex/time period group, with 95% confidence intervals.

and Late Antique periods with a great deal of overlap in the confidence intervals. This demonstrates no significant difference between these time periods for either sex.

A degree of the asymmetry of these groups may be caused by the metric sexing technique, which causes a problem for the bone lengths as it does for the stature estimations. Bone lengths are biological features that should be normally distributed in one sex of one population. The implication of a Shapiro-Wilk significance less than 0.05 is that the derivation of the material is so non-random that it cannot be taken to represent the population. To exclude the asymmetry caused by the metric sexing technique, the sexes have been plotted together for each time period in stacked histograms and error bar plots for each of the metacarpals and metatarsals to find a normal distribution that is representative of the population (even if not sex-specifically). For this to work as a means of analysing the samples, it requires the assumption that the sexes are equally represented for each variable, which cannot be determined with any certainty.

The metacarpal lengths for each time period (sexes combined) are presented in histograms (Figure 8.15) and as means with confidence intervals (Figure 8.16).

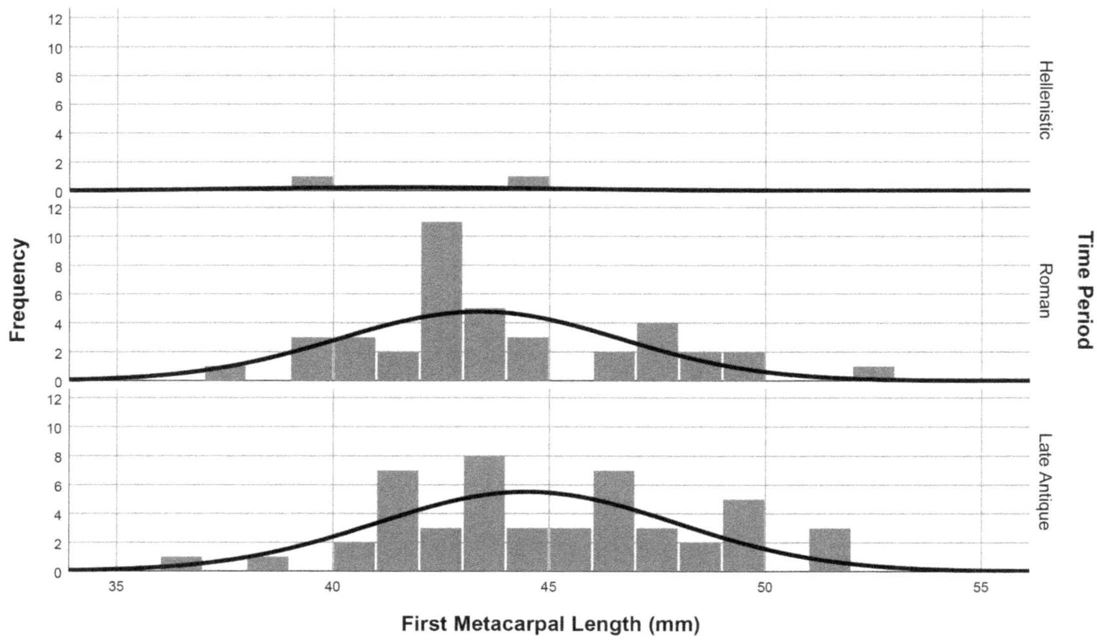

Figure 8.15. Stacked histograms showing the frequency of first metacarpal lengths for each time period group with the female and male values combined and including a normality curve to demonstrate expected values.

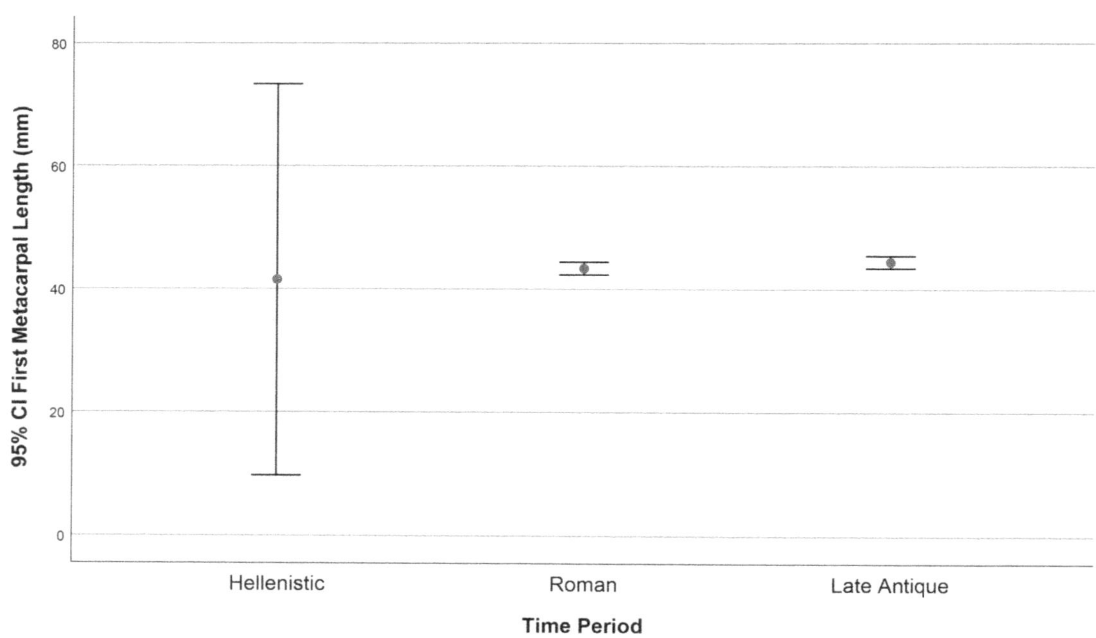

Figure 8.16. Mean first metacarpal lengths with the sexes combined for each time period group with error bar plots demonstrating 95% confidence intervals.

While they appear more symmetrical and normal in their distribution, the histograms are still a little irregular and have a number of outliers. The distribution of first metacarpal lengths for the Roman period falls just below the $p>0.05$ threshold (Shapiro-Wilk= 0.943, df=39, $p=0.046$) and the Late Antique values qualify as plausibly normal (Shapiro-Wilk= 0.972, df=48, $p=0.305$). The means and confidence intervals suggest no difference between the time periods. The Hellenistic result has extremely wide confidence intervals as it is based on only two bone lengths.

8.3.1.8. Second metacarpal

The Female Roman and Female Late Antique groups both have normal distributions of second metacarpal lengths according to the Shapiro-Wilk test, though sample sizes are small (Table 8.12). The histograms for these groups do, however, show low outliers in each case (Figure 8.17). Figure 8.18 displays the means and confidence intervals for these groups and suggests there is no difference in lengths between the time periods for females. The male results are displayed in these same graphs and the Shapiro-Wilk scores do not suggest normal distributions for either the Roman or Late Antique groups. The histograms for the male groups suggest a high degree of asymmetry, with the bars more stacked at the lower end (negative skew). The Male Late Antique mean is higher than the Male Roman mean but there is substantial overlap in confidence intervals.

Due to the asymmetry, the time periods were compared with the sexes combined. Though these histograms did not follow the normality curve perfectly (Figure 8.19), all three time periods had normal distributions: Hellenistic (Shapiro-Wilk= 0.964, df=3, $p=0.637$), Roman (Shapiro-Wilk= 0.935, df=28, $p=0.083$), and Late Antique (Shapiro-Wilk= 0.982, df=43, $p=0.737$). This indicates that these samples could be representative of the

Table 8.12. Descriptive and normality statistics for second metacarpal lengths for each sex/time period group.

Second Metacarpal Length (mm)				95% Confidence Interval			Shapiro-Wilk (normality)		
	n	Mean	Std. Error	Lower Bound	Upper Bound	Std. Deviation	Statistic	df	Sig. (*p*)
Female Hellenistic	2	62.00	2.000	36.59	87.41	2.828			
Female Roman	8	61.06	1.351	57.87	64.26	3.821	0.864	8	0.131
Female Late Antique	14	60.79	0.757	59.15	62.42	2.833	0.877	14	0.053
Male Hellenistic	1								
Male Roman	20	67.48	0.695	66.02	68.93	3.110	0.874	20	0.014
Male Late Antique	29	69.36	0.659	68.00	70.71	3.551	0.922	29	0.034

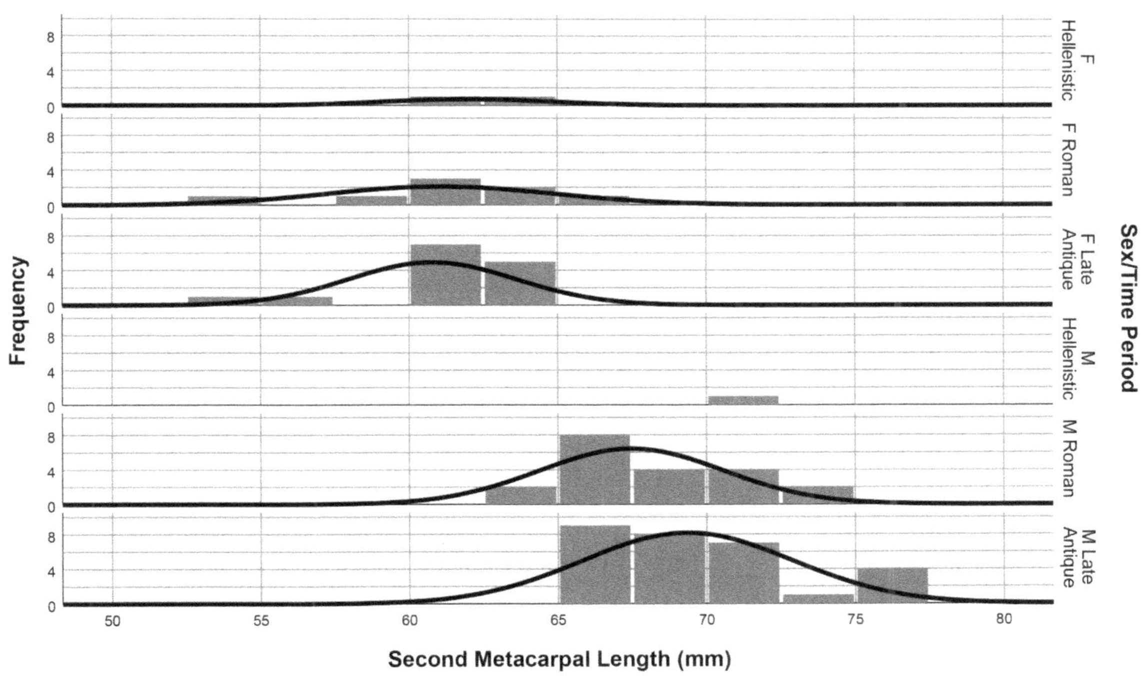

Figure 8.17. Stacked histograms showing the frequency of second metacarpal lengths for each sex/time period group and including a normality curve to demonstrate expected values.

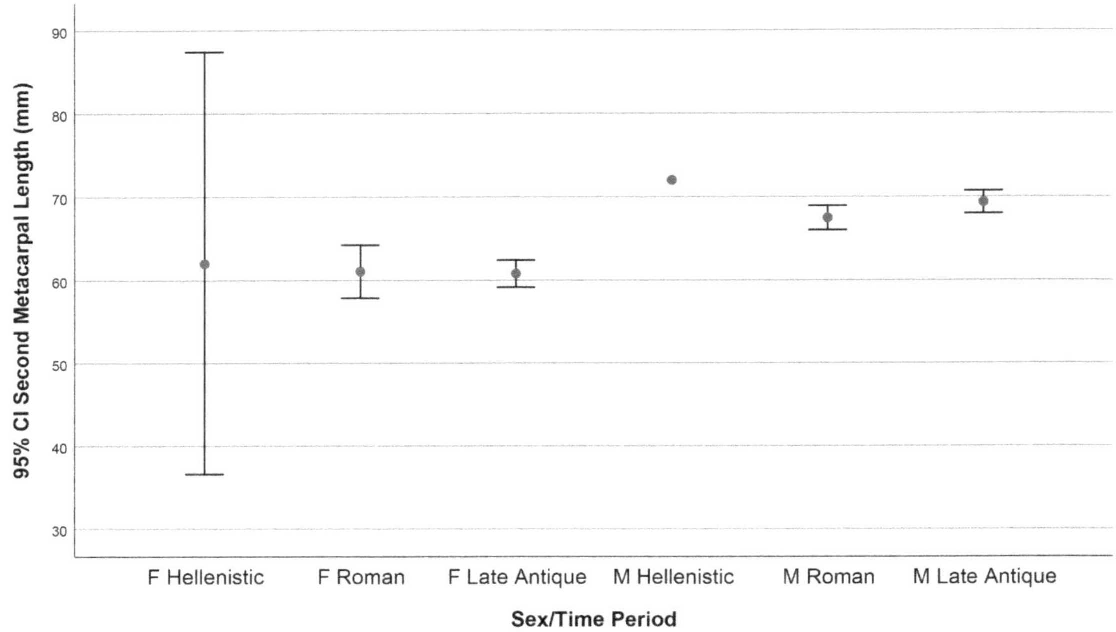

Figure 8.18. Error bar plots demonstrating mean second metacarpal lengths for each sex/time period group, with 95% confidence intervals.

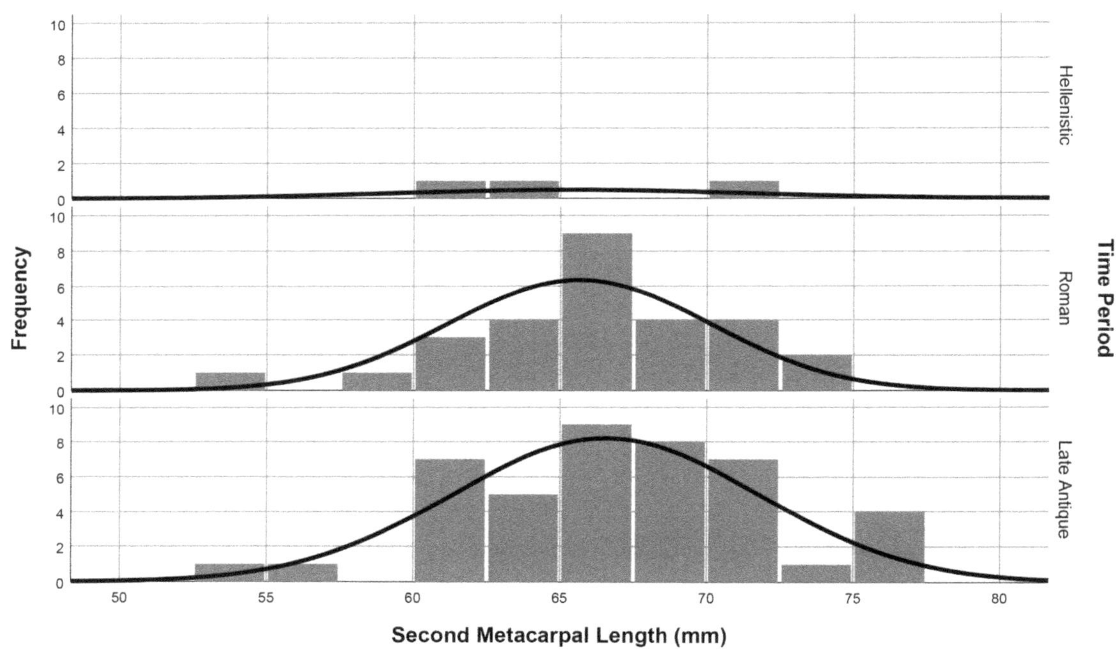

Figure 8.19. Stacked histograms showing the frequency of second metacarpal lengths for each time period group with the female and male values combined and including a normality curve to demonstrate expected values.

population. Figure 8.20 shows very similar means for all three time periods, indicating no significant difference.

8.3.1.9. Third metacarpal

The Female and Male Late Antique groups have Shapiro-Wilk p>0.05 scores suggesting that they could have normal distributions of third metacarpal lengths representing a random sample (Table 8.13). However, the histograms do not have bars that match very closely for any of the categories (Figure 8.21), suggesting it is unlikely these results are representative of the population. The results displayed in Figure 8.22 indicate no significant difference in the means between time periods for either females or males.

As there is asymmetry in some of the Figure 8.21 histograms, particularly in the two female groups, the third metacarpal results were also investigated with the sexes combined for each time period. These produced

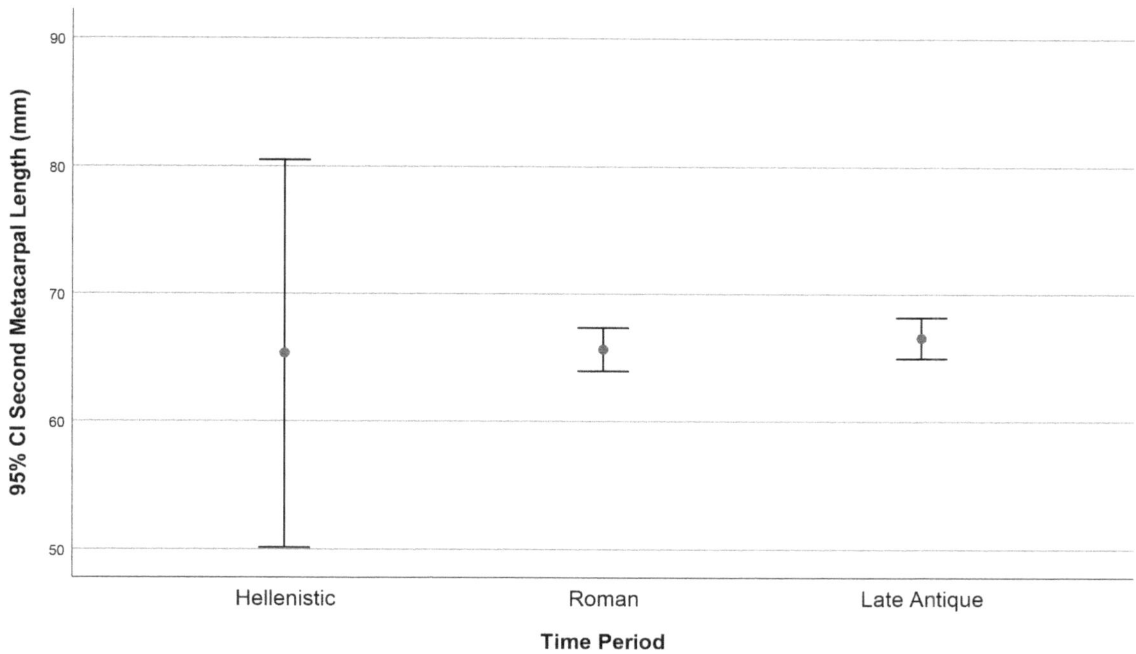

Figure 8.20. Mean second metacarpal lengths with the sexes combined for each time period group with error bar plots demonstrating 95% confidence intervals.

Table 8.13. Descriptive and normality statistics for third metacarpal lengths for each sex/time period group.

Third Metacarpal Length (mm)				95% Confidence Interval			Shapiro-Wilk (normality)		
	n	Mean	Std. Error	Lower Bound	Upper Bound	Std. Deviation	Statistic	df	Sig. (*p*)
Female Roman	22	61.61	0.544	60.48	62.75	2.554	0.896	22	0.025
Female Late Antique	22	61.27	0.447	60.34	62.20	2.097	0.920	22	0.076
Male Roman	23	67.43	0.466	66.47	68.40	2.233	0.903	23	0.030
Male Late Antique	19	68.59	0.556	67.42	69.76	2.423	0.937	19	0.237

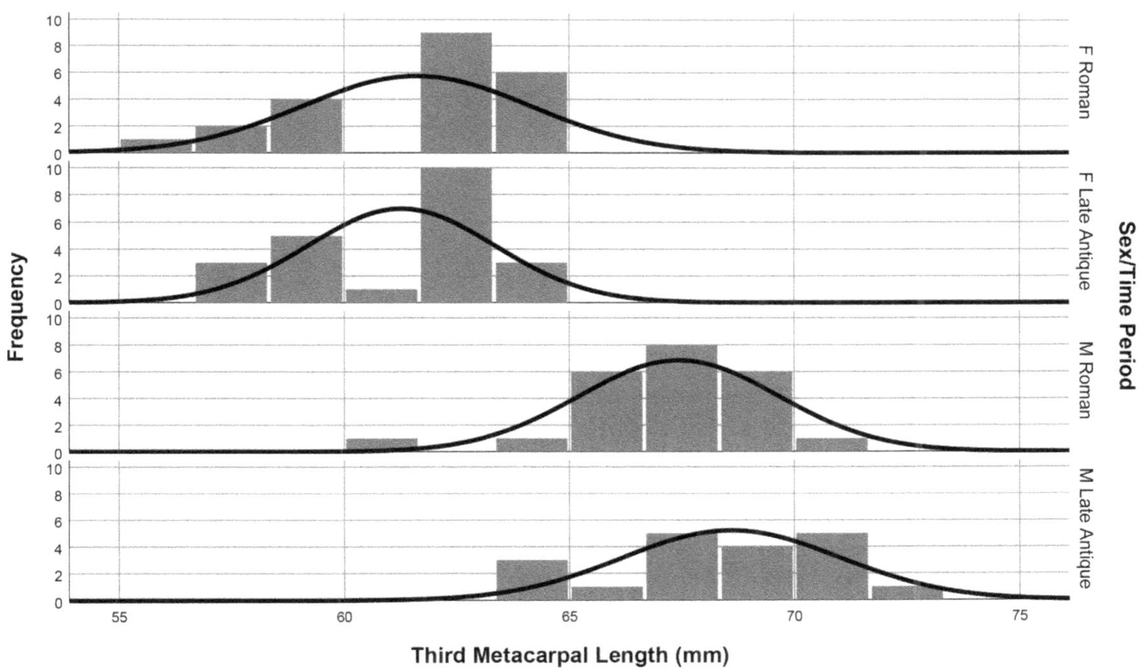

Figure 8.21. Stacked histograms showing the frequency of third metacarpal lengths for each sex/time period group and including a normality curve to demonstrate expected values.

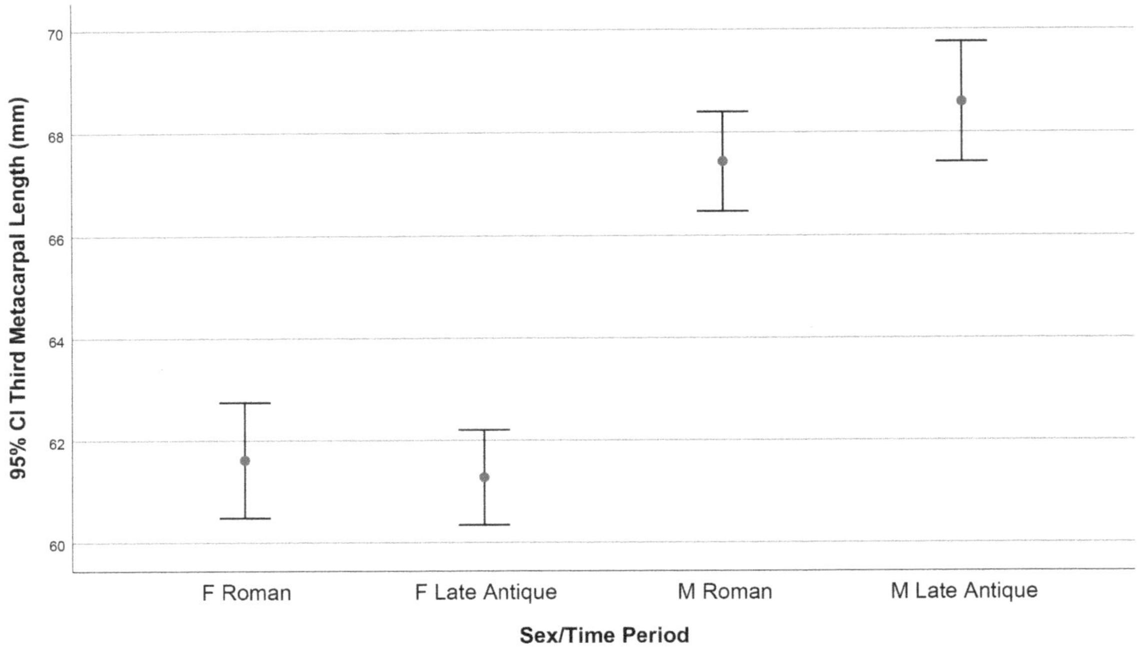

Figure 8.22. Error bar plots demonstrating mean third metacarpal lengths for each sex/time period group, with 95% confidence intervals.

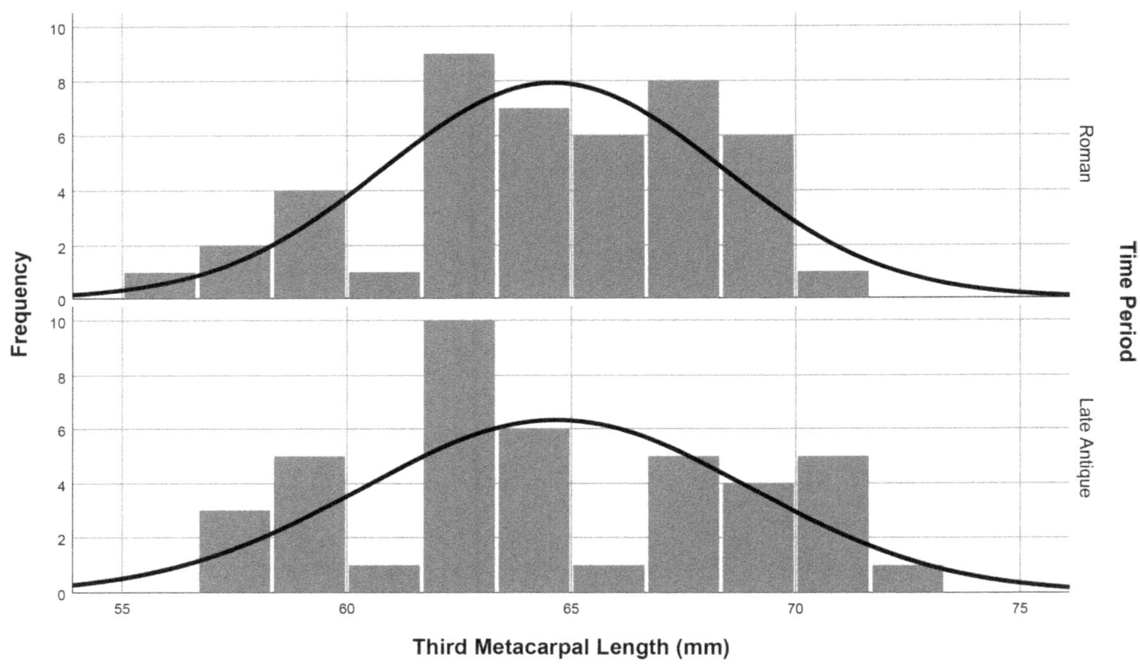

Figure 8.23. Stacked histograms showing the frequency of third metacarpal lengths for each time period group with the female and male values combined and including a normality curve to demonstrate expected values.

somewhat more normal distributions for both the Roman (Shapiro-Wilk= 0.971, df=45, p=0.314) and Late Antique (Shapiro-Wilk= 0.960, df=41, p=0.153) groups, though the normality curve on the histograms (Figure 8.23) displays that the distribution was still quite uneven. However, as a plausibly random sample, it is clear from the mean values and their confidence intervals in Figure 8.24, that there was no difference in third metacarpal lengths between the time periods.

8.3.1.10. Fourth metacarpal

Figure 8.25 shows strongly asymmetrical histograms for the fourth metacarpal lengths by sex/time period category. Except for the Male Late Antique normality result, the other groups had non-normal Shapiro-Wilk distributions (Table 8.14). Therefore, the difference in mean values displayed in Figure 8.26 cannot be taken as representative of the once-living population, which show the Late Antique

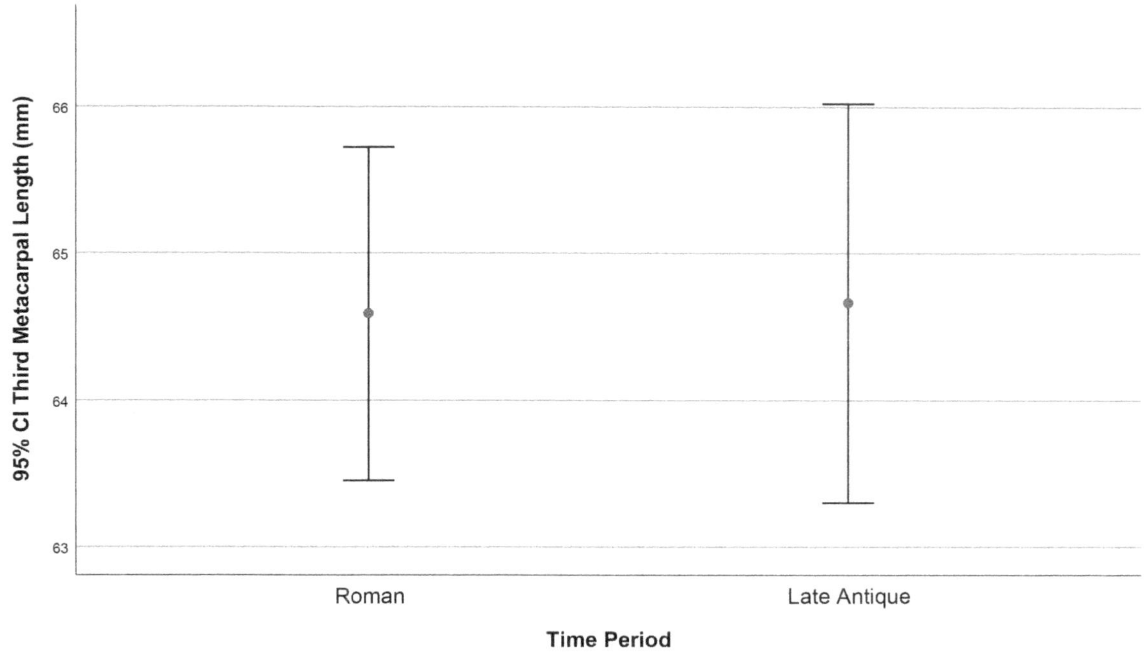

Figure 8.24. Mean third metacarpal lengths with the sexes combined for each time period group with error bar plots demonstrating 95% confidence intervals.

Table 8.14. Descriptive and normality statistics for fourth metacarpal lengths for each sex/time period group.

Fourth Metacarpal Length (mm)				95% Confidence Interval			Shapiro-Wilk (normality)		
	n	Mean	Std. Error	Lower Bound	Upper Bound	Std. Deviation	Statistic	df	Sig. (*p*)
Female Roman	20	51.80	0.622	50.50	53.10	2.783	0.872	20	0.013
Female Late Antique	15	52.81	0.613	51.50	54.13	2.374	0.799	15	0.004
Male Roman	13	57.38	0.488	56.32	58.45	1.758	0.751	13	0.002
Male Late Antique	25	59.36	0.496	58.34	60.38	2.481	0.927	25	0.072

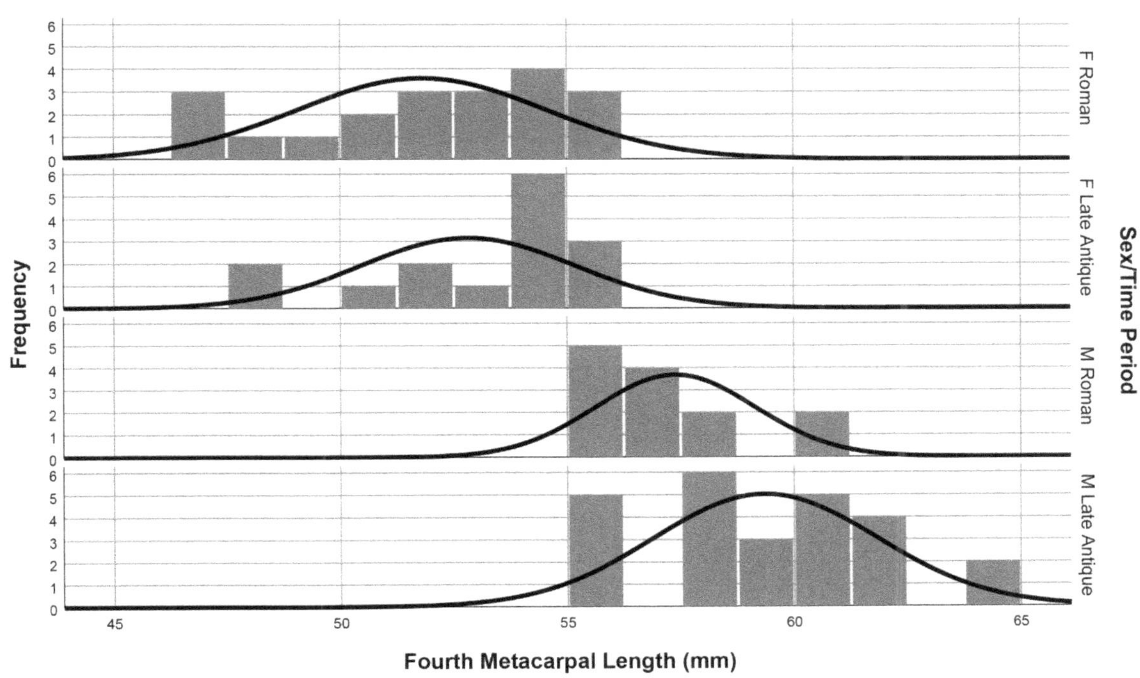

Figure 8.25. Stacked histograms showing the frequency of fourth metacarpal lengths for each sex/time period group and including a normality curve to demonstrate expected values.

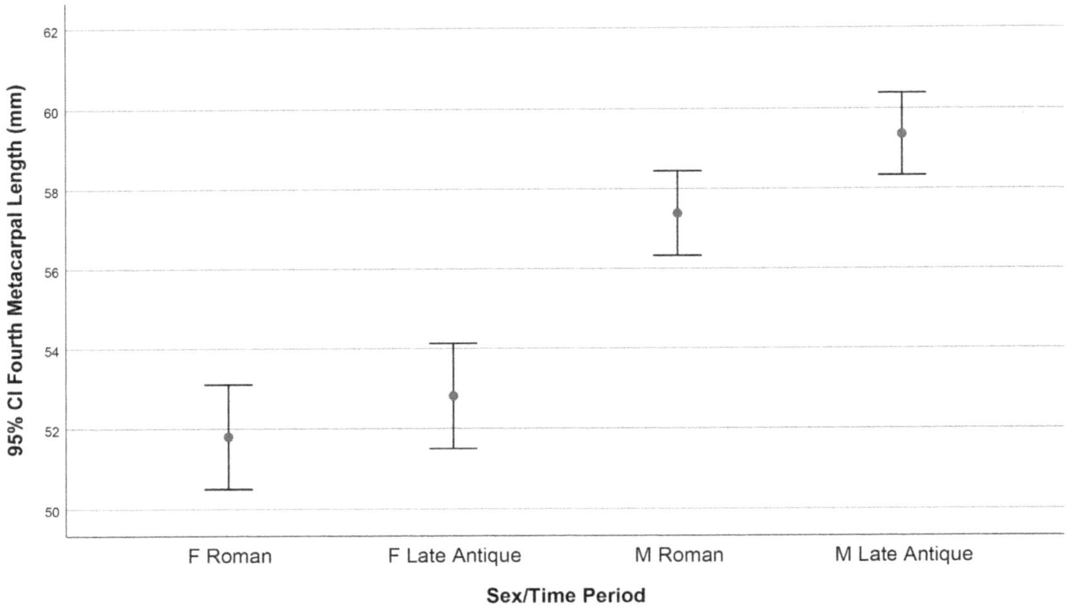

Figure 8.26. Error bar plots demonstrating mean fourth metacarpal lengths for each sex/time period group, with 95% confidence intervals.

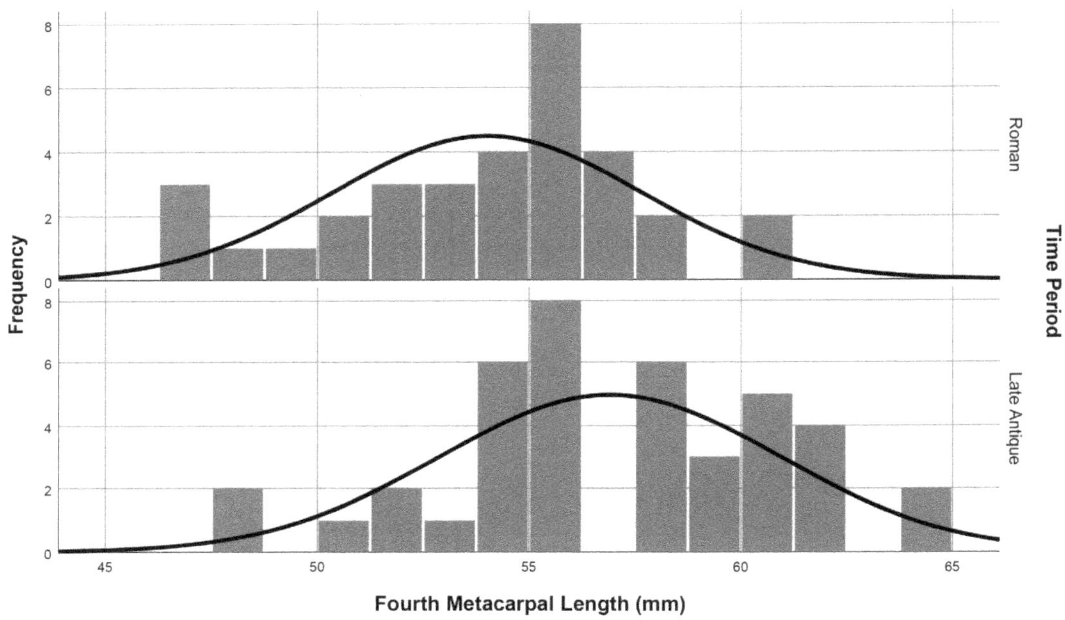

Figure 8.27. Stacked histograms showing the frequency of fourth metacarpal lengths for each time period group with the female and male values combined and including a normality curve to demonstrate expected values.

means to be higher than the Roman ones, particularly the males, with relatively little overlap in confidence intervals.

The fourth metacarpal lengths were then analysed for each time period with the sexes combined in order to remove the non-normal, asymmetrical distribution caused by the sex determination technique. Far more normal looking distributions are presented in Figure 8.27 and supported by the Shapiro-Wilk test for both the Roman (Shapiro-Wilk= 0.955, df=33, p=0.182) and Late Antique (Shapiro-Wilk= 0.970, df=40, p=0.354) groups. This means there is a plausibly random sample and the means for the Roman and Late Antique fourth metacarpal lengths can be compared in Figure 8.28. This shows the Late Antique mean to be substantially higher with no crossover in confidence intervals. A t-test was therefore employed to compare these mean values (t=−3.2, df=71, p=0.002) which produced a mean difference of −2.905, with confidence intervals of −4.716 to −1.094. As these values do not come close to or cross zero this suggests a significant difference in mean values. It is important to bear in mind that the significant difference could be caused by uneven numbers of males and females in these groups, a variable that cannot be controlled for with bilateral metric sexing as was attempted in this chapter.

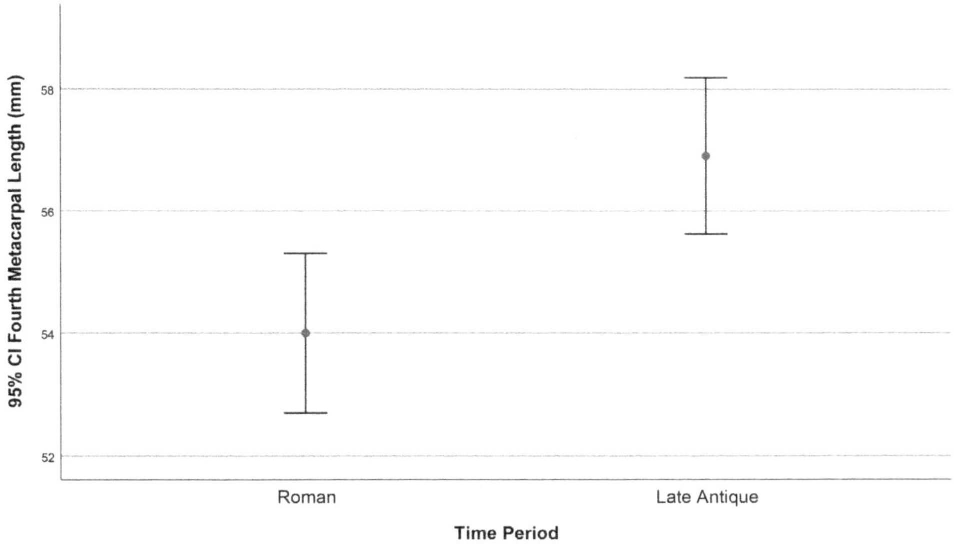

Figure 8.28. Mean fourth metacarpal lengths with the sexes combined for each time period group with error bar plots demonstrating 95% confidence intervals.

8.3.1.11. Fifth metacarpal

Although the assessment of the distribution of fifth metacarpal lengths indicates that the Female Late Antique and Male Roman could be normal, the other Shapiro-Wilk scores and the normality curves on all of the histograms do not portray very normal distributions (Table 8.15 and Figure 8.29). The comparison of the Roman and Late Antique means in Figure 8.30 show different patterns for the females and males, though in both cases there is sufficient overlap of confidence intervals to indicate no difference between the time periods for either sex.

Table 8.15. Descriptive and normality statistics for fifth metacarpal lengths for each sex/time period group.

Fifth Metacarpal Length (mm)				95% Confidence Interval			Shapiro-Wilk (normality)		
	n	Mean	Std. Error	Lower Bound	Upper Bound	Std. Deviation	Statistic	df	Sig. (*p*)
Female Roman	16	49.15	0.468	48.15	50.15	1.873	0.851	16	0.014
Female Late Antique	15	48.40	0.567	47.18	49.62	2.197	0.890	15	0.066
Male Hellenistic	1								
Male Roman	14	53.32	0.578	52.07	54.57	2.163	0.915	14	0.185
Male Late Antique	29	54.74	0.524	53.67	55.82	2.821	0.873	29	0.002

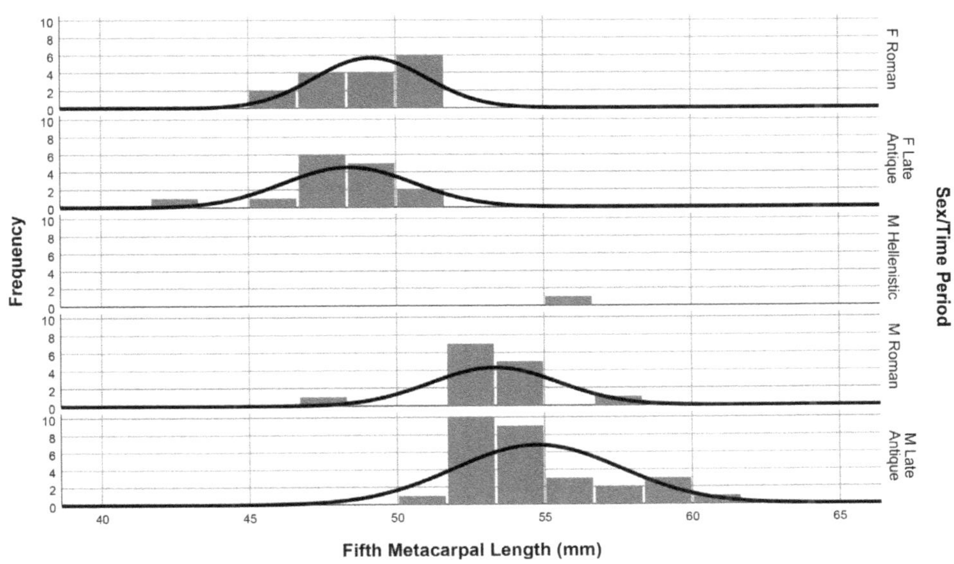

Figure 8.29. Stacked histograms showing the frequency of fifth metacarpal lengths for each sex/time period group and including a normality curve to demonstrate expected values.

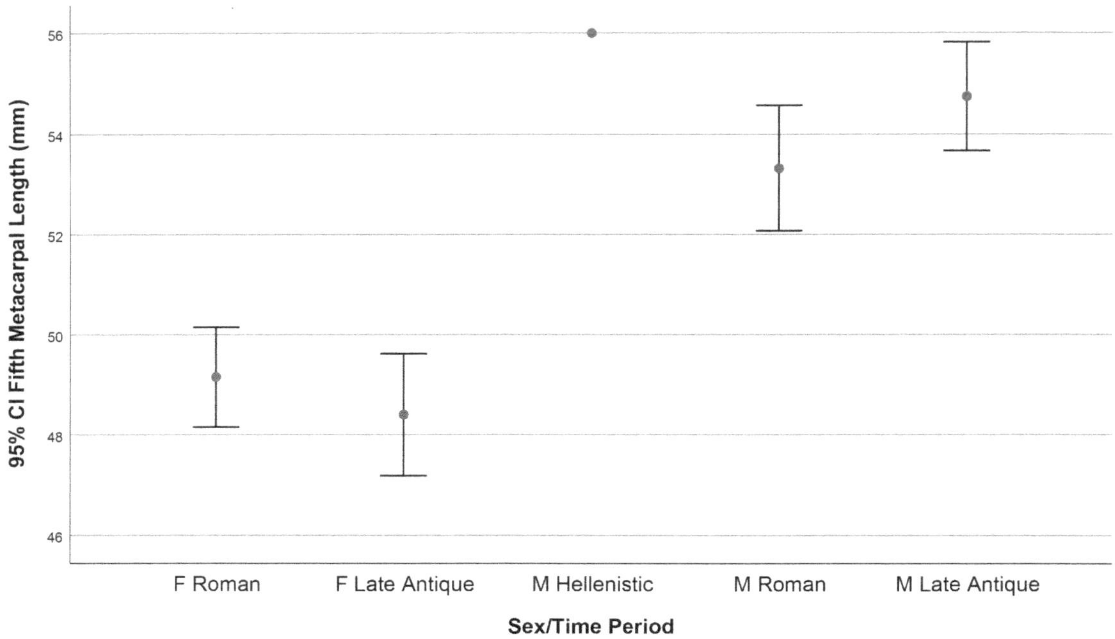

Figure 8.30. Error bar plots demonstrating mean fifth metacarpal lengths for each sex/time period group, with 95% confidence intervals.

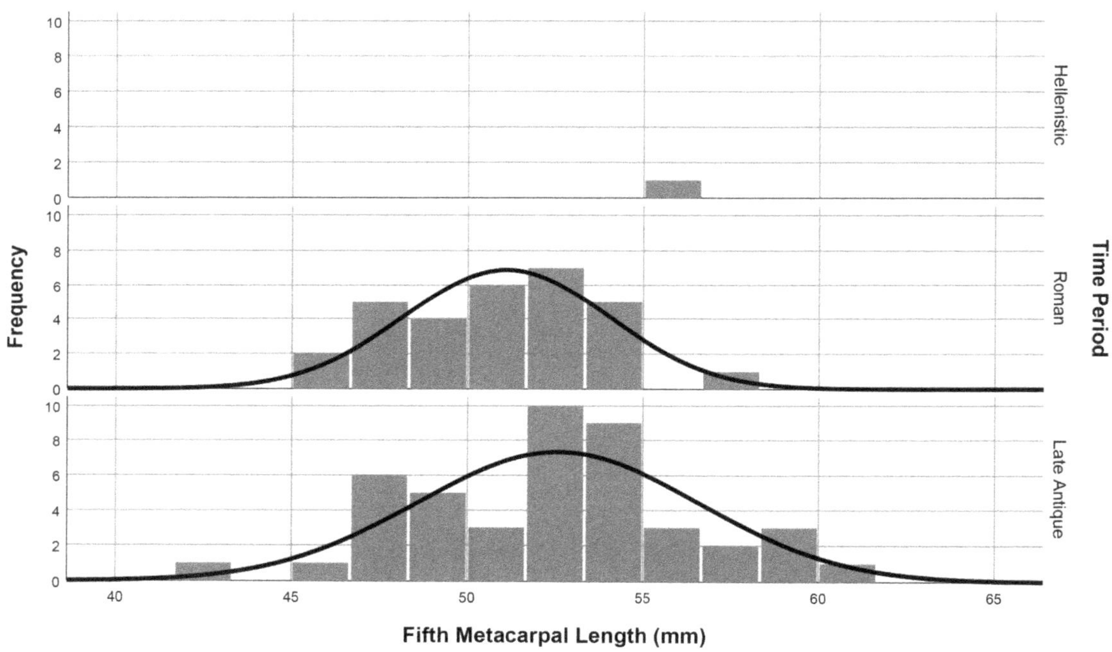

Figure 8.31. Stacked histograms showing the frequency of fifth metacarpal lengths for each time period group with the female and male values combined and including a normality curve to demonstrate expected values.

Far more normal distributions are produced when the sexes were combined for the Roman (Shapiro-Wilk= 0.974, df=30, p=0.654) and Late Antique (Shapiro-Wilk= 0.979, df=44, p=0.592) periods (Figure 8.31). Figure 8.32 shows that the Late Antique mean was higher than the Roman mean though there was overlap in the confidence intervals and a t-test confirmed that there was no significant difference in these means (t=−1.744, df=72, p=0.085, mean difference=−1.485, 95% confidence intervals −3.183 to 0.213).

8.3.1.12. First metatarsal

The metatarsals produced the largest sample sizes of measurable bones. The distributions of the bone lengths for the sex/time period categories are not normal according to the Shapiro-Wilk test with p<0.05 (Table 8.16). The histograms appear asymmetrical and there are several outlier results (Figure 8.33). The asymmetry is, again, likely due to the metric sexing technique. Figure 8.34 demonstrates that the female means were similar, with the

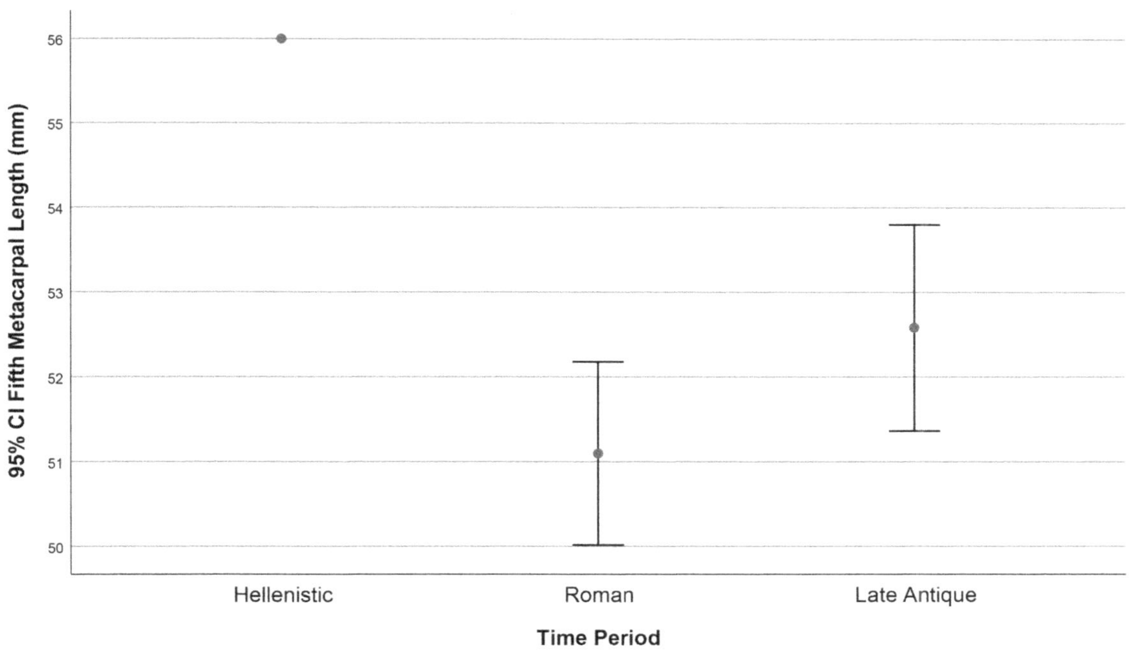

Figure 8.32. Mean fifth metacarpal lengths with the sexes combined for each time period group with error bar plots demonstrating 95% confidence intervals.

Table 8.16. Descriptive and normality statistics for first metatarsal lengths for each sex/time period group.

First Metatarsal Length (mm)				95% Confidence Interval			Shapiro-Wilk (normality)		
	n	Mean	Std. Error	Lower Bound	Upper Bound	Std. Deviation	Statistic	df	Sig. (*p*)
Female Roman	32	56.43	0.396	55.62	57.24	2.240	0.891	32	0.004
Female Late Antique	33	56.23	0.499	55.21	57.24	2.867	0.809	33	0.000
Male Roman	50	61.80	0.340	61.12	62.48	2.405	0.943	50	0.018
Male Late Antique	49	62.73	0.403	61.92	63.54	2.818	0.914	49	0.002

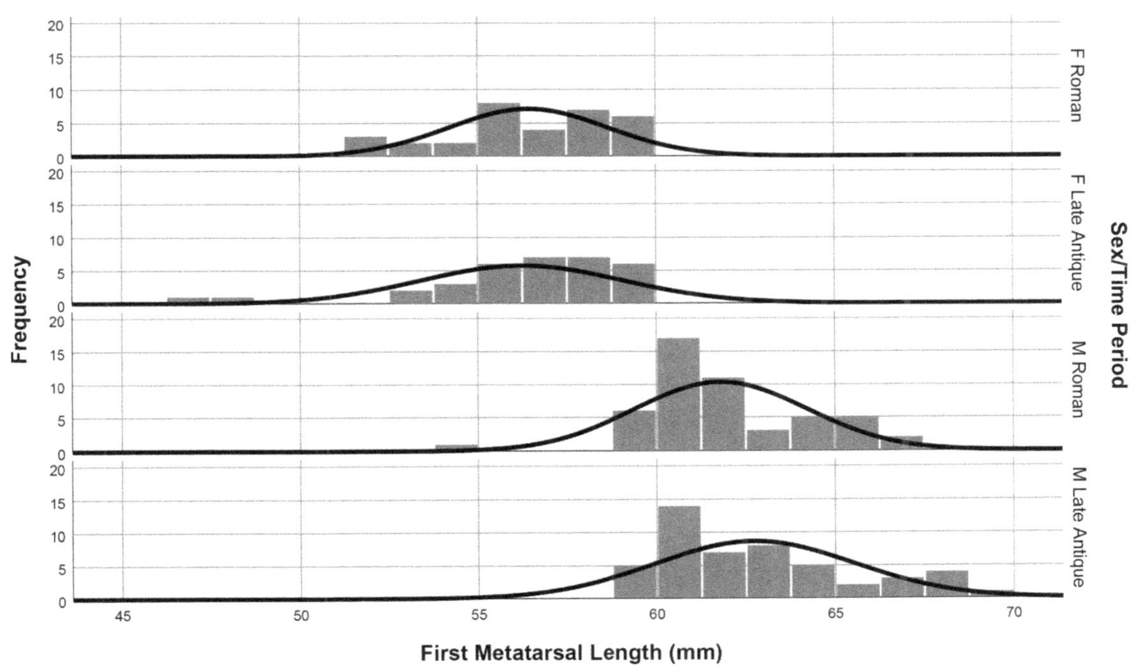

Figure 8.33. Stacked histograms showing the frequency of first metatarsal lengths for each sex/time period group and including a normality curve to demonstrate expected values.

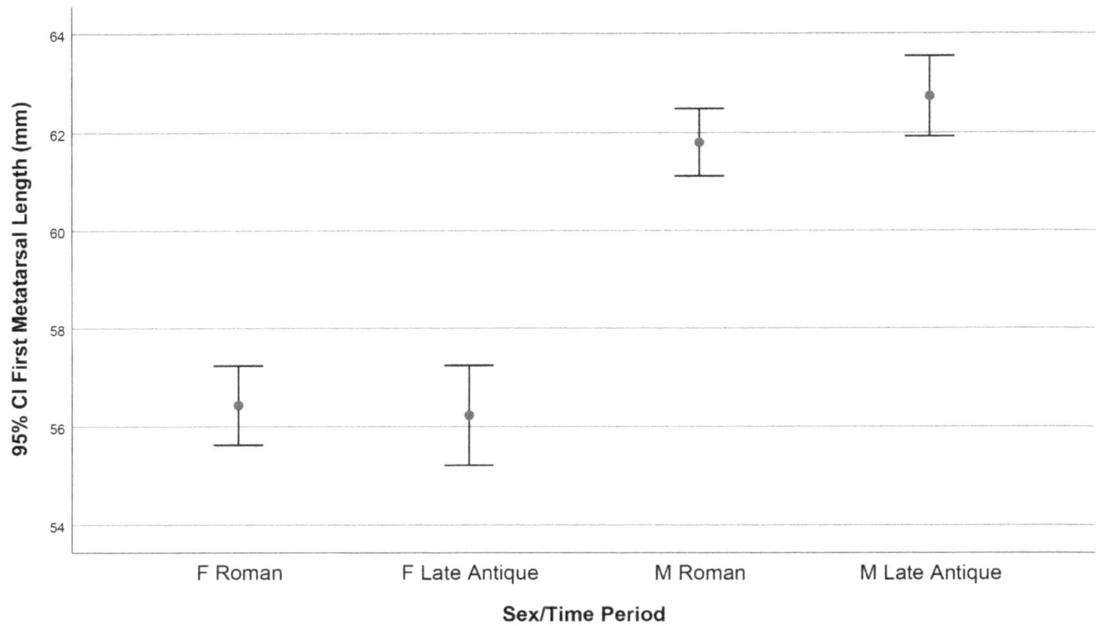

Figure 8.34. Error bar plots demonstrating mean first metatarsal lengths for each sex/time period group, with 95% confidence intervals.

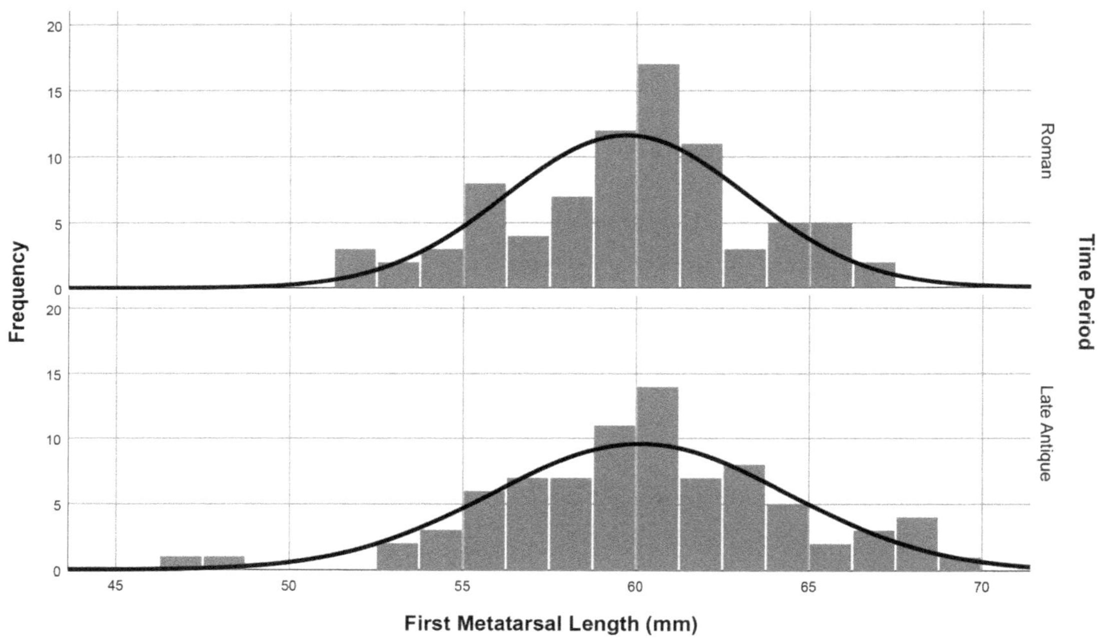

Figure 8.35. Stacked histograms showing the frequency of first metatarsal lengths for each time period group with the female and male values combined and including a normality curve to demonstrate expected values.

Late Antique result only marginally lower than the Roman mean, while the Male Late Antique mean was higher than the Roman one but with substantial overlap of confidence intervals.

The first metatarsal lengths were then compared by time period with the sexes combined. Despite the two female Late Antique outliers, the distributions of these histograms (Figure 8.35) appear quite normal, and this was supported by the Shapiro-Wilk test for the Roman (Shapiro-Wilk= 0.979, df=82, p=0.204) and Late Antique (Shapiro-Wilk= 0.975, df=82, p=0.105) groups. With a plausibly random sample established, Figure 8.36 demonstrates very little difference (0.4mm) between the Roman and Late Antique mean values with substantial overlap of confidence intervals.

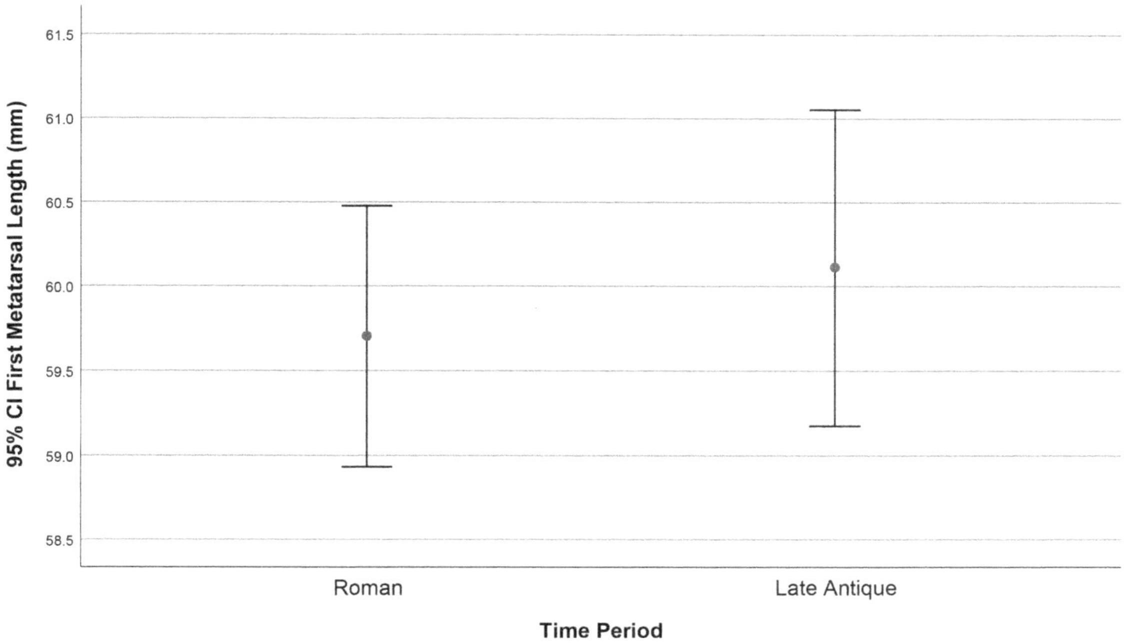

Figure 8.36. Mean first metatarsal lengths with the sexes combined for each time period group with error bar plots demonstrating 95% confidence intervals.

Table 8.17. Descriptive and normality statistics for second metatarsal lengths for each sex/time period group.

Second Metatarsal Length (mm)				95% Confidence Interval			Shapiro-Wilk (normality)		
	n	Mean	Std. Error	Lower Bound	Upper Bound	Std. Deviation	Statistic	df	Sig. (*p*)
Female Roman	32	66.31	0.545	65.20	67.42	3.084	0.917	32	0.017
Female Late Antique	25	67.36	0.512	66.31	68.42	2.560	0.853	25	0.002
Male Hellenistic	1								
Male Roman	36	75.01	0.439	74.12	75.91	2.636	0.927	36	0.020
Male Late Antique	30	76.61	0.730	75.12	78.10	3.996	0.927	30	0.041

8.3.1.13. Second metatarsal

A Shapiro-Wilk test of normality requires a significance score greater than 0.05 in order to assume a normal distribution from a random sample of the population, which was not achieved for any of the sex/time period groups for the second metatarsal lengths (Table 8.17). The asymmetry of these groups is displayed in the stacked histograms (Figure 8.37). The implication of this is that the derivation of the material is so non-random that it cannot be taken to represent the population.

The sexes combined do, however, produce normal distributions for second metatarsal lengths for both the Roman (Shapiro-Wilk=0.977, df=68, p=0.235) and Late Antique (Shapiro-Wilk=0.966, df=55, p=0.116) groups. This indicates that the asymmetry caused by the metric sexing is likely the cause of the non-normal distribution, although the histograms for the combined sexes by time period remain quite irregular compared to the normality curve (Figure 8.39). Although a random sample that is representative of the population is not guaranteed by this distribution, it is noteworthy that, for both the separate-sex (Figure 8.38) and combined-sex (Figure 8.40) comparisons of the second metatarsal lengths for the Roman and Late Antique groups, the Late Antique mean length was higher. However, a t-test demonstrates that the mean difference between the Roman and Late Antique lengths was −1.5, with 95% confidence intervals of −3.4 and 0.5, indicating that it is unlikely there is any difference between these groups.

8.3.1.14. Third metatarsal

The Male Late Antique group is the only one with a normal distribution according to the Shapiro-Wilk test

(Table 8.18), though the histogram demonstrates that it is not a neat fit for the normality curve (Figure 8.41). It also has an outlier to the lower end, representing an individual who was sexed morphologically, though if sex could be determined morphologically for more individuals, it might transpire that this was not an outlier. The histogram plots are asymmetrical due to metric sexing. The mean values show little difference between the time periods for either males and females and there is significant overlap of confidence intervals (Figure 8.42).

Due to the non-normal distribution, it is better to investigate these bone lengths with the sexes combined. The Roman distribution still looks non-normal (Shapiro-Wilk=0.962, df=66, p=0.041) with multiple peaks and outliers meaning it fails to match the normality curve on the histogram (Figure 8.43). The Late Antique distribution of lengths appeared more normal and plausibly representative (Shapiro-Wilk=0.961, df=54, p=0.078). The Late Antique mean value was higher than the Roman mean but with the extent of overlap in

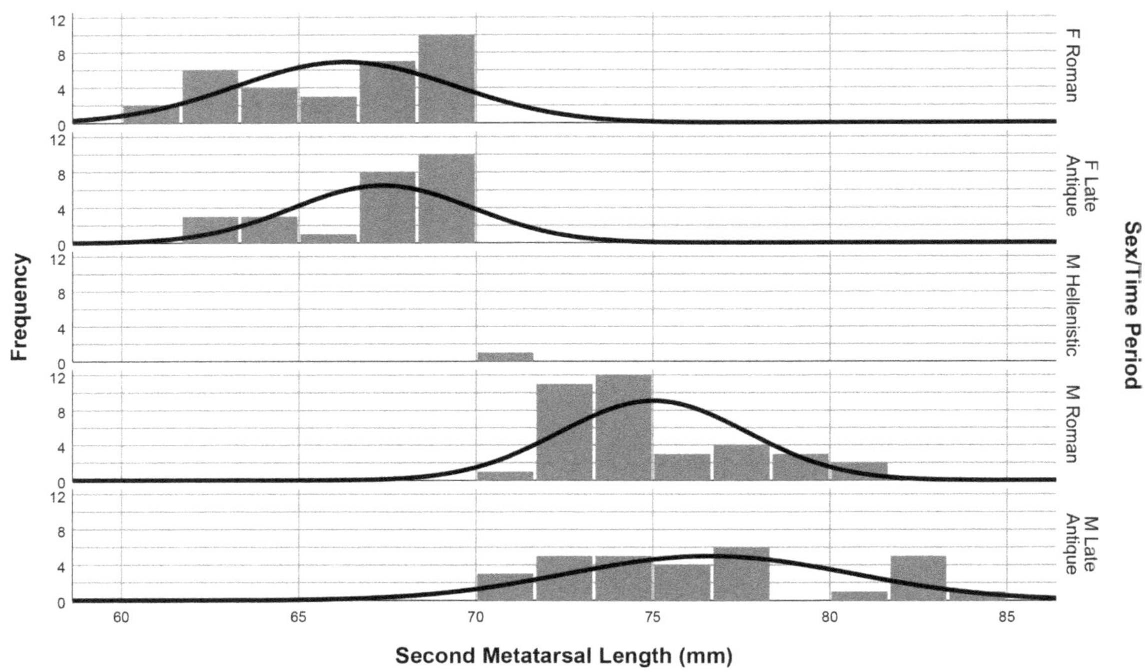

Figure 8.37. Stacked histograms showing the frequency of second metatarsal lengths for each sex/time period group and including a normality curve to demonstrate expected values.

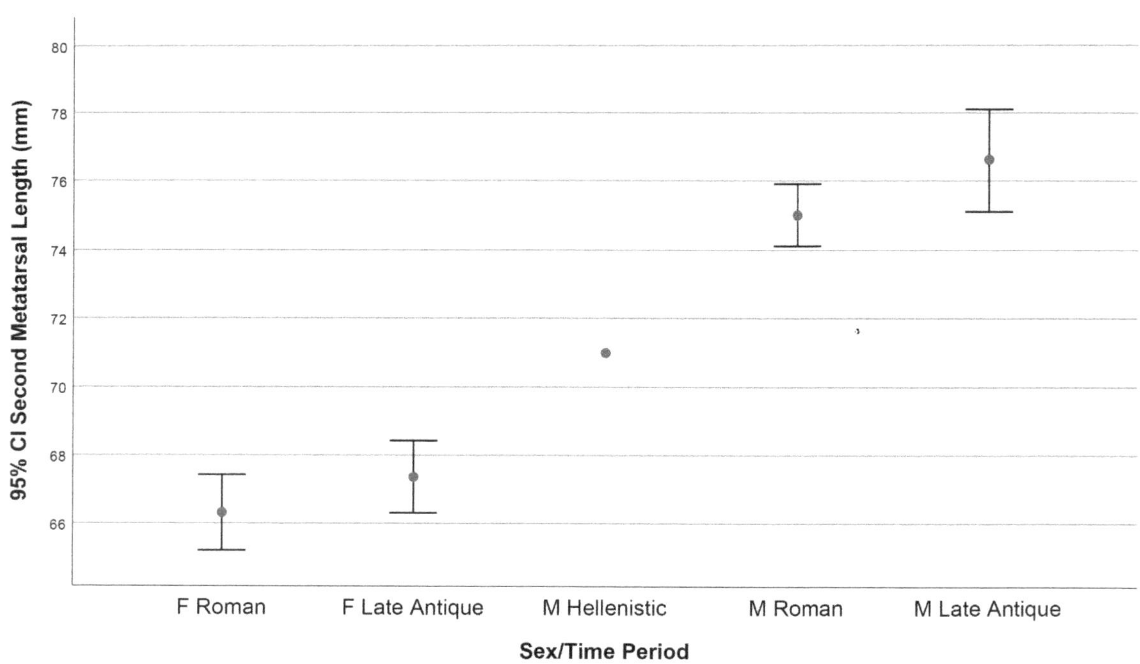

Figure 8.38. Error bar plots demonstrating mean second metatarsal lengths for each sex/time period group, with 95% confidence intervals.

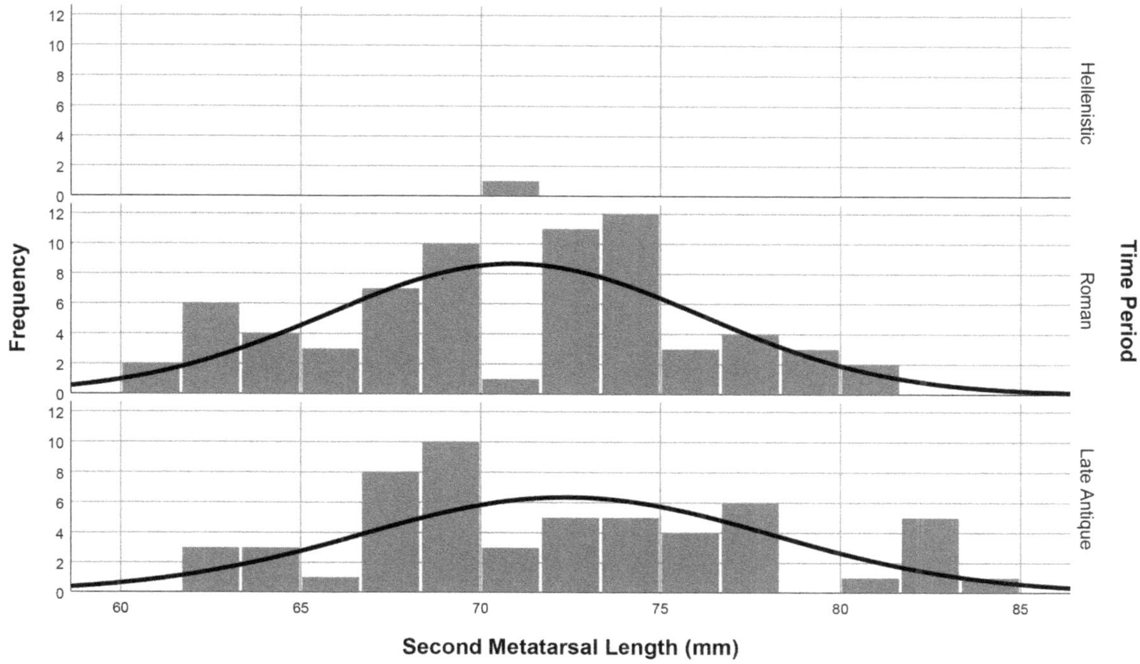

Figure 8.39. Stacked histograms showing the frequency of second metatarsal lengths for each time period group with the female and male values combined and including a normality curve to demonstrate expected values.

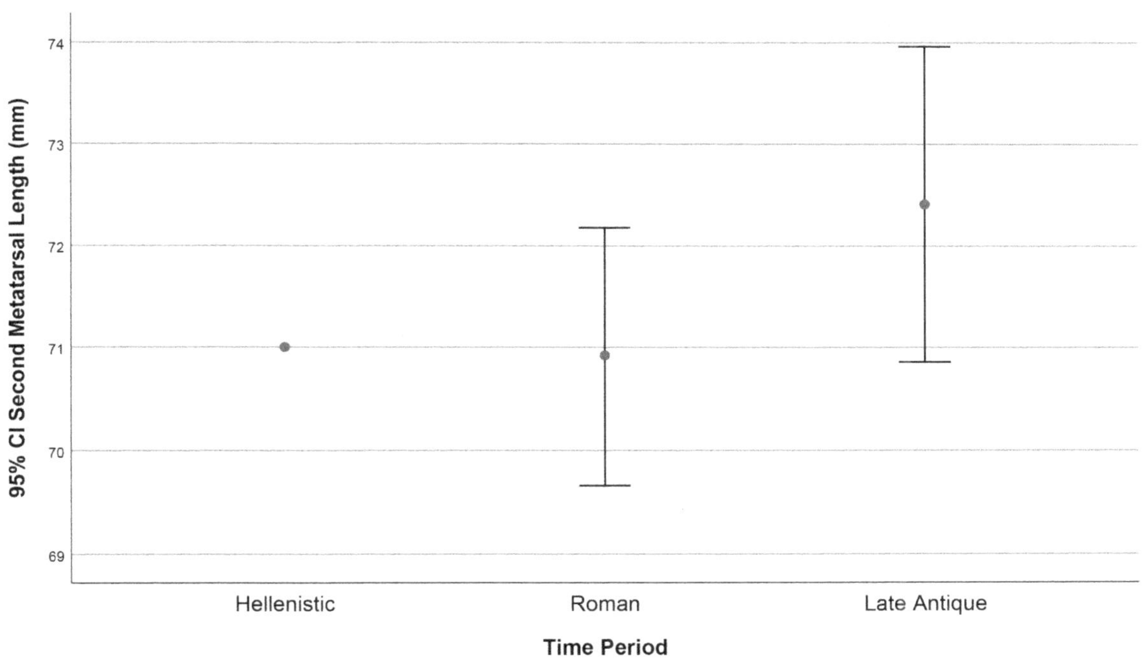

Figure 8.40. Mean second metatarsal lengths with the sexes combined for each time period group with error bar plots demonstrating 95% confidence intervals.

Table 8.18. Descriptive and normality statistics for third metatarsal lengths for each sex/time period group.

Third Metatarsal Length (mm)				95% Confidence Interval			Shapiro-Wilk (normality)		
	n	Mean	Std. Error	Lower Bound	Upper Bound	Std. Deviation	Statistic	df	Sig. (*p*)
Female Roman	30	62.87	0.667	61.50	64.23	3.655	0.875	30	0.002
Female Late Antique	21	63.76	0.881	61.92	65.59	4.035	0.709	21	0.000
Male Roman	36	71.25	0.419	70.40	72.10	2.511	0.924	36	0.017
Male Late Antique	33	72.17	0.604	70.94	73.40	3.468	0.973	33	0.559

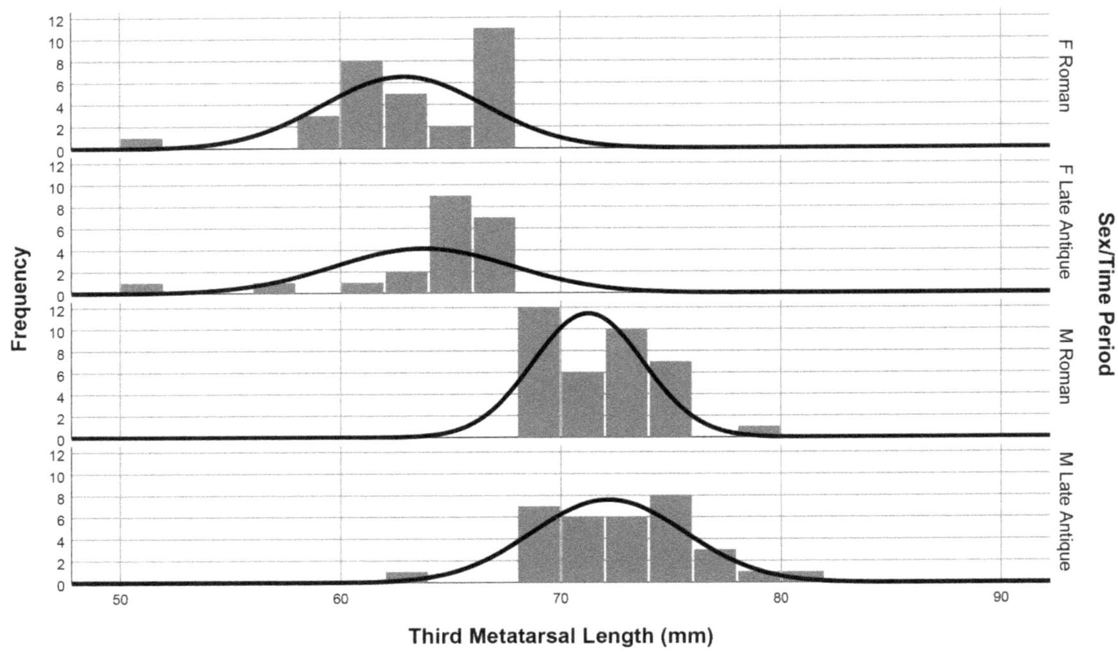

Figure 8.41. Stacked histograms showing the frequency of third metatarsal lengths for each sex/time period group and including a normality curve to demonstrate expected values.

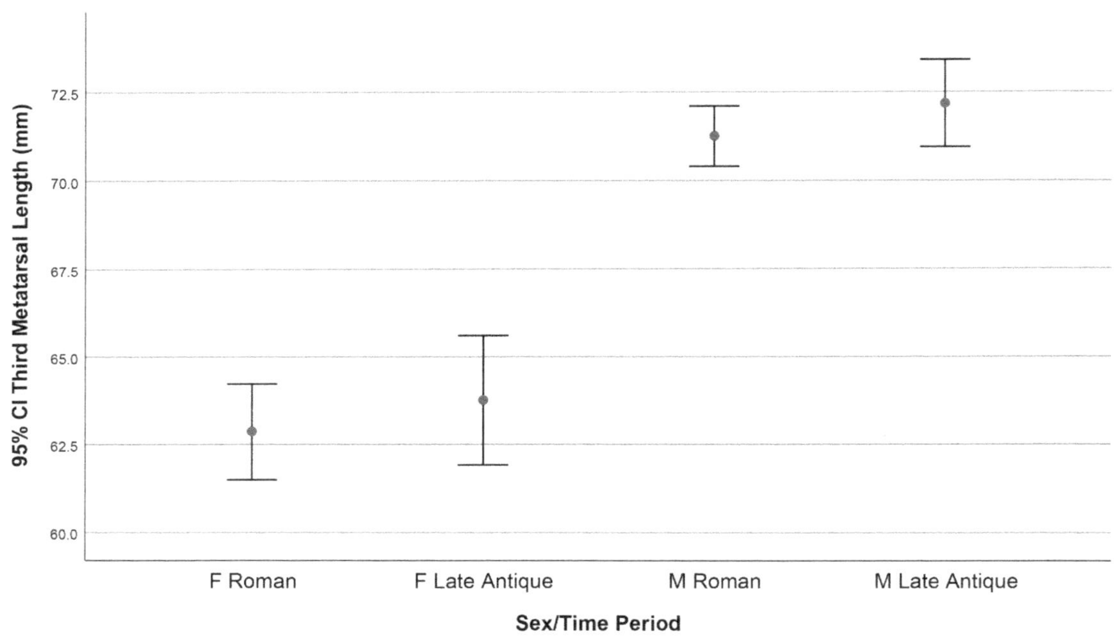

Figure 8.42. Error bar plots demonstrating mean third metatarsal lengths for each sex/time period group, with 95% confidence intervals.

the confidence intervals means there was no significant difference (Figure 8.44).

8.3.1.15. Fourth metatarsal

Although the Shapiro-Wilk scores for the two Late Antique groups indicate possible random samples, the distribution on the histograms does not appear normal for any of the sex/time period groups (Table 8.19 and Figure 8.45). The mean values presented on the error bar plots (Figure 8.46) show very similar values between the time periods for both males and females. However, due to the non-normal and asymmetrical distributions, the fourth metatarsal lengths have also been investigated with the sexes combined to compare the time periods.

Figure 8.47 shows that while these histograms have the metric sexing bias removed and appear more symmetrical in their distribution, they are still not a neat match to the normality curve. They do, however, qualify as normal

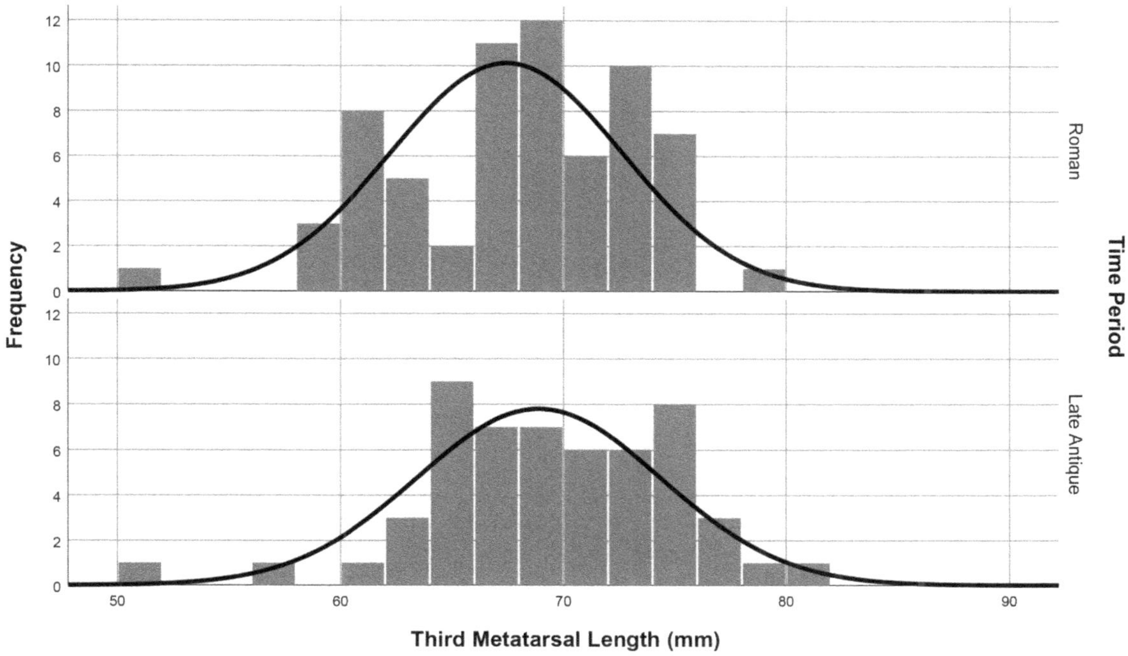

Figure 8.43. Stacked histograms showing the frequency of third metatarsal lengths for each time period group with the female and male values combined and including a normality curve to demonstrate expected values.

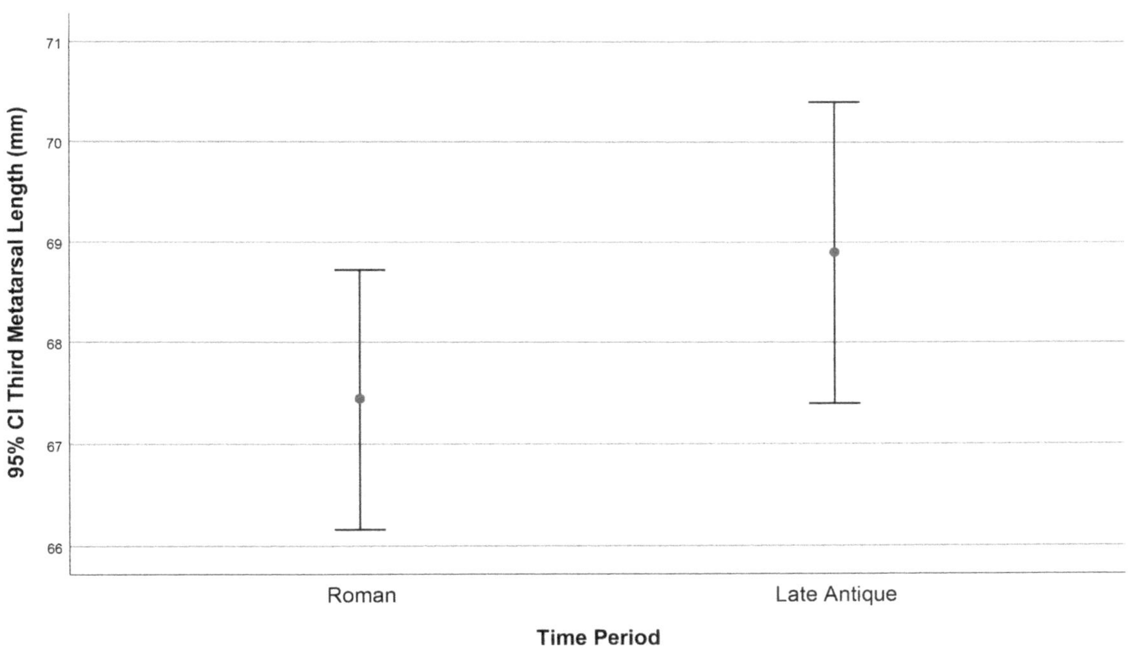

Figure 8.44. Mean third metatarsal lengths with the sexes combined for each time period group with error bar plots demonstrating 95% confidence intervals.

Table 8.19. Descriptive and normality statistics for fourth metatarsal lengths for each sex/time period group.

Fourth Metatarsal Length (mm)				95% Confidence Interval			Shapiro-Wilk (normality)		
	n	Mean	Std. Error	Lower Bound	Upper Bound	Std. Deviation	Statistic	df	Sig. (*p*)
Female Roman	17	62.53	0.543	61.38	63.68	2.239	0.882	17	0.034
Female Late Antique	15	62.99	0.504	61.91	64.07	1.952	0.890	15	0.068
Male Roman	42	68.83	0.393	68.04	69.63	2.549	0.882	42	0.000
Male Late Antique	27	68.78	0.635	67.47	70.08	3.297	0.931	27	0.073

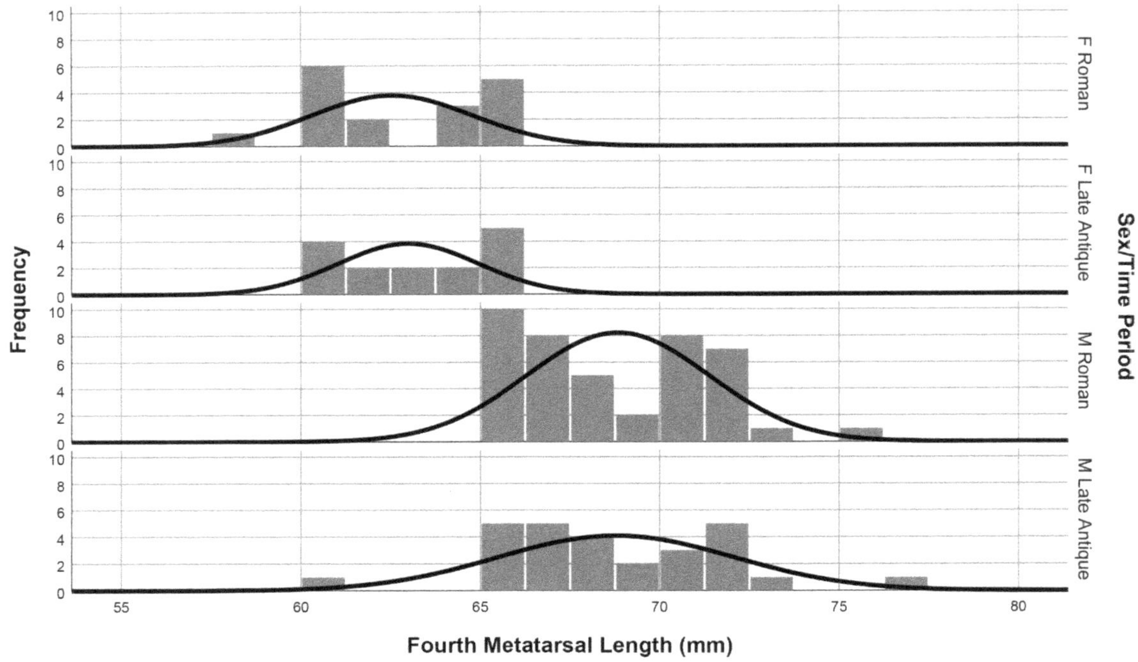

Figure 8.45. Stacked histograms showing the frequency of fourth metatarsal lengths for each sex/time period group and including a normality curve to demonstrate expected values.

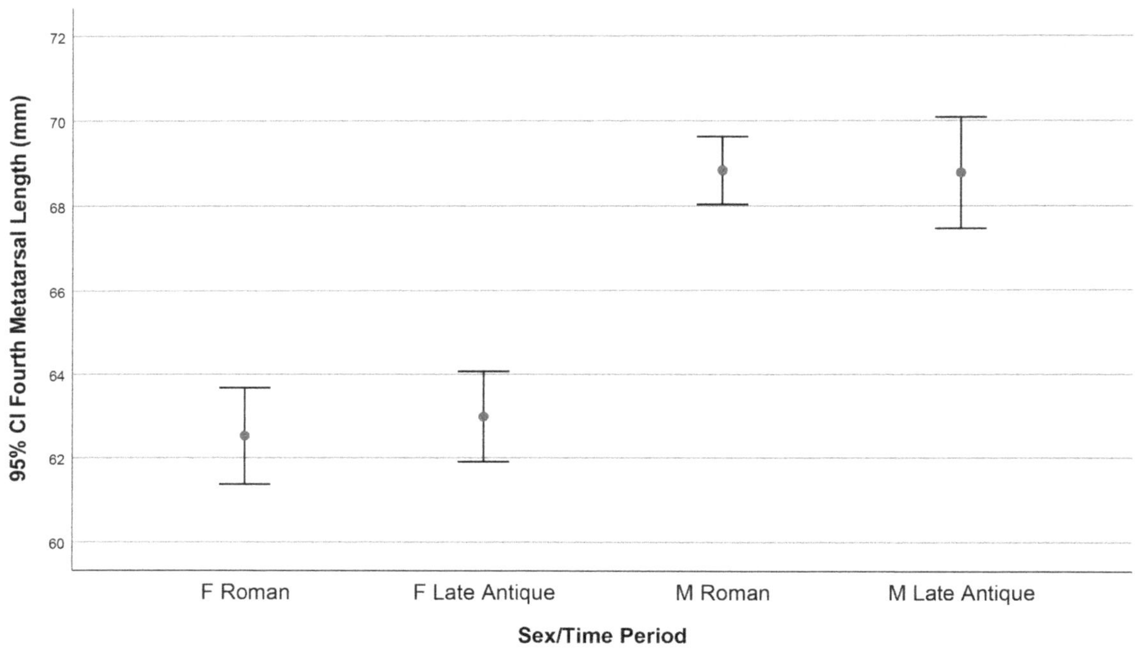

Figure 8.46. Error bar plots demonstrating mean fourth metatarsal lengths for each sex/time period group, with 95% confidence intervals.

with a $p>0.05$ in the Shapiro-Wilk test for both the Roman (Shapiro-Wilk= 0.967, df=59, $p=0.109$) and Late Antique (Shapiro-Wilk= 0.969, df=42, $p=0.312$) periods. Figure 8.48 displays very similar mean values for the two time periods with substantial overlap of the confidence intervals.

8.3.1.16. Fifth metatarsal

Other than the Late Antique Female group, the sex/time period groups had a normal enough distribution of fifth metatarsal lengths to suppose a random sample, according to the Shapiro-Wilk test (Table 8.20). However, it is clear from the histograms that none of these produced a very normal distribution and both female groups have a distinct outlier value each (Figure 8.49). Figure 8.50 shows the mean values for the sex time period groups and for both males and females there was sufficient overlap of the confidence intervals in the comparison of the time periods to suggest no significant difference.

With the sexes combined, more normal and symmetrical distributions of lengths were produced for the Roman

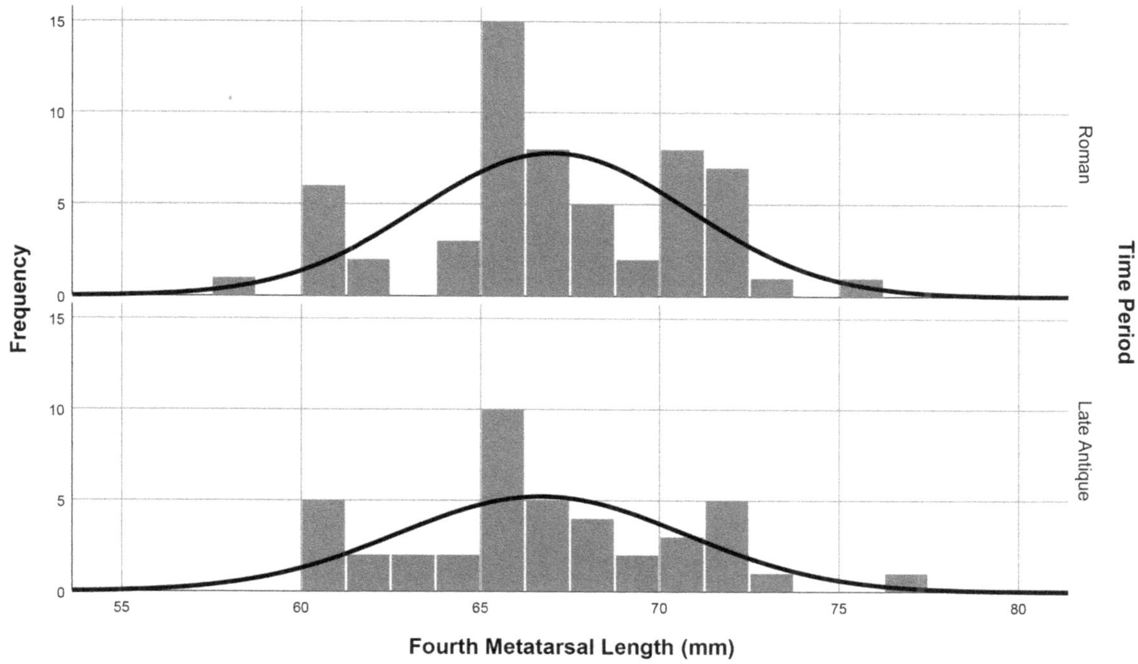

Figure 8.47. Stacked histograms showing the frequency of fourth metatarsal lengths for each time period group with the female and male values combined and including a normality curve to demonstrate expected values.

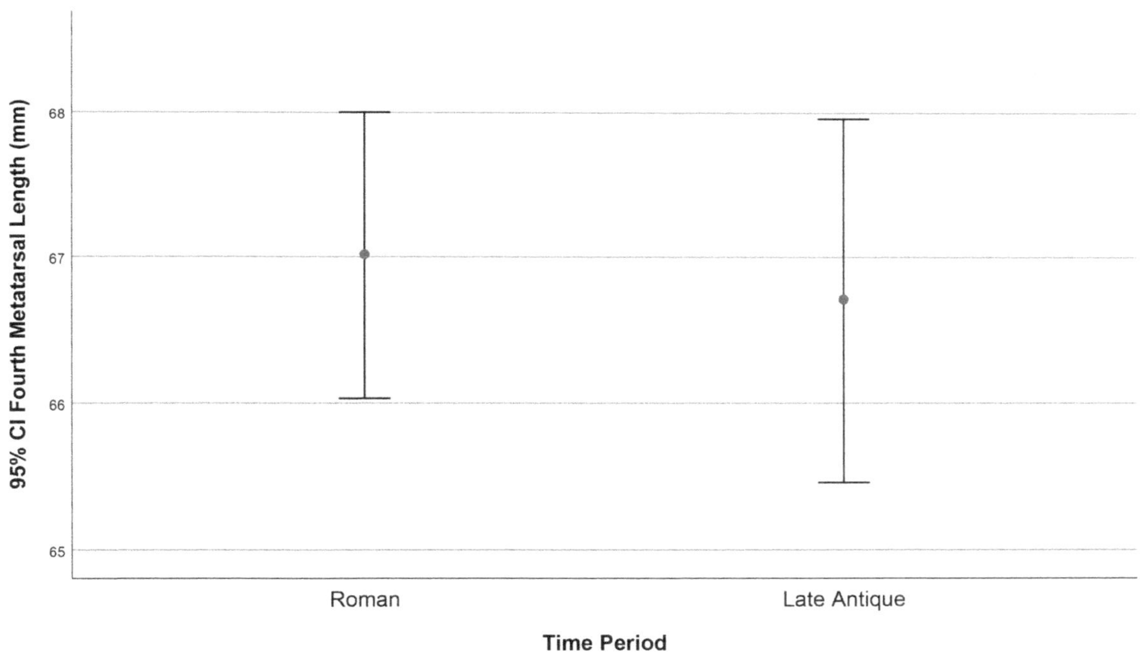

Figure 8.48. Mean fourth metatarsal lengths with the sexes combined for each time period group with error bar plots demonstrating 95% confidence intervals.

Table 8.20. Descriptive and normality statistics for fifth metatarsal lengths for each sex/time period group.

Fifth Metatarsal Length (mm)				95% Confidence Interval			Shapiro-Wilk (normality)		
	n	Mean	Std. Error	Lower Bound	Upper Bound	Std. Deviation	Statistic	df	Sig. (*p*)
Female Roman	27	63.28	0.636	61.97	64.59	3.306	0.932	27	0.078
Female Late Antique	20	62.64	0.787	60.99	64.28	3.518	0.803	20	0.001
Male Roman	29	70.03	0.529	68.95	71.12	2.847	0.966	29	0.447
Male Late Antique	30	71.19	0.612	69.94	72.44	3.353	0.933	30	0.060

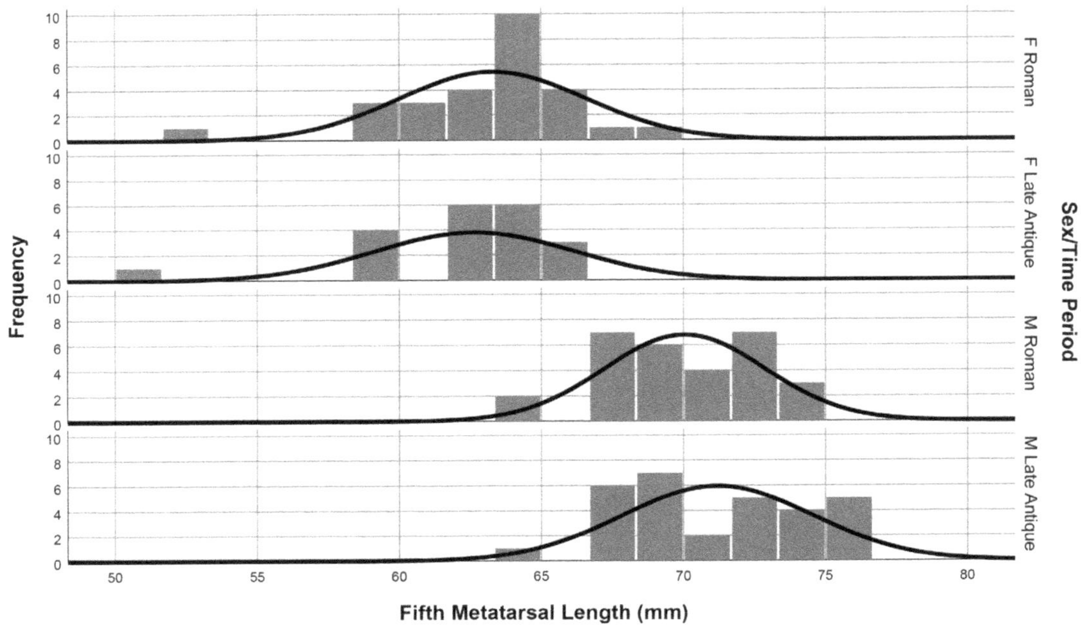

Figure 8.49. Stacked histograms showing the frequency of fifth metatarsal lengths for each sex/time period group and including a normality curve to demonstrate expected values.

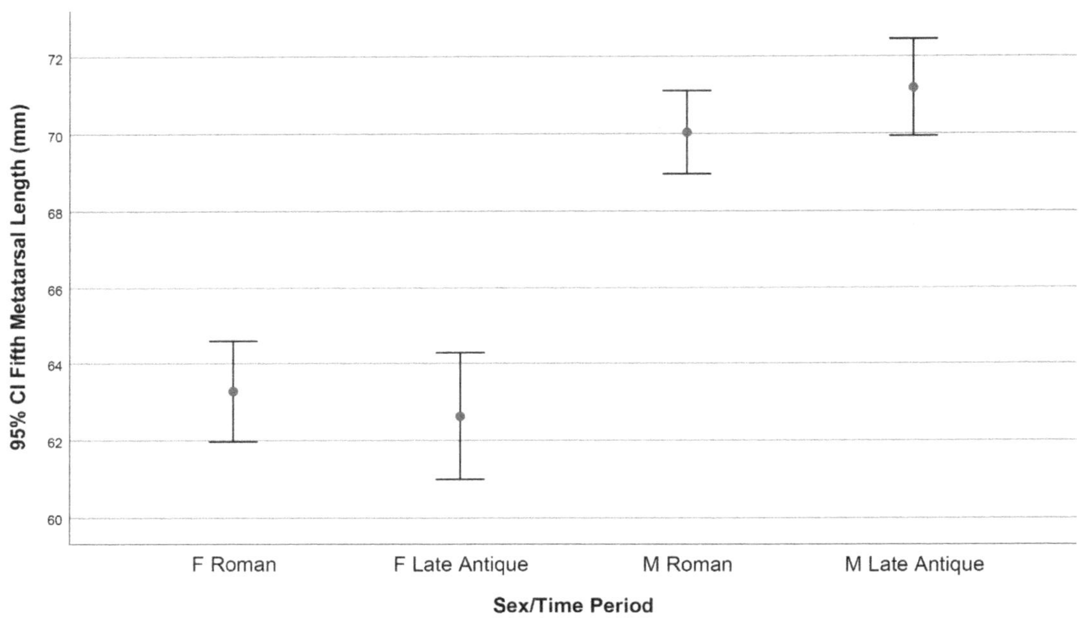

Figure 8.50. Error bar plots demonstrating mean fifth metatarsal lengths for each sex/time period group, with 95% confidence intervals.

(Shapiro-Wilk=0.974, df=56, p=0.272) and Late Antique (Shapiro-Wilk=0.961, df=50, p=0.095) periods (Figure 8.51). Figure 8.52 shows that while the Late Antique mean is slightly higher than the Roman mean, there is substantial crossover of the confidence intervals, indicating no significant difference between the time periods.

8.3.2. Tomb type

It is clear from the assessment of bone lengths by time period that the sample size for some bone types was inadequate to be representative of the population. As there are more categories of tomb type, this will reduce the sample sizes for each group further. Rather than systematically comparing the means for every bone type regardless of sample size or normality of distribution, only the larger sample sizes will be looked at in this section. The largest samples came from the metatarsals but even these were found to produce too small a sample size when the sexes were analysed separately, therefore the sexes have been combined. When any of the limb bones were plotted (both as stacked histograms and error bar plots, as before) the sample sizes were far too small to get a normal distribution or a meaningful comparison of means.

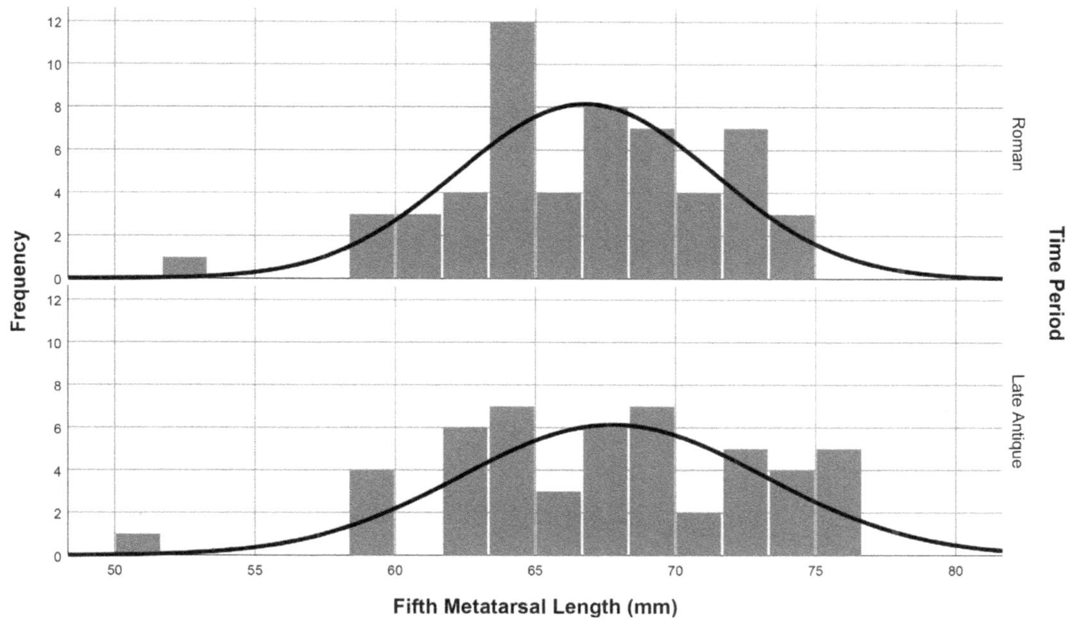

Figure 8.51. Stacked histograms showing the frequency of fifth metatarsal lengths for each time period group with the female and male values combined and including a normality curve to demonstrate expected values.

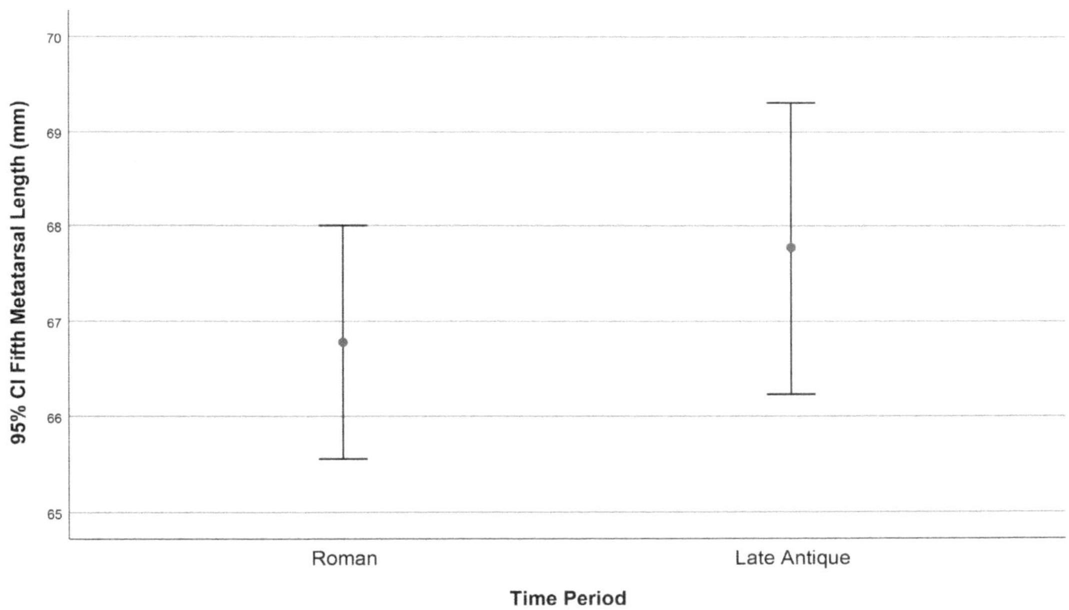

Figure 8.52. Mean fifth metatarsal lengths with the sexes combined for each time period group with error bar plots demonstrating 95% confidence intervals.

Tables 8.21–25 and Figures 8.53–62 present the metatarsal lengths data for the different tomb types. As the sexes have been combined to increase the sample size and reduce the asymmetry of the plots, each group with a large enough sample to test qualified as having a normal distribution with Shapiro-Wilk $p>0.05$ scores. In most cases, the Q-Q plots (not depicted) also support normal distributions with the lengths not deviating too far from normal. In several categories, particularly for the sarcophagus, cist, tile and pit groups, the sample sizes were too small to determine normality or to assume a representative mean. Though the normality curves on the histograms are never a perfect fit, considering the Shapiro-Wilk results, these distributions can be proposed to be a random representation of the population. In almost every case, displayed in the error bar plots for each metatarsal, there was no difference between the mean values of the different tomb type groups. The only exception to this was for the fifth metatarsal (Table 8.25 and Figure 8.62), where significant differences were confirmed by a t-test comparing the means for the built tomb and stone-lined grave groups (t=2.576, df=42, $p=0.014$, mean difference= 3.702, 95% CI= 0.802 to 6.602) and the osteothekai and stone-lined graves (t=2.310, df=55, $p=0.025$, mean difference= 4.369, 95% CI= 0.578 to 8.161). These are likely to be coincidental, false positive results as they were not detectable in any of the other bone lengths.

8.3.2.1. First metatarsal

Table 8.21. Descriptive and normality statistics for first metatarsal lengths for each tomb type group (sexes combined).

First Metatarsal Length (mm)				95% Confidence Interval			Shapiro-Wilk (normality)		
	n	Mean	Std. Error	Lower Bound	Upper Bound	Std. Deviation	Statistic	df	Sig. (*p*)
Built	49	59.77	0.507	58.75	60.78	3.546	0.964	49	0.142
Chamber	9	59.61	1.419	56.34	62.88	4.256	0.946	9	0.641
Osteotheke	78	60.07	0.493	59.09	61.05	4.356	0.975	78	0.132
Stone-lined	18	59.96	0.721	58.44	61.48	3.057	0.967	18	0.746
Sarcophagus	1								
Cist	5	58.90	1.764	54.00	63.80	3.943	0.961	5	0.817
Tile	3	60.33	2.728	48.59	72.07	4.726	0.907	3	0.407
Pit	1								

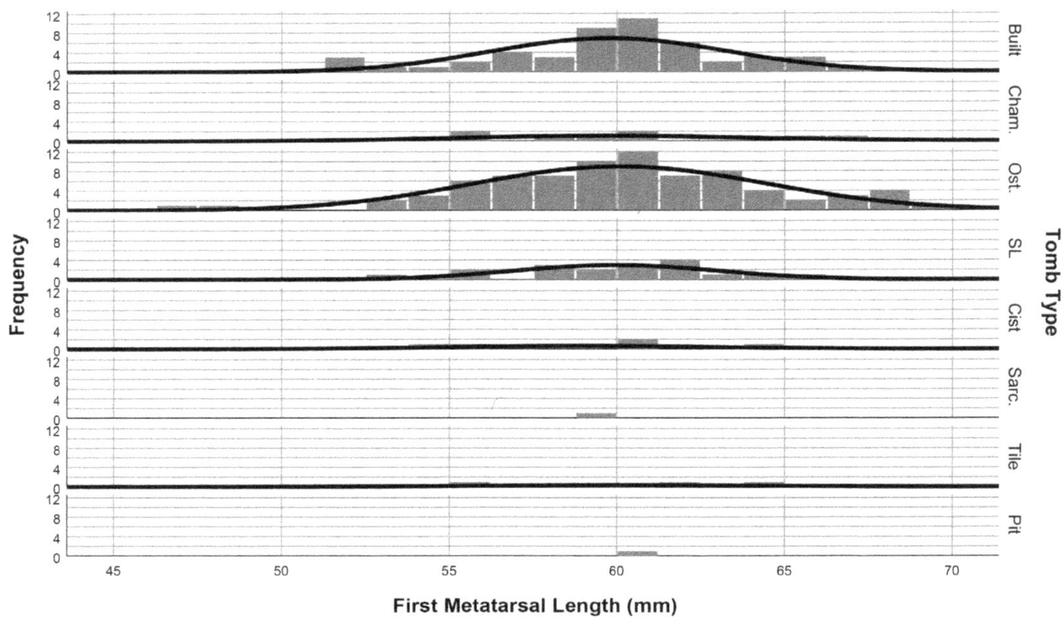

Figure 8.53. Stacked histograms showing the frequency of first metatarsal lengths for each tomb type group (sexes combined), including a normality curve to demonstrate expected values.

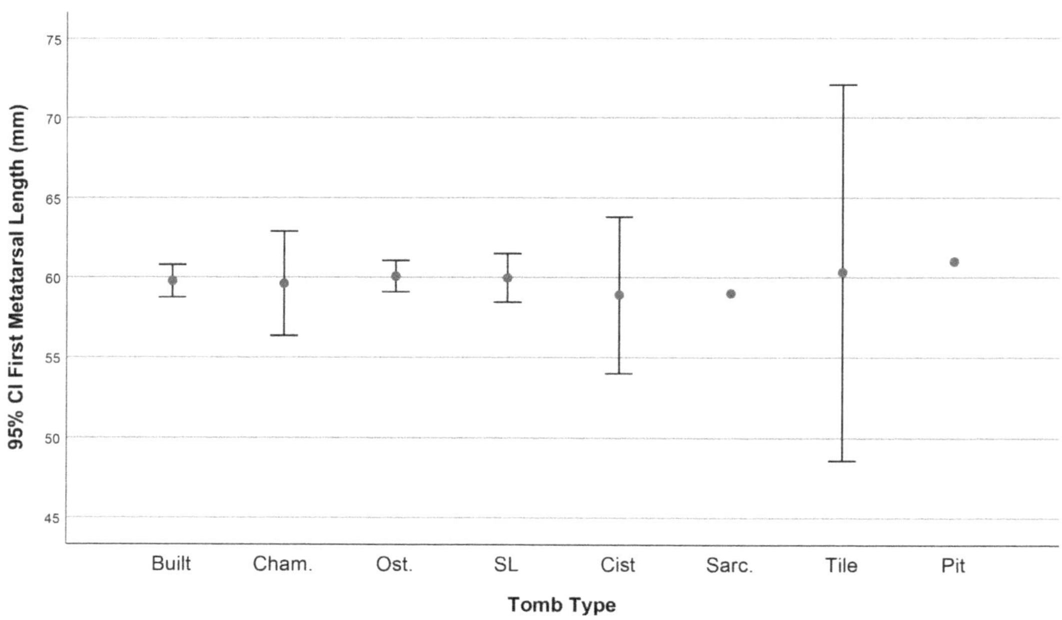

Figure 8.54. Mean first metatarsal lengths with the sexes combined for each tomb type group with error bar plots demonstrating 95% confidence intervals.

8.3.2.2. Second metatarsal

Table 8.22. Descriptive and normality statistics for second metatarsal lengths for each tomb type group (sexes combined).

Second Metatarsal Length (mm)				95% Confidence Interval			Shapiro-Wilk (normality)		
	n	Mean	Std. Error	Lower Bound	Upper Bound	Std. Deviation	Statistic	df	Sig. (*p*)
Built	43	71.41	0.748	69.90	72.92	4.907	0.965	43	0.216
Chamber	10	68.40	1.933	64.03	72.77	6.114	0.955	10	0.724
Osteotheke	53	72.35	0.804	70.73	73.96	5.852	0.960	53	0.074
Stone-lined	13	71.15	1.548	67.78	74.53	5.580	0.927	13	0.312
Cist	3	72.33	2.186	62.93	81.74	3.786	0.855	3	0.253
Pit	2	72.50	1.500	53.44	91.56	2.121			

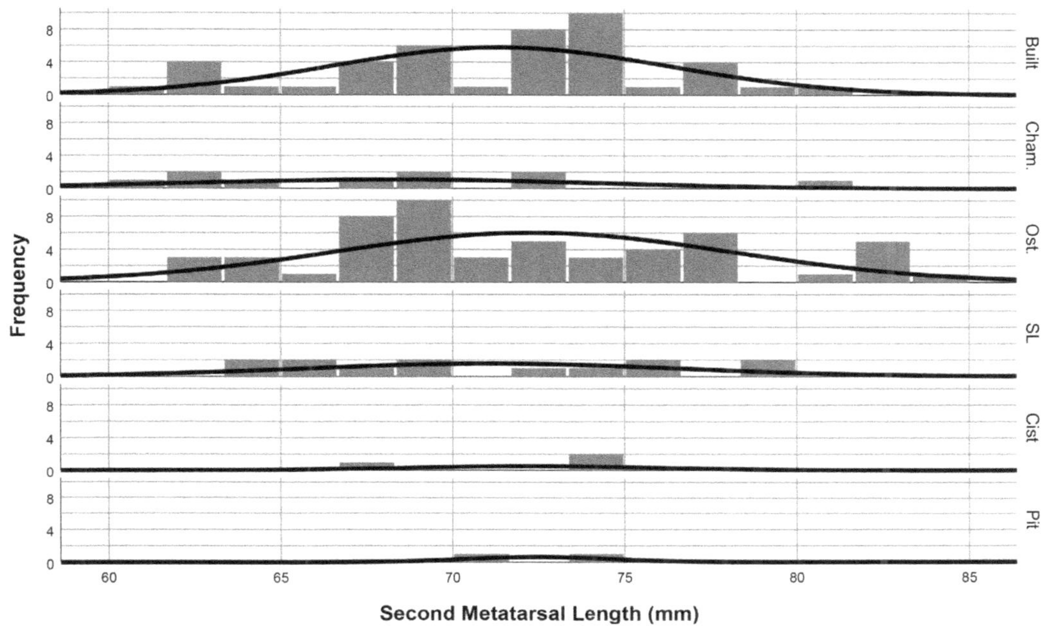

Figure 8.55. Stacked histograms showing the frequency of second metatarsal lengths for each tomb type group (sexes combined), including a normality curve to demonstrate expected values.

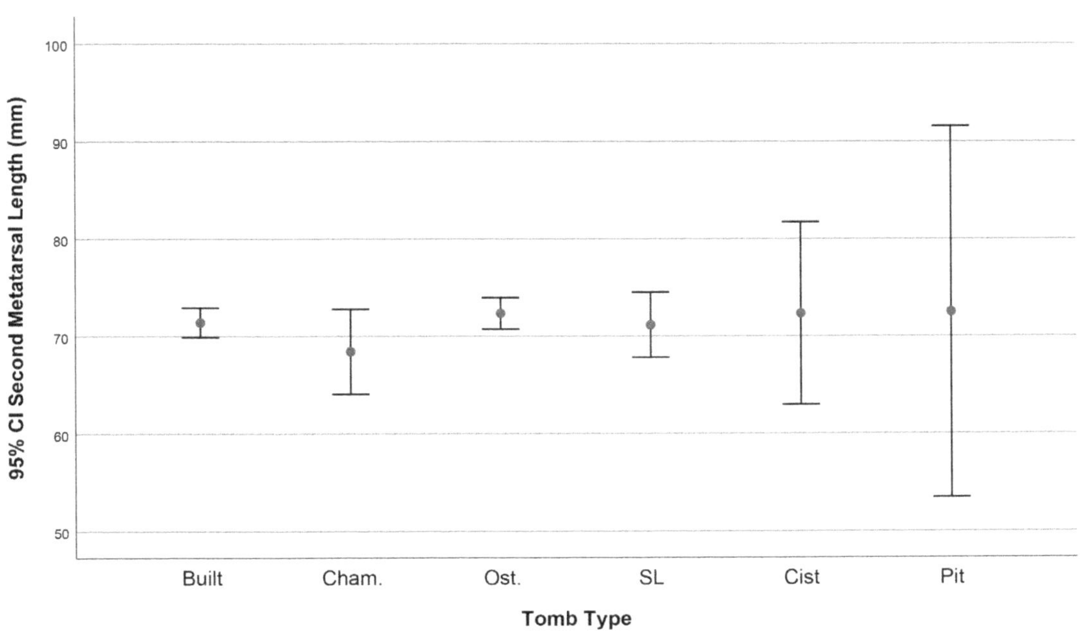

Figure 8.56. Mean second metatarsal lengths with the sexes combined for each tomb type group with error bar plots demonstrating 95% confidence intervals.

8.3.2.3. Third metatarsal

Table 8.23. Descriptive and normality statistics for third metatarsal lengths for each tomb type group (sexes combined).

Third Metatarsal Length (mm)				95% Confidence Interval			Shapiro-Wilk (normality)		
	n	Mean	Std. Error	Lower Bound	Upper Bound	Std. Deviation	Statistic	df	Sig. (*p*)
Built	40	68.23	0.662	66.89	69.56	4.185	0.958	40	0.148
Chamber	14	66.07	1.900	61.97	70.18	7.109	0.973	14	0.909
Osteotheke	53	68.92	0.766	67.38	70.45	5.578	0.961	53	0.078
Stone-lined	7	66.71	2.179	61.38	72.05	5.765	0.851	7	0.126
Cist	3	65.00	3.215	51.17	78.83	5.568	0.976	3	0.702
Tile	1								
Pit	2	71.00	3.000	32.88	109.12	4.243			

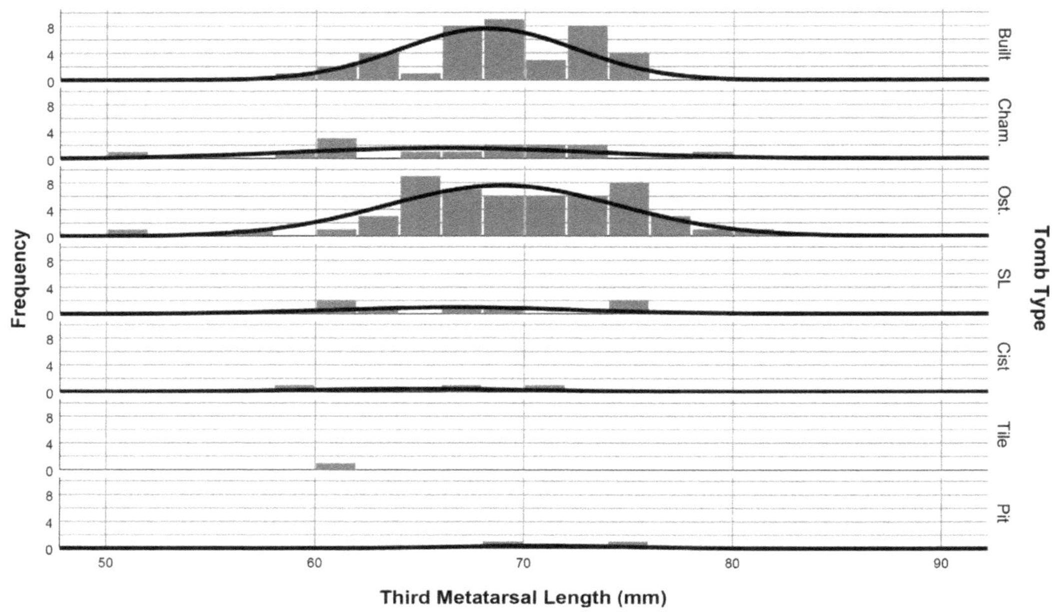

Figure 8.57. Stacked histograms showing the frequency of third metatarsal lengths for each tomb type group (sexes combined), including a normality curve to demonstrate expected values.

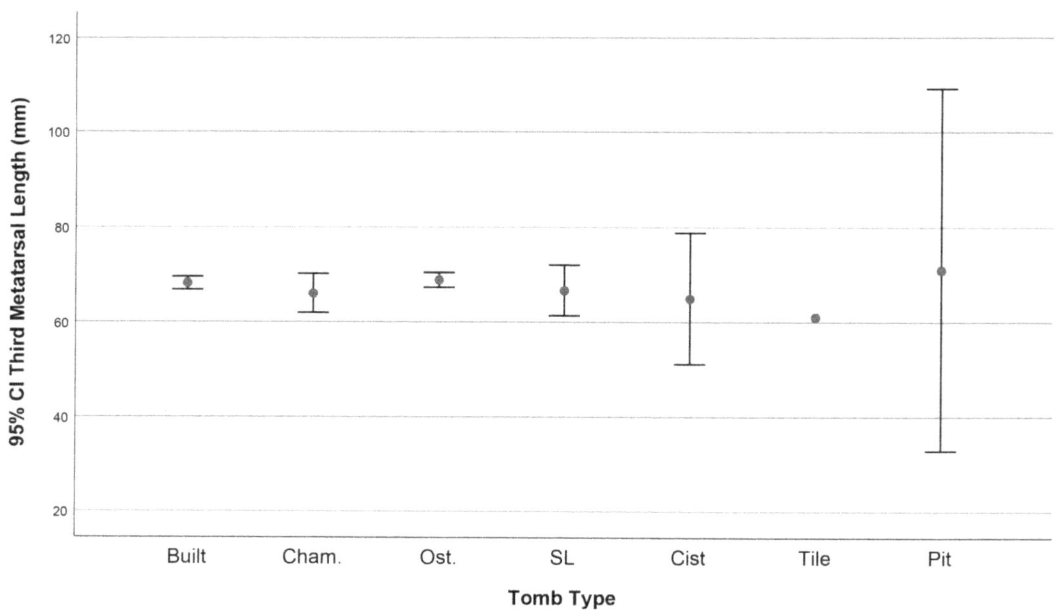

Figure 8.58. Mean third metatarsal lengths with the sexes combined for each tomb type group with error bar plots demonstrating 95% confidence intervals.

8.3.2.4. Fourth metatarsal

Table 8.24. Descriptive and normality statistics for fourth metatarsal lengths for each tomb type group (sexes combined).

Fourth Metatarsal Length (mm)				95% Confidence Interval			Shapiro-Wilk (normality)		
	n	Mean	Std. Error	Lower Bound	Upper Bound	Std. Deviation	Statistic	df	Sig. (*p*)
Built	40	66.81	0.522	65.76	67.87	3.304	0.957	40	0.127
Chamber	7	68.57	1.043	66.02	71.12	2.760	0.908	7	0.380
Osteotheke	41	66.70	0.634	65.42	67.98	4.060	0.969	41	0.318
Stone-lined	8	67.06	1.974	62.39	71.73	5.583	0.932	8	0.531
Cist	3	64.33	3.480	49.36	79.31	6.028	0.991	3	0.817
Tile	1								
Pit	1								

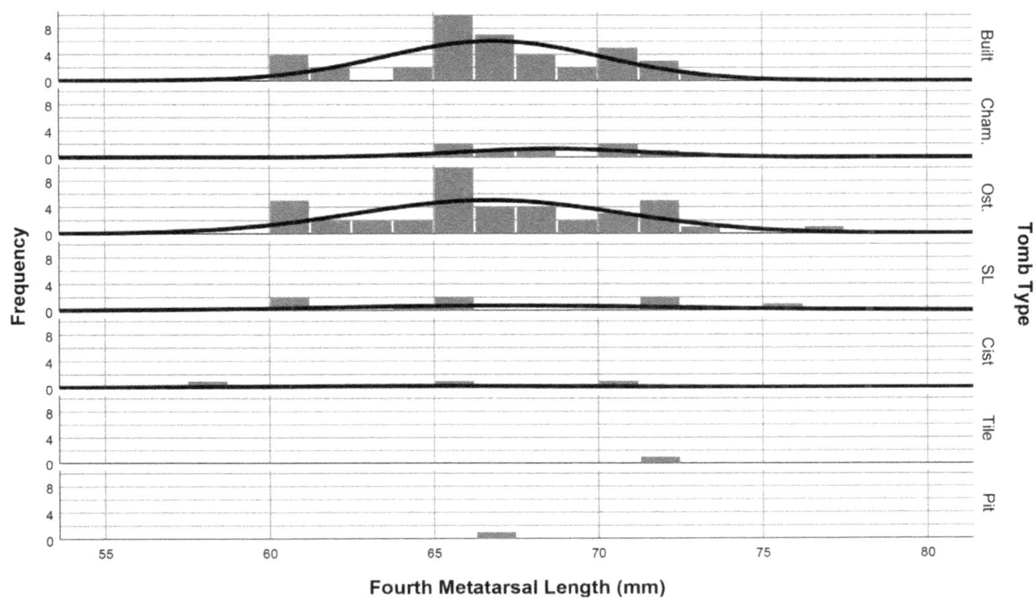

Figure 8.59. Stacked histograms showing the frequency of fourth metatarsal lengths for each tomb type group (sexes combined), including a normality curve to demonstrate expected values.

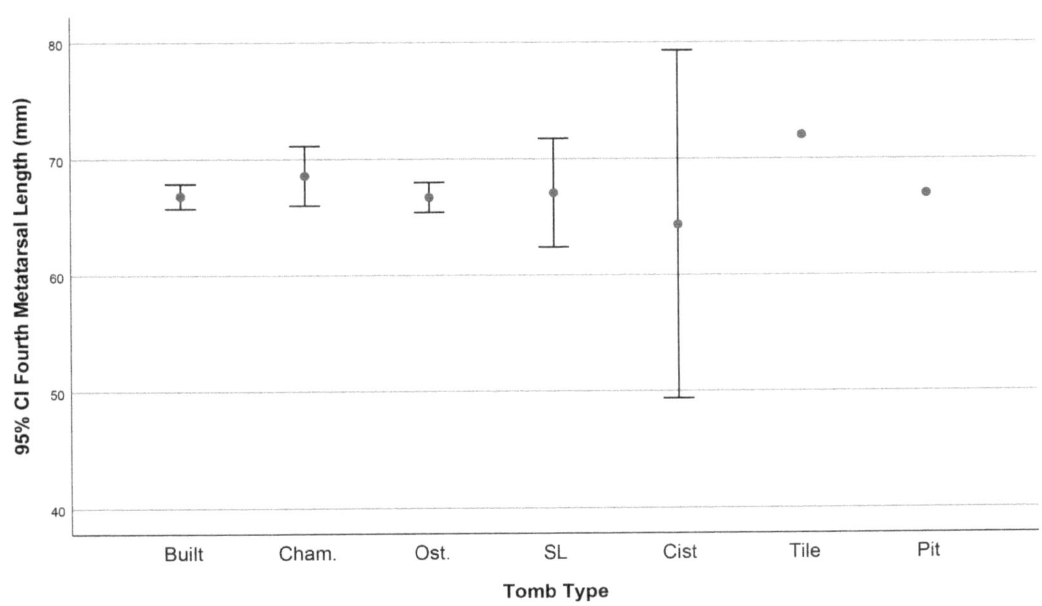

Figure 8.60. Mean fourth metatarsal lengths with the sexes combined for each tomb type group with error bar plots demonstrating 95% confidence intervals.

8.3.2.5. Fifth metatarsal

Table 8.25. Descriptive and normality statistics for fifth metatarsal lengths for each tomb type group (sexes combined).

Fifth Metatarsal Length (mm)				95% Confidence Interval			Shapiro-Wilk (normality)		
	n	Mean	Std. Error	Lower Bound	Upper Bound	Std. Deviation	Statistic	df	Sig. (p)
Built	35	67.26	0.672	65.89	68.62	3.973	0.967	35	0.363
Chamber	7	66.43	2.886	59.37	73.49	7.635	0.913	7	0.419
Osteotheke	48	67.93	0.790	66.34	69.51	5.473	0.959	48	0.093
Stone-lined	9	63.56	1.082	61.06	66.05	3.245	0.935	9	0.533
Cist	4	68.50	1.708	63.06	73.94	3.416	0.971	4	0.850
Tile	2	68.75	4.250	14.75	122.75	6.010			
Pit	1								

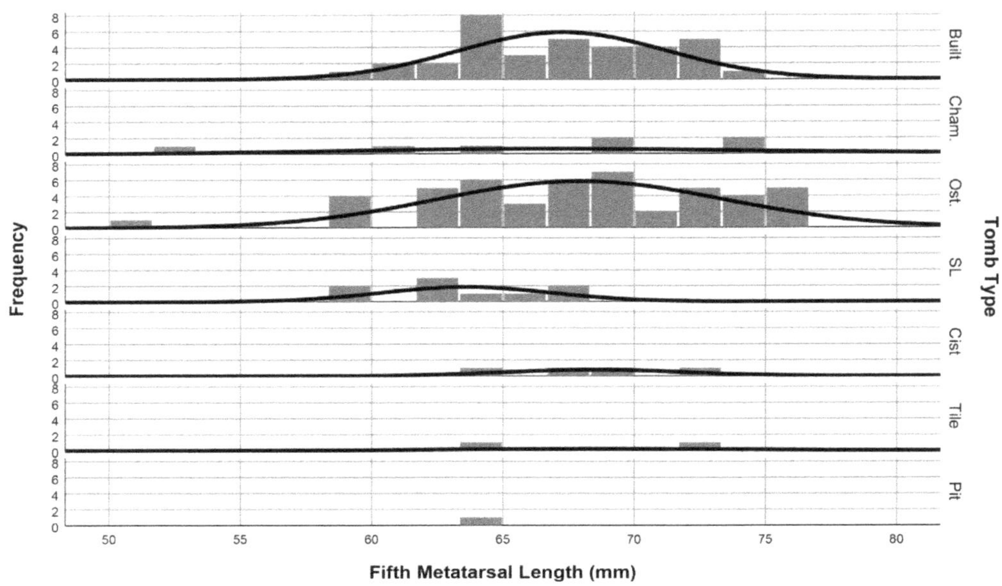

Figure 8.61. Stacked histograms showing the frequency of fifth metatarsal lengths for each tomb type group (sexes combined), including a normality curve to demonstrate expected values.

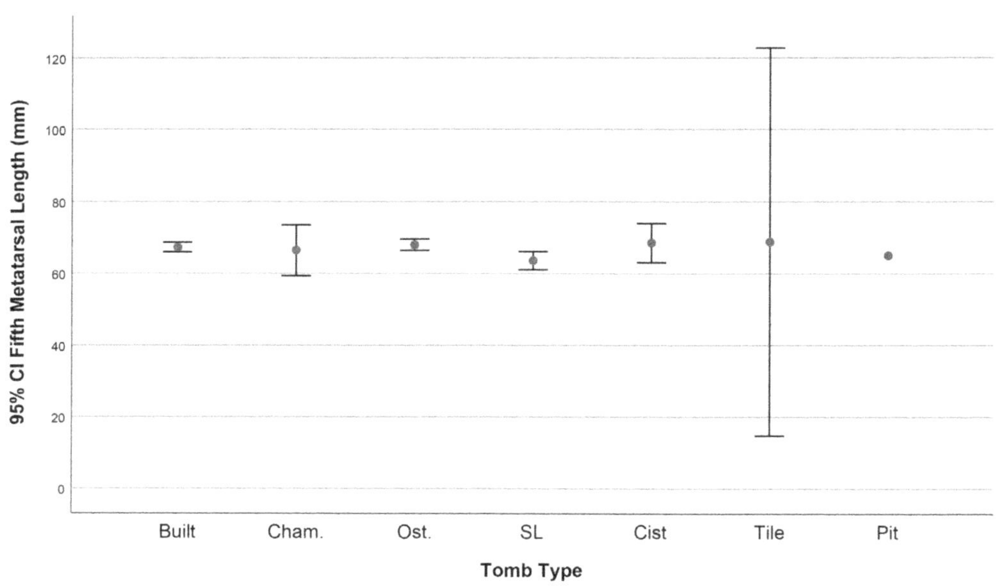

Figure 8.62. Mean fifth metatarsal lengths with the sexes combined for each tomb type group with error bar plots demonstrating 95% confidence intervals.

8.3.3. Location (cemetery)

Due to the large number of cemetery categories, reducing the sample sizes each group, the comparison of bone lengths for the different cemetery locations was approached in the same way as for the tomb types. This involved using only the metatarsals, which where the bone types with the largest samples available, and combining the sexes (which evidently cannot be determined metrically judging by the asymmetry of the single sex histograms in Section 8.3.1). The limb bones and metacarpals had far too small sample sizes for a comparison of mean values for the cemetery categories.

The data for the comparison of the metatarsal lengths between the different cemeteries and locations of the Knossos valley are presented in Tables 8.26–8.30 and Figures 8.63–8.72. Several of the cemeteries still do not have large enough sample sizes for a meaningful comparison, despite combining the sexes. The Hellenistic North Cemetery is not represented by most of the metatarsals and the Roman North Cemetery, Roman Topana tomb and Late Roman Krevatina grave are also generally too poorly represented for any meaningful analysis. For the categories that did have large enough sample sizes to apply some descriptive statistics and normality tests to, they produced Shapiro-Wilk scores of $p>0.05$ in almost every case (the third metatarsal lengths in the Late Antique North Cemetery (KFF) category were the only exception), suggesting normal distributions. However, the histograms generally showed quite ragged and spread out distributions that did not match the normality curve closely. The means and confidence intervals are presented in the error bar plots and clearly demonstrate no difference in mean metatarsal lengths between the cemetery groups. The only case were the plots looked like there might be a difference was for the fifth metatarsals (Figure 8.72) with the Roman North Cemetery mean looking noticeably lower than some of the other results (particularly the Late Roman Sanatorium and Late Antique North Cemetery (KMF) means). However, when the difference in means was tested using a t-test there were no statistically significant differences.

8.3.3.1. First metatarsal

Table 8.26. Descriptive and normality statistics for first metatarsal lengths for each cemetery group (sexes combined).

First Metatarsal Length (mm)				95% Confidence Interval			Shapiro-Wilk (normality)		
	n	Mean	Std. Error	Lower Bound	Upper Bound	Std. Deviation	Statistic	df	Sig. (*p*)
H North Cemetery	0								
R North Cemetery	2	61.00	4.000	10.18	111.82	5.657			
R Topana	2	61.75	0.750	52.22	71.28	1.061			
R Mon. Kephali	9	59.89	1.419	56.62	63.16	4.256	0.953	9	0.726
R/LR Sanatorium	67	59.73	0.416	58.90	60.56	3.407	0.970	67	0.104
LR Krevatina	3	56.83	1.922	48.56	65.10	3.329	0.953	3	0.583
LA North Cemetery (KMF)	50	59.72	0.472	58.77	60.67	3.338	0.976	50	0.404
LA North Cemetery (KFF)	31	60.72	0.991	58.70	62.75	5.515	0.935	31	0.061

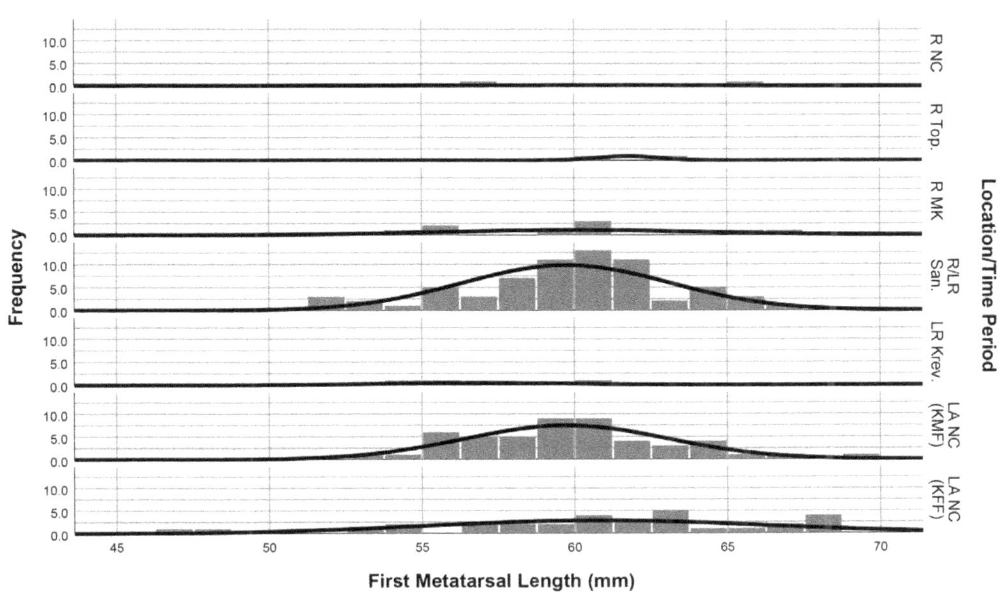

Figure 8.63. Stacked histograms showing the frequency of first metatarsal lengths for each cemetery group (sexes combined), including a normality curve to demonstrate expected values.

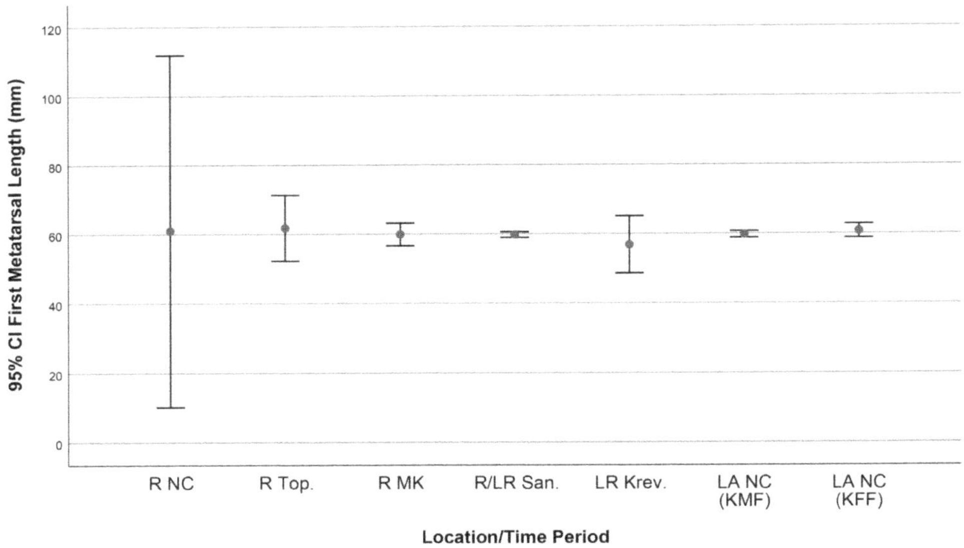

Figure 8.64. Mean first metatarsal lengths with the sexes combined for each cemetery group with error bar plots demonstrating 95% confidence intervals.

8.3.3.2. Second metatarsal

Table 8.27. Descriptive and normality statistics for second metatarsal lengths for each cemetery group (sexes combined).

Second Metatarsal Length (mm)				95% Confidence Interval			Shapiro-Wilk (normality)		
	n	Mean	Std. Error	Lower Bound	Upper Bound	Std. Deviation	Statistic	df	Sig. (*p*)
H North Cemetery	1								
R North Cemetery	1								
R Topana	2	76.25	4.250	22.25	130.25	6.010			
R Mon. Kephali	11	68.91	1.821	64.85	72.97	6.041	0.970	11	0.882
R/LR Sanatorium	53	71.32	0.668	69.98	72.66	4.867	0.970	53	0.202
LR Krevatina	2	71.50	3.500	27.03	115.97	4.950			
LA North Cemetery (KMF)	24	71.50	1.014	69.40	73.60	4.969	0.966	24	0.561
LA North Cemetery (KFF)	30	73.08	1.166	70.70	75.46	6.385	0.948	30	0.146

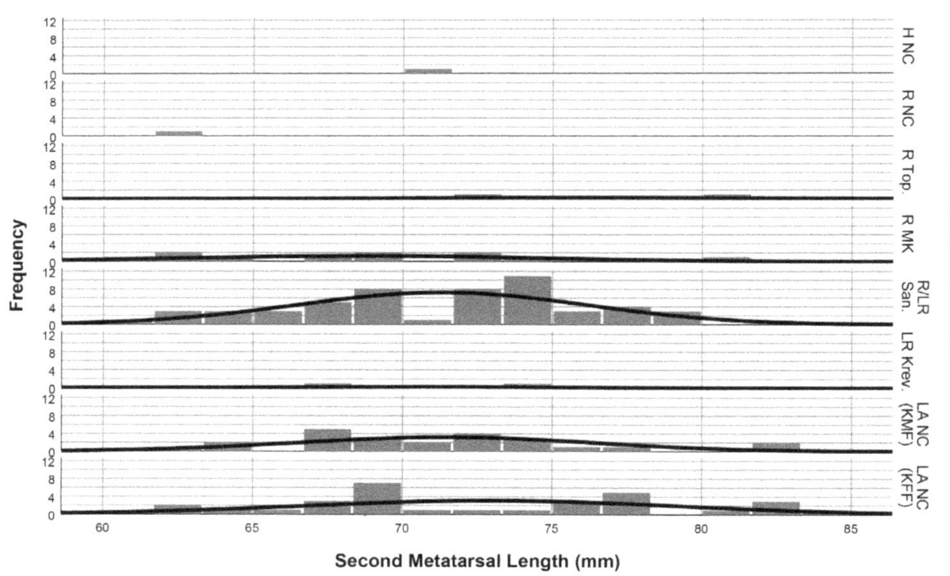

Figure 8.65. Stacked histograms showing the frequency of second metatarsal lengths for each cemetery group (sexes combined), including a normality curve to demonstrate expected values.

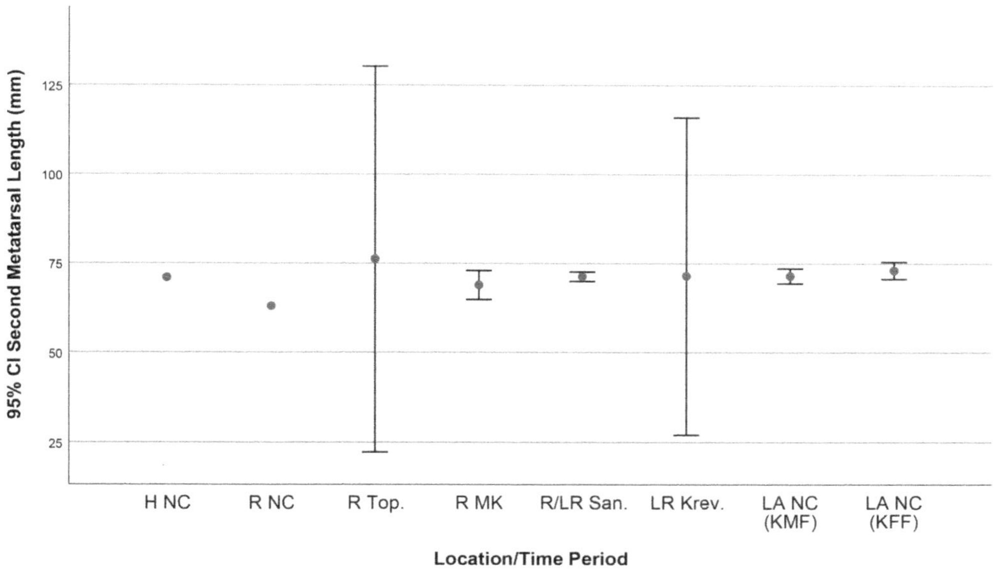

Figure 8.66. Mean second metatarsal lengths with the sexes combined for each cemetery group with error bar plots demonstrating 95% confidence intervals.

8.3.3.3. Third metatarsal

Table 8.28. Descriptive and normality statistics for third metatarsal lengths for each cemetery group (sexes combined).

Third Metatarsal Length (mm)				95% Confidence Interval			Shapiro-Wilk (normality)		
	n	Mean	Std. Error	Lower Bound	Upper Bound	Std. Deviation	Statistic	df	Sig. (*p*)
H North Cemetery	0								
R North Cemetery	2	73.00	1.000	60.29	85.71	1.414			
R Topana	1								
R Mon. Kephali	14	66.71	1.823	62.78	70.65	6.821	0.959	14	0.702
R/LR Sanatorium	47	67.49	0.674	66.13	68.85	4.620	0.954	47	0.061
LR Krevatina	3	65.00	3.215	51.17	78.83	5.568	0.976	3	0.702
LA North Cemetery (KMF)	23	68.70	1.001	66.62	70.77	4.800	0.954	23	0.349
LA North Cemetery (KFF)	30	69.08	1.129	66.77	71.39	6.184	0.915	30	0.020

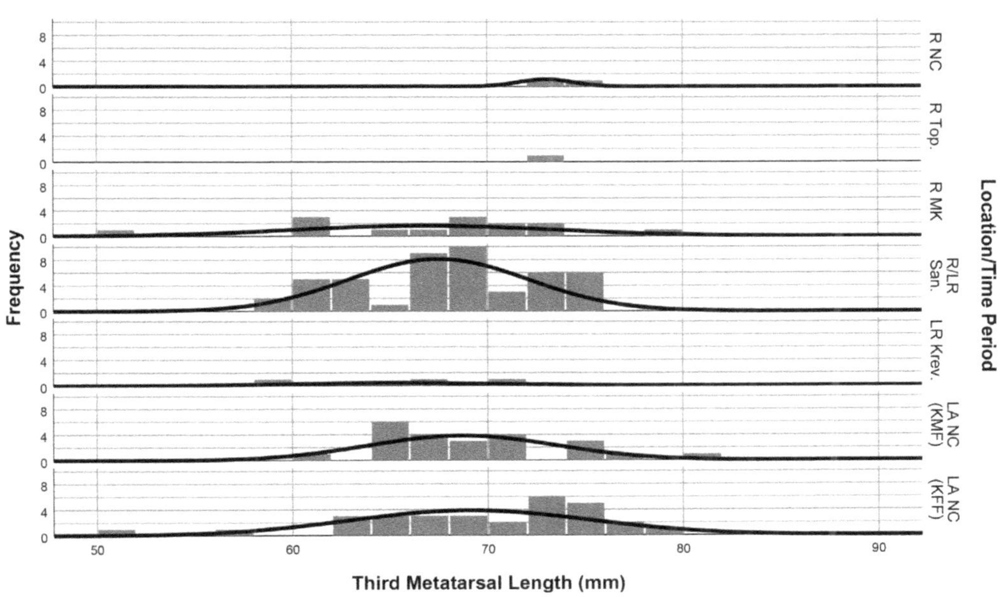

Figure 8.67. Stacked histograms showing the frequency of third metatarsal lengths for each cemetery group (sexes combined), including a normality curve to demonstrate expected values.

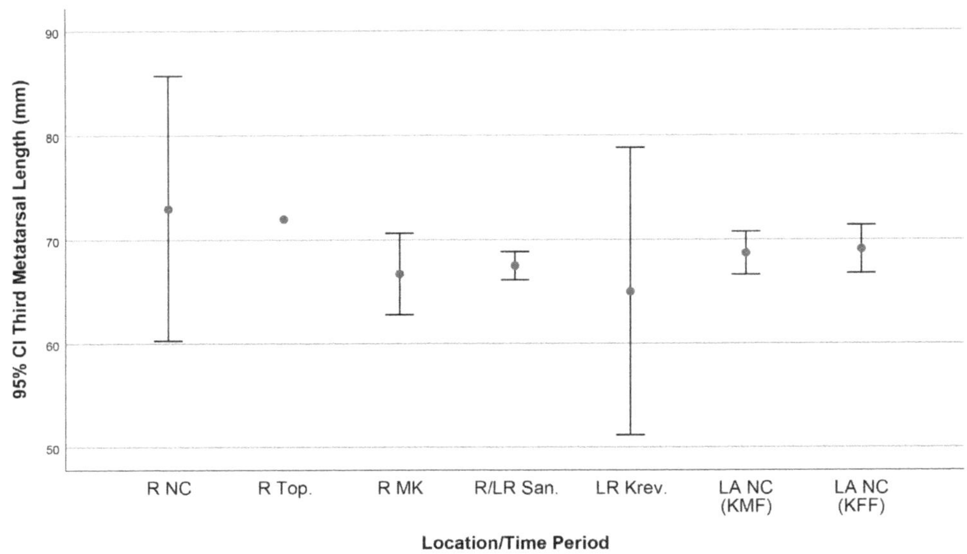

Figure 8.68. Mean third metatarsal lengths with the sexes combined for each cemetery group with error bar plots demonstrating 95% confidence intervals.

8.3.3.4. Fourth metatarsal

Table 8.29. Descriptive and normality statistics for fourth metatarsal lengths for each cemetery group (sexes combined).

Fourth Metatarsal Length (mm)				95% Confidence Interval			Shapiro-Wilk (normality)		
	n	Mean	Std. Error	Lower Bound	Upper Bound	Std. Deviation	Statistic	df	Sig. (*p*)
H North Cemetery	0								
R North Cemetery	2	66.50	0.500	60.15	72.85	0.707			
R Topana	3	68.50	2.021	59.81	77.19	3.500	0.862	3	0.274
R Mon. Kephali	8	68.38	0.925	66.19	70.56	2.615	0.903	8	0.305
R/LR Sanatorium	44	66.88	0.580	65.70	68.05	3.851	0.962	44	0.155
LR Krevatina	3	64.33	3.480	49.36	79.31	6.028	0.991	3	0.817
LA North Cemetery (KMF)	20	66.95	0.701	65.48	68.42	3.137	0.967	20	0.698
LA North Cemetery (KFF)	21	66.47	1.058	64.26	68.67	4.847	0.942	21	0.234

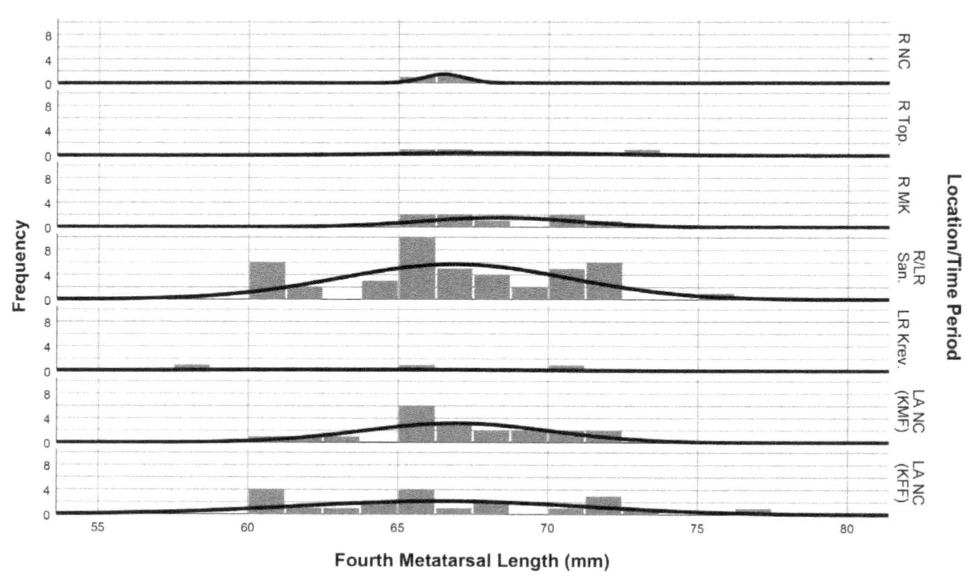

Figure 8.69. Stacked histograms showing the frequency of fourth metatarsal lengths for each cemetery group (sexes combined), including a normality curve to demonstrate expected values.

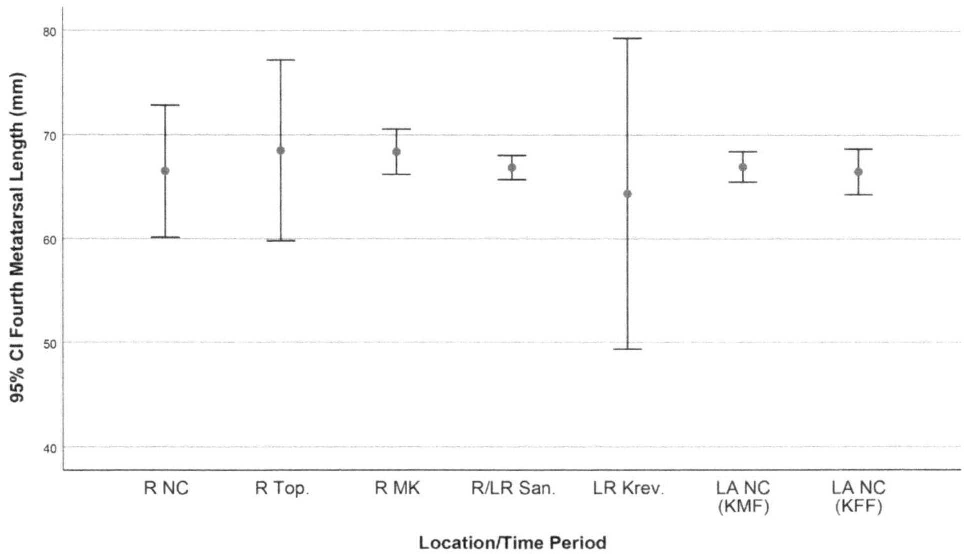

Figure 8.70. Mean fourth metatarsal lengths with the sexes combined for each cemetery group with error bar plots demonstrating 95% confidence intervals.

8.3.3.5. Fifth metatarsal

Table 8.30. Descriptive and normality statistics for fifth metatarsal lengths for each cemetery group (sexes combined).

Fifth Metatarsal Length (mm)				95% Confidence Interval			Shapiro-Wilk (normality)		
	n	Mean	Std. Error	Lower Bound	Upper Bound	Std. Deviation	Statistic	df	Sig. (*p*)
H North Cemetery	0								
R North Cemetery	4	64.63	0.239	63.86	65.39	0.479	0.863	4	0.272
R Topana	1								
R Mon. Kephali	8	66.25	2.505	60.33	72.17	7.086	0.931	8	0.530
R/LR Sanatorium	40	66.75	0.672	65.39	68.11	4.253	0.972	40	0.413
LR Krevatina	4	68.50	1.708	63.06	73.94	3.416	0.971	4	0.850
LA North Cemetery (KMF)	19	67.58	0.912	65.66	69.50	3.977	0.930	19	0.172
LA North Cemetery (KFF)	30	67.98	1.147	65.63	70.33	6.284	0.936	30	0.072

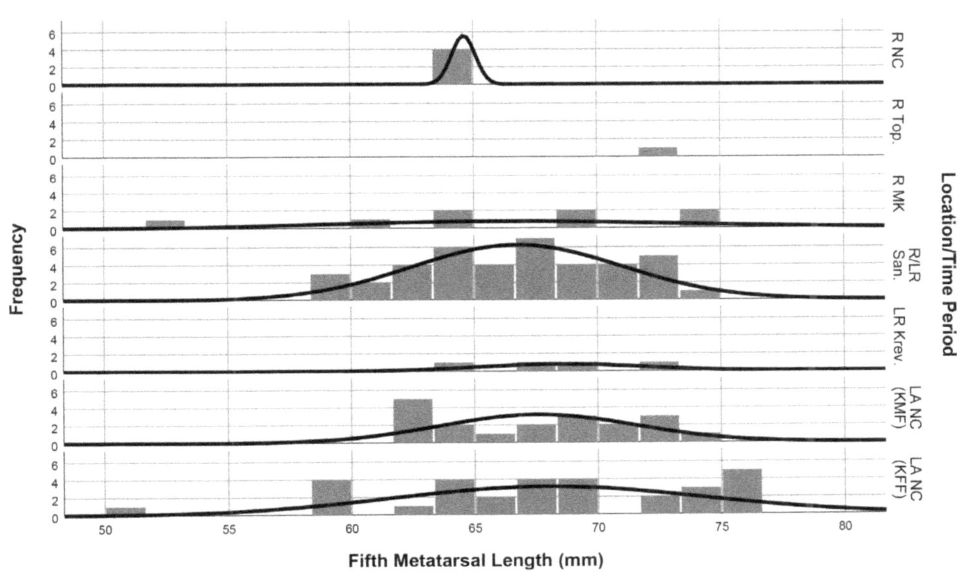

Figure 8.71. Stacked histograms showing the frequency of fifth metatarsal lengths for each cemetery group (sexes combined), including a normality curve to demonstrate expected values.

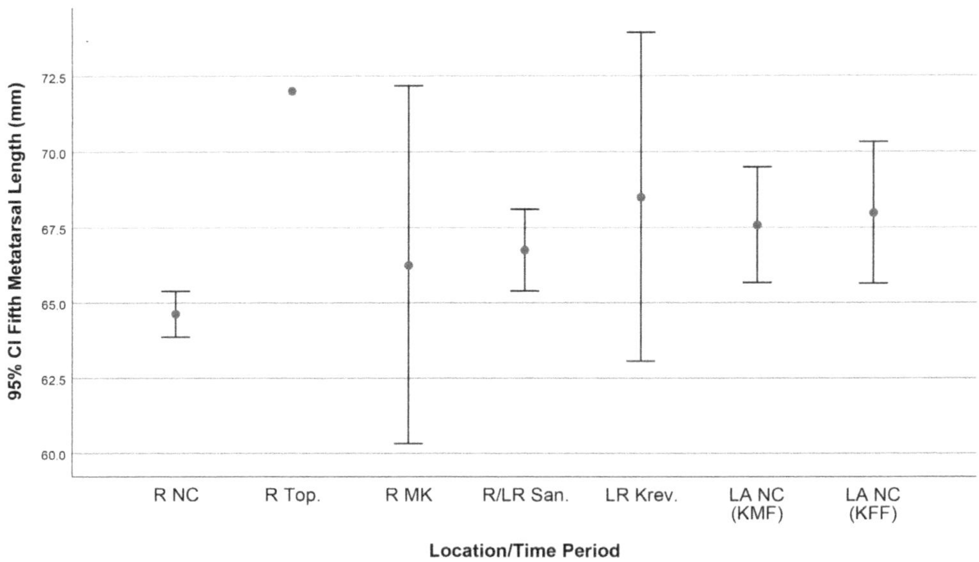

Figure 8.72. Mean fifth metatarsal lengths with the sexes combined for each cemetery group with error bar plots demonstrating 95% confidence intervals.

8.4. Stature Results

The lengths of 1194 complete long bones, metacarpals and metatarsals were used to estimate stature. In many cases a single individual is represented by multiple bones and different stature estimates, and it is often not possible to distinguish the extent of this repetition in commingled contexts. The overall mean stature estimate for females was 156.78 cm (n=505), while for males it is 171.85cm (n=689).

Stature estimation formula are sex specific, which was the primary need to attempt to determine sex metrically of all the measured bones (unlike the bone lengths which could be considered with the sexes combined). It was evident in the analysis of the bone lengths that this is not successful in producing a representative sample of a single sex within the population. It divides females and males leaving two disjointed groups of bone lengths that do not overlap, evident on the asymmetrical histograms. The following results for female and male stature estimates, by the categorical variables of time period, tomb type and cemetery groups, generally have non-normal Shapiro-Wilk scores ($p<0.05$) and asymmetrical histograms. The asymmetry caused by the metric sexing is further accentuated by using the sex-specific stature estimation formulae.

8.4.1. Time period

The stature results for females and males by time period are presented in Table 8.31. The distribution of stature results for the Hellenistic period cannot be properly assessed due to the small sample size. The Roman and Late Antique stature distributions are not normal according to the Shapiro-Wilk test and this is evident from the positive skew to the female results (Figure 8.73) and the negative skew of the male results (Figure 8.74). There is very little difference between the Roman and Late Antique Female means, though the Late Antique males had a higher mean stature estimate than the Roman males, with non-overlapping confidence intervals (Figure 8.75). A t-test proved this to be a statistically significant difference (t=−3.662, df=663.677, p=0.000, mean difference=−1.134, confidence intervals=−1.742 to −0.526). However, due to the non-normal distribution of this sample, it cannot be taken as random and may not be representative of the population.

8.4.2. Tomb type

Unlike the time period groups, some of the tomb type groups achieved a normal ($p>0.05$) Shapiro-Wilk score (Table 8.32), though in some cases this was only because there was too

Table 8.31. Descriptive and normality statistics for stature estimates for each sex/time period group.

Stature (cm)				95% Confidence Interval			Shapiro-Wilk (normality)		
	n	Mean	Std. Error	Lower Bound	Upper Bound	Std. Deviation	Statistic	df	Sig. (*p*)
F Hell.	9	155.17	2.07	150.39	159.94	6.21	0.896	9	0.230
F Roman	265	156.73	0.28	156.17	157.29	4.62	0.946	265	0.000
F LA	231	156.89	0.29	156.33	157.46	4.37	0.939	231	0.000
M Hell.	4	171.83	2.25	164.67	178.99	4.50	0.900	4	0.431
M Roman	335	171.27	0.20	170.88	171.65	3.60	0.974	335	0.000
M LA	350	172.40	0.24	171.93	172.87	4.47	0.978	350	0.000

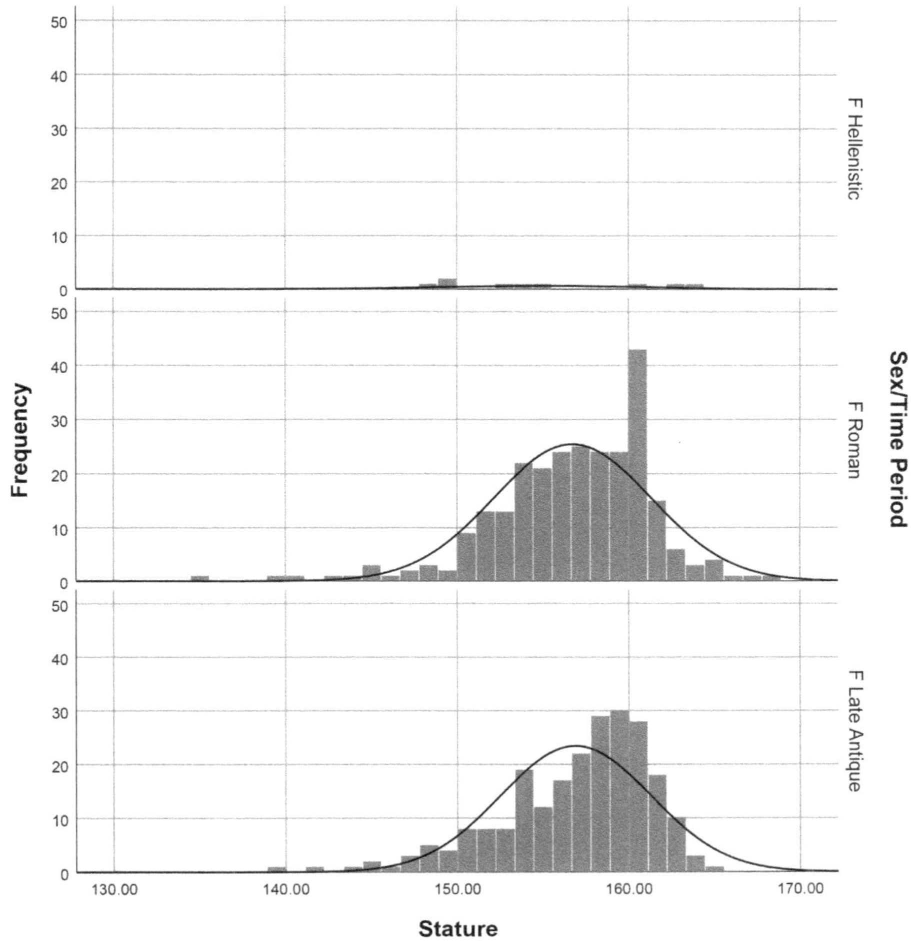

Figure 8.73. Stacked histograms showing the frequency of stature estimations for each female time period group and including a normality curve to demonstrate expected values.

small a sample size to prove otherwise. For some of the larger sample sizes, such as the osteotheke, built and chamber categories for both females and males, these non-normal statistics are caused by asymmetry, with a positive skew for females (Figure 8.76) and a negative skew for males (Figure 8.77). The normality curves do not appear to be too far from the bars of the histograms or too irregular otherwise.

For the females, there is not a large difference between the means, particularly with the majority of confidence intervals having significant overlap (Figure 8.78). However, the chamber tomb does appear to have a lower result than both the built tomb and osteotheke groups, with non-overlapping confidence intervals. Using a t-test, these differences proved to be statistically significant (though equal variances could not be assumed), for both the comparison of the built and chamber tomb groups (t=4.254, df=103.527, p=0.000, mean difference=3.227, confidence intervals= 1.723 to 4.731) and the chamber tomb and osteotheke groups (t=−3.406, df=89.564, p=0.001, mean difference=−2.474, confidence intervals= −3.917 to −1.031). As the confidence intervals do not cross zero, it is possible there is a real difference between the chamber tomb female statures and those of the built tombs and osteothekai.

There are more evident differences in mean stature for the males with the confidence intervals for a number of the tomb categories not overlapping (Figure 8.79). The six pairs of groups with statistically significant differences in means, are listed as follows:

	t	df	Sig. (2-tailed) p	Mean Difference	Std. Error Difference	95% CI Lower	95% CI Upper
Built-Osteotheke:	−5.117	466.657	0.000	−1.717	0.336	−2.377	−1.058
Built-Chamber:	−2.801	132.071	0.006	−1.379	0.492	−2.352	−0.405
Built-Cist	2.795	42.469	0.008	2.122	0.759	0.590	3.654
Chamber-Cist:	4.297	118	0.000	3.501	0.815	1.887	5.114
Osteotheke-Cist:	5.111	341	0.000	3.839	0.751	2.362	5.317
Osteotheke-Stone-lined:	2.903	370	0.004	1.716	0.591	0.554	2.879

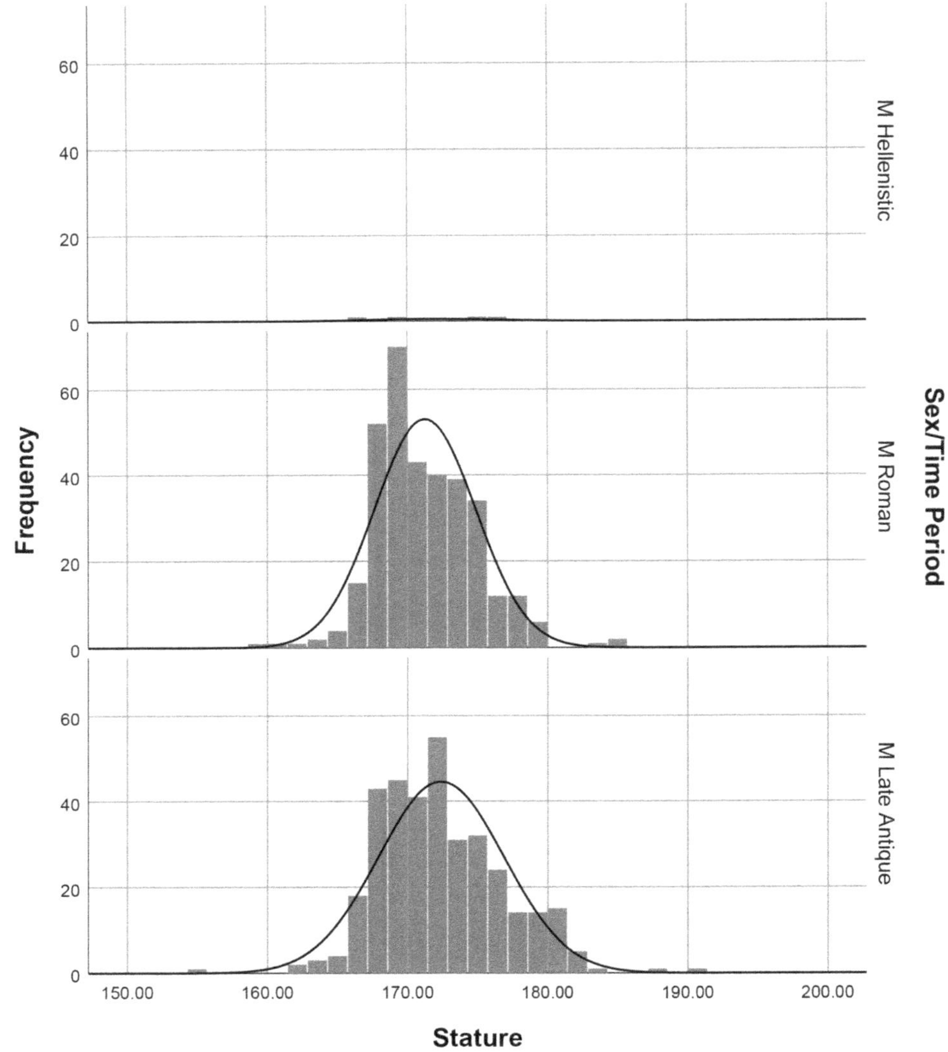

Figure 8.74. Stacked histograms showing the frequency of stature estimations for each male time period group and including a normality curve to demonstrate expected values.

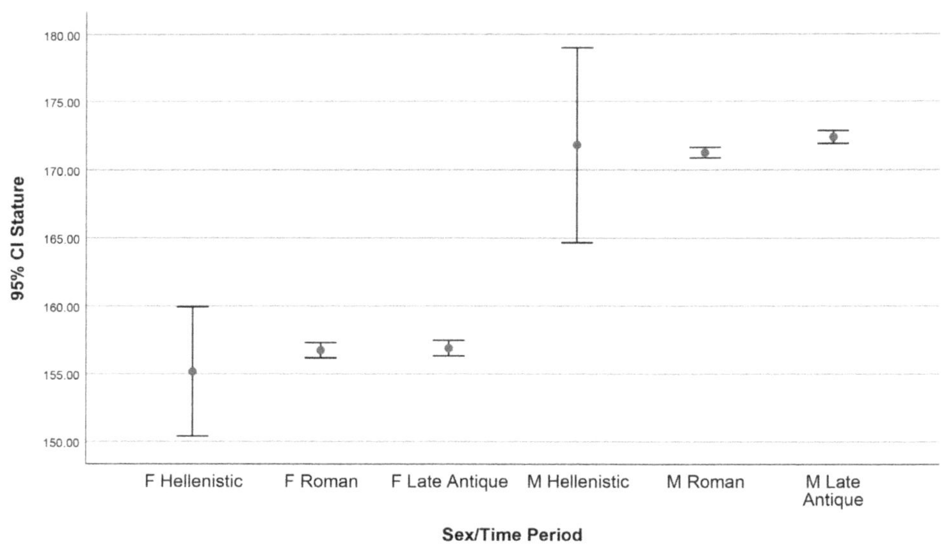

Figure 8.75. Error bar plots demonstrating mean stature estimations for each sex/time period group, with 95% confidence intervals.

Table 8.32. Descriptive and normality statistics for stature estimates for each sex/tomb type group.

Stature (cm)				95% Confidence Interval			Shapiro-Wilk (normality)		
	n	Mean	Std. Error	Lower Bound	Upper Bound	Std. Dev.	Statistic	df	Sig. (*p*)
F Built	140	157.92	0.36	157.20	158.64	4.30	0.937	140	0.000
F Chamber	65	154.69	0.67	153.36	156.02	5.37	0.902	65	0.000
F Osteotheke	213	157.17	0.29	156.59	157.74	4.23	0.929	213	0.000
F Stone-lined	35	156.02	0.62	154.76	157.27	3.66	0.952	35	0.129
F Cist	37	154.91	0.73	153.44	156.38	4.41	0.988	37	0.959
F Sarcophagus	2	158.41	2.79	123.02	193.79	3.94			
F Tile	7	155.97	1.62	152.01	159.94	4.29	0.925	7	0.511
F Pit	6	155.34	2.72	148.34	162.33	6.67	0.829	6	0.106
M Built	183	171.01	0.23	170.55	171.47	3.13	0.971	183	0.001
M Chamber	84	172.39	0.43	171.52	173.25	3.98	0.918	84	0.000
M Osteotheke	307	172.73	0.24	172.25	173.20	4.26	0.979	307	0.000
M Stone-lined	65	171.01	0.58	169.85	172.17	4.67	0.857	65	0.000
M Cist	36	168.89	0.72	167.42	170.35	4.34	0.987	36	0.944
M Sarcophagus	1								
M Tile	9	172.51	0.95	170.31	174.71	2.86	0.917	9	0.372
M Pit	4	171.49	2.03	165.01	177.96	4.07	0.837	4	0.188

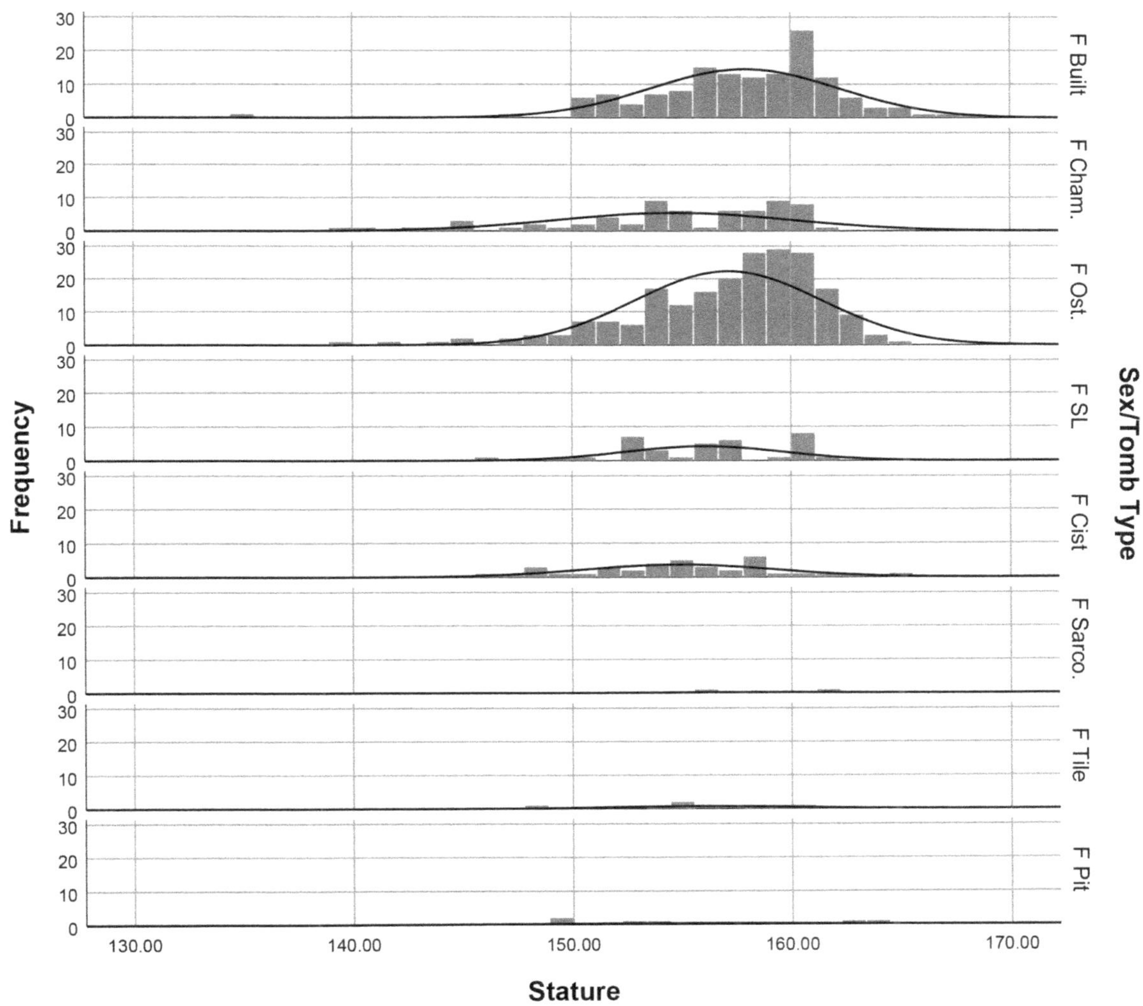

Figure 8.76. Stacked histograms showing the frequency of stature estimations for each female tomb type group and including a normality curve to demonstrate expected values.

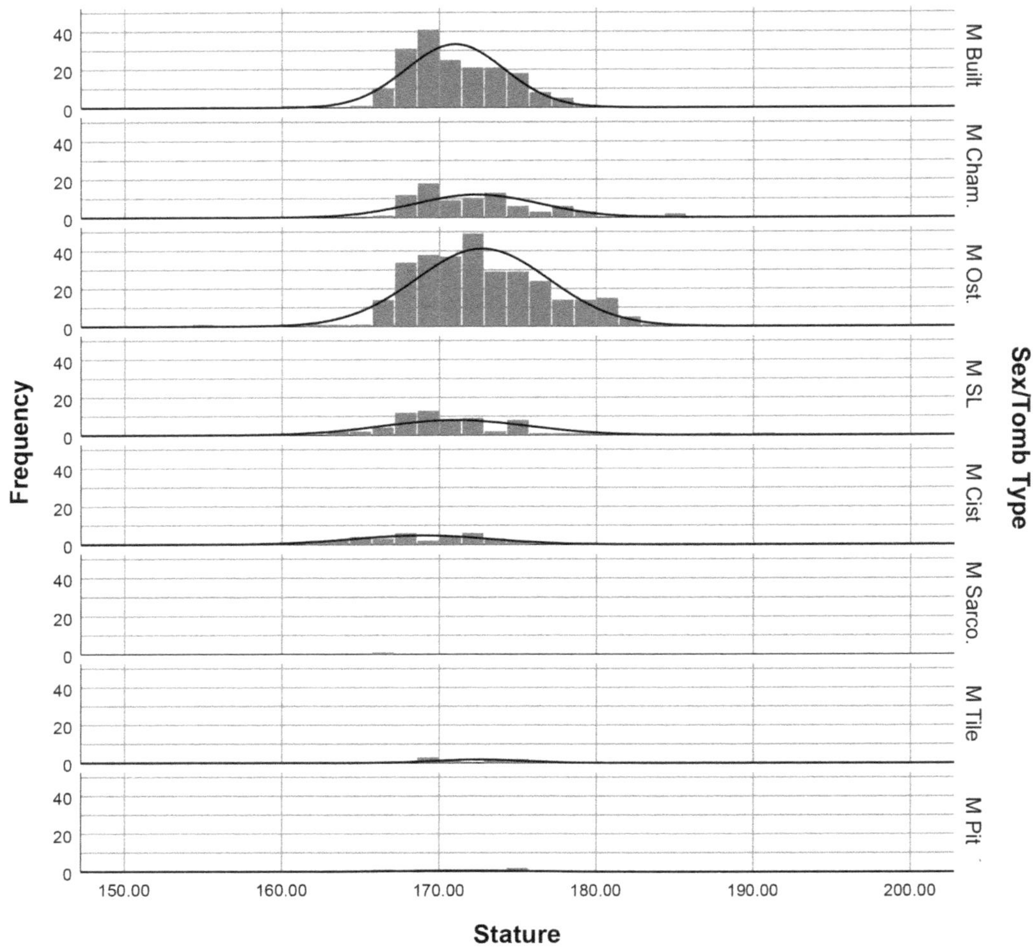

Figure 8.77. Stacked histograms showing the frequency of stature estimations for each male tomb type group and including a normality curve to demonstrate expected values.

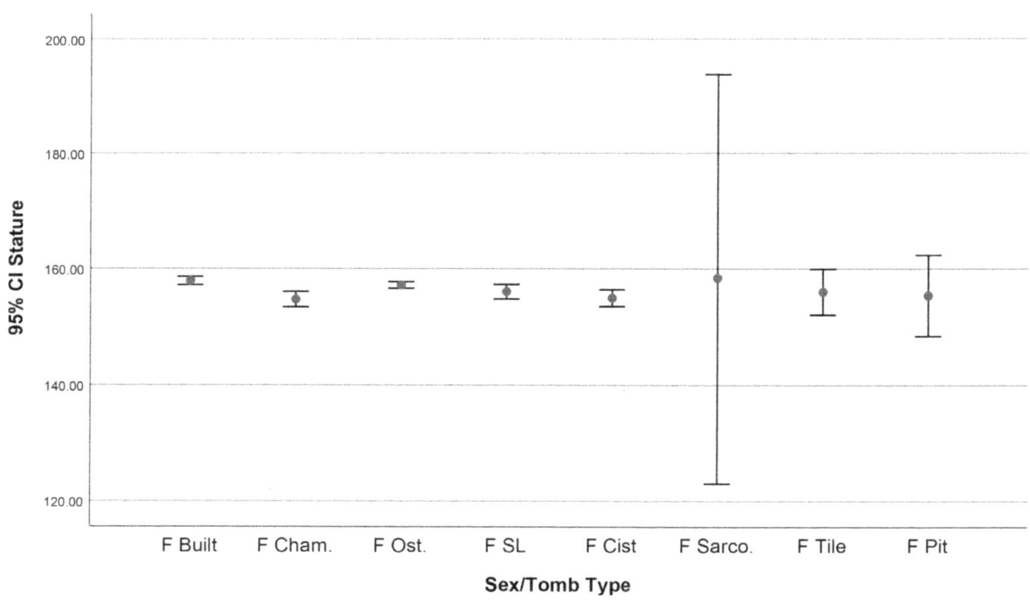

Figure 8.78. Error bar plots demonstrating mean stature estimations for each female tomb type group, with 95% confidence intervals.

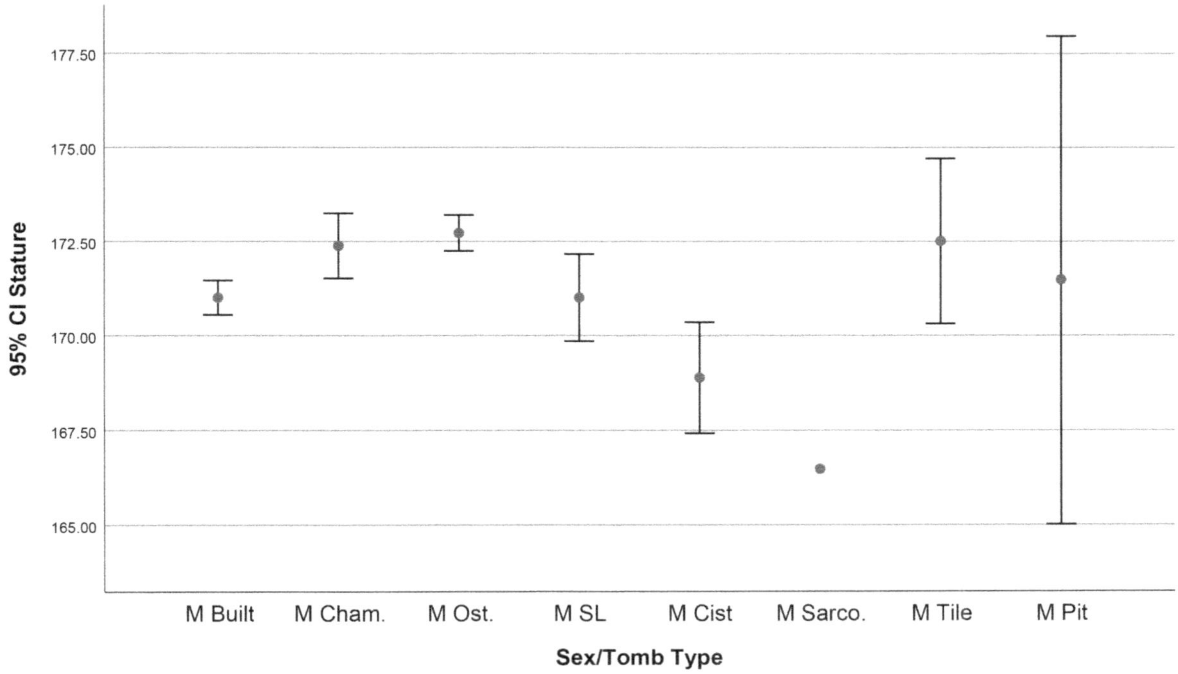

Figure 8.79. Error bar plots demonstrating mean stature estimations for each male tomb type group, with 95% confidence intervals.

Other than pairs involving the built tomb category, the variances of could be assumed to be equal. The confidence intervals in each case did not cross zero and $p<0.05$ suggesting these could be real differences. The chamber tomb and osteotheke male means were higher in each case, the former example contrasting the low female mean for the chamber tomb group and calling into question whether this was a meaningful result. The cist grave mean was low in each case, though the stature estimates were based on the bone lengths of only two individuals.

The stone-lined tomb mean male stature was significantly lower than the osteotheke mean, which was not a significant difference for the females, though the mean female stature was also higher for the osteotheke group. There was a larger sample size for the males in both of these tomb groups, suggesting it could be the more reliable result (though they did not have normal distributions). Although the built tomb mean was significantly lower than that of the osteotheke and chamber tomb groups, it was also significantly higher than the cist grave mean. This contrasts the female results for which the mean stature from the built tomb group was the highest reliable result (excluding the sarcophagus group due to sample size). This could indicate that this was not a truly significant result, or that there were different conditions for females and males.

8.4.3. Cemetery (location)

As was found to be the case for the tomb type groups, the only cemetery groups that achieve a normal Shapiro-Wilk ($p<0.05$) score are the ones with too small a sample size to prove a non-normal distribution of stature estimates (Table 8.33). The larger sample sizes display asymmetry, as observed for the previous variables, with the histograms for the female groups displaying a positive skew (Figure 8.80) and the male groups showing a negative skew (Figure 8.81), and a degree of irregularity to all of the distributions in relation to the normality curve. The male distributions for the larger samples have more regular distributions, closer to normal, with the exception of the slight negative skew.

Similar to the error bar plots for the tomb types, the cemetery error bar plots, displaying the mean stature values and their confidence intervals, the males (Figure 8.83) appear to have much greater differences in the means between the cemeteries than the females (Figure 8.82). This is also accentuated by the scale of the graph, with the wide confidence intervals of the Female Topana group extending the scale required for the female plot.

All the female mean stature estimates were within c.2cm of each other. The most substantial differences in female mean stature estimates between the cemetery

Table 8.33. Descriptive and normality statistics for stature estimates for each sex/cemetery group.

Stature (cm)				95% Confidence Interval			Shapiro-Wilk (normality)		
	n	Mean	Std. Error	Lower Bound	Upper Bound	Std. Dev.	Statistic	df	Sig. (*p*)
F H North Cemetery	9	155.17	2.07	150.39	159.94	6.21	0.896	9	0.230
F R North Cemetery	22	156.74	0.68	155.33	158.15	3.18	0.902	22	0.033
F R Topana	3	155.20	10.20	111.29	199.11	17.68	0.903	3	0.396
F R Mon. Keph.	56	155.39	0.68	154.02	156.76	5.12	0.866	56	0.000
F R/LR Sana.	159	157.33	0.34	156.65	158.00	4.29	0.971	159	0.002
F LR Krevatina	25	156.14	0.69	154.71	157.56	3.45	0.984	25	0.947
F LA North Cemetery (KMF)	110	157.43	0.36	156.71	158.14	3.77	0.943	110	0.000
F LA North Cemetery (KFF)	121	156.41	0.44	155.54	157.28	4.82	0.940	121	0.000
M H North Cemetery	4	171.83	2.25	164.67	178.99	4.50	0.900	4	0.431
M R North Cemetery	10	171.00	1.05	168.61	173.38	3.33	0.849	10	0.056
M R Topana	29	173.34	0.62	172.07	174.61	3.33	0.957	29	0.280
M R Mon. Kephali	83	172.44	0.44	171.57	173.31	3.97	0.920	83	0.000
M R/LR Sana.	186	170.73	0.22	170.30	171.16	2.99	0.967	186	0.000
M LR Krevatina	27	169.22	0.90	167.38	171.07	4.66	0.982	27	0.897
M LA North Cemetery (KMF)	152	171.63	0.35	170.93	172.33	4.36	0.932	152	0.000
M LA North Cemetery (KFF)	176	173.47	0.34	172.81	174.14	4.45	0.978	176	0.007
M LA Mon. Kephali	22	169.14	0.52	168.05	170.23	2.45	0.938	22	0.177

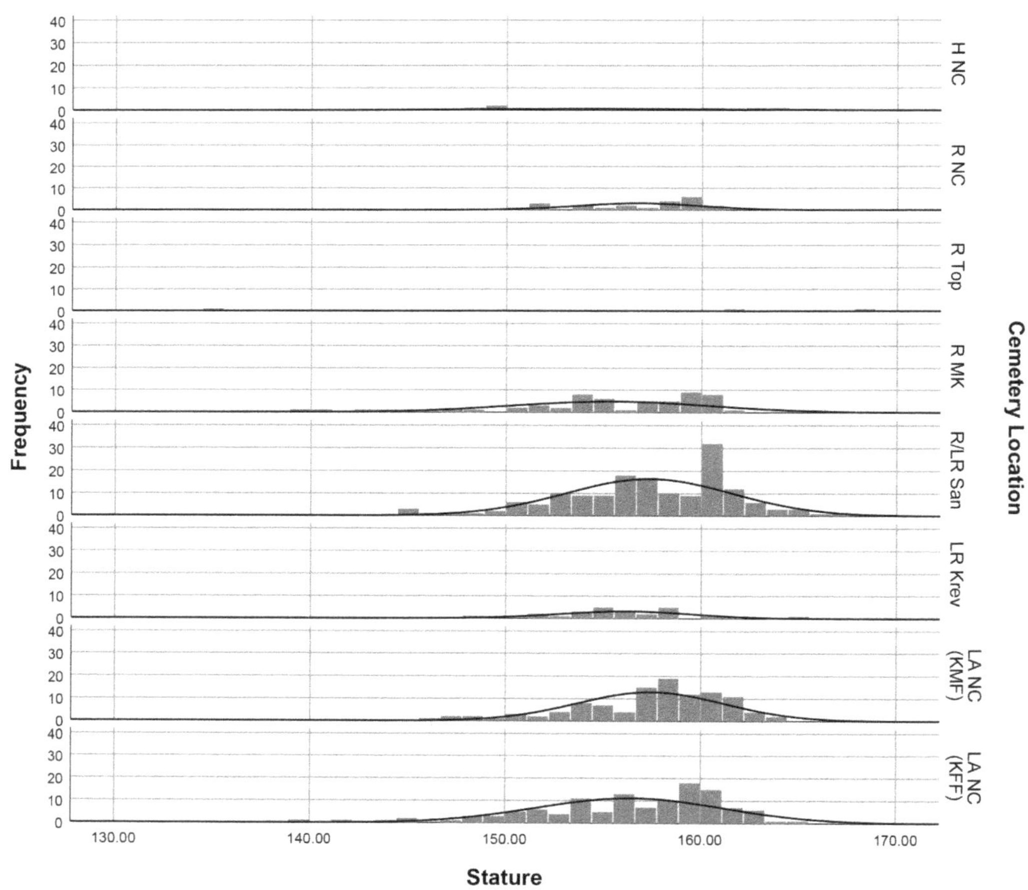

Figure 8.80. Stacked histograms showing the frequency of stature estimations for each female cemetery group and including a normality curve to demonstrate expected values.

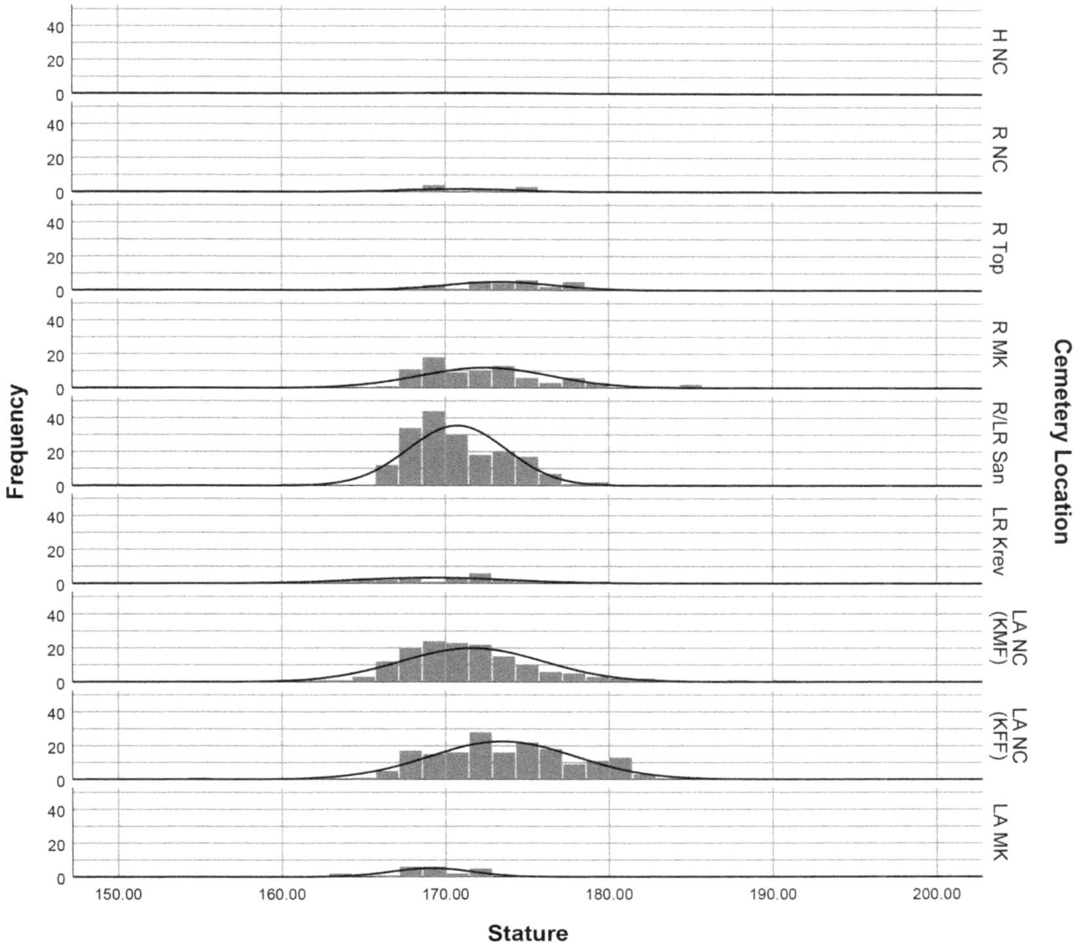

Figure 8.81. Stacked histograms showing the frequency of stature estimations for each male cemetery group and including a normality curve to demonstrate expected values.

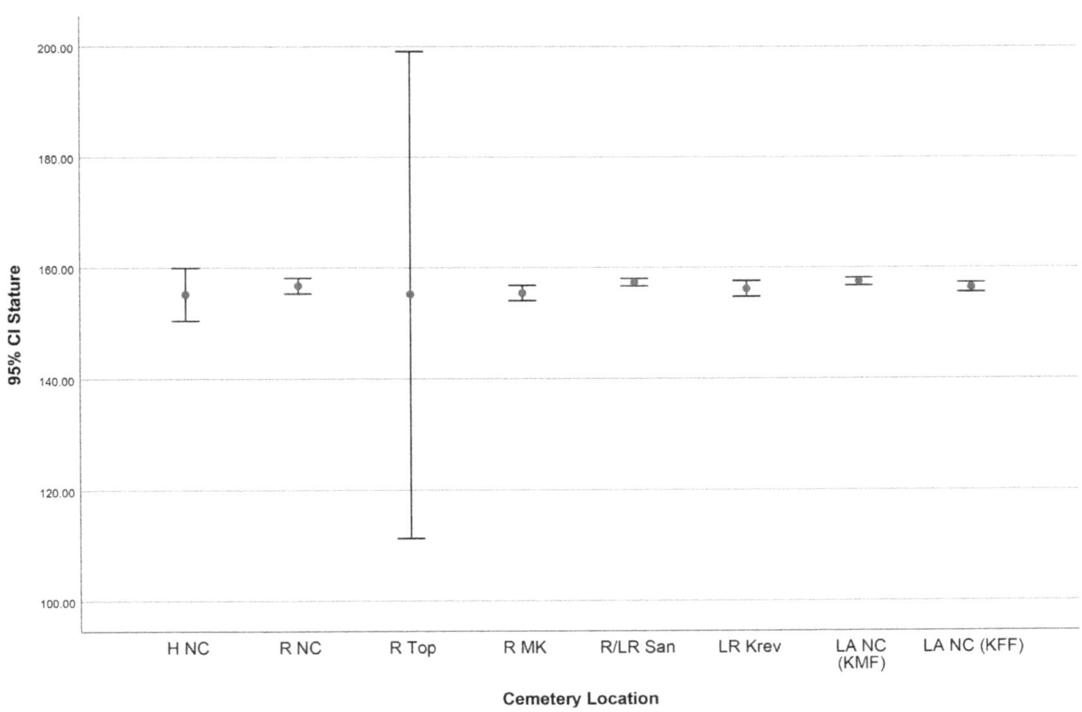

Figure 8.82. Error bar plots demonstrating mean stature estimations for each female cemetery group, with 95% confidence intervals.

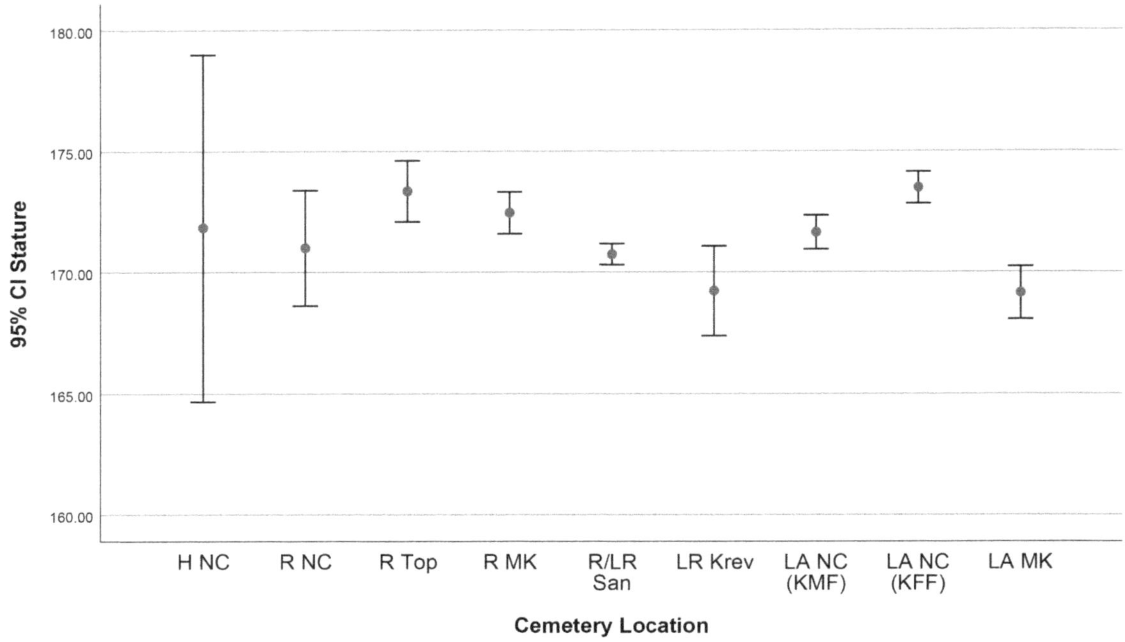

Figure 8.83. Error bar plots demonstrating mean stature estimations for each male cemetery group, with 95% confidence intervals.

groups were tested using a t-test for equality of means. The only two comparisons that produced a statistically significant result were for the Roman Monastiriako Kephali and Roman/Late Roman Sanatorium groups (t=−2.764, df=213, p=0.006, mean difference=−1.940, 95% confidence intervals= −3.324 to −0.557), and the Roman Monastiriako Kephali and Late Antique North Cemetery (KMF) groups (t=−2.640, df=86.324, p= 0.01, mean difference= −2.041, 95% confidence intervals= −3.577 to −0.504).

The male mean statures had a wider range that the females, varying by c.4cm. This produced a greater number of significant differences in means, with several examples of means that did not have overlapping confidence intervals in a comparison of the different cemetery groups (Figure 8.83). The Late Roman Krevatina and Late Antique Monastiriako Kephali groups each only represent a single tomb, the former containing two individuals and the latter only one. These both produced low mean stature estimates that were significantly different from several other cemetery groups. The other statistically significant differences, identified by a t-test, consist of the following pairs of cemetery groups:

Although both sexes produced a statistically significant result between the Roman Monastiriako Kephali (R MK) and Roman/Late Roman Sanatorium (R/LR San) groups, the R MK mean stature was lower than the R/LR San groups for females and higher for males, suggesting these significant results may be false positives and that the data may be unreliable. The male Sanatorium cemetery mean stature was, however, also significantly lower than for both the Roman Topana and Late Antique North Cemetery (KFF) groups. There was also a significant difference identified between the two different sections of the Late Antique North Cemetery, the KMF tombs (largely osteothekai) associated with the basilica church and the single osteotheke known at the KFF Fortetsa Fork. The KMF mean stature was the lower result. Although this comparison between the female mean statures from the same cemetery groups were not significantly different, the result was the opposite of the males, with the KFF female mean stature being the lower of the two. These contrasting results are more likely highlighting the unreliableness of the data, rather than significantly different conditions for females and males in these groups. Additionally, as normality could not be confirmed for the majority of these distributions, it cannot be assumed that these samples of representative of the population or of the variables being tested.

	t	df	Sig. (2-tailed) p	Mean Diff.	Std. Error Diff.	95% CI Lower	95% CI Upper
R Top- R/LR San	4.301	213	0.000	2.609	0.607	1.413	3.804
R MK- R/LR San	3.498	125.1	0.001	1.708	0.488	0.742	2.674
R/LR San- LA NC (KFF)	−6.848	304.2	0.000	−2.743	0.401	−3.532	−1.955
LA NC (KMF)- LA NC (KFF)	−3.781	326	0.000	−1.845	0.488	−2.805	−0.885

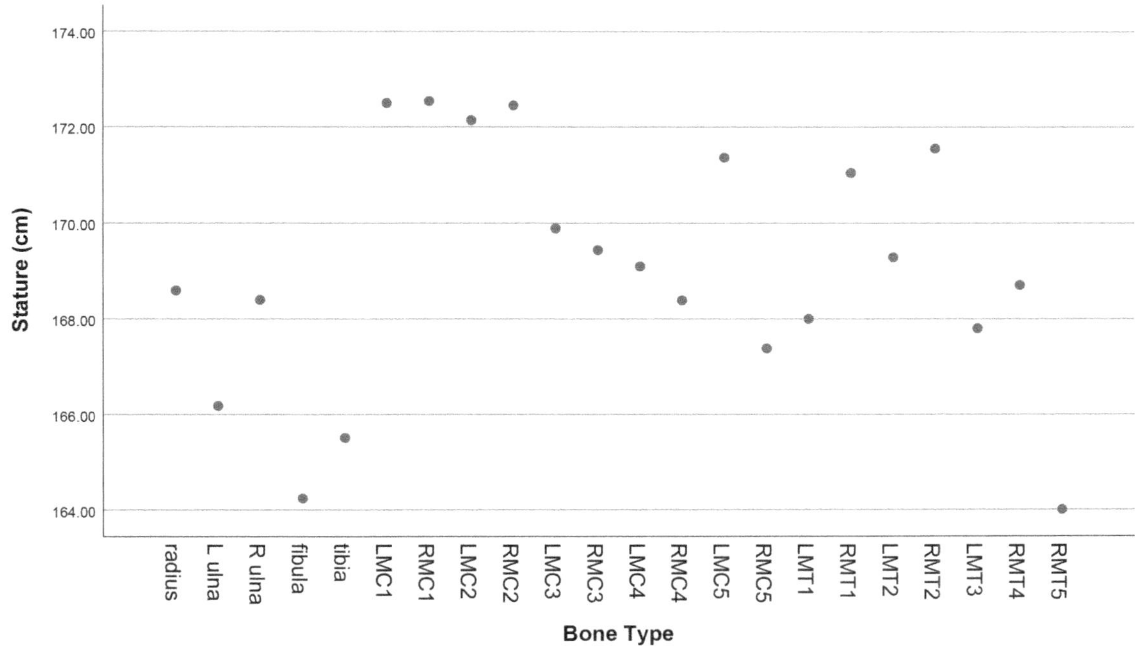

Figure 8.84. Stature estimates for a single individual (KOP/79, Unit 108, Individual 1: Late Antique, male, stone-lined grave) from each measured bone.

The Late Antique Monastiriako Kephali cemetery is represented by a burial of a single individual. Figure 8.84 gives the stature estimates from each bone available for this single individual (KOP/79, Unit 108, Individual 1). The KOP/79 individual's mean estimated stature was 169.0cm, with estimates ranging from 164.0cm (right fifth metatarsal) to 172.9cm (right first metacarpal), a difference of 8.9cm, and a standard deviation of 2.56cm. This demonstrates the wide error margin that exists for these stature estimates and how variable the stature estimates can be depending on which bone or bones are available to measure.

8.5. Discussion

8.5.1. Time period

A change in developmental conditions cannot be discerned over time from the observation of bone lengths or estimations of stature. The Hellenistic assemblage produced a disappointingly small number of intact bones suitable for measuring due to its poorer state of preservation. Thus, as with some of the other analyses, the Hellenistic sample is unreliable and is not representative of the population. In the majority of comparisons of the Roman and Late Antique periods, there was very little difference in bone lengths and (with the exception of the fourth metacarpal, which had a significantly higher Late Antique mean when the sexes were combined) none of the differences were statistically significant. For the different bone types, and often between the sexes for the same bone type, different patterns emerged as to whether the Roman or Late Antique period had the higher mean. This lack of consistency supports the fact there was no significant difference in bone lengths between these time periods.

The problems of estimating sex metrically were evident throughout the results section, producing asymmetrical distributions of bone lengths and stature estimations. This proves that this bilateral and polarised division of females and males cannot produce samples that are representative of females and males in the once living population because in a normal population there will be overlap in size of females and males. Therefore, when combining the sexes for the analysis to produce a normal distribution representative of the population, the assumption is made that females and males are roughly evenly represented. Significant differences in means, such as that of the fourth metacarpal lengths, may therefore be caused by different ratios of females to males in the samples, creating a false positive result for the variable (time period) being tested.

Although bone lengths avoid all the inherent problems that come with the stature estimation formula (discussed in the introduction to this chapter), due to the large mix of different bones being measured and small sample sizes for many of them, stature estimations were analysed as a secondary step to increase the sample size. However, it is clear from the normality tests that this data is not reliably representative of the population and the problem of metric sexing is further accentuated by the application of sex-specific formula. A difference in mean male stature values of over 1cm (greater in the later time period) was observed between the Roman and Late Antique periods, and this was a statistically significant result. However, as the data had a non-normal distribution, it cannot be assumed to be a representative result. With the largest bone length sample sizes being produced by the metatarsals, four out of the five metatarsals had longer mean lengths in the Late Antique period. Although these were not statistically significant differences, this provides some supporting evidence for the less reliable stature data that there may have been a subtle increase in bone lengths in the Late Antique period.

Despite population decline at the site and an apparent decline in conspicuous personal wealth or great public expenditure, there is potentially greater average stature in the Late Antique period, reflecting better health in the population. Such a trend has been observed in a broad-scale study of long bone lengths from approximately 10,000 individuals across the Roman Empire, which found an inverse relationship between population density and biological standard of living (Jongman *et al.* 2019).

8.5.2. Tomb type

Due to the small sample sizes for most bone lengths becoming unworkably small with the increased number of categories in the tomb type variable, only the metatarsals were analysed and only with the sexes combined. Combining the sexes enabled normal distributions to be achieved, indicating the data was reliable enough for comparisons to be made. However, the sample sizes for some of the groups, particularly the sarcophagus, cist, tile and pit groups, were too small to be representative of the population. This meant the social cross-section that this variable should have encompassed was not achieved, leaving the comparison to only include the larger and grander tomb types. The only two statistically significant results were for the comparison of the fifth metatarsal mean lengths for the built and stone-lined, and osteotheke and stone-lined groups. These were probably false positives as they were not reflected in the other bone lengths, although the latter comparison was also a significant for the comparison of male stature estimates. This suggests that there is no strong link between tomb type and bone lengths, but as the simpler tomb types are poorly represented, only certain societal groups are represented in this analysis.

Stature estimates were employed again in an attempt to boost the sample size. However, this produces non-normal distributions in most cases due to the metric sexing issue. It is noteworthy that the osteothekai appear to produce fairly consistently high mean results for both the bone lengths and the female and male stature estimates. There were several significant differences in mean stature estimates identified for the comparison of the tomb types, though none of these pairs were the same for both sexes. In fact, opposite results were found to be significant for females and males for the comparison of the built and chamber tomb groups, with the built mean being higher for females and the chamber mean higher for males. It could be the case that the social groups being buried in these tomb types (both quite elaborate Roman tomb forms in use during the 1st-2nd centuries AD) experienced greater disparity in wellbeing between females and males, potentially in the form of differential access to foodstuffs or division of labour meaning varied exposure to disease. However, it is more likely that these are false positive results, particularly considering the non-normal distributions of the data. The built tombs were the most elaborate burial structures but they do not seem to have had significantly improved developmental conditions (at least not amongst the males) compared to the contemporary individuals from the chamber tombs nor the later osteotheke burials.

The significant difference noted between the osteotheke and stone-lined groups for the fifth metatarsal lengths, was also significant for the male stature estimates. There is not a great deal of difference in the construction of these two tomb types, but the osteothekai are later in date than the majority of stone-lined tombs. The osteothekai are largely associated with the KMF basilica church, while the majority of stone-lined tombs were from the Sanatorium (KSM) site to the east. It could be the case that there was a social difference or temporal change in the developmental conditions of these burial groups. There is some suggestion that developmental conditions were not equal for all tomb type (social) groups and that, particularly in the early Roman period there may be differences in male and female conditions. However, as the more reliable data (bone lengths) show no significant differences and the stature estimate data are potentially unrepresentative (and are inconsistent between females and males) no real differences in developmental conditions can be ascertained for the different groups of society represented by the tomb type groups.

8.5.3. Cemetery (location)

The cemeteries were analysed in the same way as the tomb types, using only the metatarsals for the bone lengths and combining the sexes to maximise the sample size. Nevertheless, the sample sizes for some cemeteries (Hellenistic North Cemetery, Roman North Cemetery, Roman Topana and Late Roman Krevatina) were still too small to produce useful results. For the cemetery groups with larger sample sizes, distributions of bone lengths were largely normal and the results can therefore considered to most likely be reliable. There was very little difference between the mean bone lengths for the cemetery groups and there were no statistically significant differences.

Again, when stature estimates were employed to increase the sample size, non-normal distributions were produced. Some differences could be observed between the cemetery groups, with more sizable differences for the males. However, as with the tomb type data, the statistically significant t-test results are cancelled out by the non-normal data distributions and inconsistencies in comparisons of cemetery groups between females and males.

8.5.4. Comparative material and sex differences

Looking back to the comparative material in Table 8.1 in the introduction to this chapter, the Knossos results from all time periods are amongst some of the tallest stature estimations. Stature has been a much more frequently published measure compared to the raw bone length data, despite the issues surrounding the appropriateness of using formulae based on potentially inappropriate populations. With mean male heights in every time period over 171cm, similar to Bisel and Angel's (1985) tallest group in their assessment of stature from Neolithic through to Medieval Greece, this suggests comparatively good developmental conditions across these time periods at Knossos. In a comparison with early modern stature records, often available for males from military records, these Knossian male stature values were generally not matched until the later 20th century in much of Europe, demonstrating better developmental conditions than in Medieval and Early Modern Europe (Kron 2005, 75). The Knossos female mean results are less outstanding in comparison to the comparative material available. While the Knossos males appear to have attained higher heights in comparison to the available published stature estimates for Greek assemblages, the females do not appear to have reached quite the same levels, suggesting the possibility of difference in developmental conditions (potentially diet) between females and males. However, the small sample sizes from these comparative studies (particularly the Lerna Hollow and Gortyn females) mean that this may be a false impression and the relative discrepancy between females and males should not be further emphasised, with both sexes appearing to reach optimal heights in comparison to the majority of other samples available for similar time periods in Greece.

8.6. Conclusion

The stature data are weak, not only on principle, due to the formulae being based on potentially inappropriate populations and similar inherent problems, but also because the data distributions were non-normal, suggesting a non-random sample that cannot be taken to be representative of the population. The bilateral metric sex estimation caused problems with producing a normal dataset for both the bone lengths and the stature estimations. Combining the sexes enabled groups of bone lengths with normal distributions for the variables under investigation. Bone lengths are therefore the better data to use for this analysis but unfortunately each bone type is not comparable to another and sample sizes were very small for most bone types, leaving the analysis to depend largely on the metatarsals. The metatarsal lengths data produced normal distributions for the variable categories, establishing that these were random samples that can be taken as representative of the population. This would suggest that there were no significant differences between the time periods, tomb types and cemeteries that had sample sizes large enough to make the assessment. Unfortunately, this excludes some key variables, including the Hellenistic period, all of the simplest tomb forms and several cemeteries or burial locations.

Besides the methodological problems concerning stature estimation (discussed in Sections 8.1 and 8.2.4), there are also problems in the correlation between stature and developmental conditions, which are also discussed in the introduction (8.1). The main issue with using either bone lengths or stature to reflect on developmental conditions and wellbeing, primarily in the form of access to nutrition and exposure to disease, is that stature is c.80% genetically controlled, with a wide and varied range of environmental conditions (including diet and disease) making up the rest (McEvoy and Visscher 2009). A large migrant population might be genetically taller or shorter, thus it is possible that the difference between two groups identified either by time period or tomb type might be genetically different rather than having significantly different environmental conditions. The most likely group that would be affected by a large incoming and genetically distinct population is the early Roman assemblage, and unfortunately, due to the poor preservation of the Hellenistic sample, a comparison of the Hellenistic-Roman transition with establishment of the colony is not possible.

Although there is the consideration of genetic and other variables playing a role, it has been well-established in the research literature that insufficient nutrition and unhygienic living conditions inhibits growth, leading to shorter limb bone lengths and lower adult statures in comparison to those raised in more favourable developmental conditions. Therefore, while other factors, such as genetics and hormonal imbalances, should be considered, the most likely variables affecting growth rate, bone lengths and stature across a population group are environmental, particularly diet and disease. However, while this has been established for the limb bones, it is not clear whether it applies as noticeably to the metatarsals or other bones of the body.

There is an expectation of change across this major transition between the Hellenistic and Roman periods but unfortunately this data cannot give the definition that the impact of the socio-economic change filtered down to basic living standards and quality of life, regarding access to nutrition and exposure to disease. However, the better condition of the Roman and Late Antique material allowed for a sample that does demonstrate how the later transition affected the lives and development of the people of Knossos. With the reduction of population size throughout the later Roman and Late Antique periods, it is unlikely that there were significant numbers of incomers, which allows the exclusion of one variable (genes) for consideration. The increase in average stature in the Late Antique period for both females and males, as well as a slight increase for some of the bone lengths with larger sample sizes, may suggest an improvement in living conditions but these were not significant differences.

9

Conclusion

9.1. Aims

This study has investigated how the social, political, economic and cultural changes that took place at Knossos over a period of c. 1000 years affected the health and lifestyle of the population through the study of the human skeletal remains. Conversely, it has considered whether the analysis of the human skeletal remains could clarify or contribute to the discussion of some of the unknown or debated details of the nature of some of these broad-scale changes and the impact they had on the population at Knossos. These topics include the transition from the Hellenistic period with its predominantly subsistence economy to an economy more dependent on trade when Knossos became well-connected within the shipping networks of the Roman period (Chaniotis 1999). The significance of changes in the economy in the later Roman and Late Antique periods are also considered. Though some changes are suggested by the pottery assemblages on Crete and in the Cretan exports seen elsewhere in the later Roman and Late Antique periods, imports continue to make up a significant proportion of pottery assemblages at several Cretan sites demonstrating that trade remained important (Gallimore 2016, 185; Yangaki 2016). There was also a change from being a state frequently at war with its neighbouring states, and then resisting Roman invasion, to a period of peace when Knossos was formally recognised as a Roman colony and integrated into the Roman Empire. The refoundation of Knossos as a Roman colony has raised the question of the impact of colonisation, as well as (crucially) whether there was immigration of colonists on a significant scale. Knossos experienced some key differences to other cities on Crete due to its strong opposition to the Roman invasion and its position as a Roman colony. Christianity was introduced to Knossos from as early as the 2nd century and was evident on a monumental scale from the early 5th century. This study of health and diet can demonstrate the impact that Christianity had on the lives of the people and the nature of some of its practices or customs at Knossos.

Knossos was an important urban centre, though of changing scales of significance, throughout this time period. Though previous studies have demonstrated how change has been manifested in the urban fabric and material culture at the site, this study of health and diet – using a palaeodemographic and palaeoepidemiological approach – has demonstrated the impact of change on a human level, giving insight into aspects of daily life and wellbeing.

9.2. The Hellenistic Period

An interesting demographic picture emerges from the Hellenistic assemblage. The small numbers of sub-adult burials and complete absence of any single individual burials of neonates, infants or children is likely to be due to different burial practices for sub-adults, with another burial location likely. While an underrepresentation of sub-adults is noted for many sites in Greece (Lagia 2007, 294; Dimakis 2019), there is evidence for separate burial locations for children (particularly neonates and infants), at Athens, Eretria and Messene for the Hellenistic period (Houby-Nielsen 2000; Chenal-Velarde 2006; Lagia 2007; Bourbou and Themelis 2010; Guimier-Sorbets and Morizot 2010; Moschonissioti 2010; Liston and Rotroff 2012; Liston *et al.* 2018) as well as the exceptional child cemetery at Kylindra on Astypalaia in use from c. 750 BC until AD 100 (Clement *et al.* 2009; Hillson 2009; Michalaki-Kollia *et al.* 2010). Considering the nature of the excavations at Knossos, it is also likely that the remains of some of these individuals were not collected and that conditions were not favourable for the preservation of these more fragile bones. During the KMF excavation, many sherds of large vessels were observed in the digger fill (Coldstream and Catling 1996) which could be the remnants of child pot burials, found elsewhere in Crete in the Hellenistic period for neonate (or perinatal) burials (Guyon 2008, 103). Pot burials on Crete were found both in isolated areas of cemeteries and within individual and collective burials. A range of vessel types were used, including an amphora at Rhokka and a beehive at Chania (Platon 1960, 515; Andreadaki-Vlazaki 1997, 1014), suggesting re-use of available receptacles rather than a purpose-specific urn, and indicating a lack of investment in these burials.

Another feature of the demographic profile of the assemblage was that females were significantly more numerous than males, with two-thirds of individuals of identified sex being female. Considering there was no strict segregation of the sexes in the burial sphere (one-third of the assemblage being male is not a negligible number) and there are no known parallels for social segregation of burial location by sex at Hellenistic sites, this may indicate that a significant number of males died and were buried away from Knossos. This seems to support the traditional image of many prime age males being away from the polis as mercenaries in wars throughout the Hellenistic Greek world or engaged in local wars with neighbouring poleis on Crete or nearby islands such as Rhodes and Kos (Perlman 1999). Though both Perlman (1999) and Erickson (2010) challenge the notion of males on the island being reduced to negligible numbers by piracy and mercenary service, this skeletal assemblage does suggest a significant imbalance in the presence of females and males in the burial sphere at Knossos. Few other Hellenistic skeletal assemblages have been studied from Crete but a mass grave of young adult males at Chania (Bourbou and Niniou-Kindeli 2009) would support the suggestion that those killed in warfare were not returned to their poleis for burial or, if returned, were buried separately in such mass graves. The Hadra hydria cinerary urns at Alexandria in Egypt have also been interpreted as burials of Cretan mercenaries due to the provenance of the vessels, the use of cremation for non-local burials, and some having inscriptions identifying the occupants as foreign officials and mercenaries (Callaghan and Jones 1985; Enklaar 1985; 1986; Landvatter 2013). The sex imbalance in the skeletal assemblage is supported by the evidence for alternative male burial customs (the mass grave and cremated abroad) in suggesting that a sizeable proportion of the male population were absent from Knossos, likely engaged in a variety of affairs including diplomacy, 'piracy' and mercantile activities, mercenary service and warfare. Due to their mobile lives they are often absent from the local record in death.

The Hellenistic assemblage is unlikely to be completely representative of the full cross-section of society – on top of the demographic shortcomings – as judged by the burial contexts, due to the absence of any elaborate graves in terms of either tomb type or burial goods. Although it also seems unlikely that tomb form was an important means of expressing social status or wealth since the vast majority of tombs on Crete were pit, tile or cist graves (Guyon 2008). Nevertheless, the graves represented by the assemblage at Knossos are particularly poor being predominantly pits with a very small number of tile graves. It is possible that some of the unstudied or unexcavated rock-cut tombs are of Hellenistic date (e.g. *KS2*:154–56) and there was a possible Hellenistic cist grave reported from the Fortetsa cemetery, though the terminology used is questionable (Brock 1957, 85). A dozen *hypogea* (underground rock-cut chamber tombs with vaulted ceilings, 6–14 *loculi* for inhumations, and stepped or sloping *dromoi* leading to entrances consisting of a lintel, door jambs and blocking slab) have been discovered at Chania from the Hellenistic period. Due to the rarity of such tombs on Crete and their similarity in form (though much simpler and more basic) to tombs at Alexandria, it is possible that these could be the tombs of foreign merchants or of Cretans who have seen such tombs while abroad (Empereur and Nenna 2001; 2003; Venit 2002, 37–65; Hellmann 2006, 296–99; Guyon 2008; Guimier-Sorbets and Michaelides 2009; Nenna 2009). These differ from the more common rock-cut chamber tombs, such as those known from Roman Knossos and known only from Polyrhenia and Phaistos in the Hellenistic period (Savignoni 1901; Hatzi-Vallianou 1995), as they are not cut into the slope of a cliff or hill (Hellmann 2006, 292; Guyon 2008, 107). The only other tomb forms known from Hellenistic Crete that are more elaborate than the basic pit and tile graves, are cist graves in a variety of materials and construction styles (stone slabs, tiles, small stones, masonry blocks and spolia) (Guyon 2008, 102) and a built funerary monument at Phaistos. The suggestion of other tomb types at Knossos and the existence of more elaborate tombs elsewhere on Crete support the fact that the Knossos skeletal assemblage may not represent the highest status individuals in the community. A degree of social diversity amongst the Knossos pit and tile graves is, however, indicated by the grave goods. Many graves had either no grave goods or only one or two poorly-fired unguentaria, but some graves had a greater wealth, diversity and quality of grave goods, including a variety of shapes of pottery, glass vessels, metal vessels and utensils, coins, bronze, silver and gold jewellery (KMF/78 notebooks; Callaghan n.d.; Brock 1957, 40, 59, 100, 199). It seems likely that there was only modest differentiation in the burial sphere in Hellenistic Crete and the representation in the graves at Knossos does not seem atypical so it is unlikely that the graves for the skeletal assemblage represent only individuals of the lowest social status. However, with small numbers of more elaborate tombs known elsewhere on the island (admittedly largely only at Chania) and with gold and other prestige items known in larger quantities, including finer items such as golden wreath crowns,[24] elsewhere on the island, it seems possible that the uppermost social classes are not represented in the assemblage and that such more elaborate burials are thus far missing from the archaeological record at Knossos. It is also possible that the very lowest members of society (the enslaved) are not represented.

The diet at Hellenistic Knossos, as in all periods at the site, was a predominantly C3 plant-based diet supplemented by terrestrial protein. This would mean a diet that was composed of staples such as wheat or barley, alongside meat, dairy or eggs. The animal protein element of the diet seems to have been less frequently consumed than in later Roman and Late Antique times, indicated by lower nitrogen isotope signatures ($\delta^{15}N$). One possible fish-eating individual from a Late Hellenistic or possibly Early Roman tile grave (S22: Young Adult, unknown sex) could indicate a recent incomer to the site, or – considering the mobile nature of the male population – potentially a recently returned individual after years of absence, having come from somewhere where fish made a significant contribution to the diet or employed in a seafaring occupation. Future work including a variety of isotopic analyses could give better insight into this individual's provenience (strontium and oxygen) and extent of fish consumption (sulphur), and intra-tooth sequential dentine isotope samples could be taken for investigating short term changes in diet. There was a difference between female and male diets identified in the isotopic results, particularly in the nitrogen isotopes (a difference of 0.5‰ in mean $\delta^{15}N$ values) demonstrating that males had greater access to meat than females. Significant differences between female and male dental disease (caries, calculus and antemortem tooth loss) support the isotope results in suggesting significantly different diets between the sexes. The dental diseases show a different aspect of the diet and indicate that, in addition to having more meat in their diets, males also had greater quantities of cariogenic foodstuffs (starches or sugars) or were consuming carbohydrates more frequently. The

[24] Golden wreath crowns are known from Kissamos, Chania, Gortyn, Chersonissos and Lato (Guyon 2008, 129).

latter would mean more eating events (meals or snacks) throughout the day, suggesting different dining practices and eating habits. This may indicate that the *syssitia* (communal dining) was both habitual and widespread throughout the (at least male citizen) population, rather than only occasionally for festivals as has been surmised (Chaniotis 1999, 185–86), or that there was some form of daily social segregation in eating arrangements between the sexes, which could be explained by males eating away from the home for work during the day or for periods of time.

The Hellenistic assemblage produced remarkably low levels of caries and calculus compared to the later time periods at Knossos. While poor surface preservation may have exaggerated these low results, this cannot be the sole reason for the low frequency of observations of these dental conditions. This indicates that the Hellenistic diet was more diverse than a basic carbohydrate diet (as supported by the isotopic evidence for a meat component) but nor did it contain large amounts of sugars from fruit or honey. This refutes the notion of the *syssitia* as an aristocratic custom (Willetts 1955, 20–21) and rather suggests an egalitarian society, potentially with public land, public ownership of livestock and citizens paying a contribution from their private agricultural produce towards the provision of communal meals. However, this 'egalitarian' society would presumably have been limited to the citizen body, but the lack of sugary foodstuffs in the diet may suggest a degree of restraint in the reigning in of decadence. The (admittedly very limited numbers of) stature estimations indicate that these Hellenistic individuals reached optimal heights in comparison with contemporary Greek stature estimations and were superior to most pre-modern standards. This demonstrates that the diet was nutritionally adequate for good physical development.

The Hellenistic assemblage had the highest levels of osteoarthritis and entheseal changes for any of the time periods and also high levels of intervertebral disc disease (though the Late Antique assemblage had the highest result in this category). The assemblage was more female dominated than male but the results for both sexes show that males and females were engaged in manual labour, causing the early onset of these degenerative conditions in an assemblage that consisted predominantly of Young Adults. Additionally, the males had significantly higher prevalences of osteoarthritis than the females and with different patterns of the condition affecting joints through the body, demonstrating a division of labour between the sexes.

9.3. The Roman Period

The Roman assemblage has a better demographic representation than the Hellenistic assemblage, with sub-adults of all age groups represented and making up over a third of the minimum number of individuals (MNI). There was a shift in burial practices during the Early Roman period towards communal or family burials with larger numbers of individuals of all ages, though this was not an immediate change after the Roman conquest or establishment of the colony, with the first evidence dating to the mid-1st century AD. Amongst the adults of identified sex, males and females were almost equally represented, with only marginally more males. A larger proportion of adults were represented in the Middle and Old Adult age categories suggesting longer life expectancies in the Roman period. Elsewhere in Crete and mainland Greece, it has been observed at some sites that the Roman period brought a general decline in health, based on factors such as age-at-death, stature and pathological lesions (Bisel and Angel 1985, 203; Bourbou 2005, 102; Kirkpatrick Smith 2013, 148), though there are no studies that have compared the population across the Hellenistic and Roman periods at a single site. This decline has been blamed broadly on unhygienic living conditions (overcrowding, poor sanitation), malnutrition and endemic disease (Morris 1992, 72; Kron 2005, 68). This would have been relevant to the city of Rome due to the scale of immigration but would have had variable applicability throughout the cities of the Empire and there does not appear to have been a decrease in hygiene standards at Knossos compared to the Hellenistic period based on the age-at-death or bone length data.

In terms of the representation of a cross-section of society, the Roman assemblage represents the greatest diversity of different tomb forms. This diversity is in part due to the temporal changes in tomb types with the earliest years of the Roman period appearing to show no changes from the Hellenistic period, with all known burials prior to c.AD 50 being simple pit and tile graves, to the extent that it is likely that some of the burials assigned to the Hellenistic period may actually be Early Roman in date. Additionally, the majority of known tombs of the later 3rd century onwards (into Late Antiquity) at Knossos are various types of stone-lined tomb,[25] though tile graves also appear to have remained a common tomb type (Frend and Johnston 1962; Hood and Smyth 1981; Sweetman and Grigoropoulos 2010). Of the tomb types in use from the 1st to 3rd centuries AD, the skeletal assemblage does not include individuals from the grandest of the built tombs known from Knossos, such as the mausoleum or 'altar tomb' with a Latin inscription from the North Cemetery and several other mausolea (monumental built tombs) in the vicinity (Grammatikaki 2004; Vasilakis 2004; Guyon 2008, 116) or the so-called 'Tomb of Caiaphas' reported by early travellers to have been a monumental mausoleum. The assemblage also does not represent a large number of the simplest tomb types (two pit graves, six tile graves), therefore certain groups within society may be under-represented. Initially it was assumed, with the diversity of tomb types and burial goods, that it was likely that a better cross-section of society was documented for this time period than the earlier or later periods. However,

[25] The terminology is variable – 'cist grave', 'stone-lined tomb', 'osteotheke' – but so too are the construction techniques, materials and burial usage within the categories. See Section 3.4.

with a better understanding that the lack of diversity in the Knossos burial forms of the Hellenistic and Late Antique periods was not atypical for Crete, the burial diversity in the Roman period may demonstrate a more hierarchical society at this time and a more established elite class, at least in terms of how they chose to represent their dead in the burial sphere. Although the very grandest of the monumental, above-ground, masonry-built mausolea are not represented, there were several tombs in this 'Built' category. The rock-cut chamber tombs ('Chamber' category) also appear to be comparably elaborate in construction and in terms of burial goods being plentiful and diverse in at least some cases. Additionally, simple graves are also present (though few and containing fewer individuals), suggesting a broad range of society being represented by the skeletal material.

While the core staples in the diet likely remained the same between the Hellenistic and Roman periods, the principal difference in diets detected from the stable isotope analysis was a shift in the average carbon isotope signatures ($\delta^{13}C$). This could represent the introduction of a C4 plant at the site or could demonstrate the regular inclusion of low trophic level fish in small quantities in the diet. Millet is known to have been a minority cereal crop at some sites in Greece since the beginning of the 2nd millennium BC (Valamoti 2016, 52), and is attested in both the archaeological record and written sources throughout the Roman Empire, though generally regarded as a second-class crop for the poor or livestock (Dalby 2003, 218; Murphy 2016). Other than in the phytolith record from the Middle Neolithic (Efstratiou *et al.* 2004) and the mention of a discovery by Evans from the storerooms of the Bronze Age Palace (Evans 1935, 622; Livarda and Kotzamani 2013, 11), millet has not been identified in the – as yet limited – archaeobotanical record for other time periods at Knossos (Warren 1981, 92; Jones 1984; Livarda 2012; Nitsch *et al.* 2019), but there are no contemporary studies at Knossos for the time frame of the present project (none later than the Protogeometric period). Millet could be grown in dry conditions that would not have suited wheat, therefore with the shift towards a drier climate during the Roman period, millet may have been introduced as a secondary crop. Millet is known to have been cultivated in Campania (Spurr 1983) and it could have been transferred to the 'Capuan territories' as a back-up crop at the time this land to the south of Knossos was granted to Capua by Augustus (Baldwin Bowsky 1997). While millet is known at Roman sites in Greece, including Sparta (Waywell *et al.* 1997, 425) and Corinth (Willet 2012, 132), archaeobotanical studies at most sites have not been extensive enough to track a detailed history of the spread of millet in Greece. Considering the name of Kenchreai, the port of Corinth and known from written sources since the Classical period[26], derives from the Ancient Greek word for millet (κεχρί, Conder 1830), it is likely the crop was well-known in the Corinthia from a much earlier date rather than introduced in Roman times. Though an elevation in nitrogen isotope values might have been expected in comparison with the Hellenistic sample if fish was the cause of the elevation in the carbon isotope values, due to the wide-ranging values produced by seafood and river fish, low trophic level fish in small quantities are also a very plausible explanation. Another fish-eating outlier individual (S31, in addition to the Hellenistic individual) is likely to indicate a recent incomer to the site or may show that fish consumption was becoming more common at Knossos and represent a personal preference by someone who could get regular access to seafood. The possible introduction of new foods into the diet demonstrates that the better connectivity that Knossos enjoyed in the Roman period enabled at least some of its inhabitants to expand their horizons and experience a more diverse diet.

Dental disease (caries and antemortem tooth loss) was at its worst in the Roman period. The difference between the Hellenistic and Roman caries results was statistically highly significant demonstrating a substantial increase in cariogenic foodstuffs. The historic record supports a change in dining practices as the *syssitia* did not endure into the Roman period on Crete. With the change in the economy in the Roman period, a greater variety of foods would have been available through trade (Chaniotis 1999), potentially also to a wider segment of the population. The bulk staples of the diet would still have been locally produced but the dental evidence suggests new (potentially considered to be luxury) additions to the diet, likely in the form of sugars, such as fruit and honey. A relatively high sugar diet is also supported by the caries patterning within the zones of the teeth, which showed caries onset was frequently prior to the exposure of the dentine through wear or the root margin through continuous eruption. The pattern of lower caries prevalence in the simpler tomb forms also supports the theory that the cariogenic agent causing this increase in the disease in Roman teeth was sugars as opposed to starches from cereals (common in both periods). It was the individuals buried in the more complex tomb types that suffered most from caries.

Honey production is thought to have been common and widespread on Crete in the Roman period (Francis 2006; 2016). Whether due to climate change, intensified trade, or new tastes or customs relating to food and dining (potentially linked to intensified contacts through trade), increased fruit consumption may also have contributed to the rise in dental caries. In a comparison of rural and urban sites in Roman Britain, the urban individuals had higher caries rates which was suggested to be due to the richer Roman cuisine, including processed and sweetened foods, in comparison with the more modest rural diet (Rohnbogner and Lewis 2016). However, these foods existed on Crete since much earlier times, and the Roman processing and preservation techniques, such as drying fruit or preserving it in honey, had been commonplace throughout the Greek world for centuries (Curtis 2009, 384). The earliest evidence for ceramic beehives on Crete comes from a 2nd century BC context at Knossos (Homann-Wedeking 1950), though they have been found abundantly

[26] *IG* IV2, 1 103; Thucydides 4.42-4, 8.10, 20, 23; Xenophon *Hellenika* 4.5.1, 6.5.51, 7.1.17, 41, 7.4.5; Pseudo Scylax 55.

in Early Roman contexts from rescue excavations in the upper village (Sweetman and Grigoropoulos 2010). Although such finds are rare from the Hellenistic period, organic beehives may have been used, as described by Roman agricultural writers like Columella and Varro, which would leave no sign in the archaeological record (Francis 2016, 84).

There were no distinguishable differences in female and male diets from the isotopic results. However, males did have higher levels of dental disease, particularly for cavities prevalence. This suggests that there remained a division in the dining habits of society at least in the form of differential access for females and males to the luxury, high-sugar additions to the diet. As mentioned above, these foods were only (or at least more readily) available to higher status individuals buried in the built and chamber tombs. The greater difference in female and male stature estimates in the built and chamber tombs may suggest a greater disparity in wellbeing and access to good nutrition between the sexes of the upper social classes. No other social divisions in diet could be identified by cemetery location or north/south region of the valley.

There was a lower prevalence of joint disease and entheseal changes in the Roman assemblage compared to the Hellenistic period. This may be partially due to the majority of the assemblage coming from the more ostentatious tombs which represented a higher status group who may have had physically less demanding lifestyles. The built tombs had the lowest prevalences of osteoarthritis, intervertebral disc disease and entheseal changes and the chamber tomb prevalences were lower than average for the joint diseases. The osteoarthritis results in particular showed statistically significant differences between the simple and complex tomb forms. A division of labour or activities between the sexes was evident, with males having higher prevalences of the joint diseases and entheseal changes than females. Different patterns of joints affected throughout the body can also be detected, such as females having higher prevalences of elbow, wrist and hip osteoarthritis. It has been proposed in Chapter 7 that the lower levels of joint disease in the Roman period, and particularly in individuals from the more elaborate tombs, may represent a more established elite class and hierarchical society and a greater variety of occupations available. Peace on the island in the Roman period meant that new, smaller settlements were able to be established as have been observed in the surveys by Sanders (1982) and Hayden (2005, 333) on Crete, and it is possible that there was a movement out of the city by some labourers to farmsteads. However, in an urban settlement the size of Knossos it is likely there would still have been some farm labourers residing in the urban area (it is estimated that 80–90% of the population in the Roman world would have been engaged in agricultural work (Erdkamp 2012, 246)), in addition to labourers required for the building projects and other urban tasks, therefore it is likely this proportion of the population is underrepresented in the skeletal assemblage.

The changes that are evident at Knossos can be understood in terms of greater connectivity, resulting in a 'global' consciousness and a compression of geographic space, which takes us beyond the outdated theories of Romanisation (which embodies the dichotomies of Roman-Native, core-periphery and Italy-provinces), post-colonial narratives of indigenous trajectories of change and identity, and world systems models (that implicitly assume cultural homogenisation over time advocating too broad and general an approach to account for the regional and local variations in material culture) (Pitts and Versluys 2015a, 6–10). This connectivity or globalisation approach, considered by Pitts and Versluys (2015a) the most appropriate model to apply in order to understand the diverse, multicultural, connected Roman world, has already been discussed by Sweetman (2007) in relation to Knossos. The changes in tomb and burial type are not directly an adoption of a foreign burial type due to the presence of migrants. Rather there is a move towards display in the burial sphere and towards large, communal tombs resulting from evolving priorities in the expression of identity (affected by memory and connectivity), in terms of status, wealth, and family connections. However, the medium for that expression (the architecture, material culture, funerary rites, and treatment of the body) is a locally produced culmination of factors. Continuity (memory) and innovation (connectivity) can be seen side by side and are interconnected. Continuity can be noticed particularly in the inhumation rites, continued use of pre-Roman cemeteries (as well as new cemeteries) and in some of the grave goods. The new tomb types, the monumental built tombs and rock-cut chamber tombs, have predecessors elsewhere on the island, if not potentially at Knossos in the case of the chamber tombs, and in turn these have forerunners in Kos, Samos, Rhodes, Cyprus, Asia Minor, the Near East and Egypt (Fedak 1990; Moretti 2006, 298–99; Konrad 2007; Guyon 2008, 109; de Jong 2017), showing that intensified connections were not only with Italy, nor were they bilateral but rather part of a complex network. The built tombs vary in form and appear to have potential predecessors in both the East and West, but they may also have incorporated local building styles as no strict model form appears to be followed for many of these tombs (Grammatikaki 2004; Vasilakis 2004). The free-standing mausolea, which are common throughout the eastern Roman Empire, are often referred to as a Roman tomb type, but there were free-standing mausolea known throughout the Hellenistic world (Fedak 1990; Moretti 2006; Faber *et al.* 2007). Globalisation theory can also be applied to understanding the changes in diet. Due to the export market for honey, honey production increased, which also resulted in local consumption increasing. However, availability was not the only factor in increased honey consumption. The evolving dining practices due to changes in the expression of wealth and social status meant that elite members of society would have wanted to be seen to be consuming prestige foodstuffs. In this case, connectivity has affected both demand for a product but also attitudes towards the product.

There does not appear to be clear evidence for a sizeable influx of migrants at Knossos with its formal refoundation as a colony, beyond the magistrates attested in the epigraphic record (Sanders 1982), though in such a well-connected situation they can be notoriously difficult to detect. The increased connectivity combined with local characteristics and decision-making provide ample explanation for changes in lifestyle and material culture. However, further investigation of provenience could be conducted in the future on the human skeletal remains.

9.4. The Late Antique Period

The demographic composition of the Late Antique assemblage was similar to that of the Roman period, with all age categories represented and a better representation of sub-adults, at almost 40% of the MNI. The adult age group distribution was also quite similar to the Roman period, with a slightly smaller proportion of Old Adults but a larger proportion in the Middle Adult category. The largest adult age category remained the Young Adults. A comparison of the proportions of the sub-adult age categories shows more children and adolescents are present in the Late Antique assemblage, while the Roman MNI had larger proportions of infants and neonates. High infant mortality is to be expected in any ancient society, but larger numbers of deaths later in childhood as well as the dearth of individuals reaching Old Adulthood may indicate a deterioration in conditions for the preservation of life, such as poorer nutrition and increased disease. However, these minor differences between the Roman and Late Antique assemblages are not statistically significant and there does not appear to be any great change in the factors affecting life expectancy across these centuries. Additionally, the increase in mean estimated stature, particularly for males, from the Roman to Late Antique periods indicates a possible improvement in nutritional status and hygiene conditions (or other factors influencing disease), though this difference between the Roman and Late Antique males was not detectable in the bone length data.

The Late Antique assemblage is represented largely by osteotheke burials. Nearly all the later Roman (Sanatorium cemetery and Krevatina cist) and Late Antique burials were in stone-lined tombs (osteothekai, cists or generically referred to as stone-lined) of various construction types, numbers of individuals, and – potentially – funerary practices. It seems likely that excavators did not fully understand the uses of these tombs in terms of primary and secondary burial rites and were sometimes careless in their assignation of terminology. In many cases they did not provide adequate descriptions which would enable a better classification and understanding of burial practices to be determined from the excavation notebooks or publications (Frend and Johnston 1962; Catling *et al.* 1976; Sweetman and Becker 2005; Sweetman and Grigoropoulos 2010). For the KMF cemetery, published from the excavation notebooks by Sweetman and Becker (2005), there are some good descriptions of the existing tomb architecture with all tombs consisting of a cutting into the kouskouras and stone-lining (whether with slabs, masonry blocks, spolia or fieldstones). When tomb categories for the present project were chosen, it was assumed these distinctions were purposeful (see Section 3.4). However, as the research has progressed and particularly with the discovery of photographs for some of the tombs recently received by the BSA Archives from the Catling estate, in addition to those previously received from Jill Carrington Smith,[27] it seems less likely that these differences were meaningful. There appears to be little difference between 'cist' Tomb 309 (Figure 3.9) and 'stone-lined grave' Tomb 12 (Figure 3.10), while the construction of the osteothekai, such as Tomb 244 (Figures 3.23–24) and the KFF osteotheke (Figures 3.21–22), was highly variable.

The variation in construction styles may suggest a degree of diversity of social status, but it is not clear from the burial types how extensive a cross-section of society is represented. There are tile graves (of likely Late Antique date) known from Knossos, not represented in the skeletal assemblage, and it is likely that both pit and tile graves would have remained a common burial type in this time period at Knossos. There appears to be a conservatism in tomb form, which may suggest the elite class was no longer so established (a less hierarchical society) or that expression of status in the burial sphere may have changed towards a more modest and less differentiated portrayal of the dead and investment may have been channelled towards the church as a means of expressing status. A similar conservatism in tomb forms seems to occur across Crete, with a similar range of tombs known from Eleutherna, Gortyn, Kissamos (Diamantis 2004; Stampolidis 2004a; di Vita 2010). The majority of tombs represented by the Late Antique skeletal assemblage, and known from Knossos in this time period, are associated with the KMF basilica. The KFF osteotheke was also in the area of the North Cemetery but it may have been part of a different burial group at this time, rather than part of a spatially continuous cemetery. The only other Late Antique tomb represented by the skeletal assemblage was the KOP tomb, which was an individual burial in a substantially built stone-lined tomb of large slabs and blocks (Figures 3.19–20).

A noteworthy difference can be identified in the diet between the Early Roman, Late Roman and Late Antique periods with an increase in the carbon and nitrogen isotope values, representing an increase in fish consumption. Fish tanks are known from Roman Crete (Davaras 1974; 1975; Nakassis 1987; Francis 2010; Mourtzas 2012a; 2012b) and it is likely that fish would always have been an option in the diet at Knossos. Some sources attest to a taboo surrounding the consumption of marine life in antiquity, though paradoxically it is also described as a luxury, prestige food (Gallant 1985; Purcell 1995). The increase in

[27] This is still not a complete archive of excavation photographs. Photo reference codes in the excavation notebooks and photo logbooks kept by both Hector Catling and Jill Carrington Smith (in the BSA Archives) indicate that some photographs are still missing.

fish in the diet is likely to be connected to Christian fasting practices which required abstention from meat on many days but allowed the consumption of seafood (Dembińska 1985; Talbot 1987; Thomas and Hero 2000; Harlow and Smith 2001; Müldner and Richards 2005; Bourbou 2010, 158). People in the Late Antique period do not appear to have suffered nutritionally nor to have had significantly improved nutritional status as there were no significant differences in bone lengths or life expectancy (though there was a statistically significant increase in mean male stature estimates from the Roman to Late Antique periods, possibly suggesting a slight improvement for males). The 3rd–4th century stone-lined tombs from the Sanatorium cemetery had the most elevated average isotope values, particularly the nitrogen (mean $\delta^{15}N$) signature. These are thought to have been early Christian burials and at least some of them are thought to have been tombs for some quite important, high-status individuals due to the foundation of a basilica church on the site and its inclusion of Tomb 8 into its structure. Unfortunately, the collagen was not well enough preserved from the Tomb 8 individual (S23) to be analysed.

The prevalence of caries and antemortem tooth loss decreases in the Late Antique period but there is an increase in the occurrence of calculus.[28] The forgoing of luxury foods as a part of the Christian dietary regimen may have meant that people avoided the high-sugar foods that had potentially been the cause of the rise in caries in the Early Roman period. The connection between dietary change and religious doctrine has been made at a number of locations across Europe with the introduction of Christianity (Garvie-Lok 2001; Polet and Katzenberg 2003; Müldner and Richards 2005; Salamon *et al.* 2008; Rutgers *et al.* 2009; Reitsema *et al.* 2010; 2016; Bourbou *et al.* 2011; Baldoni *et al.* 2016; López-Costas and Müldner 2016). If this interpretation of a religious cause for the dietary changes in the later Roman and Late Antique periods at Knossos is correct, this would support that there was a sizeable Christian community at Knossos, as is already attested by the presence of at least three basilica churches at the site and suggested in written texts, which mention archbishops and a Knossian representation at ecumenical councils (Frend and Johnston 1962, 186; Sweetman 2004a, 322). It would also confirm that Christianity had a tangible impact on the daily life and diet of the population.

In the Late Antique skeletal assemblage there was an increase in the prevalence of osteoarthritis, intervertebral disc disease and Schmorl's nodes, though a decrease in the prevalence of entheseal changes compared to the sample for the Roman period. No consistent patterns or significant differences could be identified in comparing the KOP tomb individual with the North Cemetery assemblage or amongst individuals from the different osteothekai. There was, however, a difference detected between the sexes for osteoarthritis. Unusually, females had a higher prevalence than males, though there are concerns about the numbers and types of joints available for sex-specific analysis (Section 7.3.1.2). Compared to the Roman period, the males showed a statistically significant decrease in osteoarthritis, while the female rates increased. This shows that while there was still a division of labour between the sexes, there may have been some differences in activity type compared to the Roman period.

9.5. Limitations and Future Directions

The limitations of this study, in terms of sample size and the preservation of diagnostic characteristics, are a consequence of the fragmentary nature, poor condition of the material, and poor storage conditions, exacerbated by variable record keeping. These are problems experienced by all archaeological studies of legacy material to a greater or lesser extent. This study has demonstrated the value of revisiting material from old excavations alongside their archival records, though in its frustrations and limitations also highlights the importance of good practices in methodology and recording during excavation, followed by prompt study and publication of the material, with specialists involved in every stage of the process. This situation is changing but is still not standard practice in archaeology in Greece.

Future work could be done towards a better understanding and standardised terminology of tomb types during this period on Crete. This is difficult due to the state of preservation and the state of records (from early travellers' observations to excavation notes). Guyon's (2008) thesis has done a great deal of work towards this goal for the Hellenistic and Roman periods but his work has not been published.[29] Guyon sticks rigidly to Moretti's (2006) categorisation of tomb forms devised broadly for tombs across the Greek world rather than considering the features of the Cretan tombs independently and grouping them by features found commonly and important to Cretan self-representation or the representation of the dead. It is also important to identify when social changes impacted on tomb form, which Guyon's study often does not consider in grouping the Hellenistic and Roman periods together.

To further investigate the impact of a Roman, possibly Campanian, presence at the colony of Knossos and consider the scale of in-migration to the site in the Early Roman period, further skeletal analyses could be conducted to pursue these research questions, such as strontium and oxygen isotope analysis on tooth enamel and the study of heritable non-metric dental traits. Large samples of reasonably well-preserved skeletal remains would be necessary to put forward a convincing argument. The identification of skeletal material coming from tombs likely to belong to the first generation of the colony would

[28] Calculus prevalence was at its highest in the Late Antique period, but the aetiology of calculus is not well understood and it may not be primarily or directly diet related.

[29] Guyon's (2008) PhD thesis is available in microform in the libraries of the University of Rennes 2, the National Institute of History of Art at Paris (Jacques Doucet Collections), and the French School at Athens.

be particularly useful and this may be possible from the tombs excavated by Grammatikaki (1991; 1993; 1997; 2004; 2006), as well as the more recent excavations by Rousaki (2016) in the area of the North Cemetery. Such a study could be expanded to other sites in Crete to compare the impact of immigration at various site types and consider the significance of colony status.

9.6. Conclusion

The results demonstrate that in addition to the impacts on the official administration, cultural tastes, and urban fabric of the city, the effects of the broad-scale social, political and economic changes filtered right down into the everyday lives of people affecting their fundamental wellbeing and way of life. Some differences were subtle, and others remain unexplained, but patterns across the various analyses demonstrate a significant change between the Hellenistic and Roman assemblages. This included increased adult life expectancy, a diversification of diet, and the greater visibility of a non-labouring group or even an elite class, potentially with some farmworkers and labourers moving away from the city or being buried further out or in less clearly recognisable graves. These changes likely reflect the general increased connectivity of Knossos and other Cretan cities within Mediterranean networks and peace and prosperity across the island, rather than being a direct result of Knossos becoming a Roman colony. However, to establish this clearly will require comparable analyses at contemporary cities in Crete.

The impact, speed and scale of change at different cities in the Early Roman period varied greatly due to their different local characteristics. Gortyn in particular, but also Ierapetra and other port-towns and cities along the south coast, had a resident population of Roman merchants prior to the Roman invasion (Baldwin Bowsky 1994, 25; Gallimore 2015, 44). Therefore, there was a more gradual transition occurring from earlier in the Hellenistic period, and a faster change to becoming a Roman provincial city (adopting new architectural forms and material culture) after the Roman invasion of Crete, than is evident at Knossos. On mainland Greece there was also a diversity of changes at different cities. Corinth was sacked during the Roman invasion in 146 BC and therefore it needed to rebuild in order to thrive (commercially and culturally, to attract trade and migrants) as a city and then as a Roman colony, established in 44/43 BC (Wiseman 1979; Williams 1993; Walbank 1997; Romano 2005). Patras had gained in importance after the sack of Corinth, becoming the main port in the region for ships coming from the Roman west and also became a Roman colony in 14 BC (Rizakis 1988). At both these sites cremation burials are found from the second half of the 1st century BC (Corinth)/beginning of the 1st century AD (Patras) to the mid-2nd century AD (Palmer 1964; Rife 1999; Thomas 2005; Dijkstra 2013, 56; Dijkstra and Moles forthcoming) and Latin inscriptions were more common than Greek during the same period (Kent 1966, 18–19; Rizakis 1989; Millis 2010, 23–30; Dijkstra 2015, 168–72). This was different from Knossos where Latin was adopted but Greek remained more common amongst the known inscriptions. Cremations are not known at any site on Crete in the Hellenistic or Roman periods (Guyon 2008, 177–78). Differences between the burials at Corinth and its port at Kenchreai demonstrate that communities with separate histories, economic and political roles, and demographic compositions had different trajectories for the manifestation of cultural change under the Roman Empire (Rife 2007, 100, 111). Large scale political and economic changes also did not affect all levels of society equally, particularly in terms of the impact on health and diet. In cities where there was an urban elite, highly visible in the burial sphere (and in the archaeological record), it is this section of society that prospered and would have had an improved diet and living conditions, while relatively little is likely to change for the urban poor.

The later transition into Late Antiquity is a more gradual socio-economic change and this is also reflected in the less substantial differences in health and lifestyle indicators at Knossos. Age-at-death profiles were remarkably similar to the Roman period, though average stature increased slightly, suggesting an improvement in living conditions in terms of hygiene standards and nutrition. An increase in joint disease may reflect a change to a more subsistence level of living with fewer non-farming occupants, reflecting a less hierarchical society. This may represent the diminishing of an elite class or simply the movement of high-status people away from Knossos to coastal Heraklion, which superseded Knossos as the major centre for north-central Crete from the Late Antique period until today. A smaller elite group of clergy or church patrons may have remained resident at Knossos. The relative conservatism in tomb form and monumentalisation of church buildings suggests changing attitudes towards priorities for social and capital investment. The increase in marine protein consumption in this period may reflect both less pressure on resources and the adoption of a Christian dietary regimen.

The changes that occurred in the later Roman Empire due to economic decline, invading forces, the division of the Empire into East and West, and the spread of Christianity also had a diverse range and chronology of impacts. Some factors of change, such as earthquakes and epidemics, would have had varying scales of impact in different localities (Stathakopoulos 2004). Diversity would therefore be expected in the impacts on society but there appears to be a degree of uniformity in some of the discernible changes which may be due to the strength of Christian doctrine and reorganisation of political institutions, breaking the provinces up into dioceses, integrating politics and religion in the formation of ecclesiastical governments and every city having a bishop (Limberis 2005, 444). Large numbers of basilicas were constructed across Greece (Sweetman 2017), and conservatism in tomb architecture is found in the disappearance of the elaborate, above-ground mausolea known from the Early Roman period, with pit, tile and stone-lined graves predominating from the 4th century in Crete, Greece and Asia Minor (Poulou-Papadimitriou *et al.* 2012; Wenn *et al.*

2017). Cities on Crete continued to prosper during the Late Antique period and there appears to have been continuity of settlement, certainly amongst the larger centres, though several surveys have documented an increase of sites (Gallimore 2016, 184). There were churches constructed in locations where there is no evidence (as yet) for a sizeable Roman settlement (Sweetman 2017, 215). Over 90 churches were constructed on Crete in the 5th and 6th centuries demonstrating Crete's connectedness within the Christian world (Sweetman 2017, 211). Trade continued to thrive with higher proportions of imported amphorae than in the Roman period in assemblages at Eleutherna, Gortyn and Ierapetra (Gallimore 2016, 185). Although the main grain route from Egypt was now directed towards Constantinople, Crete remained an important stopping point and was still active and connected within the networks of the Late Antique Mediterranean, though the church architecture, mosaics and material culture indicate stronger connections with the East than the West (Sweetman 2004a, 316). Like the construction of churches and spread of a more rigid burial form (east-west orientation, with the head to the west facing east, extended on their back with the hands on the abdomen, and no grave goods for single inhumations, and the use of osteothekai for collective or secondary burials), the rise in fish consumption seems to be a clear sign of the spread and impact of Christianity. Though fish consumption is known in the Roman period, there is a distinct rise in numbers of fish-eating individuals across Europe and the Mediterranean in this period, particularly at inland sites such as Knossos and Eleutherna on Crete, at Sourtara in Northern Greece, and a smaller proportion of the sampled population at Messene in the Peloponnese (Bourbou 2010, 146). Stathakopoulos (2004) observed that in communities across the Empire that suffered a significant death toll from plague epidemics, the surviving population often thrived economically and nutritionally afterwards due to the easing of pressure on resources. The same would occur if there was no longer significant in-migration, as appears to be the case at Knossos as Heraklion gradually became the dominant centre in the region. Though the population size of Knossos declined during this period, it remained a well-connected and economically sucessful city.

This book has detailed the osteological study of the population of Knossos across almost 1000 years of occupation. It has been the first study of its kind for these periods on Crete in terms of the combination of the size of the assemblage, the temporal coverage, and in its integrated, bottom-up approach. It has created a social history for the people of Knossos by taking an interdisciplinary approach to the application of methods and integrating different lines of evidence. In presenting the osteological evidence and interpretations, it has shown the value of how much new information can be added to the interpretation of the archaeological and historical record using these sorts of analyses. Osteoarchaeology even now remains under-exploited discipline for this period and region. It has also highlighted the value of utilising legacy assemblages of material that have been neglected from old excavations. Through the careful analysis of this material and its nuanced interpretation, this study has presented detailed evidence for the health, diet, wellbeing and lifestyle of individuals who once lived and died at Knossos. It has considered these interpretations on a population level for an understanding of the impact of social changes on society across this time period.

Bibliography

Abu-Taleb, Noha Saleh, and Dina Mohamed El Beshlawy. 2015. "Mandibular Ramus and Gonial Angle Measurements as Predictors of Sex and Age in an Egyptian Population Sample: A Digital Panoramic Study." *Journal of Forensic Research* 6: 308.

Adams, Bradley J., and Lyle W. Konigsberg. 2008. "How Many People? Determining the Number of Individuals Represented by Commingled Human Remains." In *Recovery, Analysis, and Identification of Commingled Human Remains*, Totowa, NJ: Humana Press, 241–55.

Adams, Bradley J., and Lyle W. Konigsberg. 2004. "Estimation of the Most Likely Number of Individuals from Commingled Human Skeletal Remains." *American Journal of Physical Anthropology* 125(2): 138–51.

Agelarakis, Anagnostis P., and Argiro Agelarakis. 1989. "The Paleopathological Evidence at Polystylon, Abdera." *Byzantinische Forschungen* 14: 9–25.

Ager, Sheila L. 1994. "Hellenistic Crete and ΚΟΙΝΟΔΙΚΙΟΝ." *Journal of Hellenic Studies* 114: 1–18.

Alberici, Lisa A., and Mary Harlow. 2007. "Age and Innocence: Female Transitions to Adulthood in Late Antiquity." *Hesperia Supplements* 41: 193–203.

Alcock, Susan E. 2002. *Archaeologies of the Greek Past: Landscape, Monuments and Memories*. Cambridge: Cambridge University Press.

Alexiou, Stylianos. 1957. "Ανασκφαί Τον Ξένων Αρχαιολογικών Σχολών." *Κρητικά Χρονικά*: 340–43.

———. 1966. "Η Αρχαιολογική Κίνηση Έν Κρήτη Κατά Το 1966." *Κρητικά Χρονικά* Κ: 319–26.

———. 1967. "Αρχαιότητες Και Μνημεία Κεντρικής Και Ανατολ. Κρήτη: Μικραί Σκαφικαί Έρευναι Και Περισυλλογή Αρχαιοτήτων." *Αρχαιολογικών Δελτίων* 22 (Χρονικα Β2): 486.

———. 1968. *Guide To The Archaeological Museum Of Heraclion*. Athens: General Direction of Antiquities and Restoration.

———. 1969. "Κρήτη. Περισυλλογή Αρχαίων Και Ελ Ασσονές Ανασκαφές." *Το Έργων τνς Αρχαιολογικής Εταιρείας*: 190–92.

———. 1973. "Η Αρχαιολογική Κίνησις Έν Κρήτη Κατά Το 1973." *Κρητικά Χρονικά* 25: 464.

Ambrose, Stanley H., and Lynette Norr. 1993. "Experimental Evidence for the Relationship of the Carbon Isotope Ratios of Whole Diet and Dietary Protein to Those of Bone Collagen and Carbonate." In *Prehistoric Human Bone: Archaeology at the Molecular Level*, eds. Joseph B Lambert and Gisela Grupe. Berlin, Heidelberg: Springer, 1–37.

Andreadaki-Vlazaki, Maria. 1992. "Σταυρωμένος Χαμαλευρίου Οικόπεδο Ψαρρού." *Αρχαιολογικόν Δελτίον* 47 (Β2 Χρονικά): 590–91.

———. 1997. "Χανιά." *Αρχαιολογικόν Δελτίον* 52 (Β2 Χρονικά [2003]): 1004–12.

———, ed. 2009. *Khania (Kydonia): A Tour to Sites of Ancient Memory*. Chania: Ministry of Culture and Tourism - 25th Ephorate of Prehistoric and Classical Antiquities.

Andrews, Peter, and Silvia Bello. 2006. "Pattern in Human Burial Practice." In *The Social Archaeology of Funerary Remains*, Oxbow Books, 14–29.

Andronikos, Manolis. 1984. *Vergina: The Royal Tombs and the Ancient City*. Athens: Ekdotike Athenon.

Angel, J. Lawrence. 1946. "Skeletal Change in Ancient Greece." *American Journal of Physical Anthropology* 4(1): 69–98.

———. 1971a. "Early Neolithic Skeletons from Çatal Hüyük: Demography and Pathology." *Anatolian Studies* 21: 77–98.

———. 1971b. *Lerna Volume II: The People*. Princeton: American School of Classical Studies at Athens.

Apostolakou, Vili. 1995. "Το Ελληνιστικό – Ρωμαϊκό Νεκροταφείο Αγ. Νικολάου." In *Πεπραγμένα Ζ΄ Διεθνούς Κρητολογικού Συνεδρίου*, Rethymnon, 33–40.

———. 1997. "Ιεράπετρα: Θέση Παραμυθίας (Οικόπεδο Α. Και Δ. Μαλλιωτάκη)." *Αρχαιολογικόν Δελτίον* 52 (Β2 Χρονικά): 1047–48.

———. 2011. "Ρωμαϊκοί Καμαροσκεπείς Τάφοι Της Ιεράπυτνας." In *Πεπραγμένα Ι΄ Διεθνούς Κρητολογικού Συνεδρίου τ. Α4*, 337–54.

Arcella, D., L. Ottolenghi, A. Polimeni, and Catherine Leclercq C. 2002. "The Relationship between Frequency of Carbohydrates Intake and Dental Caries: A Cross-Sectional Study in Italian Teenagers." *Public Health Nutrition* 5(4): 553–60.

Arden, N., and M. Nevitt. 2006. "Osteoarthritis: Epidemiology." *Best Practice & Research Clinical Rheumatology* 20(1): 3–25.

Armelagos, George J., and Dennis P. Van Gerven. 2003. "A Century of Skeletal Biology and Paleopathology: Contrasts, Contradictions, and Conflicts." *American Anthropologist* 105: 53–64.

Baer, Paul N., Robert M. Stephan, and Carl L. White. 1961. "Studies on Experimental Calculus Formation in the Rat I. Effect of Age, Sex, Strain, High Carbohydrate, High Protein Diets." *Journal of Periodontology* 32(3): 190–96.

Balasse, Marie, Andrew B. Smith, Stanley H. Ambrose, and Steven R. Leigh. 2003. "Determining Sheep Birth Seasonality by Analysis of Tooth Enamel Oxygen Isotope Ratios: The Late Stone Age Site of Kasteelberg (South Africa)." *Journal of Archaeological Science* 30(2): 205–15.

Baldoni, Marica, Alessandra Nardi, Gundula Muldner, Roberta Lelli, Micaela Gnes, Francesca Ferraresi, Valentina Meloni, Pamela Cerino, Simone Greco, Guglielmo Manenti, Micaela Angle, Olga Rickards, and Cristina Martínez-Labarga. 2016. "Archaeo-Biological Reconstruction of the Italian Medieval Population of Colonna (8th–10th Centuries CE)." *Journal of Archaeological Science: Reports* 10: 483–94.

Baldwin Bowsky, Martha W. 1994. "Cretan Connections: The Transformation of Hierapytna." *Cretan Studies* 4: 1–45.

———. 1995. "Roman Crete: No Provincial Backwater." In *Seventh International Cretological Congress, Rethymno 1991*, 41–67.

———. 1997. "Knossos and Campania the Critical Connection." In *Preliminary Publication XI International Congress of Greek and Latin Epigraphy, Rome, 18-24 September 1997*, Rome, 479–87.

———. 1999. "The Business of Being Roman: The Prosopographical Evidence." In *From Minoan Farmers to Roman Traders: Sidelights on the Economy of Ancient Crete*, ed. Angelos Chaniotis. Stuttgart: Franz Steiner Verlag, 305–47.

———. 2002. "Colonia Iulia Nobilis Cnosus Creta." In *11th International Congress of Classical Studies, Kavala, 24–30 August 1999*, 75–89.

———. 2004a. "From Traders to Landowners and the Imperial Cult: Acculturation in Roman Gortyn." In *Creta Romana e Protobizantina. Atti Del Congresso Internazionale (Iraklion, 23–30 Settembre 2000)*, Padua: Bottega D'Erasmo, 33–47.

———. 2004b. "Of Two Tongues: Acculturation at Roman Knossos." In *Colonie Romane Nel Mondo Greco*, eds. G. Salmeri, A. Raggi, and A. Baroni. Rome: L'Erma di Bretschneider, 94–150.

———. 2006. "From Capital to Colony: Five New Inscriptions from Roman Crete." *The Annual of the British School at Athens* 101: 385–426.

———. 2011. "Colonia Iulia Nobilis Cnosus, the First 100 Years: The Evidence of Italian Sigillata Stamps." In *Roman Colonies in the First Century of Their Foundation*, Oxford: Oxbow Books, 117–34.

Banou, E. 1997. "Ηράκλειο." *Αρχαιολογικόν Δελτίον* 52 (Χρονικά Β'2): 985.

———. 2002. "Αμπελοκηποι." *Κρητική Εστία* 9: 307–14.

Bard, H. 2003. "Physiopathologie, Réparation, Classification Des Tendinopathies Mécaniques." In *Tendons et Enthèses*, eds. H. Bard *et al.* Montpellier: Sauramps Médical, 165–178.

Barnes, Ethne. 2003. "The Dead Do Tell Tales." In *Corinth XX: The Centenary: 1896–1996*, Princeton: The American School of Classical Studies at Athens, 435–43.

Bass, William M. 1995. *Human Osteology: A Laboratory and Field Manual of the Human Skeleton.* 4th ed. Columbia: Missouri Archaeological Society.

Bassett, Steven. 1992. *Death in Towns: Urban Responses to the Dying and the Dead, 100–1600.* Leicester: Leicester University Press.

Bedwin, Owen. 1992. "Appendix 1: The Animal Bones." In *Knossos: From Greek City to Roman Colony. Excavations at the Unexplored Mansion II*, ed. L. Hugh Sackett. Oxford: British School at Athens; Thames and Hudsen; Alden Press, 491–92.

Beer, Michael. 2010. *Taste or Taboo: Dietary Choices in Antiquity*. Totnes: Prospect Books.

Belcastro, Giovanna, Elisa Rastelli, Valentina Mariotti, Chiara Consiglio, Fiorenzo Facchini, and Benedetta Bonfiglioli. 2007. "Continuity or Discontinuity of the Life-Style in Central Italy during the Roman Imperial Age-Early Middle Ages Transition: Diet, Health, and Behavior." *American Journal of Physical Anthropology* 132(3): 381–94.

Bell, Lynne S., Glenda Cox, and Judith Sealy. 2001. "Determining Isotopic Life History Trajectories Using Bone Density Fractionation and Stable Isotope Measurements: A New Approach." *American Journal of Physical Anthropology* 116(1): 66–79.

Bello, Silvia M., Aminte Thomann, Michel Signoli, Olivier Dutour, and Peter Andrews. 2006. "Age and Sex Bias in the Reconstruction of Past Population Structures." *American Journal of Physical Anthropology* 129(1): 24–38.

Bello, Silvia M., and Peter Andrews. 2006. "The Intrinsic Pattern of Preservation of Human Skeletons and Its Influence on the Interpretation of Funerary Behaviours." In *The Social Archaeology of Funerary Remains*, eds. Rebecca Gowland and Christopher Knüsel. Oxford: Oxbow Books, 1–13.

Benton, Sylvia. 1937. "Herakles and Eurystheus at Knossos." *The Journal of Hellenic Studies* 57(01): 38–43.

Bernard, Seth G. 2016. "Food Distributions and Immigration in Imperial Rome." In *Migration and Mobility in the Early Roman Empire*, eds. Elio Lo Cascio and Laurens Ernst Tacoma. Brill, 50–71.

Bielicki, T. 1986. "Physical Growth as a Measure of the Economic Well-Being of Populations: The Twentieth Century." In *Human Growth: A Comprehensive Treatise. Volume 3: Methodology and Ecological, Genetic, and Nutritional Effects on Growth*, eds. Frank Falkner and J.M. Tanner. New York: Plenum Press, 283–305.

Bisel, Sara C., and J. Lawrence Angel. 1985. "Health and Nutrition in Mycenaean Greece: A Study in Human Skeletal Remains." In *Contributions to Aegean Archaeology: Studies in Honor of William A. McDonald*, ed. N.C. Wilkie and W.D.E. Coulson. Minneapolis, 197–210.

Blackman, David J. 1997. "Archaeology in Greece 1996–97." *Archaeological Reports* 43: 1–125.

Blackman, David J., Julian Baker, and Nicholas Hardwick. 1998. "Archaeology in Greece 1997–98." *Archaeological Reports* (44): 1–136.

Blackman, David J., and Keith Branigan. 1975. "An Archaeological Survey on the South Coast of Crete, between the Ayiofarango and Chrisostomos." *The Annual of the British School at Athens* 70: 17–36.

Boardman, John. 1967. "The Khaniale Tekke Tombs, II." *The Annual of the British School at Athens* 62: 57–75.

Bocherens, H., and D. Drucker. 2003. "Trophic Level Isotopic Enrichment of Carbon and Nitrogen in Bone Collagen: Case Studies from Recent and Ancient Terrestrial Ecosystems." *International Journal of Osteoarchaeology* 13(1–2): 46–53.

Bocquet-Appel, Jean-Pierre. 2008. *Recent Advances in Palaeodemography : Data, Techniques, Patterns*. Springer.

Bocquet-Appel, Jean-Pierre, and Claude Masset. 1982. "Farewell to Paleodemography." *Journal of Human Evolution* 11(4): 321–33.

Bogaard, Amy, Rebecca Fraser,Tim H. E. Heaton, Michael Wallace, Petra Vaiglova, Michael Charles, Glynis Jones, Richard P. Evershed, Amy K. Styring, Niels H. Andersen, Rose Marie Arbogast, László Bartosiewicz, Armelle Gardeisen, Marie Kanstrup, Ursula Maier, Elena Marinova, Lazar Ninov, Marguerita Schäfer, Elisabeth Stephan, 2013. "Crop Manuring and Intensive Land Management by Europe's First Farmers." *PNAS* 110(31): 12589–94.

Bonfiglioli, B., P. Brasili, and M.G. Belcastro. 2003. "Dento-Alveolar Lesions and Nutritional Habits of a Roman Imperial Age Population (1st–4th c. AD): Quadrella (Molise, Italy)." *HOMO - Journal of Comparative Human Biology* 54(1): 36–56.

Bonsall, Laura. 2014. "A Comparison of Female and Male Oral Health in Skeletal Populations from Late Roman Britain: Implications for Diet." *Archives of Oral Biology* 59(12): 1279–1300.

Bonsall, Laura, and Catriona Pickard. 2015. "Stable Isotope and Dental Pathology Evidence for Diet in Late Roman Winchester, England." *Journal of Archaeological Science: Reports* 2: 128–40.

Bonsall, Laura, Catriona Pickard, and Kathleen McSweeney. 2015. "Stable Isotope Reconstruction of Diet in the Ancient Greek Colony of Mesembria (Nessebar, Bulgaria)." Poster Presentation at UK Archaeological Sciences Conference, Durham University, Durham.

Borbonus, Dorian. 2014. *Columbarium Tombs and Collective Identity in Augustan Rome*. Cambridge: Cambridge University Press.

Bourbou, Chryssi. 2005. "Biological Status in Hellenistic and Roman Elites in Western Crete (Greece)." *Eres* 13: 87–110.

———. 2009. "To Live and Die in a Turbulent Era: Bioarchaeological Analysis of the Early Byzantine (6th-7th Centuries AD) Population from Sourtara Galaniou Kozanis (Northern Greece)." *Dumbarton Oaks Papers* 63: 221–34.

———. 2010. *Health and Disease in Byzantine Crete (7th-12th Centuries AD)*. Farnham: Ashgate Publishing.

Bourbou, Chryssi, Benjamin T. Fuller, Sandra J. Garvie-Lok, and Michael P. Richards. 2013. "Nursing Mothers and Feeding Bottles: Reconstructing Breastfeeding and Weaning Patterns in Greek Byzantine Populations (6th–15th Centuries AD) Using Carbon and Nitrogen Stable Isotope Ratios." *Journal of Archaeological Science* 40(11): 3903–3913.

Bourbou, Chryssi, Benjamin T. Fuller, Sandra J. Garvie-Lok, and Michael P. Richards. 2011. "Reconstructing the Diets of Greek Byzantine Populations (6th-15th Centuries AD) Using Carbon and Nitrogen Stable Isotope Ratios." *American Journal of Physical Anthropology* 146(4): 569–81.

Bourbou, Chryssi, and Sandra Garvie-Lok. 2015. "Bread, Oil, Wine, and Milk : Feeding Infants and Adults in Byzantine Greece." In *Archaeodiet in the Greek World: Dietary Reconstruction from Stable Isotope Analysis*, eds. Anastasia Papathanasiou, Michael P. Richards, and Sherry C. Fox. Princeton: American School of Classical Studies at Athens, 171–94.

Bourbou, Chryssi, and Vanna Niniou-Kindeli. 2009. "A Hellenistic Mass Burial in the City of Chania, Crete (Greece). What Can We Infer about the Fate of the Individuals Buried?" In *Vers Une Anthropologie Des Catastrophes, Acts Du 9eme Journées Anthropologique de Valbonne (Valbonne, 22–24 May 2007)*, eds. L Buchet, C Rigeade, I Seguy, and M Signoli. Antibes: Editions APDCA/INED, 273–83.

Bourbou, Chryssi, and Michael P. Richards. 2007. "The Middle Byzantine Menu: Palaeodietary Information from Isotopic Analysis of Humans and Fauna from Kastella, Crete." *International Journal of Osteoarchaeology* 17(1): 63–72.

Bourbou, Chryssi, and Petros G. Themelis. 2010. "Child Burials at Ancient Messene." In *L'Enfant et La Mort Dans l'Antiquité I. Nouvelles Recherches Dans Les Nécropoles Grecques. Le Signalement Des Tombes d'enfants. Actes de La Table Ronde Internationale Organisée à Athènes, École Française d'Athènes, 29–30 Mai 2008*, Paris: De Boccard, 111–28.

Bourbou, Chryssi, and Agathoniki Tsilipakou. 2009. "Investigating the Human Past of Greece during the 6th-7th Centuries A.D." In eds. Lynne A. Schepartz, Sherry C. Fox, and Chryssi Bourbou. *New Directions in the Skeletal Biology of Greece Hesperia Supplement* 43: 121–36.

Boz, Başak, and Lori D. Hager. 2014. "Making Sense of Social Behavior from Disturbed and Commingled Skeletons: A Case Study from Çatalhöyük, Turkey." In *Commingled and Disarticulated Human Remains*, New York, NY: Springer New York, 17–33.

Brandt, J. Rasmus, Erika Hagelberg, Gro Bjørnstad, and Sven Ahrens, eds. 2017. *Life and Death in Asia Minor in Hellenistic, Roman, and Byzantine Times : Studies in Archaeology and Bioarchaeology*. Oxford: Oxbow Books.

Branigan, Keith. 1987. "Ritual Interference with Human Bones in the Mesara Tholoi." *Aegaeum* 1: 43–51.

Bridge, G. 2009. "Urbanism." In eds. Rob Kitchin and Nigel B.T., *International Encyclopedia of Human Geography*. Oxford: Elsevier, 106–11.

Brill, W.J. 1977. "Biological Nitrogen Fixation." In eds. N. Kretchmer and W. Robertson, *Human Nutrition: Readings from Scientific American*. San Francisco: W.H. Freeman and Company, 18–27.

Brock, James K. 1957. *Fortetsa. Early Greek Tombs near Knossos (The British School at Athens Supplementary Paper 2)*. Cambridge: Cambridge University Press.

Bronner, Felix. 2008. "Metals in Bone." In *Principles of Bone Biology*, Elsevier, 515–31.

Brothwell, Don R. 1989. "The Relationship of Tooth Wear to Ageing." In ed. Mehmet Yaşar Işcan, *Age Markers in the Human Skeleton*. Springfield, IL: Charles C. Thomas, 303–316.

Brothwell, Don R. 1981. *Digging up Bones*. London: British Museum (Natural History).

Brunt, P. A. 1971. *Italian Manpower, 225 B.C.-A.D. 14*. Oxford: Oxford University Press.

Buikstra, Jane E., and Lane A. Beck, eds. 2006. *Bioarchaeology: The Contextual Analysis of Human Remains*. Burlington: Elsevier.

Buikstra, Jane E, and Douglas H Ubelaker. 1994. *Standards for Data Collection from Human Skeletal Remains*. Fayetteville: Arkansas Archeological Survey Research Series No. 44.

Byers, Steven N. 2016. *Introduction to Forensic Anthropology*. 5th ed. London; New York: Routledge.

Byers, Steven N., K Akoshima, and B Curran. 1989. "Determination of Adult Stature from Metatarsal Length." *American Journal of Physical Anthropology* 79(3): 275–79.

Cadogan, Gerald, Eleni Hatzaki, and Andonis Vasilakis. 2004. *Knossos: Palace, City, State*. London: British School at Athens.

Callaghan, Peter J. 1980. "The Trefoil Style and Second-Century Hadra Vases." *The Annual of the British School at Athens* 75: 33–47.

Callaghan, Peter J., Hector W. Catling, Elizabeth A. Catling, David Smyth, Antony J.S. Spawforth, and Sheilagh Wall. 1981. "Knossos 1975: Minoan Paralipomena and Post-Minoan Remains." *The Annual of the British School at Athens* 76: 83–108.

Callaghan, Peter J., J. Nicolas Coldstream, and Jonathan H. Musgrave. 1981. "Knossos: An Early Greek Tomb on Lower Gypsadhes Hill." *The Annual of the British School at Athens* 76: 141–65.

Callaghan, Peter J., and Richard E. Jones. 1985. "Hadra Hydriae and Central Crete: A Fabric Analysis." *The Annual of the British School at Athens* 80: 1–17.

Callaghan, Peter J. 1978. "KRS 1976: Excavations at a Shrine of Glaukos, Knossos." *The Annual of the British School at Athens* 73: 1–30.

———. 1981. "The Little Palace Well and Knossian Pottery of the Later Third and Second Centuries B.C." *The Annual of the British School at Athens* 76: 35–58.

———. 1992. "Archaic to Hellenistic Pottery." In *Knossos: From Greek City to Roman Colony. Excavations at the Unexplored Mansion II*, ed. L. Hugh Sackett. London: British School at Athens, 89–136.

———. n.d. *North Cemetery Unpublished Manuscript*. drafted c.1985, typed and edited by Todd Whitelaw 2014.

Cankardeş-Şenol, Gonca. 2007. "Stamped Amphora Handles Found in the Rescue Excavations of CEAlex in Alexandria." In *Amphores D'Égypte. De La Basse Époque à L'époque Arabe*, eds. Sylvie Marchand and Antigone Marangou. Cairo: Institut français d'archéologie orientale, 33–56.

Capasso, L., K. A. R. Kennedy, and C. A. Wilczack. 1999. *Atlas of Occupational Markers on Human Remains*. Teramo: Edigrafital S.p.A.

Cardoso, F. Alves, and C.Y. Henderson. 2009. "Enthesopathy Formation in the Humerus: Data from Known Age-at-Death and Known Occupation Skeletal Collections." *American Journal of Physical Anthropology* 141(4): 550–60.

Carington Smith, Jill. 1982. "A Roman Chamber Tomb on the South-East Slopes of Monasteriaki Kephala, Knossos." *The Annual of the British School at Athens* 77: 255–93.

Carington Smith, Jill, and Sheilagh Wall. 1994. "A Late Hellenistic Wine Press at Knossos." *The Annual of the British School at Athens* 89: 359–376.

De Caro, Stefano. 1993. "Vino Di Cnosso Dei. Campani: Un Nuovo Documento Epigrafico per La Storia Del Vino Cretese in Età Romana." *Annuario della Scuola Atene* 70–71: 307–12.

Carrier, Caroline. 2018. "Cnossos de l'époque Classique à l'époque Impériale (Ve Siècle Avant J.-C - Ier Siècle Après J.-C.). Étude de Numismatique et d'Histoire." Unpublished PhD thesis, Université Paris-Sorbonne.

Catling, Hector W. 1977a. "The Knossos Area, 1974–1976." *Archaeological Reports* 23: 3–23.

———. 1983. "Archaeology in Greece, 1982–83." *Archaeological Reports* 29: 3–62.

———. 1984. "Archaeology in Greece, 1983–84." *Archaeological Reports* 30: 3–70.

Catling, Hector W., David Smyth, Jonathan H. Musgrave, and Glynis Jones. 1976. "An Early Christian Osteotheke At Knossos." *The Annual of the British School at Athens* 71: 25–47.

Catling, Hector W. 1977b. "Archaeology in Greece, 1976–77." *Archaeological Reports* 24: 3–69.

———. 1979. "Knossos, 1978." *Archaeological Reports* (25): 43–58.

Catling, Hector W., Cressida Ridley, Jill Carington Smith, David Smyth, and Archie W. Dunn. 1982. "Knossos 1978: Roman Finds at the Venezeleion." *The Annual of the British School at Athens* 77: 59–64.

Cavanagh, William G. 1978. *KMF Excavation Notebook 16*. Unpublished.

Cavanagh, William G., and Michael Curtis. 1998. "Post-Minoan Crete: Proceedings of the First Colloquium on Post-Minoan Crete Held by the British School at Athens and the Institute of Archaeology, University College London, 10–11 November 1995." *British School at Athens Studies* (2).

Chamberlain, Andrew T. 2006. Cambridge Manuals in Archaeology *Demography in Archaeology*. Cambridge: Cambridge University Press.

Chaniotis, Angelos. 1999. "Milking the Mountains: Economic Activities on the Cretan Uplands in the Classical and Hellenistic Period." In ed. Angelos Chaniotis, *From Minoan Farmers to Roman Traders: Sidelights on the Economy of Ancient Crete*. Stuttgart: FranzSteiner Verlag, 181–220.

———. 2005. "Inscribed Instrumenta Domestica and the Economy of Hellenistic and Roman Crete." In *Making, Moving, and Managing. The New World of Ancient Economies*, eds. Z.H. Archibald, J.K. Davies, and V. Gabrielsen. Oxford: Oxbow, 92–116.

Chapman, Anne E. 1968. "Some First Century B.C. Bronze Coins of Knossos." *The Numismatic Chronicle (1966-)* 8: 13–26.

Chenal-Velarde, Isabelle. 2006. "Food, Rituals? The Exploitation of Dogs from Eretria (Greece) During the Helladic and Hellenistic Periods." In eds. Lynn M. Snyder and Elizabeth A. Moore, *Dogs and People in Social, Working, Economic or Symbolic Interaction*. Oxford: Oxbow, 24–31.

Chevrollier, François. 2016. "From Cyrene to Gortyn. Notes on the Relationships between Crete and Cyrenaica under Roman Domination (1st c. BC to 4th c. AD)." In eds. Jane E. Francis and Anna Kouremenos, *Roman Crete: New Perspectives*. Oxford: Oxbow, 11–26.

Cho, Helen, Sam D. Stout, and Thomas A. Bishop. 2006. "Cortical Bone Remodeling Rates in a Sample of African American and European American Descent Groups from the American Midwest: Comparisons of Age and Sex in Ribs." *American Journal of Physical Anthropology* 130(2): 214–26.

Ciocci, A. 1987. "Diffuse Idiopathic Skeletal Hyperostosis (DISH) and Situs Viscerum Inversus. Report of a Single Case." *Clinical and experimental rheumatology* 5(2): 159–60.

Ciranni, R., and G. Fornaciari. 2003. "Luigi Boccherini and the Barocco Cello: An 18th Century Striking Case of Occupational Disease." *International Journal of Osteoarchaeology* 13(5): 294–302.

Clement, Anna F., and Simon W. Hillson. 2012. "Intrapopulation Variation in Macro Tooth Wear Patterns-a Case Study from Igloolik, Canada." *American Journal of Physical Anthropology* 149(4): 517–24.

Clement, Anna F., Simon W. Hillson, and Maria Michalaki-Kollia. 2009. "The Ancient Cemeteries of Astypalaia, Greece." *Archaeology International* 12: 17–21.

Coldstream, J. Nicolas. 1960. "Knossos." *Αρχαιολογικόν Δελτίον* 16 (Χρονικά Β'2): 263–66.

———. 1968. "Fortetsa." *Αρχαιολογικόν Δελτίον* 23 (Χρονικά Β'2): 412.

———. 1973. *Knossos: The Sanctuary of Demeter*. London: British School at Athens.

———. 1999. "Knossos 1951–61: Classical and Hellenistic Pottery from the Town." *The Annual of the British School at Athens* 94: 321.

Coldstream, J. Nicolas, and Hector W. Catling. 1996. *Knossos North Cemetery: Early Greek Tombs*. London: British School at Athens.

Coldstream, J. Nicolas, L. Jonas Eiring, and Gary Forster. 2001. *Knossos Pottery Handbook: Greek and Roman*. London: British School at Athens.

Coldstream, J. Nicolas, George L. Huxley, and V.E.S. Webb. 1999. "Knossos: The Archaic Gap." *The Annual of the British School at Athens* 94: 289–307.

Conder, Josiah. 1830. *The Modern Traveller, Volume the Sixteenth, Greece, Vol. II*. London: James Duncan.

Cook, J. M. 1952. "Archaeology in Greece, 1951." *The Journal of Hellenic Studies* 72: 92–112.

Corti, Maria Chiara, and Chiara Rigon. 2003. "Epidemiology of Osteoarthritis: Prevalence, Risk

Factors and Functional Impact." *Aging Clinical and Experimental Research* 15(5): 359–63.

Cosmopoulos, Michael B., Haskel J. Greenfield, and Deborah Ruscillo. 2003. "Animal and Marine Remains from the New Excavations at Eleusis: An Interim Report." In eds. Eleni Kotjabopoulou, Yannis Hamilakis, Paul Halstead, Clive Gamble and Paraskevi Elefanti, *Zooarchaeology in Greece: Recent Advances*: 145–52. London: British School at Athens.

Cox, Glenda, and Judith Sealy. 1997. "Investigating Identity and Life Histories: Isotopic Analysis and Historical Documentation of Slave Skeletons Found on the Cape Town Foreshore, South Africa." *International Journal of Historical Archaeology* 1(3): 207–24.

Craig, Oliver E., Marco Biazzo, Tamsin C. O'Connell, Peter Garnsey, Cristina Martinez-Labarga, Roberta Lelli, Loretana Salvadei, Gianna Tartaglia, Alessia Nava, Lorena Renò, Antonella Fiammenghi, Olga Rickards, and Luca Bondioli. 2009. "Stable Isotopic Evidence for Diet at the Imperial Roman Coastal Site of Velia (1st and 2nd Centuries AD) in Southern Italy." *American Journal of Physical Anthropology* 139(4): 572–83.

Cross, Marita, Emma Smith, Damian Hoy, Sandra Nolte, Ilana Ackerman, Marlene Fransen, Lisa Bridgett, Sean Williams, Francis Guillemin, Catherine L Hill, Laura L Laslett, Graeme Jones, Flavia Cicuttini, Richard Osborne, Theo Vos, Rachelle Buchbinder, Anthony Woolf, and Lyn March. 2014. "The Global Burden of Hip and Knee Osteoarthritis: Estimates from the Global Burden of Disease 2010 Study." *Annals of the rheumatic diseases* 73(7): 1323–30.

Crowe, Fiona, Alessandra Sperduti, Tamsin C. O'Connell, Oliver E. Craig, Karola Kirsanow, Paola Germoni, Roberto Macchiarelli, Peter Garnsey, and Luca Bondioli. 2010. "Water-Related Occupations and Diet in Two Roman Coastal Communities (Italy, First to Third Century AD): Correlation between Stable Carbon and Nitrogen Isotope Values and Auricular Exostosis Prevalence." *American Journal of Physical Anthropology* 142(3): 355–66.

Curtis, Robert I. 2009. "Food Processing and Preparation." In *The Oxford Handbook of Engineering and Technology in the Classical World*, ed. John Peter Oleson. Oxford: Oxford University Press, 369–92.

Dalby, Andrew. 1996. *Siren Feasts: A History of Food and Gastronomy in Greece*. London: Routledge.

———. 2003. *Food in the Ancient World from A to Z*. London; New York: Routledge.

Davaras, Costis. 1968. "Περιοχή Μονής Οδηγητρίας." *Αρχαιολογικόν Δελτίον* 23 (B2 Χρονικά): 405.

———. 1974. "Rock-Cut Fish Tanks in Eastern Crete." *The Annual of the British School at Athens* 69: 87–93.

———. 1975. "A Rock-Cut Fish Tank near Hierapetra." *Αρχαιολογικόν Δελτίον* 30A: 149–54.

———. 1987. "Ρωμαϊκό Νεκροταφείο Αγίου Νικολάου." *Αρχαιολογική Εφημερίς* 1985: 130–216.

Davidson, James N. 1997. *Courtesans and Fishcakes: The Consuming Passions of Classical Athens*. Chicago: University of Chicago Press.

Deines, Peter. 1980. "The Isotopic Composition of Reduced Organic Carbon." In *The Terrestrial Environment, A Handbook of Environmental Isotope Geochemistry*, Elsevier, 329–406.

Dembińska, Maria. 1985. "Diet: A Comparison of Food Consumption between Some Eastern and Western Monasteries in the 4th–12th Centuries.' *Byzantion* 55(2): 431–62.

DeNiro, Michael J., and Samuel Epstein. 1978. "Influence of Diet on the Distribution of Carbon Isotopes in Animals." *Geochimica et Cosmochimica Acta* 42(5): 495–506.

Deniro, Michael J., and Margaret J. Schoeniger. 1983. "Stable Carbon and Nitrogen Isotope Ratios of Bone Collagen: Variations within Individuals, between Sexes, and within Populations Raised on Monotonous Diets." *Journal of Archaeological Science* 10(3): 199–203.

DeNiro, Michael J. 1987. "Stable Isotopy and Archaeology." *American Scientist* 75(2): 182–91.

van Deursen, L.L., J. Patijn, J.R. Durinck, R. Brouwer, J.R. van Erven-Sommers, and B.J. Vortman. 1999. "Sitting and Low Back Pain: The Positive Effect of Rotary Dynamic Stimuli during Prolonged Sitting." *European spine journal : official publication of the European Spine Society, the European Spinal Deformity Society, and the European Section of the Cervical Spine Research Society* 8(3): 187–93.

Diamantis, Nikitas. 1998. "Επιγραφές Από Το Παλαιοχριστιανικό Νεκροταφείο Της Κισάμου." *Αρχαιολογικών Δελτίων* 53 (Μελέτες): 313–30.

———. 2004. "Το Παλαιοχριστιανικό Νεκροταφείο Της Κισάμου." In *Creta Romana e Protobizantina. Atti Del Congresso Internazionale (Iraklion, 23–30 Settembre 2000)*, Padova: Bottega D'Erasmo, 383–95.

Dijkstra, Tamara M. 2013. "Colonia Augusta Achaica Patrensis: Grafveld En Identiteit in Een Romeinse Kolonie in Griekenland." *Tijdschrift voor Mediterrane Archeologie* 50: 53–59.

———. 2015. "Burial and Commemoration in the Roman Colony of Patras." In *Processes of Cultural Change and Integration in the Roman World*, Leiden: Brill, 154–74.

———. 2019. "From Polis to Colonia: Death, Burial, and Society in Hellenistic and Roman Patras." Unpublished PhD thesis, University of Groningen.

Dijkstra, Tamara M., and Anna C. Moles. forthcoming. "Changing Burial Practices at Patras and Knossos:

The Impact of Migration in the Early Roman Period." *Pharos*.

Dimakis, Nikolas. 2016. *Social Identity and Status in the Classical and Hellenistic Northern Peloponnese: The Evidence from Burials*. Oxford: Archaeopress.

———. 2019. "Burial and Commemoration of Children in Hellenistic Greece." In *Griechishe Nekropolen. Neue Forschugen Und Funde [Beiträge Zur Archäologie Griechenlands 5]*, eds. H. Frielinghaus, J. Stroszeck, and P. Valavanis. Möhnesee: Bibliopolis, 287–305.

Dobney, K., and K Reilly. 1988. "A Method for Recording Archaeological Animal Bones: The Use of Diagnostic Zones." *Circaea* 5(2): 79–96.

Donahue, John. 2018. "Roman Meals in Their Domestic and Wider Settings." In *The Routledge Handbook of Diet and Nutrition in the Roman World*, eds. Paul Erdkamp and Claire Holleran. Routledge, 93–100.

Dotsika, Elissavet, Dimitra Ermioni Michael, Efstathios Iliadis, Petros Karalis, and Georgios Diamantopoulos. 2018. "Isotopic Reconstruction of Diet in Medieval Thebes (Greece)." *Journal of Archaeological Science: Reports* 22: 482–91.

Drosinou, Paraskevi. 1992. "Ανασκαφικές Εργασίες. Νομός Χανίων. Κίσαμος. Οικόπεδο Αλέξ. Και Γεώργιου Ραϊσάκη." *Αρχαιολογικόν Δελτίον* 47 (B2 Χρονικά): 579–81.

Dupras, Tosha L. 1999. "Dining in the Dakhleh Oasis, Egypt: Determination of Diet Using Documents and Stable Isotope Analysis." McMaster University.

Dupras, Tosha L., Henry P. Schwarcz, and Scott I. Fairgrieve. 2001. "Infant Feeding and Weaning Practices in Roman Egypt." *American Journal of Physical Anthropology* 115(3): 204–12.

Dupras, Tosha L., and Matthew W. Tocheri. 2007. "Reconstructing Infant Weaning Histories at Roman Period Kellis, Egypt Using Stable Isotope Analysis of Dentition." *American Journal of Physical Anthropology* 134(1): 63–74.

Efstratiou, Nikos, Alexandra Karetsou, Eleni S. Banou, and Despina Margomenou. 2004. "The Neolithic Settlement of Knossos: New Light on an Old Picture." In *Palace, City, State. British School at Athens Studies*, eds. Gerald Cadogan, Eleni Hatzaki, and Andonis Vasilakis. British School at Athens, 39–49.

Eiring, L. Jonas. 2000. "Knossos at the Turn of the Millennium: Romanitas and Pottery." *Rei Cretariae Romanae Fautorum* 26: 197–203.

———. 2001. "Hellenistic Knossos: The Pottery." Unpublished PhD thesis, University of Sydney.

———. 2004. "The Earliest Italian Sigillata at Knossos." In *Early Italian Sigillata*, eds. J. Poblome, P. Talloen, R. Brulet, and Marc Waelkens. Leuven: Peeters, 71–72.

Ekroth, Gunnel. 2007. "Meat in Ancient Greece: Sacrificial, Sacred or Secular?" *Food & History* 5: 249–72.

Empereur, Jean-Yves, Antigone Marangou A, and Nikos Papadakis. 1992. "Recherches Sur Les Amphores Crétoises (III)." *Bulletin de correspondance hellénique* 116(2): 633–48.

Empereur, Jean-Yves, and Marie-Dominique Nenna. 2001. *Nécropolis 1*. Le Caire: Institut français d'archaeologie orientale.

———. 2003. *Nécropolis 2*. Le Caire: Institut français d'archéologie orientale.

Engels, Donald. 1990. *Roman Corinth: An Alternative Model for the Classical City*. Chicago: University of Chicago Press.

Enklaar, Arnold. 1985. "Chronologie et Peintres de Hydries de Hadra." *BABESCH - Bulletin Antieke Beschaving* 60: 106–51.

———. 1986. "Les Hydres de Hadra." *BABESCH - Bulletin Antieke Beschaving* 61: 41–65.

Erdkamp, Paul. 2012. "Urbanism." In *The Cambridge Companion to the Roman Economy*, Cambridge Companions to the Ancient World, ed. Walter Scheidel. Cambridge: Cambridge University Press, 241–65.

Erdkamp, Paul, and Claire Holleran. 2018. *The Routledge Handbook of Diet and Nutrition in the Roman World*. Abingdon: Routledge.

Erickson, Brice L. 2010. *Crete in Transition: Pottery Styles and Island History in the Archaic and Classical Periods*. Hesperia Supplement 45, Princeton.

Eshed, Vered, Avi Gopher, and Israel Hershkovitz. 2006. "Tooth Wear and Dental Pathology at the Advent of Agriculture: New Evidence from the Levant." *American Journal of Physical Anthropology* 130(2): 145–59.

Evans, Arthur J. 1906. *The Prehistoric Tombs of Knossos: The Cemetery of Zafer Papoura: The Royal Tomb of Isopata*. London: B. Quaritch.

———. 1928. *The Palace of Minos at Knossos Vol. II Part I*. London: MacMillan and Co.

———. 1930. *The Palace of Minos at Knossos Vol. III*. London: MacMillan and Co.

———. 1935. *The Palace of Minos: A Comparative Account of the Successive Stages of the Early Cretan Civilization as Illustred by the Discoveries at Knossos Vol. 4 (2)*. London.

Evans, J.A., C.A. Chenery, and A.P. Fitzpatrick. 2006. "Bronze Age Childhood Migration of Individuals near Stonehenge, Revealed by Strontium and Oxygen Isotope Tooth Enamel Analysis." *Archaeometry* 48(2): 309–21.

Faber, Andrea, Peter Fasold, Manuela Struck, and Marion Witteyer, eds. 2007. *Körpergräber Des 1.–3. Jahrhunderts in Der Römischen Welt: Internationales*

Kolloquium, Frankfurt Am Main, 19.–20. November 2004. Frankfurt: Archäologisches Museum Frankfurt.

Fedak, Janos. 1990. *Monumental Tombs of the Hellenistic Age: A Study of Selected Tombs from the Pre-Classical to the Early Imperial Era*. Toronto: University of Toronto Press.

Felson, David T. 2003. "Epidemiology of Osteoarthritis." In *Osteoarthritis*, eds. K.D. Brandt, M. Doherty, and L.S. Lohmander. Oxford: Oxford University Press, 9–16.

Fiorin, Elena, Pere Ibáñez-Gimeno, Douglas H. Ubelaker, Albert Isidro, and Assumpció Malgosa. 2017. "The Population of Can Reiners. Demography and Life Conditions on Mallorca (Balearic Islands, Spain) during the Middle Ages." *Journal of Archaeological Science: Reports* 15: 120–31.

Fogel, Robert W., Stanley L. Engerman, Roderick Floud, Gerald Friedman, Robert A. Margo, Kenneth Sokoloff, Richard H. Steckel, T. James Trussell, Georgia Villaflor, and Kenneth W. Wachter. 1983. "Secular Changes in American and British Stature and Nutrition." *Journal of Interdisciplinary History* 14(2): 445.

Food and Nutrition Board of the Institute of Medicine. 2005. *Dietary Reference Intakes for Energy, Carbohydrate, Fiber, Fat, Fatty Acids, Cholesterol, Protein, and Amino Acids (Macronutrients)*. Washington, D.C.: National Academies Press.

Forster, Gary. 2009. "Roman Knossos: The Pottery in Context. A Presentation of Ceramic Evidence Provided by the Knossos 2000 Project (1993–95)." Unpublished PhD thesis, University of Birmingham.

Fox Leonard, Sherry. 1997. "Comparative Health from Paleopathological Analysis of the Human Skeletal Remains Dating to the Hellenistic and Roman Periods, from Paphos, Cyprus and Corinth, Greece." Unpublished PhD thesis, University of Arizona.

Fox, Sherry. 2005. "Health in Hellenistic and Roman Times: The Case Studies of Paphos, Cyprus and Corinth, Greece." In *Health in Antiquity*, ed. Helen King. London; New York: Routledge, 59–82.

Francis, Jane E. 2006. "Beehives and Beekeeping in Graeco-Roman Sphakia." In *Πεπραγμένα Θ΄ Διεθνούς Κρητολογικού Συνεδρίου Ελούντα, 1–6 Οκτωβρίου 2001.*, eds. Th. Detorakis and S. Papadaki-Oekland. Heraklion, 379–89.

———. 2010. "A Re-Evaluation of Rock-Cut Fish Installations in Roman Crete." *Creta Antica* 11: 255–77.

———. 2016. "Apiculture in Roman Crete." In *Roman Crete: New Perspectives*, eds. Jane E. Francis and Anna Kouremenos. Oxford: Oxbow, 83–100.

Fraser, P.M. 1969. "Archaeology in Greece, 1968–69." *Archaeological Reports* 15: 3–39.

Fraser, Rebecca A., Amy Bogaard, Tim Heaton, Michael Charles, Glynis Jones, Bent T. Christensen, Paul Halstead, Ines Merbach, Paul R. Poulton, Debbie Sparkes, and Amy K. Styring. 2011. "Manuring and Stable Nitrogen Isotope Ratios in Cereals and Pulses: Towards a New Archaeobotanical Approach to the Inference of Land Use and Dietary Practices." *Journal of Archaeological Science* 38(10): 2790–2804.

Frederiksen, Martin. 1984. *Campania*. London: British School at Rome.

French, E. B. 1994. "Archaeology in Greece 1993–1994." *Archaeological Reports* 40: 3–84.

Frend, W.H.C., and David E. Johnston. 1962. "The Byzantine Basilica Church at Knossos." *The Annual of the British School at Athens* 57: 186–238.

Fuller, Benjamin T., T.I. Molleson, D.A. Harris, L.T. Gilmour, and R.E.M. Hedges. 2006. "Isotopic Evidence for Breastfeeding and Possible Adult Dietary Differences from Late/Sub-Roman Britain." *American Journal of Physical Anthropology* 129(1): 45–54.

Fully, G. 1956. "Une Nouvelle Méthode de Détermination de La Taille." *Annales de Médecine Légale* 35: 266–273.

Gagarin, Michael, and Paula J. Perlman. 2016. *The Laws of Ancient Crete c.650–400 BCE*. Oxford. Oxford University Press.

Gallant, T.W. Thomas. 1985. *A Fisherman's Tale*. Ghent: Miscellanea Graeca 7.

Gallimore, Scott. 2015. *An Island Economy: Hellenistic and Roman Pottery from Hierapytna, Crete*. New York: Peter Lang.

———. 2016. "Crete's Economic Transformation in the Late Roman Empire." In *Roman Crete: New Perspectives*, eds. Jane E. Francis and Anna Kouremenos. Oxford: Oxbow, 175–88.

Garcia, Jaume, and Climent Quintana-Domeque. 2007. "The Evolution of Adult Height in Europe: A Brief Note." *Economics & Human Biology* 5(2): 340–49.

Garland, Robert. 2013. "Children in Athenian Religion." In *The Oxford Handbook of Childhood and Education in the Classical World*, eds. Judith Evans Grubbs and Tim Parkin. Oxford: Oxford University Press, 207–26.

Garnsey, Peter. 1988. *Famine and Food Supply in the Graeco-Roman World*. Cambridge: Cambridge University Press.

———. 1999. *Food and Society in Classical Antiquity*. Cambridge: Cambridge University Press.

Garnsey, Peter, and Richard P. Saller. 2014. *The Roman Empire: Economy, Society and Culture*. London: Bloomsbury.

Garvie-Lok, Sandra J. 2001. "Loaves and Fishes: A Stable Isotope Reconstruction of Diet in Medieval Greece." Unpublished PhD thesis, University of Calgary.

Garvin, Heather M., Nicholas Passalacqua, Natalie M. Uhl, Desina R. Gipson, Rebecca S. Overbury, and Luis L. Cabo. 2012. "Developments in Forensic Anthropology: Age-at-Death Estimation." In *A Companion to Forensic Anthropology*, ed. Dennis Dirkmaat. Chichester: Blackwell, 202–23.

Gavrilaki, Eirini. 2004. "Νεκροταφείο Ρωμαϊκών Χρόνων Στην Αργυρούπολη Ρεθυμνης." In *Creta Romana e Protobizantina. Atti Del Congresso Internazionale (Iraklion, 23–30 Settembre 2000)*, Padova: Bottega D'Erasmo, 301–12.

Van Gerven, Dennis P., and George J. Armelagos. 1983. "'Farewell to Paleodemography?' Rumors of Its Death Have Been Greatly Exaggerated." *Journal of Human Evolution* 12(4): 353–60.

Giorgi, Elisabetta. 2016. *Archeologia Dell'acqua a Gortina Di Creta in Età Protobizantina.* Oxford: Archaeopress.

Girotti, M., and T. Doro Garetto. 1999. "Studio Odontologico Sulla Popolazione." In *San Michele Di Trino (VC). Dal Villaggio Romano Al Castello Medievale, Volume 2*, ed. M.M. Negro Ponzi Mancini. Florence: All'insegna del Giglio, 732–38.

Gnes, Micaela, Marica Baldoni, Lorenza Marchetti, Francesco Basoli, Donatella Leonardi, Antonella Canini, Silvia Licoccia, Flavio Enei, Olga Rickards, and Cristina Martínez-Labarga. 2018. "Bioarchaeological Approach to the Study of the Medieval Population of Santa Severa (Rome, 7th–15th Centuries)." *Journal of Archaeological Science: Reports* 18: 11–25.

Gondicas, Daphné. 1984. *Recherches Sur La Crète Occidentale de l'époque Géométrique à La Conquête Romaine. Inventaire Des Sources Archéologiques et Textuelles, Position Du Problème.* Amsterdam: A.M. Hakkert.

Grammatikaki, Eva. 1991. "Ανασκαφικές Εργασίες. Κνωσός." *Αρχαιολογικόν Δελτίον* 46 (Χρονικά Β'2): 391–94.

———. 1992. "Ανασκαφικές Εργασίες. Κνωσός." *Αρχαιολογικόν Δελτίον* 47 (Χρονικά Β'2): 556–58.

———. 1993. "Ανασκαφικές Εργασίες. Περιοχή Κνωσού." *Αρχαιολογικόν Δελτίον* 48 (Χρονικά Β'2): 445–50.

———. 1996. "Ανασκαφικές Εργασίες. Κνωσός." *Αρχαιολογικόν Δελτίον* 51 (Χρονικά Β'2): 624–30.

———. 1997. "Ανασκαφικές Εργασίες. Κνωσός." *Αρχαιολογικόν Δελτίον* 52 (Χρονικά Β'2): 987–89.

———. 2004. "Ταφικά Μνημεία Κνωσού." In *Palace, City, State. British School at Athens Studies*, eds. Gerald Cadogan, Eleni Hatzaki, and Adonis Vasilakis. London: British School at Athens, 465–72.

———. 2006. "Ελληνιστικά Νεκροταφεία Της Κνωσού." In *Πεπραγμένα Θ' Διεθνούς Κρητολογικού Συνεδρίου, Ελούντα 1–6 Οκτωβρίου 2001, Α5. Αρχαία Ελληνική Και Ρωμαϊκή Περίοδος*, Heraklion: Εταιρία Κρητικών Ιστορικών Μελετών, 25–41.

Grammatikaki, Eva, and Nikos Litinas. 2000. "Μαγικός Κατάδεσμος." *Eulimene* 1: 61–69.

Grant, Michael. 1946. *From Imperium to Auctoritas: A Historical Study of Aes Coinage in the Roman Empire, 49 B.C.–A.D. 14.* Cambridge: Cambridge University Press.

Griffin, Rebecca, Martin Pitts, Richard Smith, and Alan Brook. 2011. "Inequality at Late Roman Baldock, UK: The Impact of Social Factors on Health and Diet." *Journal of Anthropological Research* 67(4): 533–56.

Grmek, Mirko D. 1989. *Diseases in the Ancient Greek World.* Baltimore: John Hopkins University Press.

Grotle, Margreth, Kare B. Hagen, Bard Natvig, Fredrik A. Dahl, and Tore K. Kvien. 2008. "Obesity and Osteoarthritis in Knee, Hip and/or Hand: An Epidemiological Study in the General Population with 10 Years Follow-Up." *BMC musculoskeletal disorders* 9: 132.

Grubbs, Judith Evans, and Tim Parkin. 2013. "Introduction." In *The Oxford Handbook of Childhood and Education in the Classical World*, eds. Judith Evans Grubbs and Tim Parkin. Oxford: Oxford University Press, 1–15.

Guarducci, Margarita, ed. 1935. "Cnosos." In *Inscriptiones Creticae I. Opera et Consilio Friderici Halbherr Collectae*, Roma: La Libreria dello Stato, 45–82.

Guimier-Sorbets, Anne-Marie, and Demetrios Michaelides. 2009. "Alexandrian Influences on the Architecture and Decoration of the Hellenistic Tombs of Cyprus." In *Egypt and Cyprus in Antiquity, Nicosie, 2003*, eds. Demetrios Michaelides, Vasiliki Kassianidou, and Robert S. Merrillees. Oxford: Oxbow, 216–33.

Guimier-Sorbets, Anne-Marie, and Yvette Morizot. 2010. 12 *L'Enfant et La Mort Dans l'Antiquité I.* 1st ed. Editions de Boccard.

Guyon, Django. 2008. "Sépultures et Nécropoles Crétoises Aux Époques Hellénistique et Impériale : Documentation Archéologique, Anthropologie Funéraire et Perspectives Sociologiques." Université Rennes 2.

Hadler, Nortin M., Dennis B. Gillings, Harold R. Imbus, Peter M. Levltln, Diane Makuc Peter, D. Utsinger, William J. Yount, Derwood Slusser, and Nancy Moskovitz. 1978. "Hand Structure and Function in an Industrial Setting Influence of Three Patterns of Stereotyped, Repetitve Usage." *Arthritis and Rheumatism* 21(2).

Haggis, Donald C. 1996. "The Port of Tholos in Eastern Crete and the Role of a Roman Horreum along the Egyptian 'Corn Route.'" *Oxford Journal of Archaeology* 15(2): 183–209.

Halstead, Paul. 2008. "Between a Rock and a Hard Place: Coping with Marginal Colonisation in the Later Neolithic and Early Bronze Age of Crete and the Aegean." In *Escaping the Labyrinth: The Cretan Neolithic in Context,* eds. Valasia Isaakidou and Peter D. Tompkins. Oxford: Oxbow Books.

Harlow, Mary, and Wendy Smith. 2001. "Between Fasting and Feasting: The Literary and Archaeobotanical Evidence for Monastic Diet in Late Antique Egypt." *Antiquity* 75(290): 758–68.

Hassett, Brenna R. 2014. "Missing Defects? A Comparison of Microscopic and Macroscopic Approaches to Identifying Linear Enamel Hypoplasia." *American Journal of Physical Anthropology* 153(3): 463–72.

Hatzfeld, Jean. 1919. *Les Trafiquants Italiens Dans l'Orient Hellénique*. Paris: Bocard.

Hatzi-Vallianou, Despoina. 1989. "Κεντρική Κρήτη." *Αρχαιολογικών Δελτίων* 44 (B2 Χρονικά): 429–46.

———. 1995. "Λαξευτοί Τάφοι Στην Επαρχία Πυργιωτίσσης. Τα Παραδείγματα Φαιστού Και Ματάλων." In *Πεπραγμένα Του Ζ' Διεθνούς Κριτολογικού Συνέδριο A2*, Ρέθυμνο, 1007–34.

Hawkins, R.J., P.A. Main, and D. Locker. 1997. "The Normative Need for Tooth Extractions in Older Adults in Ontario, Canada." *Gerodontology* 14(2): 75–82.

Hayden, Barbara J. 2005. *Reports on the Vrokastro Area, Eastern Crete. Vol. III, The Vrokastro Regional Survey Project Sites and Pottery*. Philadelphia: University Museum Monograph 123.

Hayden, Barbara J., Jennifer A. Moody, and Oliver Rackham. 1992. "The Vrokastro Survey Project, 1986–1989: Research Design and Preliminary Results." *Hesperia: The Journal of the American School of Classical Studies at Athens* 61(3): 293–353.

Hayes, J. W. 1971. "Four Early Roman Groups from Knossos." *The Annual of the British School at Athens* 66.

———. 1983. "The Villa Dionysos Excavations, Knossos: The Pottery." *The Annual of the British School at Athens* 78: 97–169.

———. 2001. "Early Christian Pottery from Knossos: The 1978–1981 Finds from the Knossos Medical Faculty Site." *The Annual of the British School at Athens* 96: 431–54.

Heaton, T. H. E. 1987. "The 15N/14N Ratios of Plants in South Africa and Namibia: Relationship to Climate and Coastal/Saline Environments." *Oecologia* 74(2): 236–46.

Hedges, Robert E.M., John G. Clement, C. David L. Thomas, and Tamsin C. O'Connell. 2007. "Collagen Turnover in the Adult Femoral Mid-Shaft: Modeled from Anthropogenic Radiocarbon Tracer Measurements." *American Journal of Physical Anthropology* 133(2): 808–16.

Hedges, Robert E.M., and Linda M. Reynard. 2007. "Nitrogen Isotopes and the Trophic Level of Humans in Archaeology." *Journal of Archaeological Science* 34(8): 1240–51.

Hekster, O., G. Kleijn, and Daniëlle Slootjes, eds. 2007. *Crises and the Roman Empire. Proceedings of the Seventh Workshop of the International Network Impact of Empire (Nijmegen, June 20–24, 2006)*. Leiden: Brill.

Hellmann, Marie-Christine. 2006. *L'architecture Grecque: Tome 2, Architecture Religieuse et Funéraire*. Paris: A&J Picard.

Henneberg, R.J., and Maciej Henneberg. 2003. "The Diet of the Metapontine Popultion as Reconstructed from the Physical Remains." In *Living of the Chora: Diet and Nutrition at Metaponto*, ed. Joseph C. Carter. Austin: University of Texas at Austin, 29–36.

Henneberg, R.J., F.D. Pate, and M. Henneberg. 1999. "Stable Isotope Analysis of the Diet of the Inhabitants of the Ancient Greek Colony of Metaponto in Italy 7th-2nd c. BCE." *American Journal of Physical Anthropology Supplement* 28: 150.

Hershkovitz, I., L. Bedford, L. M. Jellema, and B. Latimer. 1996. "Injuries to the Skeleton Due to Prolonged Activity in Hand-to-Hand Combat." *International Journal of Osteoarchaeology* 6(2): 167–78.

Hillson, Simon W. 1996. *Dental Anthropology*. Cambridge: Cambridge University Press.

———. 2001. "Recording Dental Caries in Archaeological Human Remains." *International Journal of Osteoarchaeology* 11(4): 249–89.

———. 2005. *Teeth.* (2nd edition). Cambridge: Cambridge University Press.

———. 2008a. "Dental Pathology." In *Biological Anthropology of the Human Skeleton*, eds. Mary Anne Katzenberg and S.R. Saunders. Hoboken, New Jersey: John Wiley & Sons, 301–40.

———. 2008b. "The Current State of Dental Decay." In *Technique and Application in Dental Anthropology*, eds. Joel D. Irish and Greg C. Nelson. Cambridge: Cambridge University Press, 111–35.

———. 2009. "The World's Largest Infant Cemetery and Its Potential for Studying Growth and Development." In *New Directions in the Skeletal Biology of Greece*, eds. L Schepartz, S Fox, and C Bourbou. Princeton: American School of Classical Studies at Athens, 137–54.

Hillson, Simon W., Clark Spencer Larsen, Başak Boz, M. A. Pilloud, J. W. Sadvari, and Sabrina C. Agarwal. 2013. "The Human Remains I: Interpreting Community Structure, Health, and Diet in Neolithic Çatalhöyük." In *Humans and Landscapes of Çatalhöyük: Reports from the 2000–2008 Seasons*, ed. Ian Hodder. Los Angeles: Cotsen Archaeology Institute, 339–96.

Hillson, Simon W. 2014. *Tooth Development in Human Evolution and Bioarchaeology*. Cambridge: Cambridge University Press.

Hitch, Sarah. 2015. "Sacrifice." In *A Companion to Food in the Ancient World*, eds. John Wilkins and Robin Nadeau. Chichester, UK: John Wiley & Sons Ltd, 335–47.

Hobson, B. 2009. *Latrinae et Foricae: Toilets in the Roman World*. London: Duckworth.

Hobson, Keith A., Ray T. Alisauskas, and Robert G. Clark. 1993. "Stable-Nitrogen Isotope Enrichment in Avian Tissues Due to Fasting and Nutritional Stress: Implications for Isotopic Analyses of Diet." *The Condor* 95(2): 388.

Hodge, Harold C., and S. Wah Leung. 1950. "Calculus Formation." *Journal of Periodontology* 21(4): 211–21.

Hoefs, Jochen. 2009. *Stable Isotope Geochemistry*. 6th ed. Berlin: Springer.

Hogarth, D. G. 1900. "Knossos. Summary Report of the Excavations in 1900: II. Early Town and Cemeteries." *The Annual of the British School at Athens* 6: 70–85.

Homann-Wedeking, Betty. 1950. "A Kiln Site at Knossos." *The Annual of the British School at Athens* 45: 165–92.

Hood, M. Sinclair F. 1957. "Archaeology in Greece, 1957." *Archaeological Reports* 4: 3–25.

———. 1958. "Archaeology in Greece, 1958." *Archaeological Reports* 5: 3–24.

———. 1962. "Archaeology in Greece, 1961–62." *Archaeological Reports* 8: 3–31.

Hood, M. Sinclair F., and John Boardman. 1957. "A Hellenic Fortification Tower on the Kefala Ridge at Knossos." *The Annual of the British School at Athens* 52: 224–30.

Hood, M. Sinclair F., and David Smyth. 1981. British School at Athens Supplementary Volume 14 *Archaeological Survey of the Knossos Area*. London: British School at Athens.

Hoppa, Robert D., and T.N. Garlie. 1998. "Secular Changes in the Growth of Toronto Children during the Last Century." *Annals of Human Biology* 25(6): 553–61.

Hoppa, Robert D. 2002. "Paleodemography: Looking Back and Thinking Ahead." In *Paleodemography*, eds. Robert D. Hoppa and James W. Vaupel. Cambridge: Cambridge University Press, 9–28.

Hoppa, Robert D., and James W. Vaupel. 2002. *Paleodemography: Age Distributions from Skeletal Samples*. Cambridge: Cambridge University Press.

Houby-Nielsen, Sanne. 2000. "Child Burials in Ancient Athens." In *Children and Material Culture*, ed. Joanna R. Sofaer Derevenski. London: Routledge, 151–66.

Hunt, David R., and John Albanese. 2005. "History and Demographic Composition of the Robert J. Terry Anatomical Collection." *American Journal of Physical Anthropology* 127(4): 406–17.

Huskinson, Janet. 2000. *Experiencing Rome: Culture, Identity and Power in the Roman Empire*. Routledge in association with Open University Press.

Hutchinson, R.W. 1936. "Knossos Correspondence 1930–39 (Handwritten Reports)." BSA Archive.

Hutchinson, R. W., and John Boardman. 1954. "The Khaniale Tekke Tombs." *The Annual of the British School at Athens* 49: 215–28.

Ibrahim, Mahrous A., Azza H. Elelemi, Mostafa S. Ibrahim, and Altaf H. Bandy. 2017. "Adult Stature Estimation from Radiographically Determined Metatarsal Length in Egyptian Population." *Journal of Forensic Radiology and Imaging* 11: 28–32.

Ioannidou-Karetsou, Alexandra. 1974. "Νομός Ηρακλείου. Γόρτυς." *Αρχαιολογικών Δελτίων* 29 (Χρονικά Β3): 889–96.

Isaakidou, Valasia. 2004. "Bones from the Labyrinth: Faunal Evidence for Management and Consumption of Animals at Neolithic and Bronze Age Knossos, Crete." Unpublished PhD Thesis Institute of Archaeology University College London.

Issakidou, Valasia, Paul Halstead, Elizabeth Stroud, Anaya Sarpaki, Eleni Hatzaki, Erika K. Nitsch, and Amy Bogaard. 2022. "Changing Land Use and Political Economy at Neolithic and Bronze Age Knossos, Crete: Stable Carbon (Δ13C) and Nitrogen (Δ15N) Isotope Analysis of Charred Crop Grains and Faunal Bone Collagen." *Proceedings of the Prehistoric Society* 88: 155–91.

Ivison, Eric A. 1996. "Burial and Urbanism at Late Antique and Early Byzantine Corinth (c. AD 400–700)." In *Towns in Transition. Urban Evolution in Late Antiquity and the Early Middle Ages*, eds. Neil J. Christie and Simon T. Loseby. Aldershot: Scolar Press, 99–125.

Jackes, Mary. 2011. "Representativeness and Bias in Archaeological Skeletal Samples." In *Social Bioarchaeology*, Oxford, UK: Wiley-Blackwell, 107–46.

Jansen, G. C. M., Ann Olga Koloski-Ostrow, and E. M. Moorman, eds. 2011. *Roman Toilets: Their Archaeology and Cultural History*. Leuven: Peeters Press.

Jeffery, L. H. 1949. "Comments on Some Archaic Greek Inscriptions." *The Journal of Hellenic Studies* 69: 25–38.

Jochum, K.P., and J. Enzweiler. 2014. "Reference Materials in Geochemical and Environmental Research." *Treatise on Geochemistry*: 43–70.

Jones, Glynis. 1984. "Appendix 1: The LM II Plant Remains." In *The Minoan Unexplored Mansion at*

Knossos, eds. Mervin R Popham *et al.* Oxford: The British School at Athens. Supplementary Volumes, No. 17, 303–6.

de Jong, Lidewijde. 2017. *The Archaeology of Death in Roman Syria: Burial, Commemoration, and Empire.* Cambridge: Cambridge University Press.

Jongman, Willem M. 2007a. "Gibbon Was Right: The Decline and Fall of the Roman Economy." In *Crises and the Roman Empire. Proceedings of the Seventh Workshop of the International Network Impact of Empire (Nijmegen, June 20–24, 2006)*, eds. O. Hekster, G. Kleijn, and Daniëlle Slootjes. Leiden: Brill, 183–99.

———. 2007b. "The Early Roman Empire: Consumption." In *The Cambridge Economic History of the Greco-Roman World*, eds. Walter Scheidel, Ian Morris, and Richard P. Saller. Cambridge: Cambridge University Press, 592–618.

Jongman, Willem M., Jan P.A.M. Jacobs, and Geertje M. Klein Goldewijk. 2019. "Health and Wealth in the Roman Empire." *Economics & Human Biology* 34: 138–50.

Jurmain, Robert. 1977. "Stress and the Etiology of Osteoarthritis." *American Journal of Physical Anthropology* 46(2): 353–65.

———. 1980. "The Pattern of Involvement of Appendicular Degenerative Joint Disease." *American Journal of Physical Anthropology* 53(1): 143–50.

Jurmain, Robert, Francisca Alves Cardoso, Charlotte Henderson, and Sébastien Villotte. 2012. "Bioarchaeology's Holy Grail: The Reconstruction of Activity." In *A Companion to Paleopathology*, Oxford, UK: Wiley-Blackwell, 531–52.

Kamp, Kathryn A. 2001. "Where Have All the Children Gone?: The Archaeology of Childhood." *Journal of Archaeological Method and Theory* 8: 1–34.

Kanta, Athanasia, and Ioanna Serpetsidaki. 2015. "Το Έργο Της ΚΓ′ Εφορείας Προϊστορικών Και Κλασικών Αρχαιοτήτων Κατά Τα Έτη 2011–2013." In *Αρχαιολογικό Έργο Στην Κρήτη 3: Proceedings of the 3rd Meeting Rethymnon, 5–8 December 2013*, 53–70.

Karageorghis, Vassos. 1985. *Ετήσια Έκθεση Του Τμήματος Αρχαιοτήτων Για Το Έτος 1985.*

Karetsou, Alexandra. 1974. "Κρήτη. Περισυλλογή Αρχαίων Και Ελάσσονες Αβασκαφές." *Το Έργων τνς Αρχαιολογικής Εταιρείας*: 117.

———. 1976. "Αρχαιότητες Και Μνημεία Κεντρικής Κρήτης. Ανασκαφές Εργασίες." *Αρχαιολογικόν Δελτίον* 31 (Χρονικά Β'2): 354–60.

———. 1978. "Εφορεία Προϊστορικών Και Κλασικών Αρχαιοτήτων Ηρακλείου." *Αρχαιολογικόν Δελτίον* 33 (Χρονικά Β'2): 352–59.

Karligkioti, Anna, Kerasia Douni, Maria Mexi, Panagiota Michailidi, and Efthymia Nikita. 2023. "Approaching Life (in)Equality and Social Transformations in Eastern Attica from the Classical to the Roman Era." *Journal of Archaeological Science: Reports* 47: 103819.

Karsten, Jordan K., Sarah E. Heins, Gwyn D. Madden, and Mykhailo P. Sokhatskyi. 2015. "Dental Health and the Transition to Agriculture in Prehistoric Ukraine: A Study of Dental Caries." *European Journal of Archaeology* 18(4): 562–79.

Katzenberg, Mary Anne. 2008. "Stable Isotope Analysis: A Tool for Studying Past Diet, Demography, and Life History." In *Biological Anthropology of the Human Skeleton*, eds. Mary Anne Katzenberg and Shelley R Saunders. Hoboken, New Jersey: John Wiley & Sons, 413–42.

Keenleyside, Anne, Henry Schwarcz, and Kristina Panayotova. 2006. "Stable Isotopic Evidence of Diet in a Greek Colonial Population from the Black Sea." *Journal of Archaeological Science* 33(9): 1205–15.

Keenleyside, Anne, Henry Schwarcz, Lea Stirling, and Nejib Ben Lazreg. 2009. "Stable Isotopic Evidence for Diet in a Roman and Late Roman Population from Leptiminus, Tunisia." *Journal of Archaeological Science* 36(1): 51–63.

Kelly, Amanda. 2013. "Roman Bathhouses on Crete as Indicators of Cultural Transition: The Dynamics of Roman Influence." *Bulletin of the Institute of Classical Studies. Supplement* (120): 131–67.

Kemkes-Grottenthaler, A., F. Löbig, and F. Stock. 2002. "Mandibular Ramus Flexure and Gonial Eversion as Morphologic Indicators of Sex." *HOMO - Journal of Comparative Human Biology* 53(2): 97–111.

Kennedy, Larkin Frost. 2016. "The Busy Cemeteries of Late Antique Corinth: Geographic Identification of Migrants vs Locals, and the Characterization of a 6th-8th Century City." Unpublished PhD thesis: Texas A&M University.

Kent, John Harvey. 1966. *Corinth XIII.3 The Inscriptions, 1926–1950.* Princeton.

Kieser, J.A., C.B. Preston, and W.G. Evans. 1983. "Skeletal Age at Death: An Evaluation of the Miles Method of Ageing." *Journal of Archaeological Science* 10(1): 9–12.

Killgrove, Kristina, and Robert H. Tykot. 2013. "Food for Rome: A Stable Isotope Investigation of Diet in the Imperial Period (1st–3rd Centuries AD)." *Journal of Anthropological Archaeology* 32(1): 28–38.

———. 2018. "Diet and Collapse: A Stable Isotope Study of Imperial-Era Gabii (1st–3rd Centuries AD)." *Journal of Archaeological Science: Reports* 19: 1041–49.

King, Anthony C. 1999. "Diet in the Roman World: A Regional Inter-Site Comparison of the Mammal Bones." *Journal of Roman Archaeology* 12: 168–202.

———. 2001. "The Romanization of Diet in the Western Empire: Comparative Archaeozoological Studies." In

Italy and the West, Comparative Issues in Romanization, eds. S. Keay and N. Terrenato. Oxford: Oxbow Books, 210–23.

Kirkpatrick Smith, Susan. 2013. "Bodies of Evidence: Skeletal Analysis in Roman Greece and Cyprus." In *A Companion to the Archaeology of the Roman Republic*, Chichester: Blackwell Publishing, 141–54.

Klaus, Haagen D., Clark Spencer Larsen, and Manuel E. Tam. 2009. "Economic Intensification and Degenerative Joint Disease: Life and Labor on the Postcontact North Coast of Peru." *American Journal of Physical Anthropology* 139(2): 204–21.

van Klinken, G.J. 1999. "Bone Collagen Quality Indicators for Palaeodietary and Radiocarbon Measurements." *Journal of Archaeological Science* 26(6): 687–95.

Knüsel, Christopher J., and Alan K. Outram. 2004. "Fragmentation: The Zonation Method Applied to Fragmented Human Remains from Archaeological and Forensic Contexts." *Environmental Archaeology* 9: 85–97.

Kolhe, Ravindra, Monte Hunter, Siyang Liu, Ravirajsinh N. Jadeja, Chetan Pundkar, Ashis K. Mondal, Bharati Mendhe, Michelle Drewry, Mumtaz V. Rojiani, Yutao Liu, Carlos M. Isales, Robert E. Guldberg, Mark W. Hamrick, and Sadanand Fulzele. 2017. "Gender-Specific Differential Expression of Exosomal MiRNA in Synovial Fluid of Patients with Osteoarthritis." *Scientific Reports* 7(1): 2029.

Koloski-Ostrow, Ann Olga. 2015. *The Archaeology of Sanitation in Roman Italy*. University of North Carolina Press.

Konrad, Michaela. 2007. "Gräber Und Bestattungssitten in Den Römischen Provinzen Syria, Osrhoene Und Mesopotamia: Einheimische Und Fremde Zwischen Orientalischem Und Römischem Grabbrauch." In *Körpergräber Des 1.–3. Jahrhunderts in Der Römischen Welt. Internationales Kolloquium Frankfurt Am Main, 19.–20. November 2004*, eds. Andrea Faber, Peter Fasold, Manuela Struck, and Marion Witteyer. Frankfurt am Main: Schriften des Archäologischen Museums Frankfurt 21, 77–97.

Korhonen, Kalle. 2011. "Language and Identity in the Roman Colonies of Sicily." In *Roman Colonies in the First Century of Their Foundation*, Oxbow Books, 7–31.

Kotsonas, Antonis. 2016. "Greek and and Roman Knossos: The Pioneering Investigations of Minos Kalokairinos." *The Annual of the British School at Athens* 111: 299–324.

———. 2018. "Homer, The Archaeology of Crete and the 'Tomb of Meriones' at Knossos." *The Journal of Hellenic Studies* 138: 1–35.

Kron, Geoffrey. 2005. "Anthropometry, Physical Anthropology, and the Reconstruction of Ancient Health, Nutrition, and Living Standards." *Historia: Zeitschrift für Alte Geschichte* 54(1): 68–83.

———. 2012. "Nutrition, Hygiene, and Mortality. Setting Parameters for Roman Health and Life Expectancy Consistent with Our Comparative Evidence." In *L'impatto Della "peste Antonina*, ed. E. Lo Cascio. Bari: Edipuglia, 193–252.

———. 2018. "Comparative Perspectives on Nutrition and Social Inequality in the Roman World." In *The Routledge Handbook of Diet and Nutrition in the Roman World*, eds. Paul Erdkamp and Claire Holleran. London: Routledge, 272.

Kwok, Cynthia S. 2015. "Moving Beyond Childhood: Reconstructing Dietary Life Histories of Bronze Age and Byzantine Greeks Using Stable Isotope Analysis of Dental and Skeletal Remains." Unpublished PhD thesis, University of Calgary.

Kwok, Cynthia S., and Anne Keenleyside. 2015. "Baby Bones, Food, and Health : Stable Isotope Evidence for Infant Feeding Practices in the Greek Colony of Apollonia Pontica (5th-3rd Centuries B.C.)." In *Archaeodiet in the Greek World: Dietary Reconstruction from Stable Isotope Analysis*, eds. Anastasia Papathanasiou, Michael P. Richards, and Sherry C. Fox. Princeton: American School of Classical Studies at Athens, 147–70.

Kyle McIllvaine, Britney. 2012. "Greek Colonization of the Balkans: Bioarchaeological Reconstruction of Behavior and Lifestyle during Corinthian Colonial Expansion into Ancient Apollonia, Albania." Unpublished PhD thesis: Ohio State University.

Kyle McIllvaine, Britney, Lynne A. Schepartz, and Clark Spencer Larsen. 2016. "Mother City and Colony: Bioarchaeological Evidence of Stress and Impacts of Corinthian Colonisation at Apollonia, Albania." *International Journal of Osteoarchaeology* 26(6): 1067–77.

Lagia, Anna. 2007. "Notions of Childhood in the Classical Polis: Evidence from the Bioarchaeological Record." *Hesperia Supplements* 41: 293–306.

———. 2014. "Health Inequalities in the Classical City. A Biocultural Approach to Socioeconomic Differentials in the Polis of Athens during the Classical, Hellenistic and Imperial Roman Periods." In *Corps, Travail et Statut Social: L'apport de La Paléoanthropologie Funéraire Aux Sciences Historiques*, ed. Anne-Catherine Gilles. Villeneuve d'Ascq: Presses universitaires du Septentrion, 95–115.

———. 2015. "Diet and the Polis: An Isotopic Study of Diet in Athens and Laurion during the Classical, Hellenistic, and Imperial Roman Periods." In *Archaeodiet in the Greek World: Dietary Reconstruction from Stable Isotope Analysis*, eds. Anastasia Papathanasiou, Michael P. Richards, and Sherry C. Fox. Princeton: American School of Classical Studies at Athens, 119–46.

Lagia, Anna, Anastasia Papathanasiou, and Sevi Triantaphyllou. 2014. "The State of Approaches to Archaeological Human Remains." In *Archaeological Human Remains: Global Perspectives*, eds. Barra O'Donnabhain and María Cecilia Lozada. Heidelberg: Springer, 105–26.

LaMotta, Vince M., and Michael B. Schiffer. 2005. "Archaeological Formation Processes." In *Archaeology: The Key Concepts*, eds. Colin Renfrew and Paul Bahn. London: Routledge, 121–27.

Landvatter, Thomas Peter. 2013. "Identity, Burial Practice, and Social Change in Ptolemaic Egypt." University of Michigan.

Lanfranco, Luis Pezo, and Sabine Eggers. 2010. "The Usefulness of Caries Frequency, Depth, and Location in Determining Cariogenicity and Past Subsistence: A Test on Early and Later Agriculturalists From the Peruvian Coast." *American Journal of Physical Anthropology* 143(1): 75–91.

Langdon, Susan. 2007. "The Awkward Age: Art and Maturation in Early Greece." *Hesperia Supplements* 41: 173–91.

Larsen, Clark Spencer, J. Craig, L. E. Sering, Margaret J. Schoeninger, K. F. Russell, D.L. Hutchinson, and M. A. Williamson. 1995. "Cross Homestead: Life and Death on the Midwestern Frontier." In *Bodies of Evidence: Reconstructing History through Skeletal Analysis*, ed. Anne L. Grauer. New York: Wiley–Liss, 139–159.

Larsen, Clark Spencer. 2015. *Bioarchaeology: Interpreting Behavior from the Human Skeleton.* 2nd ed. Cambridge: Cambridge University Press.

———. 2018. "Bioarchaeology in Perspective: From Classifications of the Dead to Conditions of the Living." *American Journal of Physical Anthropology* 165(4): 865–78.

Larsen, Clark Spencer, and Dale L. Hutchinson. 1999. "Osteopathology of Carson Desert Foragers: Reconstructing Prehistoric Lifeways in the Western Great Basin." In *Prehistoric Lifeways in the Great Basin Wetlands: Bioarchaeological Reconstruction and Interpretation*, eds. Brian E. Hemphill and Clark Spencer Larsen. Salt Lake City: University of Utah Press.

Ledger, Marissa L., Friederike Stock, Helmut Schwaiger, Maria Knipping, Helmut Brückner, Sabine Ladstätter, and Piers D. Mitchell. 2018. "Intestinal Parasites from Public and Private Latrines and the Harbour Canal in Roman Period Ephesus, Turkey (1st c. BCE to 6th c. CE)." *Journal of Archaeological Science: Reports* 21: 289–97.

Lee-Thorp, Julia A., Judith C. Sealy, and Nikolaas J. van der Merwe. 1989. "Stable Carbon Isotope Ratio Differences between Bone Collagen and Bone Apatite, and Their Relationship to Diet." *Journal of Archaeological Science* 16(6): 585–99.

Leigh, R. Wood. 1935. "Notes on the Somatology and Pathology of Ancient Egypt." *The Journal of the American Dental Association (1922)* 22(2): 199–222.

Lembessi, Angeliki. 1975a. "Αρχαιότητες Και Μνημεία Δυτικής Κρήτης, Ανασκαφές." *Αρχαιολογικόν Δελτίον* 30 (Χρονικά Β'2): 341–42.

———. 1975b. "Ελάσσονος Κλιμάκος Ανασκαφαί Εις Κεντρική Κρήτη." *Πρακτικά της εν Αθήναις Αρχαιολογικής Εταιρείας*: 518–20.

———. 1975c. "Κρήτη. Περισυλλογή Αρχαίων Και Ελ Ασσονές Ανασκαφές." *Το Έργων τηνς Αρχαιολογικής Εταιρείας*: 199–202.

———. 1977. "Αρχαιότητες Και Μνημεία Κεντρικής Κρήτης." *Αρχαιολογικόν Δελτίον* 32 (Χρονικά Β'2): 314–19.

Lengsfeld, M., A. Frank, D.L. van Deursen, and P. Griss. 2000. "Lumbar Spine Curvature during Office Chair Sitting." *Medical Engineering & Physics* 22(9): 665–69.

Lewis, Jesica Jayd Harrison. 2015. "The Warrior's Banquet: Syssitia in Ancient Crete." Unpublished MA thesis, North Carolina State University.

Lieverse, A R. 1999. "Diet and the Aetiology of Dental Calculus." *International Journal of Osteoarchaeology* 9(4): 219–32.

Lightfoot, Christopher. 2017. "Christian Burials in a Pagan Context at Amorium." In *Life and Death in Asia Minor in Hellenistic, Roman and Byzantine Times: Studies in Archaeology and Bioarchaeology*, eds. J. Rasmus Brandt, Erika Hagelberg, Gro Bjørnstad, and Sven Ahrens. Oxford: Oxbow, 188–95.

Lightfoot, Emma, B. Boneva, P.T. Miracle, Mario Šlaus, and Tamsin C. O'Connell. 2011. "Exploring the Mesolithic and Neolithic Transition in Croatia through Isotopic Investigations." *Antiquity* 85(327): 73–86.

Lightfoot, Emma, Mario Šlaus, and Tamsin C. O'Connell. 2012. "Changing Cultures, Changing Cuisines: Cultural Transitions and Dietary Change in Iron Age, Roman, and Early Medieval Croatia." *American Journal of Physical Anthropology* 148(4): 543–56.

Lilimbaki-Akamati, Maria, and Nikolaos Akamatis. 2014. *Ανατολικό Νεκροταφείο Πέλλας Ανασκαφικές Περίοδοι 1991–2007*. Thessaloniki: Ministry of Culture and Sport.

Lillie, Malcolm C. 1996. "Mesolithic and Neolithic Populations of Ukraine: Indications of Diet from Dental Pathology." *Current Anthropology* 37(1): 135–42.

Lillie, Malcolm C., and Michael P. Richards. 2000. "Stable Isotope Analysis and Dental Evidence of Diet at the Mesolithic–Neolithic Transition in Ukraine." *Journal of Archaeological Science* 27(10): 965–72.

Limberis, Vasiliki. 2005. "Ecclesiastical Ambiguities: Corinth in the Fourth and Fifth Centuries." In

Urban Religion in Roman Corinth: Interdisciplinary Approaches, eds. Daniel N. Schowalter and Steven J. Friesen. Cambridge, MA: Harvard Theological Studies, Harvard Divinity School, 443–57.

Lippolis, Enzo. 2016. "Roman Gortyn: From Greek Polis to Provincial Capital." In *Roman Crete. New Perspectives*, eds. Jane E. Frances and Anna Kouremenos. Oxford: Oxbow, 155–74.

Lippolis, Enzo, Rita Sassu, Chiara Giatti, and Luigi Maria Caliò. 2015. "Gortys. Archaeological Excavations of New Mausoleums in the Praetorium Area." In *Αρχαιολογικο Εργο Κρητης 3, Πρακτικά Της 3ης Συνάντησης Ρέθυμνο, 5–8 Δεκεμβρίου 2013*, 537–52.

Liston, Maria A., Susan I. Rotroff, and Lynn M. Snyder. 2018. *The Agora Bone Well*. Hesperia S. Princeton: American School of Classical Studies at Athens.

Liston, Maria A, and Susan I Rotroff. 2012. *Babies in the Well: Archeological Evidence for Newborn Disposal in Hellenistic Greece*. eds. Judith Evans Grubbs and Tim Parkin. Oxford: Oxford University Press.

Livarda, Alexandra. 2012. "The Archaeobotanical Evidence of the Late Bronze Agre and Protogeometric Occupation under the Villa Dionysus, Knossos, Crete, and an Overview of the Protogeometric Data of Greece." *The Annual of the British School at Athens* 107: 189–209.

———. 2014. "Archaeobotany in Greece." *Archaeological Reports* 60: 106–16.

Livarda, Alexandra, and Georgia Kotzamani. 2013. "The Archaeobotany of Neolithic and Bronze Age Crete: Synthesis and Prospects." *The Annual of the British School at Athens* 108: 1–29.

Long, Austin. 1995. "From the Editor: Good-Bye to Pee Dee Belemnite and Standard Mean Ocean Water." *Radiocarbon* 37(1): iii.

López-Costas, Olalla, and Gundula Müldner. 2016. "Fringes of the Empire: Diet and Cultural Change at the Roman to Post-Roman Transition in NW Iberia." *American Journal of Physical Anthropology* 161(1): 141–54.

Lösch, Sandra, Negahnaz Moghaddam, Karl Grossschmidt, Daniele U. Risser, and Fabian Kanz. 2014. "Stable Isotope and Trace Element Studies on Gladiators and Contemporary Romans from Ephesus (Turkey, 2nd and 3rd Ct. AD) - Implications for Differences in Diet." *PLoS ONE*.

Loth, Susan R., and Maciej Henneberg. 1996. "Mandibular Ramus Flexure: A New Morphologic Indicator of Sexual Dimorphism in the Human Skeleton." *American Journal of Physical Anthropology* 99(3): 473–85.

Lovejoy, C. Owen. 1985. "Dental Wear in the Libben Population: Its Functional Pattern and Role in the Determination of Adult Skeletal Age at Death." *American Journal of Physical Anthropology* 68(1): 47–56.

Lovejoy, C. Owen, Richard S. Meindl, Robert P. Mensforth, and Thomas J. Barton. 1985. "Multifactorial Determination of Skeletal Age at Death: A Method and Blind Tests of Its Accuracy." *American Journal of Physical Anthropology* 68(1): 1–14.

Lovejoy, C. Owen, Richard S. Meindl, Thomas R. Pryzbeck, and Robert P. Mensforth. 1985. "Chronological Metamorphosis of the Auricular Surface of the Ilium: A New Method for the Determination of Adult Skeletal Age at Death." *American Journal of Physical Anthropology* 68(1): 15–28.

Lubell, David, Mary Jackes, Henry Schwarcz, Martin Knyf, and Christopher Meiklejohn. 1994. "The Mesolithic-Neolithic Transition in Portugal: Isotopic and Dental Evidence of Diet." *Journal of Archaeological Science* 21(2): 201–16.

Luff, Rosemary M. 2007. "Monastic Diet in Late Antique Egypt: Zooarchaeological Finds from Kom El-Nana and Tell El-Amarna, Middle Egypt." *Environmental Archaeology* 12(2): 161–74.

Lukacs, John R. 1996. "Sex Differences in Dental Caries Rates With the Origin of Agriculture in South Asia." *Current Anthropology* 37(1): 147–53.

———. 2007. "Dental Trauma and Antemortem Tooth Loss in Prehistoric Canary Islanders: Prevalence and Contributing Factors." *International Journal of Osteoarchaeology* 17(2): 157–73.

———. 2011. "Sex Differences in Dental Caries Experience: Clinical Evidence, Complex Etiology." *Clinical Oral Investigations* 15(5): 649–56.

Luttmann, Alwin, Matthias Jäger, Barbara Griefahn, G. Caffier, F. Liebers, and U. Steinberg. 2003. *Protecting Workers' Health Series No. 5: Preventing Musculoskeletal Disorders in the Workplace*. World Health Organisation (WHO).

Mandel, Irwin D. 1974. "Biochemical Aspects of Calculus Formation." *Journal of Periodontal Research* 9.

———. 1990. "Calculus Formation and Prevention: An Overview." *Compendium for Continuing Education in Dentistry, Supplemental* 8: 235–41.

Mandel, Irwin D., and Robert H. Thompson. 1967. "The Chemistry of Parotid and Submaxillary Saliva in Heavy Calculus Formers and Non-Formers." *Journal of Periodontology* 38(4): 310–15.

Manolis, Sotiris K., Constantine Eliopoulos, Christos G. Koilias, and Sherry C. Fox. 2009. "Sex Determination Using Metacarpal Biometric Data from the Athens Collection." *Forensic Science International* 193(1–3): 130.e1-130.e6.

Manzi, Giorgio, Loretana Salvadei, Alessandro Vienna, and Pietro Passarello. 1999. "Discontinuity of Life Conditions at the Transition from the Roman Imperial Age to the Early Middle Ages: Example from Central Italy Evaluated by Pathological Dento-Alveolar

Lesions." *American Journal of Human Biology* 11(3): 327–41.

Marangou-Lerat, Antigone. 1995. *Le Vin et Les Amphores de Crète: De l'époque Classique à l'époque Impériale*. Paris: Etudes crétoises 30.

Marangou, Antigone. 1999. "Wine in the Cretan Economy." In *From Minoan Farmers to Roman Traders: Sidelights on the Economy of Ancient Crete*, ed. Angelos Chaniotis. Stuttgart: Franz Steiner Verlag, 269–78.

Marean, Curtis W., Yoshiko Abe, Peter J. Nilssen, and Elizabeth C. Stone. 2001. "Estimating the Minimum Number of Skeletal Elements (MNE) in Zooarchaeology: A Review and a New Image-Analysis GIS Approach." *American Antiquity* 66(2): 333–48.

Margaritis, Evi. 2015a. "Agricultural Production and Domestic Activities in Rural Hellenistic Greece." In *The Ancient Greek Economy*, eds. Edward M. Harris, David M. Lewis, and Mark Woolmer. Cambridge: Cambridge University Press, 187–204.

———. 2015b. "Cultivating Classical Archaeology: Agricultural Activities, Use of Space and Occupation Patterns in Hellenistic Greece." In *Classical Archaeology in Context: Theory and Practice in Excavation in the Greek World*, Berlin; Boston: Walter de Gruyter, 333–56.

Margerison, Beverley J., and Christopher J. Knüsel. 2002. "Paleodemographic Comparison of a Catastrophic and an Attritional Death Assemblage." *American Journal of Physical Anthropology* 119(2): 134–43.

Margolis, H.C. 1990. "An Assessment of Recent Advances in the Study of the Chemistry and Biochemistry of Dental Plaque Fluid." *Journal of Dental Research* 69(6): 1337–42.

Markoulaki, Stavroula. 1996. "Λισος." *Κρητική Εστία* 5(1994–1996): 238–41.

———. 2009. "Ανασκαφή 'Πάρκο Ειρήνης Και Φιλίας' (Οδός Α Παπανδρέου) / 'Peace and Friendship of People Park' Excavation (A. Papandreou St.)." In *Χανιά (Κυδώνια) Περιήγηση Σε Χώρους Αρχαίας Μνήμης / Khania (Kydonia) A Tour to Sites of Ancient Memory*, ed. Μαρία Ανδρεαδάκη-Βλαζάκη. Chania: Ministry of Culture and Tourism - 25th Ephorate of Prehistoric and Classical Antiquities, 108–13.

Markoulaki, Stavroula, and Vanna Niniou-Kindeli. 1982. "Ελληνιστικός Λαξευτός Τάφος Χανίων, Ανασκαφή Οικοπέδου Μαθιουλάκη." *Αρχαιολογικών Δελτίων* 37 (Μελέτες Α): 8–119.

———. 2009. "Ανασκαφή 'Εμμ. Μαθιουλάκη' (Οδός Γ. Χατζηδάκη 31) / 'Mathioulaki Emm.' Excavation (31, G. Khatzidaki St.)." In *Χανιά (Κυδώνια) Περιήγηση Σε Χώρους Αρχαίας Μνήμης / Khania (Kydonia) A Tour to Sites of Ancient Memory*, ed. Maria Andreadaki-Vlazaki. Chania: Ministry of Culture and Tourism - 25th Ephorate of Prehistoric and Classical Antiquities, 128–35.

Marshall, I. Howard., and Philip Towner. 1999. *The Pastoral Epistles*. London: T & T Clark.

Masotti, S., N. Onisto, M. Marzi, and E. Gualdi-Russo. 2013. "Dento-Alveolar Features and Diet in an Etruscan Population (6th–3rd c. B.C.) from Northeast Italy." *Archives of Oral Biology* 58(4): 416–26.

Mays, S. 2016. "Estimation of Stature in Archaeological Human Skeletal Remains from Britain." *American Journal of Physical Anthropology* 161(4): 646–55.

McConnan Borstad, Courtney, Sandra Garvie-Lok, and Dora Katsonopoulou. 2018. "Diet at Ancient Helike, Achaea, Greece Based on Stable Isotope Analysis: From the Hellenistic to the Roman and Byzantine Periods." *Journal of Archaeological Science: Reports* 18: 1–10.

McCormick, M. 2001. *Origins of the European Economy. Communications and Commerce. A.D. 300–900.* Cambridge: Cambridge University Press.

McEvoy, Brian P., and Peter M. Visscher. 2009. "Genetics of Human Height." *Economics & Human Biology* 7(3): 294–306.

McKern, Thomas, and T.D. Stewart. 1957. *Skeletal Changes in Young American Males: Analysed from the Standpoint of Age Identification*. Natick, Massachusetts: Quartermaster Research and Development Center.

Meadows, L., and R. L. Jantz. 1992. "Estimation of Stature from Metacarpal Lengths." *Journal of Forensic Sciences* 37(1): 147–54.

Megaw, A. H. S. 1936. "Archaeology in Greece, 1935–1936." *The Journal of Hellenic Studies* 56: 135–58.

———. 1967. "Archaeology in Greece, 1966–67." *Archaeological Reports* 13: 3–24.

———. 1984. "A Cemetery Church with Trefoil Sanctuary in Crete." In *Actes Du Xe Congrès International d'Archéologie Chrétienne (II) Thessaloniki 28th September – 4th October 1980*, Thessaloniki, 321–29.

Meindl, Richard S., and C. Owen Lovejoy. 1985. "Ectocranial Suture Closure: A Revised Method for the Determination of Skeletal Age at Death Based on the Lateral-Anterior Sutures." *American Journal of Physical Anthropology* 68(1): 57–66.

Meindl, Richard S., C. Owen Lovejoy, Robert P. Mensforth, and Lydia Don Carlos. 1985. "Accuracy and Direction of Error in the Sexing of the Skeleton: Implications for Paleodemography." *American Journal of Physical Anthropology* 68(1): 79–85.

Merbs, C. F. 1983. *Patterns of Activity-Induced Pathology in a Canadian Inuit Population*. Ottawa: National Museums of Canada.

van der Merwe, Nikolaas J. 1982. "Carbon Isotopes, Photosynthesis, and Archaeology: Different Pathways of Photosynthesis Cause Characteristic Changes in Carbon Isotope Ratios That Make Possible the Study of Prehistoric Human Diets." *American Scientist* 70(6): 596–606.

van der Merwe, Nikolaas J., and J.C. Vogel. 1978. "13C Content of Human Collagen as a Measure of Prehistoric Diet in Woodland North America." *Nature* 276(5690): 815–16.

Michael, Dimitra, and Sotiris K. Manolis. 2014. "Using Dental Caries as a Nutritional Indicator, in Order to Explore Potential Dietary Differences between Sexes in an Ancient Greek Population." *Mediterranean Archaeology and Archaeometry* 14(2): 237–48.

Michalaki-Kollia, Maria, Anne-Marie Guimier-Sorbets, and Yvette Morizot. 2010. "Un Ensemble Exceptionnel d'enchytrismes de Nouveau-Nés, de Foetus et de Nourrissons Découvert Dans l'île d'Astypalée, En Grèce:" In *L'Enfant et La Mort Dans l'Antiquité I*, Nouvelles recherches dans les nécropoles grecques. Le signalement des tombes d'enfants, Editions de Boccard, 161–206.

Miles, A.E.W. 1963. "Dentition in the Estimation of Age." *Journal of Dental Research* 42(1): 255–63.

Millis, Benjamin W. 2010. "The Social And Ethnic Origins Of The Colonists In Early Roman Corinth." In *Corinth in Context: Comparative Studies on Religion and Society*, eds. Steve Friesen, Dan Schowalter, and James Walters. Leiden: Brill, 13–36.

Milner, George R., and Jesper L. Boldsen. 2012. "Estimating Age and Sex from the Skeleton, a Paleopathological Perspective." In *A Companion to Paleopathology*, Oxford, UK: Wiley-Blackwell, 268–84.

Ministry of Culture (ΥΠΠΟ). 1997. *Το Έργο Του Υπουργείου Πολιτισμού Στον Τομέα Της Πολιτιστικής Κληρονομιάς*.

Mitchell, Piers D. 2017. "Human Parasites in the Roman World: Health Consequences of Conquering an Empire." *Parasitology* 144(01): 48–58.

Moles, Anna C. 2012. "A Stable Isotope Analysis Study for Dietary Reconstruction at the Multi-Period Site of Mesembria on the Black Sea." Unpublished MSc thesis, University of Edinburgh.

———. 2023. "Dental Disease Reflects Differential Diets and Changes in Consumption over Time at Knossos." *International Journal of Osteoarchaeology*: 1–14.

———. Forthcoming. "The Spread of New Burial Practices in Early Roman Crete." In *The Networks of Roman Crete*, ed. Nadia Coutsinas. Turnhout: Brepols.

Moles, Anna C., Hazel Reade, Anne Lise Jourdan, and Rhiannon E. Stevens. 2022. "Stable Isotopes Reveal Dietary Shifts Associated with Social Change in Hellenistic, Roman and Late Antique Knossos." *Journal of Archaeological Science: Reports* 45: 103609.

Moody, Jennifer. 2016. "The Roman Climate: Was It Really Different?" In *Roman Crete: New Perspectives*, eds. Jane E. Francis and Anna Kouremenos. Oxford: Oxbow.

Moretti, Jean-Charles. 2006. "L'architecture Funéraire En Grèce Continentale Sous Le Haut-Empire." In *L'architecture Funéraire Monumentale: La Gaule Dans l'Empire Romain. Actes Du Colloque de Lattes, 11–13 Octobre 2001*, eds. Jean-Charles Moretti and Dominique Tardy. Paris: Edition du Comité des travaux historique et scientifiques, 99–123.

Morley, Neville. 1996. *Metropolis and Hinterland : The City of Rome and the Italian Economy, 200 BC-AD 200*. Cambridge University Press.

Morris, Ian. 1992. *Death-Ritual and Social Structure in Classical Antiquity*. Cambridge: Cambridge University Press.

Moschonissioti, Sophia. 2010. "Child Burials at the Seaside Cemetery of Ancient Mende." In *L'Enfant et La Mort Dans l'Antiquité I*, Nouvelles recherches dans les nécropoles grecques. Le signalement des tombes d'enfants, eds. Anne-Marie Guimier-Sorbets and Yvette Morizot. Editions de Boccard, 207–26.

Mountrakis, Constantine, Constantine Eliopoulos, Christos G. Koilias, and Sotiris K. Manolis. 2010. "Sex Determination Using Metatarsal Osteometrics from the Athens Collection." *Forensic Science International* 200(1–3): 178.e1-178.e7.

Mourtzas, N.D. 2012a. "Archaeological Indicators for Sea Level Change and Coastal Neotectonic Deformation: The Submerged Roman Fish Tanks of the Gulf of Matala, Crete, Greece." *Journal of Archaeological Science* 39(4): 884–95.

———. 2012b. "Fish Tanks of Eastern Crete (Greece) as Indicators of the Roman Sea Level." *Journal of Archaeological Science* 39(7): 2392–2408.

Müldner, Gundula, and Michael P. Richards. 2005. "Fast or Feast: Reconstructing Diet in Later Medieval England by Stable Isotope Analysis." *Journal of Archaeological Science* 32(1): 39–48.

Murphy, Charlene. 2016. "Finding Millet in the Roman World." *Archaeological and Anthropological Sciences* 8(1): 65–78.

Musgrave, Jonathan H., and S. P. Evans. 1981. "By Strangers Honor'd: A Statistical Study of Ancient Crania from Crete, Mainland Greece, Cyprus, Israel and Egypt." *Journal of Mediterranean Anthropology and Archaeology* 1: 50–107.

Musgrave, Jonathan H., and N. K. Harneja. 1978. "The Estimation of Adult Stature from Metacarpal Bone Length." *American Journal of Physical Anthropology* 48(1): 113–19.

Myburgh, J., K. Staub, F.J. Rühli, J.R. Smith, and M. Steyn. 2017. "Secular Trends in Stature of Late 20th Century

White South Africans and Two European Populations." *HOMO* 68(6): 433–39.

Mylona, Dimitra. 2003a. "Archaeological Fish Remains in Greece: General Trends of the Research and a Gazetteer of Sites." *British School at Athens Studies* 9: 193–200.

———. 2003b. "Fishing in Late Antiquity: The Case of Itanos, Crete." *British School at Athens Studies* 9: 103–10.

Nachemson, A. 1966. "The Load on Lumbar Disks in Different Positions of the Body." *Clinical Orthopaedics and Related Research* 45: 107–22.

Nafplioti, Argyro. 2007. "Population Bio-Cultural History in the South Aegean during the Bronze Age." Unpublished PhD Thesis, University of Southampton.

———. 2008. "'Mycenaean' Political Domination of Knossos Following the Late Minoan IB Destructions on Crete: Negative Evidence from Strontium Isotope Ratio Analysis (87Sr/86Sr)." *Journal of Archaeological Science* 35(8): 2307–2317.

———. 2015. "Social Variation in Middle Bronze Age Knossos: Palaeodietary Evidence." In *Minoan Archaeology. Perspectives for the 21st Century. Proceedings of the International PhD and Post-Doc Conference at Heidelberg, 23–27 March 2011*, Louvain-la-Neuve: Presses universitaires de Louvain, 213–21.

———. 2016. "Eating in Prosperity: First Stable Isotope Evidence of Diet from Palatial Knossos." *Journal of Archaeological Science: Reports* 6: 42–52.

Nakassis, Th. 1987. "Quarry and Fish Trap in Kato Zakros Bay." *Tech. J. Ed. Ministry of Culture*: 85–98.

Nappo, Dario. 2007. "The Impact of the Third Century Crisis on the International Trade with the East." In *Crises and the Roman Empire. Proceedings of the Seventh Workshop of the International Network Impact of Empire (Nijmegen, June 20–24, 2006)*, eds. O. Hekster, G. de Kleijn, and Daniëlle Slootjes. Leiden, The Netherlands: Brill, 233–44.

Van Neer, W., and A. Ervynck. 2004. "Remains of Traded Fish in Archaeological Sites: Indicators of Status, or Bulk Food?" In *Behaviour Behind Bones: The Zooarchaeology of Ritual, Religion, Status and Identity.*, eds. S. Jones O'Day, W. Van Neer, and A. Ervynck. Oxford: Oxbow Books, 203–14.

Nemeskéri, J., and Gy. Acsádi. 1970. *History of Human Life Span and Mortality*. Budapest: Akadémiai Kiadó.

Nenna, Marie-Dominique. 2009. "Modèles Alexandrins ? Apport Des Fouilles et Prospections Récentes Dans La Nécropole Occidentale d'Alexandrie à La Connaissance de l'architecture Funéraire Hellénistique et Impériale." In *Egypt and Cyprus in Antiquity, Nicosie, 2003*, eds. D. Michaelides, Vasiliki Kassianidou, and Robert S. Merrillees. Oxford: Oxbow, 176–93.

Niessen, Linda C., and Robert J. Weyant. 1989. "Causes of Tooth Loss in a Veteran Population." *Journal of Public Health Dentistry* 49(1): 19–23.

Nikita, Efthymia, Chelsey Schrock, Victoria Sabetai, and Elena Vlachogianni. 2019. "Bioarchaeological Perspectives to Diachronic Life Quality and Mobility in Ancient Boeotia, Central Greece: Preliminary Insights from Akraiphia." *International Journal of Osteoarchaeology* 29(1): 26–35.

Niniou-Kindeli, Vanna. 2004. "Ρωμαϊκή Άπτερα. Μια Πρώτη Προσέγγιση." In *Creta Romana e Protobizantina. Atti Del Congresso Internazionale (Iraklion, 23–30 Settembre 2000)*, Padova: Bottega D'Erasmo, 313–34.

———. 2005. "Απτέρα: Στερέωση - Ανάδειξη Οχύρωσης Αρχαίας Απτέρας." *Αρχαιολογικόν Δελτίον* 60 (B2, Χρονικα): 1024–27.

———. 2008. *Aptera - Απτέρα*. Chania: Ministry of Culture and Tourism - 25th Ephorate of Prehistoric and Classical Antiquities.

———. 2009. "Ανασκαφή 'Ρόβλια' (Οδός Ρενιερη 9) / 'Rovlia' Excavation (9, Renieri St.)." In *Χανιά (Κυδώνια) Περιήγηση Σε Χώρους Αρχαίας Μνήμης / Khania (Kydonia) A Tour to Sites of Ancient Memory*, ed. Μαρία Ανδρεαδάκη-Βλαζάκη. Chania: Ministry of Culture and Tourism - 25th Ephorate of Prehistoric and Classical Antiquities, 146–51.

Niniou-Kindeli, Vanna, Maria Andreadaki-Vlazaki, and Stavroula Markoulaki. 1988. "Ανασκαφικές Εργασίες - Νομός Χανίων - Πόλη Χανίων - Στρατόπεδο Ζομπανάκη (Πάρκο Ειρήνης Και Φιλίας)/Excavations in the Chania Prefecture - Chania City - Zombanakis Military Camp (Peace and Friendship Park)." *Αρχαιολογικών Δελτίων* 43 (B2 Χρονικά): 545–49.

Niniou, Vanna. 1993. "Καστέλι Κισάμου, Β΄ Δημοτικό Σχολείο." *Αρχαιολογικόν Δελτίον* 48 (B2, Χρονικά): 475–76.

Nitsch, Erika K., Glynis Jones, Anaya Sarpaki, M. Hald, and Amy Bogaard. 2019. "Farming Practice and Land Management at Knossos, Crete: New Insights from Δ13C and Δ15N Analysis of Neolithic and Bronze Age Crop Remains." In *Country in the City: Agricultural Functions of Protohistoric Urban Settlements (Aegean and Western Mediterranean)*, eds. Dominique Garcia, Raphael Orgeolet, Maia Pomadere, and Julien Zurbach. Oxford: Archaeopress, 159–74.

Nobis, Günter. 2003. "Αρχαιοζωολογιχή Μελέτη Στην Ελεύθερνα Της Κρήτης (Ανασχαφές 1994-7): Συμβολή Στον Προβληματισμό Για Την Εξάπλωση Των Άγριων Θηλαστιχών Σε Συτή Τη Ζωογεωγραφιχή Περιοχή." *British School at Athens Studies* 9: 91–102.

Novak, Mario, and Mario Šlaus. 2011. "Vertebral Pathologies in Two Early Modern Period (16th-19th Century) Populations from Croatia." *American Journal of Physical Anthropology* 145(2): 270–81.

O'Connell, Tamsin C., C.J. Kneale, N. Tasevska, and G.G.C. Kuhnle. 2012. "The Diet-Body Offset in Human Nitrogen Isotopic Values: A Controlled Dietary Study." *American Journal of Physical Anthropology* 149(3): 426–34.

O'Connor, Terence Patrick. 2004. *The Archaeology of Animal Bones*. Texas A & M University Press.

Oginni, Fadekemi Olufunmilayo. 2005. "Tooth Loss in a Sub-Urban Nigerian Population: Causes and Pattern of Mortality Revisited." *International Dental Journal* 55(1): 17–23.

Ortner, D.J., and W.G. Putschar. 1981. *Identification of Pathological Conditions in Human Skeletal Remains*. Washington, DC: Smithsonian Institution Press.

Ortolani, Giorgio. 2004. "La Fortificazione Bizantina Sull'acropoli Di Gortina." In *Creta Romana e Protobizantina. Atti Del Congresso Internazionale (Iraklion, 23–30 Settembre 2000)*, Padova: La Bottega d'Erasmo, 801–12.

Ousley, Stephen D. 1995. "Should We Estimate Biological or Forensic Stature?" *Journal of Forensic Sciences* 40(5): 768–73.

———. 2012. "Estimating Stature." In *A Companion to Forensic Anthropology*, John Wiley & Sons, Ltd, 330–34.

Palmer, Hazel. 1964. "The Classical and Roman Periods." In *Corinth XIII: The North Cemetery*, eds. Carl W. Blegen, Hazel Palmer, and Rodney S. Young. Princeton: American School of Classical Studies at Athens, 65–327.

Panagiotopoulou, Eleni, and Anastasia Papathanasiou. 2015. "Dietary Reconstruction at the Geometric Period Burial Site of Agios Dimitrios in Central Greece." In *Archaeodiet in the Greek World: Dietary Reconstruction from Stable Isotope Analysis*, eds. Anastasia Papathanasiou, Michael P. Richards, and Sherry C. Fox. Princeton: American School of Classical Studies at Athens, 105–18.

Papadimitriou, Anastasios, Dimitrios Chiotis, Georgios Tsiftis, Maria Hatzisimeon, Maria Maniati, Xenofon Krikos, Anastasia Tzonou, and Catherine Dacou-Voutetakis. 2002. "Secular Growth Changes in the Hellenic Population in the Twentieth Century." *Hormones (Athens, Greece)* 1(4): 245–50.

Papadopoulou, Eleni. 1997. "Σφακάκι Παγκαλοχωρίου: Οικόπεδο Μ. Πυργαρούση." *Αρχαιολογικόν Δελτίον* 52(B2 Χρονικά): 1034–35.

Papageorgopoulou, Christina, and Nikolaos I. Xirotiris. 2009. "Anthropological Research on a Byzantine Population from Korytiani, West Greece." In *New Directions in the Skeletal Biology of Greece*, eds. L Schepartz, S Fox, and C Bourbou. Princeton: American School of Classical Studies at Athens, 193–222.

Papathanasiou, Anastasia, Eleni Panagiotopoulou, Konstantinos Beltsios, Maria-Foteini Papakonstantinou, and Maria Sipsi. 2013. "Inferences from the Human Skeletal Material of the Early Iron Age Cemetery at Agios Dimitrios, Fthiotis, Central Greece." *Journal of Archaeological Science* 40(7): 2924–33.

Papathanasiou, Anastasia, and Michael P. Richards. 2015. "Patterns in the Carbon and Nitrogen Isotope Data through Time." In *Archaeodiet in the Greek World: Dietary Reconstruction from Stable Isotope Analysis*, eds. Anastasia Papathanasiou, Michael P. Richards, and Sherry C. Fox. Princeton: American School of Classical Studies at Athens, 195–204.

Parker Pearson, Mike. 1999. *The Archaeology of Death and Burial*. Texas A&M University Press.

Paterakis, Nektarios O. 2011. "Από Το Ρωμαϊκό Νεκροταφείο Της Κισάμου." In *Πεπραγμένα Ι΄ Διεθνούς Κρητολογικού Συνεδρίου τ. Α4*, Χανιά, 355–70.

Paton, Sara. 1991. "A Roman Corinthian Building at Knossos." *The Annual of the British School at Athens* 86: 297–318.

———. 1994. "Roman Knossos and the Colonia Julia Nobilis Cnossus." In *Knossos, a Labyrinth of History : Papers Presented in Honour of Sinclair Hood*, eds. Don Evely, Helen Hughes-Brock, and Nicoletta Momigliano. London: British School at Athens, 141–54.

———. 1998. "The Villa Dionysos at Knossos and Its Predecessors." *British School at Athens Studies* 2: 123–28.

———. 2004. "Knossos: An Imperial Renaissance." In *Knossos: Palace, City, State*, eds. Gerald Cadogan, Eleni Hatzaki, and A Vasilakis. London: British School at Athens, 451–55.

Paton, Sara, and R. M. Schneider. 1999. "Imperial Splendour in the Province: Imported Marble on Roman Crete." In *From Minoan Farmers to Roman Traders: Sidelights on the Economy of Ancient Crete*, ed. Angelos Chaniotis. Stuttgart: Franz Steiner Verlag, 279–304.

Payne, H. G. G. 1935. "Archaeology in Greece, 1934–1935." *The Journal of Hellenic Studies* 55(2): 147–71.

Peres, Tanya M. 2010. "Methodological Issues in Zooarchaeology." In *Integrating Zooarchaeology and Paleoethnobotany: A Consideration of Issues, Methods, and Cases*, eds. A.M. Van Derwarker and T.M. Peres. New York: Springer-Verlag, 15–36.

Perkins, Matthew J., Robbie A. McDonald, F. J. Frank van Veen, Simon D. Kelly, Gareth Rees, and Stuart Bearhop. 2014. "Application of Nitrogen and Carbon Stable Isotopes (δ(15)N and δ(13)C) to Quantify Food Chain Length and Trophic Structure." *PloS one* 9(3): e93281.

Perlman, Paula. 1992. "One Hundred-Citied Crete and the 'Cretan ΠΟΛΙΤΕΙΑ.'" *Classical Philology* 87: 193–205.

———. 1999. "Krētes Aei Lēistai? The Marginalization of Crete in Greek Thought and the Role of Piracy in the Outbreak of the First Cretan War." In *Hellenistic Rhodes: Politics, Culture, and Society*, eds. Vincent Gabrielsen *et al.* Aarhus: Aarhus University Press, 132–61.

Petaros, Anja, Sabrina B. Sholts, Mario Slaus, Alan Bosnar, and Sebastian K.T.S. Wärmländer. 2015. "Evaluating Sexual Dimorphism in the Human Mastoid Process: A Viewpoint on the Methodology." *Clinical Anatomy* 28(5): 593–601.

Petry, Lindsay A. 2020. "Echoes in the Bones: An Osteological Analysis of the Biological Impact of Roman Rule at Corinth, Greece." *Chronika* 10: 54–67.

Phenice, T. W. 1969. "A Newly Developed Visual Method of Sexing the Os Pubis." *American Journal of Physical Anthropology* 30(2): 297–301.

Phipps, Kathy R., and Victor J. Stevens. 1995. "Relative Contribution of Caries and Periodontal Disease in Adult Tooth Loss for an HMO Dental Population." *Journal of Public Health Dentistry* 55(4): 250–52.

Pitts, Martin, and Miguel John Versluys. 2015a. "Globalisation and the Roman World: Perspectives and Opportunities." In *Globalisation and the Roman World: World History, Connectivity and Material Culture*, eds. Martin Pitts and Miguel John Versluys. Cambridge: Cambridge University Press, 3–31.

———, eds. 2015b. *Globalisation and the Roman World.* New York: Cambridge University Press.

Platon, N. 1947. "Η Αρχαιολογική Κίνησις Εν Κρήτη Κατά Τα Έτη 1941–1947." *Κρητικά Χρονικά* A: 631–40.

———. 1959. "Η Αρχαιολογική Κίνησις Εν Κρήτη Το Έτος 1959." *Κρητικά Χρονικά* 13: 359–93.

———. 1960. "Η Αρχαιολογική Κίνησης Εν Κρήτη Το Έτος 1960." *Κρητικά Χρονικά* 14: 515.

———. 1973. "Η Αρχαιολογική Κίνησης Εν Κρήτη Το Έτος 1973." *Κρητικά Χρονικά*: 464.

Poblome, J. 2004. "Italian Sigillata in the Eastern Mediterranean." In *Early Italian Sigillata*, eds. J. Poblome, P. Talloen, R. Brulet, and Marc Waelkens. Leuven: Peeters, 17–30.

Polet, C., and Mary Anne Katzenberg. 2003. "Reconstruction of the Diet in a Mediaeval Monastic Community from the Coast of Belgium." *Journal of Archaeological Science* 30(5): 525–33.

Pollard, A.M., P. Ditchfield, E. Piva, S. Wallis, C. Falys, and S. Ford. 2012. "'Sprouting like Cockle amongst the Wheat": The St. Brice's Day Massacre and the Isotopic Analysis of Human Bones from St John's College, Oxford.'" *Oxford Journal of Archaeology* 31(1): 83–102.

Pologiorgi, Melpo. 1985. "Κίσαμος. Η Τοπογραφία Μιας Αρχαίας Πόλης Της Δυτικής Κρήτης." *Αρχαιολογικά Ανάλεκτα εξ Αθηνών* 18: 65–80.

———. 1991. "Από Το Κλασικό Και Ελληνιστικό Νεκροταφείο Της Κυδωνίας (From the Classical and Hellenistic Cemetery of Kydonia)." *Αρχαιολογικών Δελτίων* 40 (1985) (A Μελέτες): 162–77.

Popham, Mervyn. 1978. "Notes from Knossos, Part II." *The Annual of the British School at Athens* 73: 179–87.

Poulou-Papadimitriou, Natalia, Elli Tzavella, and Jeremy Ott. 2012. "Burial Practices in Byzantine Greece: Archaeological Evidence and Methodological Problems for Its Interpretation." In *Rome, Constantinople and Newly-Converted Europe:Archaeological and Historical Evidence*, eds. Maciej Salamon, Marcin Wołoszyn, Alexander Musin, and Perica Špehar. Kraków, Leipzig, Rzeszów, Warszawa: Geisteswissenschaftliches Zentrum Geschichte und Kultur Ostmitteleuropas. Instytut Archeologii i Etnologii (Polska Akademia Nauk) Uniwersytet Rzeszowski. Instytut Archeologii., 377–428.

Powell, Betty, and Jerry J. Garnick. 1978. "The Use of Extracted Teeth to Evaluate Clinical Measurements of Periodontal Disease." *Journal of Periodontology* 49(12): 621–24.

Prent, Mieke. 2005. *Cretan Sanctuaries and Cults.* Leiden: Brill.

Price, T. Douglas, Gisela Grupe, and Peter Schröter. 1994. "Reconstruction of Migration Patterns in the Bell Beaker Period by Stable Strontium Isotope Analysis." *Applied Geochemistry* 9(4): 413–17.

Propstmeier, Johanna, Olaf Nehlich, Michael P Richards, Gisela Grupe, Gundula H. Muldner, and Wolf-Rudiger Teegen. 2017. "Diet in Roman Pergamon Using Stable Isotope (C, N, S), Osteoarchaeological and Historical Data - Preliminary Results." In *Life and Death in Asia Minor in Hellenistic, Roman and Byzantine Times: Studies in Archaeology and Bioarchaeology*, eds. J Rasmus Brandt, Erika Hagelberg, Gro Bjørnstad, and Sven Ahrens. Oxford: Oxbow Books, 237–49.

Prowse, Tracy L. 2001. "Isotopic and Dental Evidence for Diet from the Necropolis of Isola Sacra (1st--3rd Centuries AD), Italy." Unpublished PhD thesis, McMaster University.

Prowse, Tracy L., Henry P. Schwarcz, Shelley Saunders, Roberto Macchiarelli, and Luca Bondioli. 2004. "Isotopic Paleodiet Studies of Skeletons from the Imperial Roman-Age Cemetery of Isola Sacra, Rome, Italy." *Journal of Archaeological Science* 31(3): 259–72.

Prowse, Tracy L., Henry P. Schwarcz, Shelley R. Saunders, Roberto Macchiarelli, and Luca Bondioli. 2005. "Isotopic Evidence for Age-Related Variation in Diet from Isola Sacra, Italy." *American Journal of Physical Anthropology* 128(1): 2–13.

Prummel, Wietske. 2003. "Animal Remains from the Hellenistic Town of New Halos in the Almirós Plain, Thessaly." *British School at Athens Studies* 9: 153–59.

Punitha, V. C., A. Amudhan, P. Sivaprakasam, and V. Rathanaprabu. 2015. "Role of Dietary Habits and Diet in Caries Occurrence and Severity among Urban Adolescent School Children." *Journal of Pharmacy & BioAllied Sciences* 7 (Suppl 1): S296–300.

Purcell, Nicholas. 1995. "Eating Fish. The Paradoxes of Seafood." In *Food in Antiquity*, eds. J. Wilkins, D. Harvey, and M. Dobson. Exeter: University of Exeter Press, 132–49.

Raab, Holly Alane. 2001. *Rural Settlement in Hellenistic and Roman Crete : The Akrotiri Peninsula.* Archaeopress.

Rau, G. H., A. J. Mearns, D. R. Young, R. J. Olson, H. A. Schafer, and I. R. Kaplan. 1983. "Animal C/C Correlates with Trophic Level in Pelagic Food Webs." *Ecology* 64(5): 1314–18.

Raxter, Michelle H., Benjamin M. Auerbach, and Christopher B. Ruff. 2006. "Revision of the Fully Technique for Estimating Statures." *American Journal of Physical Anthropology* 130(3): 374–84.

Reitsema, Laurie J., Douglas E. Crews, and Marek Polcyn. 2010. "Preliminary Evidence for Medieval Polish Diet from Carbon and Nitrogen Stable Isotopes." *Journal of Archaeological Science* 37(7): 1413–23.

Reitsema, Laurie J., Giuseppe Vercellotti, and Rosa Boano. 2016. "Subadult Dietary Variation at Trino Vercellese, Italy, and Its Relationship to Adult Diet and Mortality." *American Journal of Physical Anthropology* 160(4): 653–64.

Reitz, Elizabeth Jean, and Elizabeth S. Wing. 1999. *Zooarchaeology*. Cambridge University Press.

Rethemiotakis, Georgos. 1983. "Λύκτος Πεδιάδος." *Αρχαιολογικόν Δελτίον* 38 (Χρονικά Β'2): 354.

Ricci, Paola, Carmina Sirignano, Simona Altieri, Mariangela Pistillo, Alfonso Santoriello, and Carmine Lubritto. 2016. "Paestum Dietary Habits during the Imperial Period: Archaeological Records and Stable Isotope Measurement." *ACTA IMEKO* 5(2): 26.

Richards, Michael P., and Robert E.M. Hedges. 2008. "Stable Isotope Evidence of Past Human Diet at the Sites of the Neolothis Cave of Gerani, the Late Minoan III Cemetery of Armenoi, Grave Circles A and B at the Palace Site of Mycenae; and the Late Helladic Chamber Tombs." In *Archaeology Meets Science: Biomolecular Investigations in Bronze Age Greece*, eds. Yannis Tzedakis, Holley Martlew, and Martin Jones. Oxford: Oxbow, 220 – 230.

Richards, Michael P., and P. A. Mellars. 1998. "Stable Isotopes and the Seasonality of the Oronsay Middens." *Antiquity* 72(275): 178–84.

Rife, Joseph L. 1999. "Death, Ritual and Memory in Greek Society during the Early and Middle Roman Empire." Unpublished PhD thesis, University of Michigan.

———. 2007. "Inhumation and Cremation at Early Roman Kenchreai (Corinthia) in Local and Regional Context." In *Körpergräber Des 1.-3. Jh. in Der Römischen Welt: Internationales Kolloquium Frankfurt Am Main 19.–20. November 2004.*, eds. A. Faber, P. Fasold, M. Struck, and M. Witteyer. Frankfurt: Schriften des Archäologischen Museums Frankfurt 21, 99–120.

———. 2012. *Isthmia. Volume IX. The Roman and Byzantine Graves and Human Remains*. Princeton: The American School of Classical Studies at Athens.

Rife, Joseph L., Melissa Moore Morison, Alix Barbet, Richard K. Dunn, Douglas H. Ubelaker, and Florence Monier. 2007. "Life and Death at a Port in Roman Greece: The Kenchreai Cemetery Project 2002–2006." *Hesperia* 76: 143–181.

Ringrose, T. J. 1993. "Bone Counts and Statistics: A Critique." *Journal of Archaeological Science* 20: 121–57.

Rizakis, Athanasios D. 1997. "Roman Colonies in the Province of Achaia: Territories, Land and Population." In *The Early Roman Empire in the East*, ed. Susan E. Alcock. Oxford: Oxbow, 15–36.

———. 1988. "Le Port de Patras et Les Communications Avec l'Italie Sous La République." *Cahiers d'histoire* 33(3–4): 453–72.

———. 1989. "La Colonie Romaine de Patras En Achaie: Le Temoignane Epigraphique." In *The Greek Renaissance in the Roman Empire*, eds. Susan Walker and Avril Cameron. London: The Tenth British Museum Classical Colloquium Bulletin Supplement, no 55, University of London, 180–86.

Robb, John, Renzo Bigazzi, Luca Lazzarini, Caterina Scarsini, and Fiorenza Sonego. 2001. "Social 'Status' and Biological 'Status': A Comparison of Grave Goods and Skeletal Indicators from Pontecagnano." *American Journal of Physical Anthropology* 115(3): 213–22.

Roberts, Charlotte, Chryssi Bourbou, Anna Lagia, Sevi Triantaphyllou, and Anastasia Tsaliki. 2005. "Health and Disease in Greece: Past, Present and Future." In *Health in Antiquity*, ed. Helen King. New York: Routledge, 32–57.

Robinson, Henry S. 1959. "Pottery of the Roman Period: Chronology." *The Athenian Agora* 5: iii–149.

Robinson, Mark, and Erica Rowan. 2015. "Roman Food Remains in Archaeology and the Contents of a Roman Sewer at Herculaneum." In *A Companion to Food in the Ancient World*, eds. John Wilkins and Robin Nadeau. Chichester: John Wiley & Sons, 105–15.

Rodineau, J. 1991. "Pathogénie Des Enthésopathies Du Membre Supérieur." In *Pathologie Des Insertions et Enthésopathies*, eds. L. Simon, C. Hérisson, and J. Rodineau. Paris: Masson, 166–171.

Rogers, J., L. Shepstone, and P. Dieppe. 1997. "Bone Formers: Osteophyte and Enthesophyte Formation

Are Positively Associated." *Annals of the rheumatic diseases* 56(2): 85–90.

Rohnbogner, A., and Mary E. Lewis. 2016. "Dental Caries as a Measure of Diet, Health, and Difference in Non-Adults from Urban and Rural Roman Britain." *Dental Anthropology* 29(1): 16–31.

Rojas-Sepúlveda, Claudia, Yann Ardagna, and Olivier Dutour. 2008. "Paleoepidemiology of Vertebral Degenerative Disease in a Pre-Columbian Muisca Series from Colombia." *American Journal of Physical Anthropology* 135(4): 416–30.

Romano, David Gilman. 2005. "Urban and Rural Planning in Roman Corinth." In *Urban Religion in Roman Corinth: Interdisciplinary Approaches*, eds. Daniel N. Schowalter and Steven J. Friesen. Cambridge, MA: Harvard Theological Studies, Harvard Divinity School, 25–59.

Rousaki, Maria, Yorgos Brokalakis, Ioanna Triantafyllidis, Eirini Chrysanthakopoulou, and Dimitra Pylarinou. 2016. "Οι Πρόσφατες Ανασκαφές Στο Χώρο Του Βενιζελείου Νοσοκομείου: Οι Τάφοι Της Ρωμαϊκής Περιόδου [Poster]." In *12th International Congress of Cretan Studies, Heraklion, Crete, Greece, 21–25 September 2016*.

Rousaki, Maria, Yorgos Brokalakis, Ioanna Triantafyllidi, Eirini Chrysanthakopoulou, and Dimitra Pilarinou. 2019. "A Glimpse into the Knossian Mortuary Landscape: The Roman Tombs at the Venizeleio Hospital, from the 2014 and 2015 Excavation Seasons." In *Proceedings of the 12th International Congress of Cretan Studies (Heraklion, 21–25 September 2016)*, 1–20.

Rousaki, Maria, Yorgos Brokalakis, Ioanna Triantafyllidis, and Eirini Chrysanthakopoulou. 2019. "Ανασκάπτοντας Τις Νεκροπόλεις Της Κνωσού. Νέα Ευρήματα Από Το Ελληνορωμαϊκό Νεκροταφείο Στον Χώρο Του Βενιζελείου Νοσοκομείου." In *I. Τα Νεκροταφεία. Χωροταξική Οργάνωση - Ταφικά Έθιμα - Τελετουργίες*, eds. E. Κουντούρη and A. Γκαδόλου. Ταμείο Αρχαιολογικών Πόρων και Απαλλοτριώσεων, 505–28.

Rousaki, Maria, Ioanna Triantafyllidi, and Yorgos Brokalakis. 2020. "Νέες Ανασκαφές Στον Χώρο Του Βενιζελείου Νοσοκομείου Ηρακλείου 2014–2015." In *Αρχαιολογικό Έργο Στην Κρήτη 4 (2016)*, 281–93.

Rowan, Erica. 2017. "Bioarchaeological Preservation and Non-Elite Diet in the Bay of Naples: An Analysis of the Food Remains from the Cardo V Sewer at the Roman Site of Herculaneum." *Environmental Archaeology* 22(3): 318–36.

Rutgers, L.V. V., M. Van Strydonck, M. Boudin, and C. van der Linde. 2009. "Stable Isotope Data from the Early Christian Catacombs of Ancient Rome: New Insights into the Dietary Habits of Rome's Early Christians." *Journal of Archaeological Science* 36(5): 1127–34.

Sackett, L. Hugh, K. Branigan, P.J. Callaghan, H.W. Catling, E.A. Catling, J. Nicolas Coldstream, R.A. Higgins, M.R. Popham, J. Price, M.J. Price, and G.B. Waywel. 1992. *Knossos: From Greek City to Roman Colony : Excavations at the Unexplored Mansion II.* London: British School at Athens.

Sackett, L. Hugh, and Jonathan H Musgrave. 1976. "A New Figured Krater from Knossos." *The Annual of the British School at Athens* 71: 117–29.

Sairam, V., M. V. Geethamalika, Praveen B. Kumar, G. Naresh, and Gareema P. Raju. 2016. "Determination of Sexual Dimorphism in Humans by Measurements of Mandible on Digital Panoramic Radiograph." *Contemporary clinical dentistry* 7(4): 434–39.

Sakashita, Reiko, Masakazu Inoue, Naohiko Inoue, Qifeng Pan, and Hong Zhu. 1997. "Dental Disease in the Chinese Yin-Shang Period with Respect to Relationships between Citizens and Slaves." *American Journal of Physical Anthropology* 103(3): 401–8.

Salamon, Maciej, A. Coppa, M. McCormick, M. Rubini, R. Vargiu, and N. Tuross. 2008. "The Consilience of Historical and Isotopic Approaches in Reconstructing the Medieval Mediterranean Diet." *Journal of Archaeological Science* 35(6): 1667–72.

Sallares, R. 1991. *The Ecology of the Ancient Greek World.* Ithaca, New York: Cornell University Press.

Sanders, Ian F. 1982. *Roman Crete: An Archaeological Survey and Gazetteer of Late Hellenistic, Roman, and Early Byzantine Crete.* Warminster, Wilts. England: Aris & Phillips.

Savignoni, Luigi. 1901. "Esplorazione Archeologica Delle Province Occidentali Di Creta I–II. Topografia e Monumenti." *Monumenti Antichi* 11: 285–550.

Schaefer, Maureen, Sue Black, and Louise Scheuer. 2009. *Juvenile Osteology: A Laboratory and Field Manual.* Burlington, MA; London; San Diego: Academic Press.

Scheidel, Walter. 2009a. Princeton/Stanford Working Papers in Classics *Disease and Death in the Ancient City of Rome.*

———. 2009b. "In Search of Roman Economic Growth." *Journal of Roman Archaeology* 22: 46–70.

———. 2013. "Disease and Death." In *The Cambridge Companion to Ancient Rome*, Cambridge Companions to the Ancient World, ed. Paul Erdkamp. Cambridge: Cambridge University Press, 45–59.

Schoeninger, Margaret J. 1985. "Trophic Level Effects on 15N/14N and 13C/12C Ratios in Bone Collagen and Strontium Levels in Bone Mineral." *Journal of Human Evolution* 14(5): 515–25.

Schoeninger, Margaret J., and Michael J. DeNiro. 1982. "Carbon Isotope Ratios of Apatite from Fossil Bone Cannot Be Used to Reconstruct Diets of Animals." *Nature* 297(5867): 577–78.

———. 1984. "Nitrogen and Carbon Isotopic Composition of Bone Collagen from Marine and Terrestrial Animals." *Geochimica et Cosmochimica Acta* 48(4): 625–39.

Schour, L., and M. Massler. 1941. "The Development of the Human Dentition." *Journal of the American Dental Association* 28: 1153–1160.

Schroeder, H.E. 1969. *Formation and Inhibition of Dental Calculus*. Berne: Hans Huber Publishers.

Scotton, Paul D. 2011. "Imperial Cult and Imperial Reconciliation." In *Roman Colonies in the First Century of Their Foundation*, Oxbow Books, 75–84.

Sealy, Judith C., Richard Armstrong, and Carmel Schrire. 1995. "Beyond Lifetime Averages: Tracing Life Histories through Isotopic Analysis of Different Calcified Tissues from Archaeological Human Skeletons." *Antiquity* 69(263): 290–300.

Sealy, Judith C., Nikolaas J. van der Merwe, Julia A.Lee Thorp, and John L. Lanham. 1987. "Nitrogen Isotopic Ecology in Southern Africa: Implications for Environmental and Dietary Tracing." *Geochimica et Cosmochimica Acta* 51(10): 2707–17.

Serpetsidaki, Ioanna. 1994. "Περιοχή Κνωσού." *Αρχαιολογικόν Δελτίον* 49 (Χρονικά B'2): 698–99.

Sharma, Leena, Dipali Kapoor, and Sakeba Issa. 2006. "Epidemiology of Osteoarthritis: An Update." *Current Opinion in Rheumatology* 18(2): 147–56.

Shearer, G., D. H. Kohl, R. A. Virginia, B. A. Bryan, J. L. Skeeters, E. T. Nilsen, M. R. Sharifi, and P. W. Rundel. 1983. "Estimates of N2-Fixation from Variation in the Natural Abundance of 15N in Sonoran Desert Ecosystems." *Oecologia* 56(2–3): 365–73.

Shimada, Izumi, Ken-ichi Shinoda, Julie Farnum, Robert Corruccini, and Hirokatsu Watanabe. 2004. "An Integrated Analysis of Pre-Hispanic Mortuary Practices: A Middle Sicán Case Study." *Current Anthropology* 45(3): 369–402.

Simmons, T., R. L. Jantz, and W. M. Bass. 1990. "Stature Estimation from Fragmentary Femora: A Revision of the Steele Method." *Journal of Forensic Sciences* 35(3): 628–36.

Skordou, Maria. 2016. "Ταφικό Μνημείο Κισάμου." In *Πεπραγμένων Του IB' Διεθνούς Κρητολογικού Συνεδρίου*, Heraklion, 1–17.

———. 2020. "Λαξευτός Θαλαμωτός Τάφος Κισάμου." In *Αρχαιολογικό Έργο Κρήτης 4, Rethymno, 24–27 November 2016*, 713–25.

Slane, Kathleen W. 2017. *Corinth XXI: Tombs, Burials, and Commemoration in Corinth's Northern Cemetery*. Princeton: American School of Classical Studies at Athens.

Šlaus, Mario, Zeljka Bedic, Petra Rajic Sikanjic, Marin Vodanovic, Alka Domic Kunic, Željka Bedić, Petra Rajić Šikanjić, Marin Vodanović, and Alka Domić Kunić. 2011. "Dental Health at the Transition from the Late Antique to the Early Medieval Period on Croatia's Eastern Adriatic Coast." *International Journal of Osteoarchaeology* 21(5): 577–90.

Smith, B.H. 1984. "Patterns of Molar Wear in Hunter-Gatherers and Agriculturalists." *American Journal of Physical Anthropology* 63: 39–56.

Sofaer Derevenski, Joanna R. 2000. "Sex Differences in Activity-Related Osseous Change in the Spine and the Gendered Division of Labor at Ensay and Wharram Percy, UK." *American Journal of Physical Anthropology* 111(3): 333–54.

de Souza, Philip. 1998. "Late Hellenistic Crete and the Roman Conquest." In *Post-Minoan Crete: Proceedings of the First Colloquium on Post-Minoan Crete Held by the British School at Athens and the Institute of Archaeology, University College London, 10–11 November 1995*, London: British School at Athens, 112–16.

Spanu, Marcello. 2000. "Burial in Asia Minor during the Imperial Period with a Particular Reference to Cilicia and Cappadocia." In *Burial, Society and Context in the Roman World*, eds. John Pearce, Martin Millett, and Manuela Struck. Oxford: Oxbow Books, 169–78.

Spawforth, Antony J.S. 1996. "Roman Corinth: The Formation of a Colonial Elite." In *Proceedings of the International Colloquium on Roman Onomastics, Athens 7–9 September 1993, ΜΕΛΕΤΗΜΑΤΑ 21*, ed. A.D Rizakis. Athens: De Boccard, 167–82.

Sperduti, Alessandra, Luca Bondioli, and Peter Garnsey. 2012. "Skeletal Evidence for Occupational Structure at the Coastal Towns of Portus and Velia (1st-3rd c. A.D.)." In *More Than Just Numbers? The Role of Science in Roman Archaeology*, ed. Irene Schrüfer-Kolb. Portsmouth, Rhode Island: Journal of Roman Archaeology Supplement 91, 53–70.

Sporn, Katja. 2002. *Heiligtümer Und Kulte Kretas in Klassischer Und Hellenistischer Zeit*. Heidelberg: Verlag Archäologie und Geschichte.

Sporn, Katja. 2014. "Graves and Grave Markers in Archaic and Classical Crete." In *Cultural Practices and Material Culture in Archaic and Classical Crete*, Berlin, Boston: De Gruyter.

Spurr, M. S. 1983. "The Cultivation of Millet in Roman Italy." *Papers of the British School at Rome* 51: 1–15.

Spyridakis, Stylianos. 1970. *Ptolemaic Itanos and Hellenistic Crete*. Berkeley: University of California Press.

Spyridakis, Stylianos V. 1992. *Cretica: Studies on Ancient Crete*. New Rochelle: Aristide D. Caratzas.

Srikanth, Velandai K., Jayne L. Fryer, Guangju Zhai, Tania M. Winzenberg, David Hosmer, and Graeme Jones. 2005. "A Meta-Analysis of Sex Differences

Prevalence, Incidence and Severity of Osteoarthritis." *Osteoarthritis and Cartilage* 13(9): 769–81.

St Hoyme, L.E., and M Yaşar İşcan. 1989. "Determination of Sex and Race: Accuracy and Assumptions." In *Reconstruction of Life from the Skeleton*, eds. M Yaşar İşcan and Kenneth A R Kennedy. New York: Alan R. Liss Inc, 53–95.

Stabholz, Ayala, Itai Babayof, Alex Mersel, and Jonathan Mann. 1997. "The Reasons for Tooth Loss in Geriatric Patients Attending Two Surgical Clinics in Jerusalem, Israel." *Gerodontology* 14(2): 84–88.

Stampolidis, Nikolaos C., ed. 2004a. *Ελεύθερνα. Πόλη - Ακρόπολη - Νεκρόπολη (Eleutherna. Polis - Acropolis - Necropolis)*. Athens: Museum of Cycladic Art.

———. 2004b. "Οι Νεκροπόλεις Τον Ελληνορωμαϊκών Και Πρωτοβυζαντινών Χρόνων." In *Ελεύθερνα. Πόλη - Ακρόπολη - Νεκρόπολη*, ed. Stampolidis Nikolaos C. Athens: Museum of Cycladic Art, 138–45.

Stathakopoulos, Dionysios. 2004. *Famine and Pestilence in the Late Roman and Early Byzantine Empire : A Systematic Survey of Subsistence Crises and Epidemics*. Aldershot: Ashgate.

Steckel, R.H., P.W. Sciulli, and Jerome C. Rose. 2002. "A Health Index from Skeletal Remains." In *The Backbone of History: Health and Nutrition in the Western Hemisphere*, eds. R.H. Steckel and Jerome C. Rose. Cambridge: Cambridge University Press, 61–93.

Steele, D.G. 1970. "Estimation of Stature from Fragments of Long Limb Bones." In *Personal Identification in Mass Disasters*, ed. T.D. Stewart. Washington DC: Smithsonian Institution, 85–97.

Stephensen, Charles B. 1999. "Burden of Infection on Growth Failure." *The Journal of Nutrition* 129(2): 534S–538S.

Stevens, Rhiannon E., Emma Lightfoot, Julie Hamilton, Barry Cunliffe, and Robert E.M. Hedges. 2010. "Stable Isotope Investigations of the Danebury Hillfort Pit Burials." *Oxford Journal of Archaeology* 29(4): 407–28.

Stewart, T.D. 1979. *Essentials of Forensic Anthropology*. Springfield: Thomas.

Stinson, Sara. 2012. "Growth Variation: Biological and Cultural Factors." In *Human Biology*, Hoboken, NJ, USA: John Wiley & Sons, Inc., 587–635.

Stirland, Ann J. 2000. *Raising the Dead : The Skeleton Crew of Henry VIII's Great Ship, the Mary Rose*. Wiley.

Stiros, Stathis C., and Sofia Papageorgiou. 2001. "Seismicity of Western Crete and the Destruction of the Town of Kisamos at AD 365: Archaeological Evidence." *Journal of Seismology* 5(3): 381–97.

Suzuki, H., K. Yajima, and T. Yamanobe. 1967. *Studies on the Graves, Coffin Contents, and Skeletal Remains of the Tokugawa Shoguns and Their Families at the Zojoji Temple*. Tokyo: Tokyo University Press.

Svoronos, J.N. 1890. *Numismatique de La Crète Ancienne*. Mâcon: Protat Frères.

Swärdstedt, Torsten. 1966. "Odontological Aspects of a Medieval Population in the Province of Jämtland, Mid-Sweden." Unpublished PhD thesis, University of Lund.

Sweetman, Rebecca J. 2003. "The Roman Mosaics of the Knossos Valley." *The Annual of the British School at Athens* 98: 517–48.

———. 2004a. "Late Antique Knossos. Understanding the City: Evidence of Mosaics and Religious Architecture." *The Annual of the British School at Athens* 99: 315–54.

———. 2004b. "The Changing Nature of Knossos: Roman to Late Antique – Some Problems." In *Knossos: Palace, City, State*, eds. Gerald Cadogan, Eleni Hatzaki, and A Vasilakis. London: British School at Athens, 481–88.

———. 2006. "Knossos: Processes of Romanization." In *Πεπραγμένα Θ' Διεθνούς Κρητολογικού Συνεδρίου, Ελούντα, 1–6 Οκτωβρίου 2001 (9th International Cretological Congress. Elounda, 2001)*, Herakleion: A5, 421–34.

———. 2007. "Roman Knossos: The Nature of a Globalized City." *American Journal of Archaeology* 111(1): 61–82.

———. 2011a. "100 Years of Solitude: Colonies in the First Century of Their Foundation." In *Roman Colonies in the First Century of Their Foundation*, Oxbow Books, 1–6.

———. 2011b. "The Knossos Medical Faculty Basilica in Its Cretan Context." In *Proceedings of the 10th International Cretelogical Congress B2*, 49–67.

———. 2013. *The Mosaics of Roman Crete: Art, Archaeology and Social Change*. Cambridge: Cambridge University Press.

———. 2017. "Networks and Church Building in the Aegean: Crete, Cyprus, Lycia and the Peloponnese." *The Annual of the British School at Athens* 112: 207–66.

Sweetman, Rebecca J., and Marshall Joseph Becker. 2005. "Knossos Medical Faculty Site: Late Antique Graves and Other Remains." *The Annual of the British School at Athens* 100: 331–86.

Sweetman, Rebecca J., and Dimitris Grigoropoulos. 2010. "Roman Knossos: Discovering the City through the Evidence of Rescue Excavations." *The Annual of the British School at Athens* 105: 339–79.

Talbot, Alice-Mary. 1987. "An Introduction to Byzantine Monasticism." *Illinois Classical Studies* 12(2): 229–41.

Tanasi, Davide, Robert H. Tykot, Andrea Vianello, and Stephan Hassam. 2018. "Stable Isotope Analysis of the Dietary Habits of a Greek Community in Archaic

Syracuse (Sicily): A Pilot Study." *STAR: Science & Technology of Archaeological Research*: 1–12.

Temple, Daniel H. 2015. "Caries: The Ancient Scourge." In *A Companion to Dental Anthropology*, Hoboken, NJ: John Wiley & Sons, Inc, 433–49.

Temple, Daniel H., and Clark Spencer Larsen. 2007. "Dental Caries Prevalence as Evidence for Agriculture and Subsistence Variation during the Yayoi Period in Prehistoric Japan: Biocultural Interpretations of an Economy in Transition." *American Journal of Physical Anthropology* 134(4): 501–12.

Themelis, Petros G., and Yiannis P. Touratsoglou. 1997. *Οι Τάφοι Του Δερβενίου*. Athens: Ministry of Culture.

Theodoulou, T., B. Foley, and A. Tourtas. 2018. "Western Crete Project, 2013: Preliminary Report. Underwater Survey at Kissamos Bay and the Promontories of Rhodopos and Gramvousa." In *Diving into the Past. Underwater Archaeological Research, 1976–2014, Athens, 6th March 2015*, ed. A. Simossi. Athens: Fund of Archaeological Proceeds, 305–12.

Thomas, Christine M. 2005. "Placing the Dead: Funerary Practice and Social Stratification in the Early Roman Period at Corinth and Ephesos." In *Urban Religion in Roman Corinth: Interdisciplinary Approaches*, Cambridge, MA: Harvard Theological Studies, Harvard Divinity School, 281–306.

Thomas, J., and A.C. Hero. 2000. "Appendix B: The Regulation of Diet in the Byzantine Monastic Foundation Documents." In *Byzantine Monastic Foundation Documents, Vol. 5.*, Washington, DC: Dumbarton Oaks Research Library and Collection, 1696–1716.

Todd, T. Wingate. 1920. "Age Changes in the Pubic Bone. I. The Male White Pubis." *American Journal of Physical Anthropology* 3(3): 285–334.

Tomczyk, Jacek, Krzysztof Szostek, Iulian Komarnitki, Hanna Mańkowska-Pliszka, and Marta Zalewska. 2013. "Dental Caries and Chemical Analyses in Reconstruction of Diet, Health and Hygienic Behaviour in the Middle Euphrates Valley (Syria)." *Archives of Oral Biology* 58(6): 740–51.

Tomlinson, R. A. 1996. "Archaeology in Greece 1995–96." *Archaeological Reports* (42): 1–47.

Toynbee, Jocelyn M. C. 1971. *Death and Burial in the Roman World.* Baltimore; London: John Hopkins University Press.

Trainor, Conor P. 2019. "Polis, Colony and beyond: Urban Knossos from Archaic to Late Antique Times." *Proceedings of the 12th International Congress of Cretan Studies (Heraklion, 21–25 September 2016)* A1.

———. 2021. "The Late Hellenistic Wine Press Excavations from Knossos: The Early Iron Age, Hellenistic and Early Roman Contexts." *Annual of the British School at Athens* 116: 235–90.

Triantaphyllou, Sevi. 2001. *A Bioarchaeological Approach to Prehistoric Cemetery Populations from Central and Western Greek Macedonia.* Oxford: Archaeopress.

———. 2015. "A Stable Isotope Analysis of Skeletal Assemblages from Prehistoric Northern Greece." In *Archaeodiet in the Greek World: Dietary Reconstruction from Stable Isotope Analysis*, eds. Anastasia Papathanasiou, Michael P. Richards, and Sherry C. Fox. Princeton: American School of Classical Studies at Athens, 57–76.

———. 2018. "Managing with Death in Prepalatial Crete: The Evidence of the Human Remains." In *From the Foundations to the Legacy of Minoan Society*, eds. Maria Relaki and Yiannis Papadatos. Oxford: Oxbow Books, 141–66.

Triantaphyllou, Sevi, Michael P. Richards, Carol Zerner, and Sofia Voutsaki. 2008. "Isotopic Dietary Reconstruction of Humans from Middle Bronze Age Lerna Argolid, Greece." *Journal of Archaeological Science* 35(11): 3028–3034.

Tritsaroli, Paraskevi. 2014. "Human Remains from Pigi Athinas, Greece, 1999–2011." *Bioarchaeology of the Near East* 8: 125–37.

———. 2020. "'BODICON': BODIes of CONtact Identity Negotiations and Biocultural Effects in the Roman Colonies of Macedonia, Greece." *TMA - Tijdschrift voor Mediterrane Archeologie* 63: 52.

Tritsaroli, Paraskevi, and Chryssa Karadima. 2017. "The People of Early Byzantine Maroneia, Greece (5th–6th c. AD)." *Bioarchaeology of the Near East* 11: 29–62.

Tritsaroli, Paraskevi, and Frédérique Valentin. 2008. "Byzantine Burials Practices for Children; Case Studies Based on a Bioarchaeological Approach to Cemeteries from Greece." In *Nasciturus, Infans, Puerulus Vobis Mater Terra. La Muerte En La Infancia*, eds. F. J. Gusi, S. Muriel, and C. Olaria. Diputació de Castelló: Servei d'Investigacions Arqueològiques i Prehistòriques, 93–113.

Trotter, Mildred. 1970. "Estimation of Stature from Intact Long Bones." In *Personal Identification in Mass Disasters*, ed. T.D. Stewart. Washington, DC: Smithsonian Institution Press, 71–83.

Trotter, Mildred, and Goldine C. Gleser. 1952. "Estimation of Stature from Long Bones of American Whites and Negroes." *American Journal of Physical Anthropology* 10(4): 463–514.

———. 1958. "A Re-Evaluation of Estimation of Stature Based on Measurements of Stature Taken during Life and of Long Bones after Death." *American Journal of Physical Anthropology* 16(1): 79–123.

———. 1977. "Corrigenda to 'Estimation of Stature from Long Limb Bones of American Whites and Negroes,' American Journal Physical Anthropology (1952)."

American Journal of Physical Anthropology 47(2): 355–56.

Tsigkou, Angeliki. 2004. "Οδός Χατζηδάκη 31α (Οικόπεδο Με. Μαθιουλάκη)." *Αρχαιολογικών Δελτίων* 56–59 (2001–2004 Χρονικα Β5): 407–8.

———. 2009. "Ανασκαφή 'Μαρ. Μαθιουλάκη' (Οδός Χατζηδάκη 31α) / 'Mathioulaki Mar.' Excavation (31α, Khatzidaki St.)." In *Χανιά (Κυδώνια) Περιήγηση Σε Χώρους Αρχαίας Μνήμης / Khania (Kydonia) A Tour to Sites of Ancient Memory*, ed. Maria Andreadaki-Vlazaki. Chania: Ministry of Culture and Tourism - 25th Ephorate of Prehistoric and Classical Antiquities, 136–45.

Tzanakaki, Katerina. 2011. "Δυτικό Νεκροταφείο Απτέρας: Πρόσφατες Σωστικές Έρευνες." In *Πεπραγμένα Ι΄ Διεθνούς Κρητολογικού Συνεδρίου τ. Α4*, 375–95.

Valamoti, Soultana Maria. 2016. "Millet, the Late Comer: On the Tracks of Panicum Miliaceum in Prehistoric Greece." *Archaeological and Anthropological Sciences* 8(1): 51–63.

Vasilakis, Andonis. 1988. "Κνωσός." *Κρητική Εστία* 2: 323–24.

———. 2004. "Ρωμαϊκά Μαυσωλεία Κνωσού Και Γόρτυνας." In *Creta Romana e Protobizantina. Atti Del Congresso Internazionale (Iraklion, 23–30 Settembre 2000)*, Padova: Bottega D'Erasmo, 699–708.

Venit, Marjorie Susan. 2002. *Monumental Tombs of Ancient Alexandria: The Theater of the Dead.* Cambridge: Cambridge University Press.

Vergidou, Chryssa, Georgia Karamitrou-Mentessidi, Sofia Voutsaki, and Efthymia Nikita. 2021. "Oral Health and Its Implications on Male-Female Dietary Differences: A Study from the Roman Province of Macedonia." *Journal of Archaeological Science: Reports* 35: 102784.

———. 2022. "A Bioarcheological Contribution to the Social History of Roman Macedonia: The Pontokomi-Vrysi Site in Kozani Prefecture, Greece." *International Journal of Osteoarchaeology* 32(5): 1020–34.

Vika, Efrossini. 2011. "Diachronic Dietary Reconstructions in Ancient Thebes, Greece: Results from Stable Isotope Analyses." *Journal of Archaeological Science* 38(5): 1157–63.

Vika, Efrossini, V. Aravantinos, and Michael P. Richards. 2009. "Aristophanes and Stable Isotopes: A Taste for Freshwater Fish in Classical Thebes (Greece)?" *Antiquity* 83(322): 1076–83.

Vika, Efrossini, and Tatiana Theodoropoulou. 2012. "Re-Investigating Fish Consumption in Greek Antiquity: Results from Δ13C and Δ15N Analysis from Fish Bone Collagen." *Journal of Archaeological Science* 39(5): 1618–27.

Villotte, Sébastien. 2008. "Enthésopathies et Activités Des Hommes Préhistoriques - Recherche Méthodologique et Application Aux Fossiles Européens Du Paléolithique Supérieur et Du Mésolithique." Université Sciences et Technologies - Bordeaux.

Villotte, Sébastien, Dominique Castex, Vincent Couallier, Olivier Dutour, Christopher J Knüsel, and Dominique Henry-Gambier. 2010. "Enthesopathies as Occupational Stress Markers: Evidence From the Upper Limb." *American Journal of Physical Anthropology* 142(2): 224–34.

Villotte, Sébastien, Sandra Assis, Francisca Alves Cardoso, Charlotte Yvette Henderson, Valentina Mariotti, Marco Milella, Doris Pany-Kucera, Nivien Speith, Cynthia A. Wilczak, and Robert Jurmain. 2016. "In Search of Consensus: Terminology for Entheseal Changes (EC)." *International Journal of Paleopathology* 13: 49–55.

Virginia, Ross A., and C. C. Delwiche. 1982. "Natural 15N Abundance of Presumed N2-Fixing and Non-N2-Fixing Plants from Selected Ecosystems." *Oecologia* 54(3): 317–25.

di Vita, Antonio. 2010. *Gortina Di Creta. Quindici Secoli Di Vita Urbana.* Rome: L'Erma di Bretschneider.

Viviers, Didier. 1999. "Economy and Territorial Dynamics in Crete from the Archaic to the Hellenistic Period." In *From Minoan Farmers to Roman Traders: Sidelights on the Economy of Ancient Crete*, ed. Angelos Chaniotis. Stuttgart: Franz Steiner Verlag, 221–33.

Vogeikoff-Brogan, Natalia. 2004. "The Late Hellenistic Period in East Crete." In *Crete beyond the Palaces*, eds. Leslie Preston Day, Margaret S Mook, and James D Muhly. Philadelphia: INSTAP Academic Press, 213–20.

Walbank, Mary E. Hoskins. 1997. "The Foundation and Planning of Early Roman Corinth." *Journal of Roman Archaeology* 10: 95–130.

———. 2005. "Unquiet Graves: Burial Practices of the Roman Corinthians." In *Urban Religion in Roman Corinth: Interdisciplinary Approaches*, eds. D. N. Schowalter and S. J. Friesen. Cambridge, MA: Harvard University Press, 249 –80.

Waldron, Tony. 1992. "Unilateral Spondylolysis." *International Journal of Osteoarchaeology* 2(2): 177–81.

———. 1994. *Counting the Dead : The Epidemiology of Skeletal Populations*. John Wiley & Sons.

———. 2007. *Palaeoepidemiology: The Measure of Disease in the Human Past.* Walnut Creek, California: Left Coast Press.

———. 2009. *Palaeopathology*. Cambridge; New York: Cambridge University Press.

———. 2012. "Joint Disease." In *A Companion to Paleopathology*, Oxford, UK: Wiley-Blackwell, 513–30.

Waldron, Tony, and Juliet Rogers. 1990. "An Epidemiologic Study of Sacroiliac Fusion in Some Human Skeletal

Remains." *American Journal of Physical Anthropology* 83(1): 123–27.

Walker, P. L., and S. E. Hollimon. 1989. "Changes in Osteoarthritis Associated with the Development of a Maritime Economy among Southern California Indians." *International Journal of Anthropology* 4(3): 171–83.

Walker, Phillip L., G. Dean, and P. Shapiro. 1991. "Estimating Age from Tooth Wear in Archaeological Populations." In *Advances in Dental Anthropology*, eds. M.A. Kelley and C.S. Larsen. Chichester: Wiley-Liss, 13–31.

Walker, Phillip L., and Barry S. Hewlett. 1990. "Dental Health Diet and Social Status among Central African Foragers and Farmers." *American Anthropologist* 92(2): 383–98.

Walker, Phillip L., and Della Collins Cook. 1998. "Brief Communication: Gender and Sex: Vive La Difference." *American Journal of Physical Anthropology* 106(2): 255–59.

Wall, Sheilagh, Jonathan H. Musgrave, and Peter M. Warren. 1986. "Human Bones from A Late Minoan IB House at Knossos." *The Annual of the British School at Athens* 81: 333–88.

Wardle, Ken A. 1972. "Two Notes from Knossos." *The Annual of the British School at Athens* 67: 271–84.

Wardle, Ken A, and Diana Wardle. 2004. "Glimpses of Private Life: Roman Rock Cut Tombs of the First and Second Centuries AD at Knossos." In *Knossos: Palace, City, State*, eds. Gerald Cadogan, Eleni Hatzaki, and A Vasilakis. London: British School at Athens, 473–80.

Warren, Peter M. 1988. "Knossos: Stratigraphical Museum Excavations, 1978–82. Part IV." *Archaeological Reports* (34): 86–104.

———. 1981. "Knossos: Stratigraphical Museum Excavations, 1978–1980. Part I." *Archaeological Reports* 27: 73–92.

Wasterlain, Sofia N., Simon Hillson, and Eugénia Cunha. 2009. "Dental Caries in a Portuguese Identified Skeletal Sample from the Late 19th and Early 20th Centuries." *American Journal of Physical Anthropology* 140(1): 64–79.

Waywell, G.B., J.J. Wilkes, Roger Bland, E. Jane Sidell, Keith N. Willkinson, and Graham M. Chandler. 1997. "Excavations at Sparta: The Roman Stoa, 1988-91 Part 3." *The Annual of the British School at Athens* 92: 401–34.

Wells, Calvin. 1982. "The Human Burials." In *Cirencester Excavations II: Romano-British Cemeteries at Cirencester*, eds. Alan McWhirr, Linda Viner, and Calvin Wells. Cirencester: Cirencester Excavation Committee, Corinium Museum, 135–202.

Wenn, Camilla Cecilie, Sven Ahrens, and J. Rasmus Brandt. 2017. "Romans, Christians, and Pilgrims at Hierapolis in Phrygia: Changes in Funerary Practices and Mental Processes." In *Life and Death in Asia Minor in Hellenistic, Roman and Byzantine Times: Studies in Archaeology and Bioarchaeology*, eds. J. Rasmus Brandt, Camilla Cecilie Wenn, Gro Bjørnstad, and Sven Ahrens. Oxford: Oxbow, 196–218.

Wesolowsky, A. B. 1973. "The Skeletons of Lerna Hollow." *Hesperia* 42(3): 340.

White, T. D., and P. A. Folkens. 2005. *The Human Bone Manual*. London: Elsevier Academic Press.

Whitelaw, Todd, Maria Bredaki, and Andonis Vasilakis. 2007. "The Knossos Urban Landscape Project: Investigating the Long-Term Dynamics of an Urban Landscape." *Archaeology International* 10: 28–31.

———. 2016. *The Knossos Urban Landscape Project Report on the 2016 Study Season*. London.

———. 2017. *The Knossos Urban Landscape Project: Report on the 2017 Study Season*. London.

———. 2019. "The Long-Term Dynamics of Knossos in Context." *Proceedings of the 12th International Congress of Cretan Studies (Heraklion, 21–25 September 2016)* A1.

Whitelaw, Todd, and Conor P. Trainor. 2016. "A City in Flux: Hellenistic and Roman Knossos." In *The Enigma of Late Hellenistic and Roman Crete: Unanswered Questions. The 1st International Conference of the Colloquium on Roman Crete. University of Nottingham, 18–19 November 2016*.

Whitelaw, Todd, Andonis Vasilakis, and Maria Bredaki. 2012. "Knossos through Nine Millennia: Preliminary Perspectives from the Knossos Urban Landscape Project (2005–2011)." In *Annual Open Meeting of the British School at Athens*, Athens; Thessaloniki.

Wilkens, Barbara. 1996. "Faunal Remains from Italian Excavations on Crete." In *Pleistocene and Holocene Fauna of Crete and Its First Settlers*, ed. David S. Reese. Madison, Wisconsin: Prehistory Press, 241–62.

Wilkins, John, and S. Hill. 2006. *Food in the Ancient World*. Oxford: Blackwell Publishing.

Wilkins, John, and Robin Nadeau. 2015. "Introduction." In *A Companion to Food in the Ancient World*, eds. John Wilkins and Robin Nadeau. Chichester, UK: John Wiley & Sons, Ltd, 1–16.

Willet, Rinse. 2012. "Whirlwind of Numbers - Demographic Experiments for Roman Corinth." *Ancient Society* 42: 127–58.

Willetts, R.F. 1955. *Aristocratic Society in Ancient Crete*. London: Routledge.

Williams, Charles K. II. 1993. "Roman Corinth as a Commercial Center." In *The Corinthia in the Roman Period*, ed. Tim E. Gregory. Ann Arbor: Journal of Roman Archaeology Supplement 8, 31–46.

Winkler, Lauren A., Clark Spencer Larsen, Victor D. Thompson, Paul W. Sciulli, Dale L. Hutchinson, David Hurst Thomas, Elliot H. Blair, and Matthew C. Sanger. 2017. "The Social Structuring of Biological Stress in Contact-Era Spanish Florida: A Bioarchaeological Case Study from Santa Catalina de Guale, St. Catherines Island, Georgia." In *Colonized Bodies, Worlds Transformed: Toward a Global Bioarchaeology of Contact and Colonialism*, eds. Melissa S. Murphy and Haagen D. Klaus. Gainesville: Florida University Press, 129–62.

Wirth, Louis. 1938. "Urbanism as a Way of Life." *American Journal of Sociology* 44(1): 1–24.

Wiseman, James R. 1979. "Corinth and Rome I: 228 B.C.—A.D. 267." In *Aufstieg Und Niedergang Der Römischen Welt. 7/1. Politische Geschichte (Provinzen Und Randvölker: Griechischer Balkanraum; Kleinasien)*, Berlin, Boston: De Gruyter, 438–547.

Wong, Megan, Elise Naumann, Klervia Jaouen, and Michael P Richards. 2017. "Isotopic Investigations of Human Diet and Mobility at the Site of Hierapolis, Turkey." In *Life and Death in Asia Minor in Hellenistic, Roman and Byzantine Times: Studies in Archaeology and Bioarchaeology*, eds. J. Rasmus Brandt, Erika Hagelberg, Gro Bjørnstad, and Sven Ahrens. Oxford: Oxbow Books, 228–36.

Wood, James W., George R. Milner, Henry C. Harpending, Kenneth M. Weiss, Mark N. Cohen, Leslie E. Eisenberg, Dale L. Hutchinson, Rimantas Jankauskas, Gintautas Česnys, Mary Anne Katzenberg, John R. Lukacs, Janet W. McGrath, Eric Abella Roth, Douglas H. Ubelaker, and Richard G. Wilkinson. 1992. "The Osteological Paradox: Problems of Inferring Prehistoric Health from Skeletal Samples." *Current Anthropology* 33(4): 343–70.

Wood, James W., Darryl J. Holman, Kathleen A. O'Connor, and Rebecca J. Ferrell. 2002. "Mortality Models for Paleodemography." In *Paleodemography*, eds. Robert D. Hoppa and James W. Vaupel. Cambridge: Cambridge University Press, 129–68.

Xanthoudides, Stefanos. 1918. "Λαξευτός Οικογενειακός Τάφος Παρά Την Κνωσον." *Αρχαιολογικόν Δελτίον* 4: 18–19.

Yangaki, Anastasia. 2016. "Pottery of the 4th-Early 9th Centuries AD on Crete: The Current State of Research and New Directions." In *Roman Crete: New Perspectives*, eds. Jane E. Francis and Anna Kouremenos. Oxford: Oxbow, 199–234.

Yegül, F. K. 2010. *Bathing in the Roman World*. Cambridge: Cambridge University Press.

Zohary, Daniel, and Maria Hopf. 2000. *Domestication of Plants in the Old World*. 3rd edition. Oxford: Oxford University Press.

Zohary, Tamar, Jonathan Erez, Moshe Gophen, Ilana Berman-Frank, and Mariana Stiller. 1994. "Seasonality of Stable Carbon Isotopes within the Pelagic Food Web of Lake Kinneret." *Limnology and Oceanography* 39(5): 1030–43.

www.ingramcontent.com/pod-product-compliance
Ingram Content Group UK Ltd.
Pitfield, Milton Keynes, MK11 3LW, UK
UKHW061845041026
15591UKWH00015B/923

9 781407 360355